Application of Bioinformatics in Cancers

Application of Bioinformatics in Cancers

Special Issue Editor

Chad Brenner

MDPI • Basel • Beijing • Wuhan • Barcelona • Belgrade

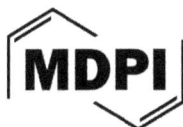

MDPI

Special Issue Editor
Chad Brenner
University of Michigan Health Systems
USA

Editorial Office
MDPI
St. Alban-Anlage 66
4052 Basel, Switzerland

This is a reprint of articles from the Special Issue published online in the open access journal *Cancers* (ISSN 2072-6694) from 2018 to 2019 (available at: https://www.mdpi.com/journal/cancers/special_issues/Bioinformatics_cancers).

For citation purposes, cite each article independently as indicated on the article page online and as indicated below:

LastName, A.A.; LastName, B.B.; LastName, C.C. Article Title. *Journal Name* **Year**, *Article Number*, Page Range.

ISBN 978-3-03921-788-5 (Pbk)
ISBN 978-3-03921-789-2 (PDF)

Contents

About the Special Issue Editor

Chad Brenner is an assistant professor in the Department of Otolaryngology-Head and Neck Surgery and Department of Pharmacology at the University of Michigan. Dr. Brenner serves as the co-director of the Head and Neck Oncology program at the University of Michigan, and his lab, the Michigan Otolaryngology and Translational Oncology lab (MiOTO), aims to identify new diagnostic tests and precision medicine therapies for cancer patients. Dr. Brenner received an undergraduate degree in biomedical engineering from the University of Michigan, Master's in Engineering degree in bioelectrical engineering and a doctorate in Cellular and Molecular Biology for his seminal contributions to molecular mechanisms of prostate cancer progression and therapeutic inhibition of the disease. Dr. Brenner's current research is focused on functional genomic, proteomic and bioinformatics approaches to study cancer to discover novel therapeutic approaches that benefit patients (precision medicine) and to help understand the mechanisms that drive cancer progression. Dr. Brenner's lab has identified novel approaches to overcome PI3K and EGFR inhibitor resistance pathways in head and neck squamous cell carcinoma as well as discovered novel driving lesions in clinically aggressive mucoepidermoid carcinomas. Current studies build on this previous work and are now focused on understanding how tumor cells and the surrounding microenvironment adapt to precision-guided therapies, including immunotherapy, with the goal of identifying new clinical trial paradigms that may benefit patients. Additional research is focused on understanding how to leverage artificial intelligence based algorithms and precision-guided therapies to improve the immune response to cancer, and if immune checkpoint inhibitors can be used to prevent cancer initiation.

Preface to "Application of Bioinformatics in Cancers"

Bioinformatics applications in cancer have rapidly evolved over the past several years. Ever since its initial implementation, next generation sequencing has altered our understanding of cancer biology, and the approaches to analyze more and more complex datasets have also become increasingly complex. Routine bioinformatics pipelines now range from those that rapidly detect and predict functional impact of molecular alterations to those that quantify changes to the tumor microenvironment. For example, several tools that analyze tumor-immune interactions have been successfully developed to assess tumor infiltrating lymphocyte content, microsatellite instability, total mutational burden and neoantigen presentation. Further complexity of integrated omics-based analysis is also now coupled with the emergence of modern machine learning and network-based approaches to analyze large datasets in the context of publicly available resources, such as the cancer genome atlas.

While much of the focus has so far been on annotating molecular alterations as well as infiltrating cell types or cell states in ideal sequencing conditions, alternative and application-specific approaches are now emerging that improve on a wide variety of established analysis techniques. These include techniques that range from improved quantification of copy number and gene expression from formalin fixed tissues as well as applications that require high sensitivity such as the quantification of tumor mutations from liquid biopsies (circulating cell free DNA). Further novel applications attempt to improve the ability to analyze the distribution and molecular impact of complicated genetic features such as repetitive or transposable endogenous elements (e.g., LINE-1) as well as exogenous genetic elements (e.g., human papilloma virus).

As we develop a better understanding of the limitations of these new informatics approaches, we can ultimately hope to apply these techniques to existing datasets and build well-annotated databases of easily accessible information that can be leveraged in multi-variable analysis pipelines. Similar to the success of SIGdb and cBioPortal, this should help yield new diagnostic and prognostic/predictive biomarkers for standard interventional modalities as well as emerging areas like immuno-oncology, and areas of unmet clinical need. This Special Issue will highlight the current state of the art in bioinformatics applications in cancer biology, and infer future prospects for improving informatics applications through artificial intelligence and machine learning approaches.

Chad Brenner
Special Issue Editor

cancers

MDPI

Editorial

Applications of Bioinformatics in Cancer

Chad Brenner [1,2,3]

[1] Department of Otolaryngology–Head and Neck Surgery, Michigan Otolaryngology and Translational Oncology Laboratory, University of Michigan Health Systems, Ann Arbor, MI 48109-0602, USA; chadbren@umich.edu; Tel.: +1-734-763-2761

[2] Department of Pharmacology, Michigan Otolaryngology and Translational Oncology Laboratory, University of Michigan Health Systems, Ann Arbor, MI 48109-0602, USA

[3] Rogel Cancer Center, University of Michigan Medical School, 1150 E. Medical Center Dr., 9301B MSRB3, Ann Arbor, MI 48109-0602, USA

Received: 22 October 2019; Accepted: 23 October 2019; Published: 24 October 2019

Keywords: bioinformatics; machine learning; artificial intelligence; Network Analysis; single-cell sequencing; circulating tumor DNA (ctDNA); Neoantigen Prediction; precision medicine; Computational Immunology

This series of 25 articles (22 original articles, 3 reviews) is presented by international leaders in bioinformatics and biostatistics. This original series of articles details emerging approaches that leverage artificial intelligence and machine learning algorithms to improve the utility of bioinformatics applications in cancer biology. Importantly, the issue also addresses the limitations of current approaches to analyzing high throughput datasets by providing support for novel methods that can be used to improve complex multi-variable analysis. For example, in order to help identify clinically meaningful genes, Shen et al. demonstrate how the implementation of a knockoff procedure can control false discovery rates in next-generation datasets with relatively small sample sizes [1]. Additionally, tools were developed and validated to address complex problems ranging from tumor heterogeneity to mutation signature analysis. For example, intertumor heterogeneity scores were characterized from >2800 tumors and used to identify genes associated with high heterogeneity including histone methyltransferase *SETD2* and DNA methyltransferase *DNMT3A*, which were then validated by CRISPR/CAS9 in experimental systems [2]. Likewise, a tool was derived to infer tumor RNA expression signatures of genes with copy loss to support gene-loss driven biomarker analysis [3], and, a weight-matrix based approach was used to highlight the distribution of APOBEC and AID-related gene signatures in multiple cancers that drive subsets of the somatic mutation spectra [4]. Together these manuscripts demonstrate how novel tools and statistical approaches are being used to refine analysis of large next generation sequencing datasets. Extending these concepts, Veronesi et al. also develop an R-script based tool box for efficient analysis of gene signatures with diagnostic and prognostic variable that highlights how tools are being rapidly adapted into easy-to-use application packages [5].

Several papers in this series also demonstrate the potential to integrate large and diverse datasets and use machine learning approaches to develop significantly improved multi-variable predictors of clinical outcome. For example, deep learning artificial intelligence-based approaches were shown to be highly effective at integrating genomic data from multiple sources using de-noising auto-encoders to curate deep features associated with breast cancer clinical characteristics and outcomes [6]. Moreover, artificial intelligence-driven classification techniques were also used on multiple independent colorectal cancer datasets to identify and verify biomarkers of diagnosis and prognosis that may have important implications for the disease [7]. As another example, the Taiwan Cancer Registry database was analyzed to evaluate the value of the Wu co-morbidity score for accuracy in assessing curative-surgery-related 90-day mortality risk and overall survival in patients with locoregionally advanced head and neck cancer [8]; and, in an alternative approach, Ferroni et al. demonstrate the utility of using machine learning-driven decision support systems to extract data from electronic health records and refine prognostic variables [9]. As an alternative approach, and to understand how gene sets may correlate with outcome, Locati et al. utilized self-organizing map approaches to curate publicly available HPV+ cancer data and inferred gene signatures associated with three biological subtypes of the disease [10]. Novel datasets comparing the molecular composition of primary colorectal cancer and brain metastases were also generated [11]. In an interesting informatics approach, analysis of steroid hormone-related gene sets in publicly available data identified steroidogenic acute regulatory protein as a potential prognostic biomarker in breast cancer [12]. Likewise, a meta-analysis of GEO and TCGA miRNA datasets led to the prioritization of candidate biomarkers of prognosis and overall survival in oral cancer [13]. Machine learning approaches were similarly used to prioritize relevant miRNAs and validate the high performance of highly ranked miRNAs in classification models, suggesting that prioritization of targets from expression data is a highly effective strategy [14]. Analysis of miRNA data using an observed survival interval was reported to overcome issues with clinical outcome associations [15]. Collectively suggesting the potential of these approaches in this new era of machine learning approaches. Finally, additional analysis of similar datasets also highlighted the role of detailed characterization of clinical characteristics in avoiding biological and the clinical outcome analysis bias in large dataset analysis was well demonstrated in the analysis of pancreatic cancer TCGA data by Nicolle et al. [16].

More broadly, machine learning-driven informatics approaches, which were demonstrated to have utility in improving statistical analysis of integrated histopathologic datasets, were implemented to analyze the TCGA lung adenocarcinoma dataset as an alternative approach to modeling outcomes [17]. Furthermore, using both the lung adenocarcinoma and hepatocellular carcinoma datasets to analyze the utility of integrated gene and imaging data, multiple individual genes, conditional on imaging features, were shown to drive significant improvement in prognosis modeling [18]. These improvements in integrated multi-feature image analysis and molecular analysis for outcome modeling suggest that complex models incorporating diverse variables may be key to making substantial improvements to clinical outcome models in the future.

Interestingly, several of the articles also highlight the ability to use emerging bioinformatic techniques, high throughput small molecule screening data, and/or outcomes data to make improved predictive models. Lu et al. leveraged a support vector machine learning algorithm to analyze datasets from the Cancer Cell Line Encyclopedia and identify a 10-gene predictive model of recurrence-free survival and overall survival in epithelial ovarian cancer, validated on two independent datasets [19]. Diverse bioinformatics approaches were used to demonstrate how Bufadienolide-like chemicals may contribute to cardiotoxicity and function as anti-neoplastic agents providing a roadmap for prioritizing the mechanisms of action of small molecules with recent informatics techniques [20]. Further, a novel pipeline was developed to predict acquired resistance to EGFR inhibition, in which the team built a meta-analysis-based, multivariate model that leveraged eight independent studies and had high predictive performance [21]. Network pharmacologic analysis was used as an approach to nominate herb-derived compounds for their potential efficacy in tumor immune microenvironment regulation and tumor prevention [22], showing the utility of informatics approaches for deconvolution of drug screening data.

The collection also includes insightful reviews discussing major bioinformatics approaches involved in the analysis of cell-free DNA sequencing data for detecting genetic mutation, copy number alteration, methylation change, and nucleosome positioning variation [23]; how bioinformatics approaches can be used to understand the functional effects of *TERT* regulation by alternative splicing [24]; and how automatic computer-assisted methods and artificial intelligence-based approaches may be leveraged for brain cancer characterization in a machine and deep learning paradigm [25].

The diversity of approaches and datasets highlighted in this collection of articles underscore the broad range of bioinformatics techniques that are being developed to answer complex questions ranging from how to better predict clinical outcomes to prioritizing lead compounds capable of disrupting the tumor-immune microenvironment. The articles collectively demonstrating the machine learning approaches can be used to make significant advances in cancer biology. Indeed, as we develop a better understanding of how different machine learning approaches are best suited to pursue critical questions as outlined in the articles of this series, we can ultimately hope to improve research efficiency and make substantial improvements to the overall health of patients.

Funding: C.B. received funding from NIH Grants U01-DE025184 and R01-CA194536 and the American Cancer Society.

Conflicts of Interest: The authors declare no conflict of interest.

References

1. Shen, A.; Fu, H.; He, K.; Jiang, H. False Discovery Rate Control in Cancer Biomarker Selection Using Knockoffs. *Cancers* **2019**, *11*, 744. [CrossRef] [PubMed]
2. de Matos, M.R.; Posa, I.; Carvalho, F.S.; Morais, V.A.; Grosso, A.R.; de Almeida, S.F. A Systematic Pan-Cancer Analysis of Genetic Heterogeneity Reveals Associations with Epigenetic Modifiers. *Cancers* **2019**, *11*, 391. [CrossRef] [PubMed]
3. Angeli, D.; Fanciulli, M.; Pallocca, M. Reverse Engineering Cancer: Inferring Transcriptional Gene Signatures from Copy Number Aberrations with ICAro. *Cancers* **2019**, *11*, 256. [CrossRef] [PubMed]
4. Rogozin, I.B.; Roche-Lima, A.; Lada, A.G.; Belinky, F.; Sidorenko, I.A.; Glazko, G.V.; Babenko, V.N.; Cooper, D.N.; Pavlov, Y.I. Nucleotide Weight Matrices Reveal Ubiquitous Mutational Footprints of AID/APOBEC Deaminases in Human Cancer Genomes. *Cancers* **2019**, *11*, 211. [CrossRef] [PubMed]
5. Veronesi, G.; Kunz, M. A Toolbox for Functional Analysis and the Systematic Identification of Diagnostic and Prognostic Gene Expression Signatures Combining Meta-Analysis and Machine Learning. *Cancers* **2019**, *11*, 1606. [CrossRef]
6. Liu, Q.; Hu, P. Association Analysis of Deep Genomic Features Extracted by Denoising Autoencoders in Breast Cancer. *Cancers* **2019**, *11*, 494. [CrossRef]
7. Zhang, X.; Sun, X.F.; Shen, B.; Zhang, H. Potential Applications of DNA, RNA and Protein Biomarkers in Diagnosis, Therapy and Prognosis for Colorectal Cancer: A Study from Databases to AI-Assisted Verification. *Cancers* **2019**, *11*, 172. [CrossRef]
8. Qin, L.; Chen, T.M.; Kao, Y.W.; Lin, K.C.; Yuan, K.S.; Wu, A.T.H.; Shia, B.C.; Wu, S.Y. Predicting 90-Day Mortality in Locoregionally Advanced Head and Neck Squamous Cell Carcinoma after Curative Surgery. *Cancers* **2018**, *10*, 392. [CrossRef]
9. Ferroni, P.; Zanzotto, F.M.; Riondino, S.; Scarpato, N.; Guadagni, F.; Roselli, M. Breast Cancer Prognosis Using a Machine Learning Approach. *Cancers* **2019**, *11*, 328. [CrossRef]
10. Locati, L.D.; Serafini, M.S.; Ianno, M.F.; Carenzo, A.; Orlandi, E.; Resteghin, C.; Cavalieri, S.; Bossi, P.; Canevari, S.; Licitra, L.; et al. Mining of Self-Organizing Map Gene-Expression Portraits Reveals Prognostic Stratification of HPV-Positive Head and Neck Squamous Cell Carcinoma. *Cancers* **2019**, *11*, 1057. [CrossRef]
11. Roussille, P.; Tachon, G.; Villalva, C.; Milin, S.; Frouin, E.; Godet, J.; Berger, A.; Emambux, S.; Petropoulos, C.; Wager, M.; et al. Pathological and Molecular Characteristics of Colorectal Cancer with Brain Metastases. *Cancers* **2018**, *10*, 504. [CrossRef] [PubMed]
12. Manna, P.R.; Ahmed, A.U.; Yang, S.; Narasimhan, M.; Cohen-Tannoudji, J.; Slominski, A.T.; Pruitt, K. Genomic Profiling of the Steroidogenic Acute Regulatory Protein in Breast Cancer: In Silico Assessments and a Mechanistic Perspective. *Cancers* **2019**, *11*, 623. [CrossRef] [PubMed]
13. Falzone, L.; Lupo, G.; La Rosa, G.R.M.; Crimi, S.; Anfuso, C.D.; Salemi, R.; Rapisarda, E.; Libra, M.; Candido, S. Identification of Novel MicroRNAs and Their Diagnostic and Prognostic Significance in Oral Cancer. *Cancers* **2019**, *11*, 610. [CrossRef] [PubMed]
14. Rehman, O.; Zhuang, H.; Muhamed Ali, A.; Ibrahim, A.; Li, Z. Validation of miRNAs as Breast Cancer Biomarkers with a Machine Learning Approach. *Cancers* **2019**, *11*, 431. [CrossRef] [PubMed]
15. Xiong, J.; Bing, Z.; Guo, S. Observed Survival Interval: A Supplement to TCGA Pan-Cancer Clinical Data Resource. *Cancers* **2019**, *11*, 280. [CrossRef]

16. Nicolle, R.; Raffenne, J.; Paradis, V.; Couvelard, A.; de Reynies, A.; Blum, Y.; Cros, J. Prognostic Biomarkers in Pancreatic Cancer: Avoiding Errata When Using the TCGA Dataset. *Cancers* **2019**, *11*, 126. [CrossRef]

17. Xu, Y.; Zhong, T.; Wu, M.; Ma, S. Histopathological Imaging(-)Environment Interactions in Cancer Modeling. *Cancers* **2019**, *11*, 579. [CrossRef]

18. Zhong, T.; Wu, M.; Ma, S. Examination of Independent Prognostic Power of Gene Expressions and Histopathological Imaging Features in Cancer. *Cancers* **2019**, *11*, 361. [CrossRef]

19. Lu, T.P.; Kuo, K.T.; Chen, C.H.; Chang, M.C.; Lin, H.P.; Hu, Y.H.; Chiang, Y.C.; Cheng, W.F.; Chen, C.A. Developing a Prognostic Gene Panel of Epithelial Ovarian Cancer Patients by a Machine Learning Model. *Cancers* **2019**, *11*, 270. [CrossRef]

20. Zhang, Y.; Tang, X.; Pang, Y.; Huang, L.; Wang, D.; Yuan, C.; Hu, X.; Qu, L. The Potential Mechanism of Bufadienolide-Like Chemicals on Breast Cancer via Bioinformatics Analysis. *Cancers* **2019**, *11*, 91. [CrossRef]

21. Kim, Y.R.; Kim, Y.W.; Lee, S.E.; Yang, H.W.; Kim, S.Y. Personalized Prediction of Acquired Resistance to EGFR-Targeted Inhibitors Using a Pathway-Based Machine Learning Approach. *Cancers* **2019**, *11*, 45. [CrossRef] [PubMed]

22. Zheng, J.; Wu, M.; Wang, H.; Li, S.; Wang, X.; Li, Y.; Wang, D.; Li, S. Network Pharmacology to Unveil the Biological Basis of Health-Strengthening Herbal Medicine in Cancer Treatment. *Cancers* **2018**, *10*, 461. [CrossRef] [PubMed]

23. Huang, C.C.; Du, M.; Wang, L. Bioinformatics Analysis for Circulating Cell-Free DNA in Cancer. *Cancers* **2019**, *11*, 805. [CrossRef] [PubMed]

24. Ludlow, A.T.; Slusher, A.L.; Sayed, M.E. Insights into Telomerase/hTERT Alternative Splicing Regulation Using Bioinformatics and Network Analysis in Cancer. *Cancers* **2019**, *11*, 666. [CrossRef]

25. Tandel, G.S.; Biswas, M.; Kakde, O.G.; Tiwari, A.; Suri, H.S.; Turk, M.; Laird, J.R.; Asare, C.K.; Ankrah, A.A.; Khanna, N.N.; et al. A Review on a Deep Learning Perspective in Brain Cancer Classification. *Cancers* **2019**, *11*, 111. [CrossRef] [PubMed]

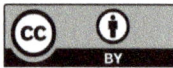

cancers

MDPI

Article

False Discovery Rate Control in Cancer Biomarker Selection Using Knockoffs

Arlina Shen [1,†], Han Fu [2,†,‡], Kevin He [2] and Hui Jiang [2,*]

[1] The Blake School, 511 Kenwood Pkwy, Minneapolis, MN 55403, USA; ahshen20@blakeschool.org
[2] Department of Biostatistics, University of Michigan, 1415 Washington Heights, Ann Arbor, MI 48109, USA; fu.607@osu.edu (H.F.); kevinhe@umich.edu (K.H.)
* Correspondence: jianghui@umich.edu; Tel.: +1-734-764-6742
† These authors contributed equally to this work.
‡ Current address: Department of Statistics, Ohio State University, 1958 Neil Ave, Columbus, OH 43210, USA.

Received: 10 May 2019; Accepted: 23 May 2019; Published: 29 May 2019

Abstract: The discovery of biomarkers that are informative for cancer risk assessment, diagnosis, prognosis and treatment predictions is crucial. Recent advances in high-throughput genomics make it plausible to select biomarkers from the vast number of human genes in an unbiased manner. Yet, control of false discoveries is challenging given the large number of genes versus the relatively small number of patients in a typical cancer study. To ensure that most of the discoveries are true, we employ a knockoff procedure to control false discoveries. Our method is general and flexible, accommodating arbitrary covariate distributions, linear and nonlinear associations, and survival models. In simulations, our method compares favorably to the alternatives; its utility of identifying important genes in real clinical applications is demonstrated by the identification of seven genes associated with Breslow thickness in skin cutaneous melanoma patients.

Keywords: cancer biomarker; diseases genes; variable selection; false discovery rate; knockoffs

1. Introduction

The discovery of biomarkers that are informative for cancer risk assessment, diagnosis, prognosis and treatment predictions is crucial. Many biomarkers have been proven to be very informative for clinical usage, with prominent examples such as BRCA1 and HER2 in breast cancer [1,2], EGFR in non-small-cell lung carcinoma [3] and PSA in prostate cancer [4]. Recent advances in high-throughput genomics make it plausible to select biomarkers from the vast number of human genes in an unbiased manner. For instance, genes associated with disease-related clinical outcomes can be identified by linking a patient's gene expression to the disease progression [5] or other disease phenotypes. Furthermore, by understanding the regulatory roles of these associated genes on various cancers, treatment strategies may be developed. For these reasons, many gene signatures have been discovered for a variety of cancers.

However, many challenges exist for the selection of genes from the high-throughput and high-dimensional expression data at a genomic scale. Besides computational challenges due to the large size of data, a critical statistical difficulty is the control of false discoveries of all identified genes mainly due to the large number of genes versus the relatively small number of patients in a typical cancer study. The conventional method for genomic data analysis is known as univariate analysis, that is, exploring the relationship of the disease-related outcomes with one gene at a time. Due to its simplicity and intuitiveness, univariate analysis has been widely used in gene selection. However, high correlations exist among genes induced by co-expression activities, and hence genes correlated with disease-related genes are also correlated with disease outcomes (a.k.a. spurious correlation). Therefore they will be selected via univariate analysis, leading to high false discoveries. Another issue of univariate analysis is its low statistical power of identifying any disease-related genes due to the multiplicity of hypothesis testing [6] as well as noise that is unaccounted for. That is, relatively fewer genes that are truly associated with the outcome will be identified from univariate analysis than that with multivariate analysis. For the reasons above, penalized multivariate analysis approaches such as the lasso regression [7] and its extensions such as penalized generalized linear models and the Cox proportional hazard model with elastic-net penalty [8,9] have been applied recently to genomic data analysis [10,11]. Nevertheless, because cross-valuation is typically used for the selection of the optimal tuning parameters, such approaches often fail to control false discoveries [12]. This aspect has been clearly illustrated in our simulations in Section 3.1.

For prediction purposes, genes with spurious correlations to the disease outcomes may be useful. However, they are unsuitable when the goal is to understand the disease etiology, or to identify potential treatment targets, where genes that are genuinely associated with the disease are required. In other words, when the number of false discoveries is high, the discoveries are not scientifically replicable. Due to the high cost to experimentally validate the selected genes, there is an urgent need to control for false discoveries in gene selection procedures. The false discovery rate (FDR) [13], defined as the expected proportion of false discoveries among all discoveries, is a widely used method to control for false discoveries in genomic studies, due to its high statistical power compared with conventional methods that control for family-wise error rates (FWER) such as the Bonferroni correction. Controlling for FDR leads to limited proportion of non-true findings among all findings produced by a given analysis and discovery procedure, which translates to reliable scientific discoveries as well as reduced attempts and costs to validate non-true findings. The importance of controlling for the false discovery rate in lasso regression has also been recognized. Recently, [12] proposed a bootstrap/resampling method to control the FDR in lasso type variable selection. The smoothness of the limiting distributions of the bootstrap, which is the standard assumption for the bootstrap, is needed for such methods [14]. In [15], a knockoff procedure was introduced to control the FDR in linear regression when the number of variables is not too large; knockoff variables are constructed to mimic the correlation structure found within the existing variables. In a follow-up paper [16], the method was further expanded to a general framework and a high-dimensional situation for Gaussian variables was studied extensively. However, there is still a gap between the generally simple knockoff framework and the complicated data structures in real world applications.

In this paper, we propose several novel strategies based on the knockoff framework for variable selection subject to control for the false discovery rate. The proposed method is general and flexible, accommodating arbitrary covariate distributions, linear and nonlinear associations, and survival models. Simulation experiments and a real data example on gene identification for Breslow thickness in skin cutaneous melanoma patients demonstrate the utility of the proposed method.

2. Methodology

In many practical situations, identification of a set of explanatory variables which are truly associated with the response is a primary interest in investigation. This is particularly true in biomedical research when genes are selected from a pool of candidate genes that are potentially associated with a disease. To assure that most of the discoveries are true and replicable, one must know whether the false discovery rate, or the expected fraction of false discoveries among all discoveries, as defined in Definition 1, is acceptable or too large. In other words, the false discovery rate in this discovery process needs to be controlled at a desirable level.

Definition 1 (False discovery). *Let S be the true set of variables associated with an outcome, and $\hat{S}$ be the set of variables selected based on a dataset. The false discovery proportion (FDP) is defined as the proportion of false discoveries among all discoveries, i.e., $FDP := |\hat{S} \setminus S| / |\hat{S}|$, where $|\cdot|$ is the size of a set, with the convention $0/0 = 0$. The false discovery rate (FDR) [13] is defined as the expectation of FDP, i.e., $FDR := E[FDP]$.*

The method proposed in this paper is based on the knockoff framework first proposed in [15] and later generalized in [16]. The knockoff framework provides a recipe for building algorithms to control for FDR in variable selection. Under certain mild conditions, the FDR can be theoretically guaranteed to be controlled at a pre-specified level. The key contribution of the knockoff framework is the introduction of the concept of knockoff variables, as defined in Definition 2.

Definition 2 (Knockoff variables). *A set of random variables* $(\widetilde{X}_1, \cdots, \widetilde{X}_p)$ *is said to be model-free knockoffs [16] for* $(X_1, \cdots, X_p)$ *with respect to response Y if they are constructed without looking at Y, and for any* $j \in \{1, \cdots, p\}$, *the pair* $(X_j, \widetilde{X}_j)$ *is exchangeable conditioned on all the other variables* $(\widetilde{X}_1, \cdots \widetilde{X}_p)$ *and* $(X_1, \cdots, X_p)$ *excluding* $(X_j, \widetilde{X}_j)$.

In layman's terms, each knockoff variable $\widetilde{X}_j$ can be considered as a "fake" duplicate of the corresponding variable X_j, in that the relationship between $\widetilde{X}_j$ and all the other variables and their knockoffs excluding X_j is indistinguishable from the relationship between X_j and all the other variables and their knockoffs excluding $\widetilde{X}_j$. Furthermore, the knockoff variables are constructed without using the outcome variable, and therefore are guaranteed not to be associated with the outcome. As a result, in a variable selection procedure, a knockoff variable $\widetilde{X}_j$ has equal chance of being selected as the "original" variable X_j when X_j is not associated with the outcome, which makes the knockoff variables robust benchmarks for FDR control. In this paper, we propose several novel strategies based on the knockoff framework for variable selection subject to control for the false discovery rate.

2.1. Construction of Model-Free Knockoff Variables

The first step for variable selection based on the knockoff framework is to construct knockoff variables. In [15,16], algorithms for constructing knockoff variables for low and high dimensional multivariate Gaussian distributions were proposed, respectively. In particular, an approximated algorithm was proposed in [16] to construct knockoffs by sampling from a multivariate Gaussian distribution with the same first two moments as that of the original variables. When the joint distribution of the original variables is known, the conditional distributions can be derived, based on which random samples can be drawn directly and can be used as knockoffs.

Although built on a multivariate Gaussian distribution, the performance of the knockoff variables constructed using the algorithm in [16] is reported to be quite robust against deviations from the Gaussian assumption, as long as the first two moments are approximated well. We also have the same observations in our experiments (See Appendix C). Therefore, we use the algorithm in [16] for the construction of knockoff variables for all the simulated and real data experiments in this paper, unless otherwise noted. Moreover, we propose another algorithm for constructing knockoff variables without the Gaussian assumption with much higher computational burden (See Appendix A), which may be used in situations when the Gaussian assumption is severely violated.

2.2. Model-Free Statistics

The knockoff framework guarantees that the FDR is controlled at a desirable level for variable selection. However, the statistical power for variable selection depends on the specific statistic being used in the knockoff framework. In [16], the lasso coefficient difference (LCD) statistic was proposed and shown to be very powerful for variable selection based on the lasso regression model. However, it assumes a linear relationship between the response variable and the predictors. When such relationship does not hold, the statistical power will be compromised. In this section, we propose two novel statistics to accommodate arbitrary relationships between the response and predictor variables, thereby realizing our goal of model-free variable selection. In contrast to the lasso regression model in [16], we incorporate machine learning techniques, such as support vector regression [17] and boosting [18], to allow for more flexible and complex model settings.

2.2.1. Difference in R-Squared (DRS) Statistic

Intuitively, variable importance can be measured by the amount of variability of the response data explained by each specific variable. In practice, we can define a statistic named difference in R-squared (DRS) based on the difference between the R^2 value achieved by the full model and that by a partial model where one predictor variable is excluded at a time. See Appendix B for details.

2.2.2. Risk Reduction in Boosting (RRB) Statistic

This statistic stems from the mboost R package which implements a functional gradient descent algorithm for model-based boosting. This method uses component-wise least squares estimates or regression trees as base-learners to optimize general risk functions. The algorithm is quite flexible in that it allows for various kinds of base-learners to be used, for example, linear, P-spline, and tree based base-learners, as well as a variety of loss functions and corresponding risk functions to be optimized. In a fitted boosting model, the accumulated in-bag risk reductions per boosting step for each base-learner or variable can be used to reflect variable importance. The amount of risk reduction can be provided by a function called varimp in the mboost R package with appealing computing efficiency. Similar to DRS, the risk reduction in boosting (RRB) statistic W_j can be constructed by the difference between the risk reduction of variable X_j and that of its corresponding knockoff $\widetilde{X}_j$. Again, W_j here attains the anti-symmetry property and a symmetric distribution under the null hypothesis. The high flexibility of the boosting method allows us to model arbitrarily complex relationships between y and $(X, \widetilde{X})$. The computational efficiency also makes this statistic favorable for our high-dimensional variable selection purpose. In our simulations, compared with the DRS statistic, we found that the RRB statistic achieves better performance in terms of FDR control and of statistical power for variable selection (See Appendix C), with much lower computational burden. Therefore, we use the RRB statistic for all the simulated and real data experiments in this paper, unless otherwise noted.

2.3. Nonlinear Screening

As genomic datasets are often high-dimensional, that is, the number of genes p is much larger than the sample size n, computing the statistics W_j for each variable X_j will take a lot of time. Here, we propose a nonlinear screening strategy to accelerate this procedure. In particular, when $2p > n$, we perform univariate fitting of y to each X_j as well as $\widetilde{X}_j$, using nonlinear regression based on B-splines. In particular, we rank all the variables and their knockoffs based on the L_2 norm of the block-wise gradient vector. The top variables are corresponding to the steepest descent directions, which minimizes the direction derivative, and hence, provides the largest decrease in the linear approximation of the objective function. We then retain the top n variables for computing their W_j's subsequently using a chosen statistic, and set the W_j's for all the remaining $2p - n$ variables to be zero. In our simulations, we found that this nonlinear screening strategy can substantially reduce computational time while maintaining the FDR control as well as statistical power for variable selection (See Appendix C). Therefore, we use this nonlinear screening strategy for all the simulated and real data experiments in this paper, unless otherwise noted.

3. Results

3.1. Simulations

We first use simulation studies to evaluate the performance of our proposed method against two other existing methods: the knockoff method with lasso coefficient difference (LCD) [16] and lasso regression [7] with cross-validation (CV), a widely used variable selection approach. In simulations, we examine several situations to demonstrate that the proposed method performs well in terms of FDR control with increased statistical power. These simulations support the usage of the proposed method for analyzing a real dataset in Section 3.2. All simulations are performed in R.

In particular, we consider three cases of linear and nonlinear associations as well as survival models. In each case, we apply our proposal of using the boosting method with P-spline base-learners to approximate linear or nonlinear associations. We use the knockoff construction algorithm introduced in [16], the RRB statistic described in Section 2.2.2, and the nonlinear screening described in Section 2.3. Specifically, we use the mboost R package to fit y against the augmented design matrix $(X, \widetilde{X})$. For fitting lasso penalized models in the knockoff with the LCD method of [16] and in lasso regression with cross-validation, we use the glmnet R package [8,9] with five-fold cross-validation for selection of the regularization parameter of lasso in simulations for linear (Section 3.1.1) and nonlinear (Section 3.1.2) associations and the Cox proportional hazards regression [19] in simulations for survival analysis (Section 3.1.3).

3.1.1. Linear Associations

The first simulation study focuses on linear associations in regression. In particular, the data were simulated from a linear regression model

$$Y = \sum_{j=1}^{p} X_j \beta_j + \varepsilon, \quad \varepsilon \sim N(0, \sigma^2), \tag{1}$$

in which $X = (X_1, \cdots, X_p)^T$ is distributed according to a p-dimensional Gaussian distribution $N(0, \Sigma)$, with the ij-th element of Σ being $\rho^{|i-j|}$, following an auto-regressive variance structure with the auto-regressive coefficient ρ. Moreover, X and ε are independent. Of p variables, we randomly choose k variables $X_{j_1}, \cdots, X_{j_k}$ and set the corresponding $\beta_{j_l} = \zeta_{j_l} A$, where A, called amplitude, is a varying magnitude given in Figure 1, ζ_{j_l} is a random sign, and $\beta_j = 0$ if $j \notin \{j_1, \ldots, j_k\}$. The amplitude represents the association strength (e.g., correlation) between a biomarker and the outcome. In this case, we simulate $p = 2000$, $k = 10$, $\rho = 0.3$, and $\sigma^2 = 1$ from (1) with sample size $n = 300$. This mimics the real data analysis in Section 3.2. We use the multivariate Gaussian distribution for its simplicity in simulating correlated covariates and the fact that the knockoff framework is robust against deviations from this distributional assumption, as long as the first two moments are approximated well [16]. Furthermore, the relationship between outcome and covariates can be arbitrary.

As suggested by Figure 1, the FDR is controlled around our target value of 20% for the proposed method (knockoff + mboost). The FDR for the knockoff + LCD method is slightly higher. In contrast, the FDR of the lasso + CV method is so high that the discovery is unreliable. All three methods have similar statistical power, and power increases and gets close to 1 as the signal strength gets stronger. A statistical power of 1 means the ideal situation that all genes that are truly associated with the outcome are identified. Although Lasso + CV has the highest power, it is not desirable for discovery, given the uncontrollable FDR levels. Thus, lasso + CV is not a suitable approach for gene selection.

As will be seen in the cases of nonlinear associations (Section 3.1.2) and survival models (Section 3.1.3), the proposed method becomes more powerful when the model assumption of linear associations is violated.

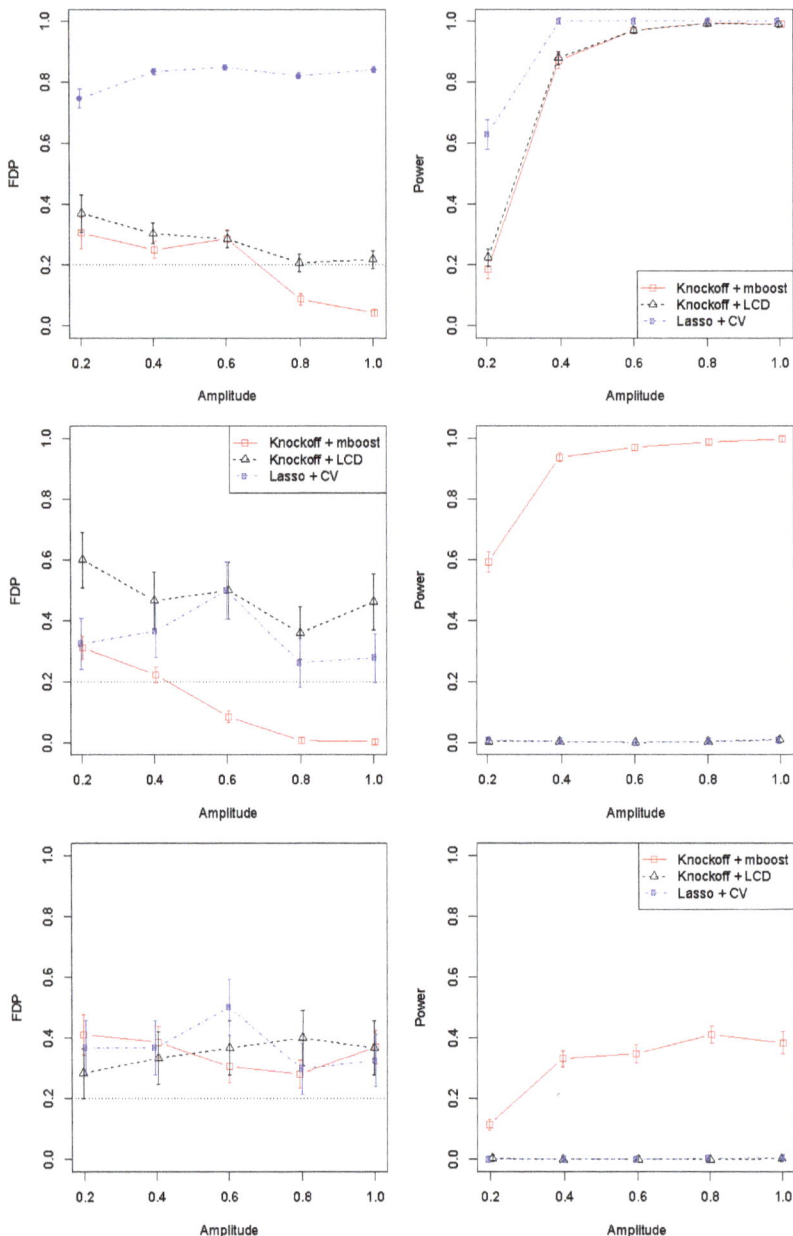

Figure 1. Simulation results for linear associations (**top panel**), nonlinear associations (**middle panel**) and survival analysis (**bottom panel**). Left panel: averaged false discovery proportion (FDP, the empirical version of FDR) and the standard error bars for knockoff variable selection with mboost (red), lasso coefficient difference (LCD) (black) and lasso regression with cross-validation (CV) (blue) as a function of amplitude (association strength (e.g., correlation) between a biomarker and the outcome) based on 30 simulation replications. The reference lines indicate the target false discovery rate of 20%. Right panel: corresponding empirical statistical power of the three methods.

3.1.2. Nonlinear Associations

Our second simulation study deals with nonlinear relationships in regression, in which we again compare the proposed knockoff + mboost method with the knockoff + LCD method of [16] as well as lasso + CV. Here, we replace $\sum_{j=1}^{p} X_j \beta_j$ in (1) by $\sum_{j=1}^{p} X_j^2 \beta_j$ to accommodate nonlinear associations. All other settings are the same as in Section 3.1.1.

As indicated in Figure 1, the FDR for the proposed method (knock + mboost) is controlled under the target value of 20%, as marked by the horizontal dotted line, whereas the FDRs for the other two methods are above the target level. In terms of statistical power, the proposed method is much better than the other two methods, which assume a linear predictor while the proposed method is more flexible without such assumptions.

3.1.3. Survival Analysis

Our third simulation study concerns the Cox proportional hazards regression [19] with a nonlinear predictor $\sum_{j=1}^{p} X_j^2 \beta_j$ as in Section 3.1.2. Specifically, we generate y from the Cox model with a baseline hazard rate equals to 0.002 and a hazard rate of censoring equals to 0.004. The event time follows a Weibull distribution with the shape parameter equals to 1 and scale parameter equals to the baseline hazard rate multiplied by the exponential of the predictor, i.e., $\exp(\sum_{j=1}^{p} X_j^2 \beta_j)$. The censoring time is also sampled from a Weibull distribution with the shape parameter equals to 1 and scale parameter equals to the hazard rate of censoring. The actual observation time is the smaller value between the event and censoring times.

As shown in Figure 1, all three methods roughly achieve the objective of controlling the FDR at the desired level of 20% with slight inflation. The proposed method exhibits much higher power than the other two as was the case in Section 3.1.2.

Based on the simulation studies, we conclude that the proposed method performs well for linear and nonlinear associations as well as survival models. In practice, we do not need to assume linear or non-linear association between the biomarkers and the outcome, and our method will identify biomarkers with high statistical power and well controlled FDR regardless of the type of association that is present in the dataset.

3.2. Cancer Data

In this section we apply our proposed method as described in Section 3.1 to a real dataset from a cancer study for the identification of genes that are associated with clinical outcomes. We investigate a skin cutaneous melanoma (SKCM) dataset, which contains the expression levels of 20,531 genes from 355 melanoma patients measured by RNA-Seq. The dataset is a part of The Cancer Genome Atlas (TCGA) project and publicly available from the TCGA data portal at https://portal.gdc.cancer.gov/. The aim is to identify a set of genes associated with the clinical variable of interest, called Breslow thickness.

Due to the large number of genes and the relatively small sample size, to expedite computation while enhancing the accuracy of identification, we apply a filtering rule to select genes whose mean expression levels exceed 1 normalized transcripts per million (TPM) and the q-value (corrected using the BH procedure [13]) from univariate correlation tests with the response less than 0.2. This leaves us 4171 genes to which to apply our method with the log-transformed Breslow thickness as the response. The predictor variables are measured in log-transformed gene expression values (in TPM).

In this case, at a target FDR of 20%, our method identifies seven genes BOLA1 (BolA Family Member 1), CLDN16 (Claudin 16), EBF2 (EBF Transcription Factor 2), KCTD16 (Potassium Channel Tetramerization Domain Containing 16), KRT14 (Keratin 14), LOC100240735 (Uncharacterized LOC100240735), and MAP4K4 (Mitogen-Activated Protein Kinase 4). In the literature, the CLDN (Claudin) gene family is known to be associated with tumor suppressor genes; for example, hypermethylation of the CLDN11 promoter occurs frequently in malignant melanoma of the skin [20], which may encode a novel melanoma-specific tumor suppressor gene [21]. CLDN16 has been found to be associated with breast [22], thyroid [23], ovarian [24] and lung [25] cancers. Our finding suggests that CLDN16 is also associated with cutaneous melanoma of the skin, which seems consistent with the role of CLDN in terms of tumor suppression. Moreover, MAP4k4 belongs to the mammalian STE20/MAP4K family, which is often overexpressed in many types of human cancer and cancer cell lines, including malignant melanoma [26], because of its crucial role in transformation, invasiveness, adhesion, and cell migration [27]. KRT14 has been found to be associated with melanoma [28]. EBF2 has been found to be associated with prostate [29], bone [30], hematological and epithelial [31] cancers. KCTD16 has been found to be associated with thyroid cancer [32], while KCTD12, a member of the KCTD family, has been found to be associated with uveal melanoma [33]. BOLA1 and LOC100240735 (an RNA gene) are not known to be associated with any malignancies. To further understand the roles of these genes in melanoma, experimental follow-up studies are needed.

As a comparison, we also run Lasso + CV on the same dataset, for which a total of 140 genes are identified. Five of the seven genes identified by Knockoff + mboost are also identified by Lasso + CV. The two genes not identified by Lasso + CV are KRT14 and LOC100240735. Given the high false discovery rates of Lasso + CV in simulations (top-left panel of Figure 1), we expect a large proportion of these 140 genes to be false positives.

Furthermore, to demonstrate the performance of our approach in non-Gaussian data, we randomly pick 500 genes and assign 10 random genes among them to be truly associated genes with the remaining 490 genes to be null genes. We then randomly assign coefficients for the 10 truly associated genes by sampling from $Uniform(1,5)$ with a random sign. To make the problem even more challenging and to demonstrate the ability of our approach working with non-quantitative data, we dichotomize the resulting linear predictor $Y = \sum_{j=1}^{p} X_j \beta_j$ at the median of its distribution so that the outcomes are binary (i.e., two groups of equal sizes). After running Knockoff + mboost at a target FDR level of 20%, a total of seven genes are identified, with five true positives and two false positives, which corresponds to an FDP of 28.6% and a statistical power of 50%.

4. Discussion

An advantage of our method is that no prior specification of the type of association (i.e., linear or non-linear) is needed, which is usually unknown for a given dataset. The knockoff construction algorithm in [16] is based on Gaussian assumption. Nevertheless, it seems robust for non-Gaussian data in our experiments. We also present a knockoff construction algorithm which does not require the Gaussian assumption in case such assumption is severely violated.

The statistical power depends both on the statistic being used and the correlation structure among covariates, which was also noted in [16]. As the correlation among covariates increases, the statistical power decreases. Therefore, a future research direction may be developing methods for the detection of highly correlated gene clusters that are associated with the outcome of interest. Furthermore, due to the high computational cost of building the knockoff variables, right now we can only practically use our method with up to around 5000 pre-selected genes. Thus, developing more efficient computational algorithms for building knockoff variables may be another future research direction.

The datasets and R programs for producing the results in this paper are available at http://www-personal.umich.edu/~jianghui/knockoff/.

5. Conclusions

The results in this paper demonstrate that our proposed approach can provide reliable false discovery rate control for variable selection in various statistical models. Such rigorous false discovery rate control is crucial for improving replicability of the findings and avoiding wasting resources for attempts to validate false discoveries. With additional enhancements, our method offers a promising avenue to identify reliable gene markers in cancer studies.

Author Contributions: Conceptualization, H.J.; methodology, K.H. and H.J.; formal analysis, A.S., H.F., K.H. and H.J.; writing-original draft preparation, A.S. and H.F.; writing-review and editing, K.H. and H.J.; supervision, K.H. and H.J.; project administration, H.J.; funding acquisition, H.J.

Funding: This research was supported in part by a startup grant from the University of Michigan and the National Cancer Institute grants P30CA046592. H.F. was supported in part by the Summer Internship Funds of Certificate in Public Health Genetics (CPHG) Program at the University of Michigan.

Acknowledgments: We thank National Cancer Institute and National Human Genome Research Institute for making the TCGA data portal available, and thank Yang Shi at Augusta University for the skin cutaneous melanoma dataset. Thanks to the reviewers for their valuable comments, and to Megan Ludwig at the UM-CMB and Kirsten Herold at the UM-SPH Writing Lab for their helpful suggestions.

Conflicts of Interest: The authors declare no conflict of interest. The funders had no role in the design of the study; in the collection, analyses, or interpretation of data; in the writing of the manuscript, or in the decision to publish the results.

Abbreviations

The following abbreviations are used in this manuscript:

FDR	False Discovery Rate
FWER	Family-Wise Error Rate
LCD	Lasso Coefficient Difference
SKCM	Skin Cutaneous Melanoma
TCGA	The Cancer Genome Atlas
TPM	Transcripts Per Million

Appendix A New Algorithm for Model-Free Knockoff Variable Construction

We propose a new algorithm for constructing knockoff variables without Gaussian assumption, by obtaining the conditional distributions empirically through regression models, regardless of the joint distribution of the covariates. Knockoff construction is independent from the response and the form of associations between response and covariates. Our proposal is to generate random samples from the conditional distributions by simply permuting the residuals, assuming that the residuals are approximately independently and identically distributed. Details of the algorithm are summarized in Algorithm A.1.

Algorithm A.1 (Algorithm for construction of model-free knockoff variables).

For each covariate X_j, $j = 1, \cdots, p$,

(1) Fit X_j on $(X_{-j}, \widetilde{X}_{1:j-1})$ with a regression model, where X_{-j} denotes $(X_1, \cdots, X_{j-1}, X_{j+1}, \cdots, X_p)$ and $\widetilde{X}_{1:j-1}$ represents existing knockoffs. No knockoffs are taken into consideration for X_1.

(2) Compute residuals $\varepsilon = (\varepsilon_1, \cdots, \varepsilon_n)$ by subtracting the predicted value for X_j from the corresponding observed values, i.e., $\varepsilon_l = X_{jl} - \hat{X}_{jl}, l = 1, \ldots, n$, where $\hat{X}_{jl}$ is the predicted value of X_{jl} by the regression model.

(3) Permute the residuals randomly, denoted by the permuted residuals $\varepsilon^* = (\varepsilon_1^*, \cdots, \varepsilon_n^*)$.

(4) Construct knockoff variable $\widetilde{X}_j$ by adding the corresponding permuted residual to the predicted value for X_j, i.e., $\widetilde{X}_{jl} = \hat{X}_{jl} + \varepsilon_l^*, l = 1, \ldots, n$.

(5) Proceed to the next covariate until all knockoffs are constructed.

Unlike [15,16], our proposed algorithm does not assume the multivariate Gaussian joint distributions of the covariates. The only requirement is the independence of the residuals, which may require an appropriate choice of regression model for fitting. For example, lasso [7] would be a good choice when X_j is linearly dependent on $(X_{-j}, \widetilde{X}_{1:j-1})$, and supervised machine learning techniques like support vector regression [17] and gradient boosting [18] are flexible enough to approximate nonlinear functional dependence. To avoid the problem of over-fitting, we may use K-fold cross-validation on test sets for prediction in subsequent calculations. Cross-validation may also help select optimal tuning parameters in the regression model and thus enable the method to be well adaptive to the observed covariate data.

Given the construction algorithm, we can generate knockoff variables from an arbitrary distribution, thus, effectively increasing the level of flexibility on the covariate distribution. For instance, for a binary response, we can simply replace the aforementioned regression models by classification models and then permute the binary response within the same prediction group to generate random samples for knockoffs.

The drawback of Algorithm A.1 is an increased computational burden. In our simulations, we noticed that the moments-based knockoff construction algorithm proposed in [16] is not very sensitive to the multivariate Gaussian assumption, and achieve similar performance as our regression-based knockoff construction algorithm in most cases (See Appendix C). Therefore, to save computing times, we use the algorithm in [16] for all the simulations and real data experiments, unless otherwise noted. Nevertheless, our regression-based knockoff construction algorithm has the potential to be used in broader scenarios, including situations when the Gaussian assumption is severely violated.

Appendix B Difference in R-Squared (DRS) Statistic

Algorithm B.1 gives the complete procedure for calculating the DRS statistics.

Algorithm B.1 (The DRS algorithm).

(1) Fit y with $(X, \widetilde{X})$ using a prediction model and obtain R^2, where $X = (X_i, \ldots, X_p)$ contains the original predictor variables and $\widetilde{X} = (\widetilde{X}_1, \ldots, \widetilde{X}_p)$ contains the corresponding knockoff variables. $(X, \widetilde{X})$ is considered as an augmented design matrix with $2p$ columns.

(2) For each variable or knockoff variable in $(X, \widetilde{X})$, $j = 1, \ldots, 2p$, fit y with $(X, \widetilde{X})$ excluding the j-th variable with the same prediction model as in step 1) and obtain R_j^2. Calculate the absolute value of the difference between the two R-squared values, $Z_j = \left| R^2 - R_j^2 \right|$, $j = 1, \ldots, 2p$, and record it as the importance score for the j-th variable (or knockoff variable).

(3) For $j = 1, \ldots, p$, the DRS statistic for X_j can be derived as $W_j = Z_j - Z_{j+p}$, that is, the difference in Z between a variable and its knockoff.

The anti-symmetry requirement for feature statistics in [16] is fulfilled by the way we construct the DRS statistic. A large positive value of W_j provides evidence that variable X_j is strongly associated with the response y, while the statistic for a null variable is equally likely to take on a small positive or negative value, i.e., to have a symmetric distribution around zero. Similar to Algorithm A.1, we can apply various prediction methods for fitting in steps (1) and (2), for example, lasso for the linear relationship between y and $(X, \widetilde{X})$, and supervised machine learning techniques such as support vector regression and gradient boosting for nonlinear associations. To avoid the problem of over-fitting, we can use K-fold cross-validation and summarize the predictive power of the models by mean squared prediction error which can produce a cross-validated R^2. Cross-validation can also help select the tuning parameters in the prediction model and thereby enable the method to be well adaptive to the observed data.

Appendix C Additional Simulations

We conduct additional simulation experiments to compare four approaches: (1) knockoff construction using Gaussian based algorithm in [16] with RRB statistics in Section 2.2.2 (named Knockoff + mboost), (2) knockoff construction using model-free algorithm in Appendix A with RRB statistics (named Model-free knockoff + mboost), (3) knockoff construction using Gaussian based algorithm with DRS statistics in Appendix B (named Knockoff + DRS), and (4) knockoff construction using Gaussian based algorithm with RRB statistics but without nonlinear screening in Section 2.3 (named Knockoff + mboost + no screening). The simulation setting is similar to that of Section 3.1.1, except that here we exponentiate each element of the design matrix X, so that the covariates follow multivariate log-normal distribution. Furthermore, to save computing time, we let $n = 100$ and $p = 100$. The comparison results are shown in Figure A1. We can see that except for Knockoff + DRS which has an inflated FDP and a lower power, all three other methods have similar performance.

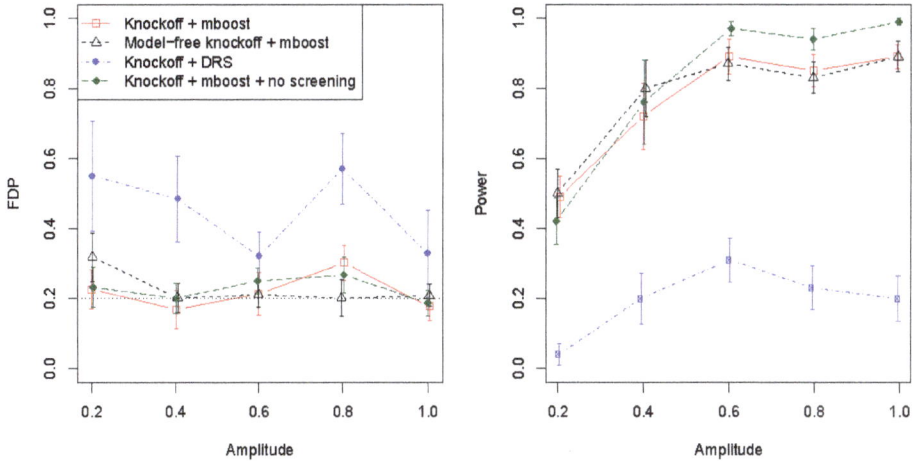

Figure A1. Simulation results for linear associations with log-normal covariates. Left panel: averaged false discovery proportion (FDP, the empirical version of FDR) and the standard error bars for knockoff variable selection with Knockoff with mboost (red), Model-free knockoff with mboost (black), Knockoff with DRS (blue) and Knockoff with mboost without screening (dark green) as a function of amplitude (association strength (e.g., correlation) between a biomarker and the outcome) based on 10 simulation replications. The reference lines indicate the target false discovery rate of 20%. Right panel: corresponding empirical statistical power of the four methods.

References

1. Miki, Y.; Swensen, J.; Shattuck-Eidens, D.; Futreal, P.A.; Harshman, K.; Tavtigian, S.; Liu, Q.; Cochran, C.; Bennett, L.M.; Ding, W.; et al. A strong candidate for the breast and ovarian cancer susceptibility gene BRCA1. *Science* **1994**, *266*, 66–71. [CrossRef] [PubMed]
2. Slamon, D.J.; Leyland-Jones, B.; Shak, S.; Fuchs, H.; Paton, V.; Bajamonde, A.; Fleming, T.; Eiermann, W.; Wolter, J.; Pegram, M.; et al. Use of chemotherapy plus a monoclonal antibody against HER2 for metastatic breast cancer that overexpresses HER2. *N. Engl. J. Med.* **2001**, *344*, 783–792. [CrossRef] [PubMed]
3. Paez, J.G.; Jänne, P.A.; Lee, J.C.; Tracy, S.; Greulich, H.; Gabriel, S.; Herman, P.; Kaye, F.J.; Lindeman, N.; Boggon, T.J.; et al. EGFR mutations in lung cancer: correlation with clinical response to gefitinib therapy. *Science* **2004**, *304*, 1497–1500. [CrossRef] [PubMed]
4. Catalona, W.J.; Smith, D.S.; Ratliff, T.L.; Dodds, K.M.; Coplen, D.E.; Yuan, J.J.; Petros, J.A.; Andriole, G.L. Measurement of prostate-specific antigen in serum as a screening test for prostate cancer. *N. Engl. J. Med.* **1991**, *324*, 1156–1161. [CrossRef]
5. Shaughnessy, J.D.; Zhan, F.; Burington, B.E.; Huang, Y.; Colla, S.; Hanamura, I.; Stewart, J.P.; Kordsmeier, B.; Randolph, C.; Williams, D.R.; et al. A validated gene expression model of high-risk multiple myeloma is defined by deregulated expression of genes mapping to chromosome 1. *Blood* **2007**, *109*, 2276–2284. [CrossRef]
6. Sun, S.; Hood, M.; Scott, L.; Peng, Q.; Mukherjee, S.; Tung, J.; Zhou, X. Differential expression analysis for RNAseq using Poisson mixed models. *Nucleic Acids Res.* **2017**, *45*, e106. [CrossRef]

7. Tibshirani, R. Regression shrinkage and selection via the lasso. *J. R. Stat. Soc. Ser. B (Methodol.)* **1996**, *58*, 267–288. [CrossRef]
8. Friedman, J.; Hastie, T.; Tibshirani, R. Regularization paths for generalized linear models via coordinate descent. *J. Stat. Softw.* **2010**, *33*, 1. [CrossRef]
9. Simon, N.; Friedman, J.; Hastie, T.; Tibshirani, R. Regularization paths for Coxars proportional hazards model via coordinate descent. *J. Stat. Softw.* **2011**, *39*, 1. [CrossRef] [PubMed]
10. Ayers, K.L.; Cordell, H.J. SNP selection in genome-wide and candidate gene studies via penalized logistic regression. *Genet. Epidemiol.* **2010**, *34*, 879–891. [CrossRef]
11. Wu, T.T.; Chen, Y.F.; Hastie, T.; Sobel, E.; Lange, K. Genome-wide association analysis by lasso penalized logistic regression. *Bioinformatics* **2009**, *25*, 714–721. [CrossRef]
12. He, K.; Zhou, X.; Jiang, H.; Wen, X.; Li, Y. False discovery control for penalized variable selections with high-dimensional covariates. *Stat. Appl. Genet. Mol. Biol.* **2018**, *17*. [CrossRef]
13. Benjamini, Y.; Hochberg, Y. Controlling the false discovery rate: A practical and powerful approach to multiple testing. *J. R. Stat. Soc. Ser. B (Methodol.)* **1995**, *57*, 289–300. [CrossRef]
14. Efron, B. Estimation and accuracy after model selection. *J. Am. Stat. Assoc.* **2014**, *109*, 991–1007. [CrossRef] [PubMed]
15. Barber, R.F.; Candès, E.J. Controlling the false discovery rate via knockoffs. *Ann. Stat.* **2015**, *43*, 2055–2085. [CrossRef]
16. Candes, E.; Fan, Y.; Janson, L.; Lv, J. Panning for gold:'model-X' knockoffs for high dimensional controlled variable selection. *J. R. Stat. Soc. Ser. B (Stat. Methodol.)* **2018**, *80*, 551–577. [CrossRef]
17. Cortes, C.; Vapnik, V. Support-vector networks. *Mach. Learn.* **1995**, *20*, 273–297. [CrossRef]
18. Friedman, J.H. Greedy function approximation: A gradient boosting machine. *Ann. Stat.* **2001**, 1189–1232. [CrossRef]
19. Cox, D.R. Regression models and life-tables. *J. R. Stat. Soc. Ser. B (Methodol.)* **1972**, *34*, 187–202. [CrossRef]
20. Gao, L.; Smit, M.A.; van den Oord, J.J.; Goeman, J.J.; Verdegaal, E.M.; van der Burg, S.H.; Stas, M.; Beck, S.; Gruis, N.A.; Tensen, C.P.; et al. Genome-wide promoter methylation analysis identifies epigenetic silencing of MAPK 13 in primary cutaneous melanoma. *Pigment Cell Melanoma Res.* **2013**, *26*, 542–554. [CrossRef]
21. Walesch, S.; Richter, A.; Helmbold, P.; Dammann, R. Claudin11 promoter hypermethylation is frequent in malignant melanoma of the skin, but uncommon in nevus cell nevi. *Cancers* **2015**, *7*, 1233–1243. [CrossRef]
22. Kuo, S.J.; Chien, S.Y.; Lin, C.; Chan, S.E.; Tsai, H.T.; Chen, D.R. Significant elevation of CLDN16 and HAPLN3 gene expression in human breast cancer. *Oncol. Rep.* **2010**, *24*, 759–766.
23. Gomez-Rueda, H.; Palacios-Corona, R.; Gutiérrez-Hermosillo, H.; Trevino, V. A robust biomarker of differential correlations improves the diagnosis of cytologically indeterminate thyroid cancers. *Int. J. Mol. Med.* **2016**, *37*, 1355–1362. [CrossRef] [PubMed]
24. Rangel, L.B.; Sherman-Baust, C.A.; Wernyj, R.P.; Schwartz, D.R.; Cho, K.R.; Morin, P.J. Characterization of novel human ovarian cancer-specific transcripts (HOSTs) identified by serial analysis of gene expression. *Oncogene* **2003**, *22*, 7225. [CrossRef] [PubMed]
25. Fan, J.; Zhu, M.; Wang, Y.; Li, Z.; Zhang, J.; Wang, L.; Sun, Q.; Dai, J.; Jin, G.; Hu, Z.; et al. Genome-wide analysis of expression quantitative trait loci identified potential lung cancer susceptibility variants among Asian populations. *Carcinogenesis* **2019**. [CrossRef]
26. Collins, C.S.; Hong, J.; Sapinoso, L.; Zhou, Y.; Liu, Z.; Micklash, K.; Schultz, P.G.; Hampton, G.M. A small interfering RNA screen for modulators of tumor cell motility identifies MAP4K4 as a promigratory kinase. *Proc. Natl. Acad. Sci. USA* **2006**, *103*, 3775–3780. [CrossRef] [PubMed]
27. Liang, J.J.; Wang, H.; Rashid, A.; Tan, T.H.; Hwang, R.F.; Hamilton, S.R.; Abbruzzese, J.L.; Evans, D.B.; Wang, H. Expression of MAP4K4 is associated with worse prognosis in patients with stage II pancreatic ductal adenocarcinoma. *Clin. Cancer Res.* **2008**, *14*, 7043–7049. [CrossRef]
28. Wang, L.X.; Li, Y.; Chen, G.Z. Network-based co-expression analysis for exploring the potential diagnostic biomarkers of metastatic melanoma. *PLoS ONE* **2018**, *13*, e0190447. [CrossRef]
29. Nikitina, A.S.; Sharova, E.I.; Danilenko, S.A.; Butusova, T.B.; Vasiliev, A.O.; Govorov, A.V.; Prilepskaya, E.A.; Pushkar, D.Y.; Kostryukova, E.S. Novel RNA biomarkers of prostate cancer revealed by RNA-seq analysis of formalin-fixed samples obtained from Russian patients. *Oncotarget* **2017**, *8*, 32990. [CrossRef]

30. Patiño-García, A.; Zalacain, M.; Folio, C.; Zandueta, C.; Sierrasesúmaga, L.; San Julián, M.; Toledo, G.; De Las Rivas, J.; Lecanda, F. Profiling of Chemonaive Osteosarcoma and Paired-Normal Cells Identifies EBF2 as a Mediator of Osteoprotegerin Inhibition to Tumor Necrosis Factor–Related Apoptosis-Inducing Ligand–Induced Apoptosis. *Clin. Cancer Res.* **2009**, *15*, 5082–5091. [CrossRef]

31. Dunwell, T.; Hesson, L.; Rauch, T.A.; Wang, L.; Clark, R.E.; Dallol, A.; Gentle, D.; Catchpoole, D.; Maher, E.R.; Pfeifer, G.P.; et al. A genome-wide screen identifies frequently methylated genes in haematological and epithelial cancers. *Mol. Cancer* **2010**, *9*, 44. [CrossRef]

32. Cai, W.Y.; Chen, X.; Chen, L.P.; Li, Q.; Du, X.J.; Zhou, Y.Y. Role of differentially expressed genes and long non-coding RNAs in papillary thyroid carcinoma diagnosis, progression, and prognosis. *J. Cell. Biochem.* **2018**, *119*, 8249–8259. [CrossRef]

33. Luo, L.; Cui, J.; Feng, Z.; Li, Y.; Wang, M.; Cai, Y.; Wu, Y.; Jin, J. Lentiviral-mediated overexpression of KCTD12 inhibits the proliferation of human uveal melanoma OCM-1 cells. *Oncol. Rep.* **2017**, *37*, 871–878. [CrossRef]

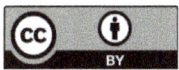

cancers

MDPI

Article

A Systematic Pan-Cancer Analysis of Genetic Heterogeneity Reveals Associations with Epigenetic Modifiers

Mafalda Ramos de Matos [1], Ioana Posa [1], Filipa Sofia Carvalho [1], Vanessa Alexandra Morais [1], Ana Rita Grosso [1,2,*] and Sérgio Fernandes de Almeida [1,*]

[1] Instituto de Medicina Molecular João Lobo Antunes, Faculdade de Medicina da Universidade de Lisboa, 1649-028 Lisboa, Portugal; mafaldarmatos@msn.com (M.R.d.M.); ioana.posa@gmail.com (I.P.); filipa.carvalho@medicina.ulisboa.pt (F.S.C.); vmorais@medicina.ulisboa.pt (V.A.M.)

[2] UCIBIO, Departamento de Ciências da Vida, Faculdade de Ciências e Tecnologia, Universidade NOVA de Lisboa, 2829-516 Caparica, Portugal

* Correspondence: argrosso@fct.unl.pt (A.R.G.); sergioalmeida@medicina.ulisboa.pt (S.F.d.A.)

Received: 12 February 2019; Accepted: 17 March 2019; Published: 20 March 2019

Abstract: Intratumor genetic heterogeneity (ITH) is the main obstacle to effective cancer treatment and a major mechanism of drug resistance. It results from the continuous evolution of different clones of a tumor over time. However, the molecular features underlying the emergence of genetically-distinct subclonal cell populations remain elusive. Here, we conducted an exhaustive characterization of ITH across 2807 tumor samples from 16 cancer types. Integration of ITH scores and somatic variants detected in each tumor sample revealed that mutations in epigenetic modifier genes are associated with higher ITH levels. In particular, genes that regulate genome-wide histone and DNA methylation emerged as being determinant of high ITH. Indeed, the knockout of histone methyltransferase SETD2 or DNA methyltransferase DNMT3A using the CRISPR/Cas9 system on cancer cells led to significant expansion of genetically-distinct clones and culminated in highly heterogeneous cell populations. The ITH scores observed in knockout cells recapitulated the heterogeneity levels observed in patient tumor samples and correlated with a better mitochondrial bioenergetic performance under stress conditions. Our work provides new insights into tumor development, and discloses new drivers of ITH, which may be useful as either predictive biomarkers or therapeutic targets to improve cancer treatment.

Keywords: cancer; intratumor heterogeneity; genomic instability; epigenetics; mitochondrial metabolism

1. Introduction

The expansion of genetically-distinct cell populations within a tumor creates a subclonal architecture that varies dynamically throughout cancer progression [1]. This acquired cancer trait, termed intratumor heterogeneity (ITH), is the substrate for Darwinian evolution to act upon, selecting subclones carrying phenotypes that favor tumor progression [2]. The outgrowth of such subclones impacts cancer development, drug resistance and tumor relapse [3–6]. Despite the key role ITH plays in cancer, important questions regarding its magnitude, origin and genetic drivers across different cancer types remain largely unanswered. By facilitating the emergence of nucleotide sequence mutations, copy-number alterations, chromosomal translocations or aneuploidies, genomic instability has been regarded as the major source of ITH [4,7–9]. However, discrepancies in the rates of genomic instability and ITH observed in previous comprehensive studies [3] suggest that additional events congregate to increase genetic heterogeneity in tumors.

Besides mutations, cancer cells invariably present with some degree of epigenetic alterations that contribute to the acquisition of the cancer hallmarks [10,11]. Indeed, there is evidence that epigenomic reprogramming plays a seminal role in tumorigenesis by creating a progenitor-like cell state that facilitates expression of driver mutations and tumor initiation [12]. High-resolution genome-sequencing efforts have identified driver mutations in genes that regulate the epigenome, namely, genome-wide chromatin and DNA methylation [13,14]. For instance, acute monocytic leukemias frequently (20.5%) carry mutations in the de novo DNA methyltransferase gene *DNMT3A*, displaying aberrant genome-wide DNA methylation profiles [15]. Ten percent of kidney renal clear cell carcinomas (KIRC) have mutations in *SETD2*, the methyltransferase responsible for trimethylation of Lys36 in histone H3 (H3K36me3), which is necessary for accurate gene expression and DNA repair [16–19]. H3K36me3 is also involved in targeting DNMT3A to chromatin [20], highlighting the finely tuned epigenetic interplay between histone and DNA methylation that is needed for normal cell function and is frequently disrupted in cancer cells.

While epigenetic deregulation in cancer arises primarily as a consequence of DNA mutations, the view that altered epigenomes may also change DNA mutation rates highlights reciprocal interactions that contribute to cancer development [14,21]. Accordingly, epigenomic disruption should favor the development of genetically-diverse tumor cell populations, fueling ITH [21]. In fact, a possible relationship between genomic and epigenomic alterations during clonal evolution of tumors has recently been suggested in esophageal squamous cell carcinoma and glioma, where high concordance was observed between the evolution of genetic and epigenetic diversification [22,23]. In this study, we reasoned that analysis of whole-exome datasets of The Cancer Genome Atlas (TCGA) would disclose patterns of covariation between specific epigenetic modifier genes and ITH levels. Our integrative pan-cancer characterization of somatic variants and ITH identified mutations in epigenetic modifier genes that display an association with increased clonal evolution across several cancer types. Experimental ablation of specific *loci* provided direct evidence that loss of *SETD2* or *DNMT3A* drives the emergence of genetically-distinct subclonal cell populations. Knockout cells showed increased mitochondrial bioenergetic performance under stress conditions, a phenotypic trait that fosters the Darwinian selection of clones. Our results provide an unprecedented pan-cancer portrait of the major determinants of ITH and an experimental validation of the role of specific epigenetic modifier genes, laying a foundation for more effective cancer prognoses and treatment.

2. Results

2.1. Genomic Instability Does Not Predict ITH in Many Cancer Types

To estimate correlations between genomic instability and ITH in different cancers, we examined 2807 tumor whole-exome sequences from 16 cancer types of TCGA. We assigned an overall genomic instability score to each tumor, defined as the number of somatic point mutations and small insertions and deletions (INDELs) ranging from 1 to 100 bp in length. The ITH score was obtained using the mutant-allele tumor heterogeneity (MATH) method (Figure 1A and Table S1) [24]. MATH evaluates the variability of the mutant-allele fractions among all tumor-specific mutated *loci*. Therefore, homogeneous tumors with high mutation incidence have a narrower distribution of mutant-allele fractions than heterogeneous tumors. In agreement with previous reports [3], we found that the degree of genomic instability is highly variable across tumors types (Figure 1A). Notably, high levels of genomic instability were not positively correlated with ITH in several tumors (Figure 1B). Individual analysis of each cancer type revealed that only thyroid carcinoma (THCA), pancreatic adenocarcinoma (PAAD) and kidney renal clear cell carcinoma (KIRC) exhibited a statistically significant positive correlation between genomic instability and ITH (Figure 1B). Moreover, we found a significant negative correlation between these two features in kidney renal papillary cell carcinoma (KIRP) and adrenocortical carcinoma (ACC) (Figure 1B). This finding suggests that factors other than increased mutability determine the development and expansion of genetically-distinct subclonal cell populations within a tumor.

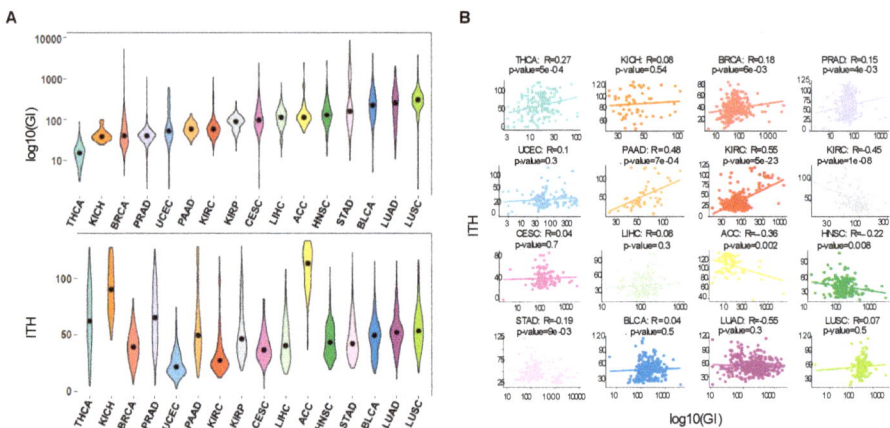

Figure 1. Pan-cancer correlations reveal that genomic instability does not predict ITH. (**A**) Distribution of genomic instability (log10 transformed) and ITH across 16 TCGA cancer types: THCA (thyroid carcinoma), KICH (kidney Chromophobe), BRCA (breast invasive carcinoma), PRAD (prostate adenocarcinoma), UCEC (uterine Corpus Endometrial Carcinoma), PAAD (pancreatic adenocarcinoma), KIRC (kidney renal clear cell carcinoma), KIRP (kidney renal papillary cell carcinoma), CESC (cervical squamous cell carcinoma and endocervical adenocarcinoma), LIHC (liver hepatocellular carcinoma), ACC (adrenocortical carcinoma), HNSC (head and neck squamous cell carcinoma), STAD (stomach adenocarcinoma), BLCA (bladder urothelial carcinoma), LUAD (lung adenocarcinoma), LUSC (lung squamous cell carcinoma). Cancers are ordered according to genomic instability levels. (**B**) Pearson correlation between genomic instability (log10 transformed) and ITH for each cancer type. Each point represents one patient and the line shows the fitted linear model.

2.2. Mutations in Epigenetic Modifier Genes Are Strong Determinants of ITH

To investigate whether epigenomic deregulation drives the development of tumors with high levels of ITH, we focused our analysis on KIRC, the cancer type with the highest frequency of mutations in epigenetic modifiers (Figure 2A). The important role of epigenomic deregulation in the development and progression of KIRC is illustrated by the finding that patients with mutations in epigenetic modifiers have worse overall survival compared to those without mutations in these genes ($p < 0.05$, log-rank test; Figure 2B). To investigate how epigenomic deregulation compares with other specific cellular processes in influencing ITH in KIRC, we analyzed significantly mutated genes grouped in broad functional categories as previously described [25]. The linear model revealed that mutations in epigenetic modifiers are the most strongly associated with high ITH in KIRC, amongst all categories of genes analyzed (Figure 2C). Moreover, the presence of mutations in epigenetic modifier genes correlates positively with increased ITH across different cancer types (Figure 2D and Table S2). Next, we aimed at identifying the individual genes that, when mutated, more accurately predict ITH. To this end, we used generalized linear models previously applied to infer the association of genetic alterations with other phenotypic variables [26]. The strongest predictor of high ITH in both KIRC alone or across several cancer types was the presence of mutations in *SETD2*, *DNMT1* and *DNTM3A* (Figure 2E). Importantly, we could model 32% of variability in KIRC ITH using only mutations in *SETD2*, *DNMT1* and *DNTM3A* (Figure 2F). The optimal model showed a significant correlation between the observed and predicted ITH levels based on the tumor mutation profiles (Figure 2F,G). These data suggest that epigenomic deregulation is an important determinant of ITH and identify mutations in *SETD2*, *DNMT1* and *DNTM3A* as candidate drivers of ITH.

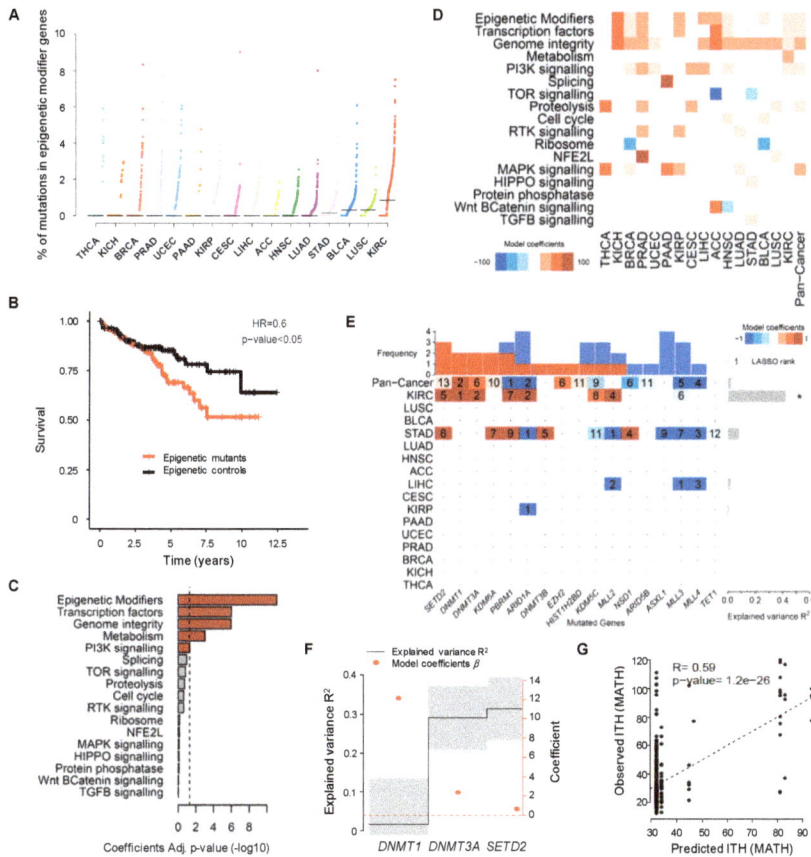

Figure 2. Driver mutations of pan-cancer ITH. (**A**) Pan-cancer analysis of the percentage of somatic mutations in epigenetic modifier genes across 16 TCGA cancer types. The vertical axis shows the percentage of mutations in epigenetic modifier genes whereas the different cancer types are ordered on the horizontal axis from the lowest to the highest percentage of mutations in these genes. (**B**) Kaplan-Meier plot comparing the survival of KIRC patients segregated according to the presence (red) or absence (black) of mutations in epigenetic modifiers. The log-rank test was used for statistical analysis. (**C**) Statistical significance ($-\log 10$ Benjamini-Hochberg Adj. *p*-value) of the linear model coefficients estimated for each gene group in KIRC. The vertical dashed line corresponds to the significance level (BH adj. *p*-value of 0.05). (**D**) Heatmap of the linear model coefficients estimated for each cancer type and gene group. Only statistically significant coefficients are represented (BH adj. *p*-value < 0.05). (**E**) Heatmap of driver mutations of ITH across several cancer types depicted by a LASSO penalized model. LASSO-selected coefficients are colored according to the effect of each standardized covariate in the optimal model. The numbers on each tile denote the order in which variables are included indicating their relative importance. The top bar plot indicates the frequency at which each driver-gene mutation occurs in the ITH fitted model. The right bar plot shows the explained variance. An asterisk (*) denotes models where the explained variance (R^2) is greater than zero by a margin of more than one standard deviation. (**F**) Variance explained by selected driver genes (black line $\pm$ 1 standard deviation) ordered by their occurrence in a LASSO penalized model for ITH in KIRC using only the mutated genes *DNMT1, DNMT3A* and *SETD2*. The optimal model maximizes the explained variance R2. The right axis indicates the effect of each standardized covariate in the optimal model (red dots). (**G**) Scatter plot of predicted and observed ITH for KIRC (Estimate and statistical significance of the Pearson correlation are presented).

2.3. Knockout of SETD2 or DNMT3A Expands the Clonal Diversity of Cancer Cell Populations

We next sought to experimentally validate the role of *SETD2*, *DNMT1* and *DNMT3A* mutations in driving the emergence of genetically-distinct subclonal cell populations. The mutations found in these genes were predicted as deleterious causing loss of function (Table S3). To recapitulate this phenotype, we employed CRISPR/Cas9 system to specifically knockout each of these genes in KIRC Caki-2 cell lines. Insertion of small INDELs at the target sites was confirmed by DNA sequencing and efficiency of gene knockout evaluated by measuring protein levels (Figure 3A). Decreased H3K36me3 levels were used as a surrogate for SETD2 depletion (Figure 3A). Importantly, knockout of DNMT1 rendered KIRC cells senescent (Figure 3B), in contrast to DNMT3A and SETD2 depletion, which were well tolerated and did not significantly affect cell proliferation (Figure 3C). This finding suggests that additional compensatory mutations are required to allow the proliferation of *DNMT1* mutant cells within tumors. Alternatively, *DNMT1* mutant clones could be selected during tumor evolution due their ability to promote carcinogenesis through the senescence-associated secretory phenotype [27–29].

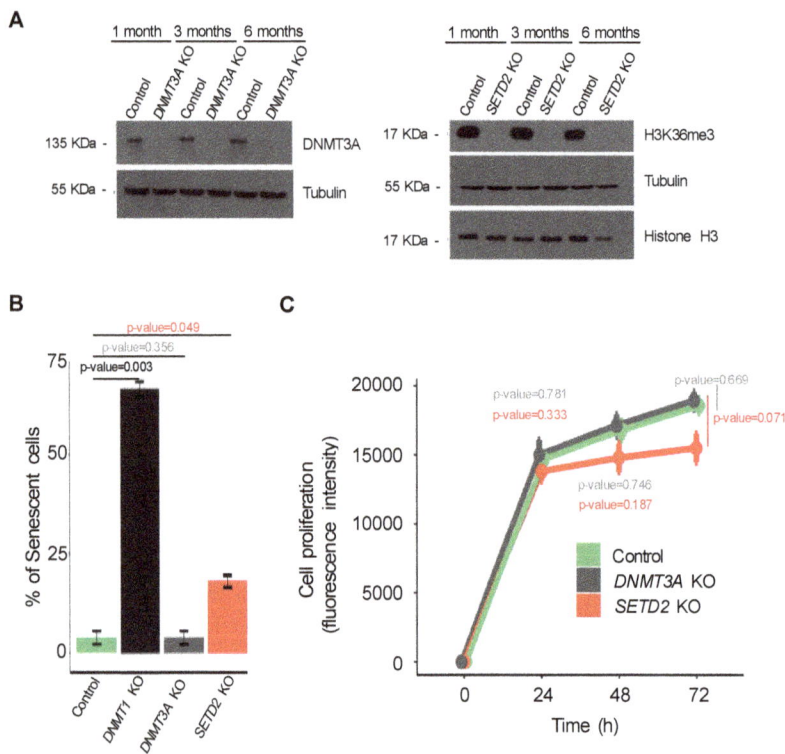

Figure 3. CRISPR/Cas9 knockout of candidate ITH-driver genes in cancer cells. (**A**) The levels of DNMT3A and H3K36me3 were estimated by western blot 1, 3 and 6 months after knockout. (**B**) The percentage of senescent cells in control and mutant conditions (*SETD2*, *DNMT1* and *DNMT3A* knockouts) was assessed by β-galactosidase staining (error bars indicate SEM; n = 3 counting regions of 150 cells/condition in triplicate; Student t-test). (**C**) The proliferation rate of the indicated cells was measured by AlamarBlue dye reduction at the indicated time points. All data are presented as mean (four technical replicates in the same experiment) ± SEM.

To investigate whether loss of *DNMT3A* or *SETD2* drives the acquisition of genetically-heterogeneous cell populations over time, we performed whole-exome sequencing of control and knockout cells cultured during 1, 3 and 6 months (Figure 4A). ITH levels of three different cell populations per experimental condition (control, *SETD2* and *DNMT3A* knockout) were measured at each time point using MATH. Compared to control cells, loss of either *SETD2* or *DNMT3A* resulted in significantly increased and comparable levels of ITH after just one month (Figure 4B and Table S4). However, while ITH rose for up to three months after *SETD2* depletion, it remained constant through time in *DNMT3A* knockout cells (Figure 4B). Bayesian cluster analysis of mutations using PyClone [30] identified 25 mutation clusters that are distributed in each cell population at a frequency that permits segregation according to the knockout gene (Figure 4C). ITH scores observed in *SETD2* and *DNMT3A* knockout cell lines were not significantly different from those determined in TCGA samples carrying *SETD2* and *DNMT3A* mutations, respectively (Figure 4D). This finding reveals that the clonal dynamics of cancer cells grown in vitro recapitulates the in vivo scenario. Altogether, these data suggest that loss of *SETD2* or *DNMT3A* drives specific patterns of clonal evolution that culminate in tumors with increased levels of ITH.

2.4. Epigenomic Deregulation Drives Favorable Metabolic Phenotypic Variation

The increased ITH observed knockout of *SETD2* or *DNMT3A* knockout suggests that new clones carrying phenotypic traits that confer selective advantage within the cell populations have expanded and were selected. In cancer cells, mitochondria play important roles in energy production, redox and calcium homeostasis, transcriptional regulation and cell death [31]. Changes in mitochondrial metabolism constitute an important source of variability for natural selection to act upon [32,33]. To test whether epigenomic deregulation drives altered mitochondrial metabolic functions, we evaluated the ability of cells to adapt to shifts in energy demands by measuring mitochondrial respiration rates using an oxygen electrode on the Seahorse platform. In this assay, the oxygen consumption rate was measured before and after the addition of inhibitors to derive parameters of mitochondrial respiration in baseline and stress conditions (Figure 5A). Basal mitochondrial respiration in knockout and parental cells was equally efficient (Figure 5B), indicating that no major intrinsic metabolic alterations were caused upon loss of either *SETD2* or *DNMT3A*. We then measured the maximal respiratory capacity and spare capacity rate (SCR) of cells challenged with the mitochondrial uncoupler FCCP and the Complex I and Complex III specific inhibitors rotenone and antimycin A, respectively. Both parameters were significantly increased in *SETD2* and *DNMT3A* knockout cells when compared to parental cells under similar conditions (Figure 5C,D). Analysis of *SETD2* and *DNMT3A* knockout cells revealed mutations in genes involved in mitochondria biogenesis and function (Table S5); however, inspection of mitochondria network in knockout cells using fluorescence confocal microscopy did not reveal any major alterations (Figure 5E). These data rule out altered morphology as a causing factor for the observed increase in the spare capacity rate. Instead, our data suggest that gain-of-function mutations in genes involved in mitochondrial function drive higher spare capacity rates in knockout cells. Such an association between epigenetics, altered nuclear DNA expression and mitochondrial function has already been demonstrated in previous studies [34]. Altogether, these data provide direct experimental evidence for the emergence of favorable characteristics in *SETD2* and *DNMT3A* depleted cells that may foster the increased number of genetically-distinct clones within the cell population.

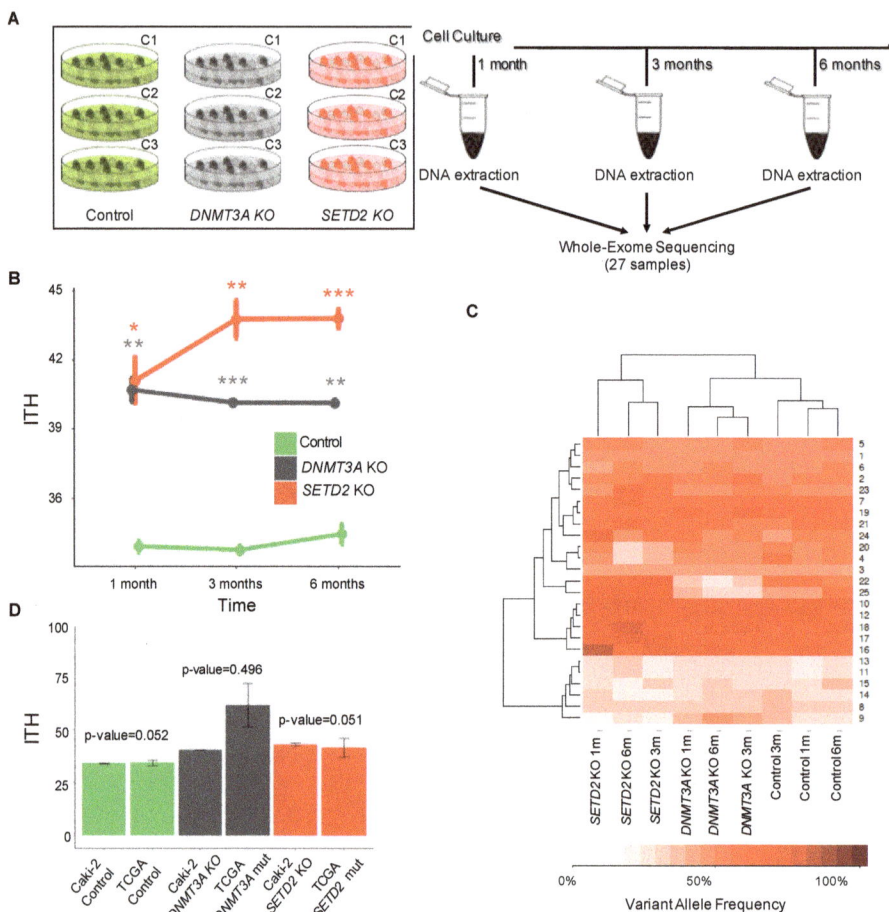

Figure 4. *SETD2* and *DNMT3A* knockout drive ITH. (**A**) Schematic representation of the experimental setup. Control and knockout cells were cultured during the indicated time periods before DNA extraction and whole-exome sequencing (WES). ITH was inspected after three independent clonal expansions (C1–C3) for each knockout at each time point. (**B**) ITH levels of *SETD2* and *DNMT3A* knockout cells after 1, 3 and 6 months. WES data of the indicated conditions were used to calculate ITH, as described in the Methods. Data from three independent clonal expansions analyzed per group are presented as mean ± SEM. Statistical analysis was a two-tailed Student's *t*-test (* $p < 0.05$, ** $p < 0.01$, *** $p < 0.001$). (**C**) Hierarchical cluster analysis of the mean variant allele frequency estimated with PyClone in control, *SETD2* and *DNMT3A* knockout cells. (**D**) Distribution and comparison of the ITH levels across KIRC patients from TCGA and Caki-2 cell lines for the indicated conditions (control, *SETD2* and *DNMT3A* knockouts). The bar graph displays mean ITH values and s.e.m. (standard error of the mean). Statistical analysis was performed with Wilcox-test but no statistical significance was observed between TCGA patients and each cell line.

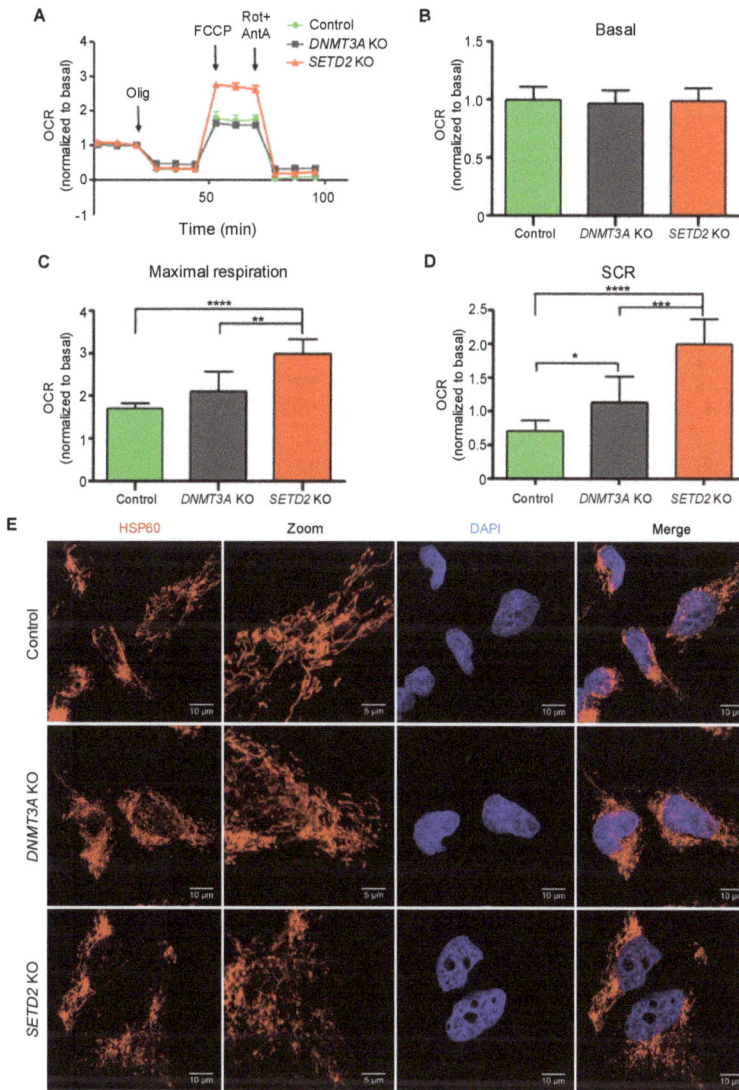

Figure 5. *SETD2* and *DNMT3A* knockout increase bioenergetic performance. Oxygen Consumption Rates (OCR) trace and respiration parameters were measured in control, *SETD2* and *DNMT3A* knockout cells. Seahorse extracellular flux measurements of OCR was normalized to basal respiration (**A**). Basal respiration (**B**), maximal respiration (**C**) and spare capacity rate (SCR) (**D**) of Caki-2 cell lines were obtain by OCR values representative of 3 independent experiments in which each data point represents replicates of three to five wells each cell line. Statistical analysis was performed using the unpaired Student's *t*-test, where * $p < 0.05$; ** $p < 0.01$; *** $p < 0.001$; **** $p < 0.0001$, data were represented as the mean $\pm$ SD. Olig: Oligomycin; FCCP; carbonyl cyanide-4-(trifluoromethoxy)phenylhydrazone; Rot+AntA; Rotenone+Antimycin A. (**E**) Mitochondria morphology of Caki-2 control, *DNMT3A* KO and *SETD2* KO cell lines. Cells were fixed and stained with the mitochondrial marker Hsp60 (red) and with the nucleus marker DAPI (blue). Cells were imaged on an inverted Zeiss LSM 880 microscope. Fiji software was used to calculate scale bar (10 µm or 5 µm for zoom-in). Selected image is representative of three independent experiments.

3. Discussion

Tumors evolve through multiple rounds of clonal expansion, diversification and selection that enable the acquisition of metabolic and bioenergetic phenotypes better adapted to the local microenvironment. Such evolutionary adaptation also accounts for therapeutic failure as drug-resistant tumor clones may be selected during therapy. High ITH is the substrate for this Darwinian model of cancer evolution and therapeutic resistance, and hence, highlights the need for further understanding of drivers and mechanisms of clonal evolution. Despite the major discrepancies observed in their covariance rates [3], genomic instability is still considered a major source of ITH [4,7–9]. In this study we show that genomic instability is not positively correlated with ITH in most cancer types. In fact, there is a significant negative correlation in some cancers, suggesting that additional processes must congregate to drive genetic heterogeneity. Our results are in agreement with previous studies, where ITH was associated with different forms of instability [35]. Recently, high concordance was observed between the evolution of genetic and epigenetic diversification in esophageal squamous cell carcinoma and in glioma, disclosing possible relationships between genomic and epigenomic alterations during the clonal evolution of tumors [22,23]. An interesting hypothesis linking DNA mutations and epigenetics in cancer is that altered DNA methylation or chromatin modifications may accelerate mutation rates. Examples of such relationship were already described. For example, abnormal DNA hypomethylation near guanine quadruplexes (G4s)-rich regions is a common signature for many DNA breakpoints associated with somatic copy-number alterations [36]. This finding suggests that DNA hypomethylation in genomic regions enriched for G4s acts as a mutagenic factor in cancer. Additionally, the genome organization into heterochromatin and euchromatin-like domains is a dominant determinant of mutation rates, as illustrated by the finding that H3K9me3 levels alone can predict over 40% of somatic mutation *loci* in human cancer samples [37]. Conversely, we and others have shown that H3K36me3 protects active coding sequences of the genome from error-prone DNA double-strand break repair mechanisms by promoting homologous recombination [17,38,39]. Together, these data establish a strong association between epigenomic deregulation—namely, DNA and histone methylation and genomic mutations, which we show play important roles during clonal evolution and genetic diversification of tumors. In fact, we found that mutations in epigenetic modifier genes are the strongest determinants of ITH amongst a panel of 17 distinct cellular pathways. Particularly, we identified and validated mutations in the methyltransferase genes *SETD2* and *DNMT3A* as potent drivers of ITH. Other epigenetic modifiers were also associated with high levels of ITH in KIRC (e.g., *PBRM1* or *KDM5C*), but correlated with lower heterogeneity in a pan-cancer analysis or in other cancer types. Our findings add direct experimental evidence to previous studies implicating SETD2 loss-of-function in mechanisms that generate ITH [40,41].

As tumor cells adapt to the environment, they acquire distinctive bioenergetic features to take advantage of available fuels. For instance, tumor cells growing in an environment rich in adipocytes could use fatty acids as a major energy source [33]. This remarkable versatility arises from clonal evolution, during which genetic heterogeneity would eventually impact the function of metabolic enzymes [32,33]. We thus reasoned that the increased ITH observed upon *SETD2* or *DNMT3A* knockout likely underpins phenotypic variations in mitochondrial metabolism upon which natural selection could act. In agreement with this, we observed that both *SETD2* and *DNMT3A* depleted cell populations have increased bioenergetic performance under stress conditions, a phenotype that was accompanied by mutations in genes involved in mitochondria function.

4. Materials and Methods

4.1. Cell Culture

Caki-2 cells (Cell Line Services, Eppelheim, Germany) that do not have *SETD2* mutations were selected as a cellular model of KIRC. Caki-2 and human embryonic kidney (HEK) 293T (ATCC, Manassas, VA, USA) cells were grown as monolayers in Dulbecco's modified Eagle medium (DMEM,

Invitrogen, Carlsbad, CA, USA), supplemented with 10% (*v/v*) FBS, 1% (*v/v*) nonessential amino acids, 1% (*v/v*) L-glutamine and 100U/mL penicillin-streptomycin and maintained at 37 °C in a humidified atmosphere with 5% CO_2.

4.2. Gene Knockout by CRISPR/Cas9

To establish knockout cell lines, we used the genome editing one vector system (lentiCRISPR-v2) (Addgene #52961). sgRNAs were designed by GenScript and the potential off-target effects was confirmed using the CRISPR tool (http://crispr.mit.edu). The following sgRNA sequences were selected: *DNMT1* CRISPR guide RNA 1: CTAGACGTCCATTCAC TTCC; *DNMT3A* CRISPR guide RNA 2: TGGCGCTCCTCCTTGCCACG and *SETD2* CRISPR guide RNA 1: AGTTCTTCTCGGTGTCCAAA. As a control we used a pCas-Scramble CRISPR Vector (SantaCruz, sc-418922). Recombinant lentiviruses were produced by co-transfecting HEK293T cells with each lentiCRISPR-v2 expression plasmid together with packaging plasmid pCMV-dR8.91 (Addgene) and the envelope plasmid pCMV-VSV-G (Addgene #8454) using Lipofectamine™ 3000 (Thermo Fisher Scientific, Waltham, MA, USA) as a transfection reagent and Opti-MEM (Invitrogen), according to the manufacturer's instructions. Infectious lentiviruses were collected 48 h after transfection. The supernatant was filtered through 0.45 μm filters (GE Healthcare, Chicago, IL, USA) and concentrated by ultra-centrifugation at 25,000 rpm, 4 °C for 90 min. Cells were infected with lentivirus at approximately 60% confluence. After 24 h, cells were incubated with 5 μg/mL of puromycin (InvivoGen, San Diego, CA, USA) for 2 days. To identify KO clones, infected cells were single-cell cloned in 96-well plates. Several clones from 96-well plates were selected and the presence of DNMT1, DNMT3A and SETD2 was verified by western blot and Sanger sequencing. Genomic DNA was extracted from each clone and a segment surrounding the *DNMT1*, *DNMT3A* and *SETD2* edited region was amplified with specific primers (Table S6). Target sites and specificity were validated using the UCSC Genome Browser (https://genome.ucsc.edu/).

4.3. Western Blot

Whole cell protein extracts were prepared by cell lysis with SDS-PAGE buffer (80 mM Tris-HCL pH 6.8, 16% glycerol, 4.5% SDS, 450 mM DTT, 0.01% bromophenol blue) with 200 U/mL benzonase (Sigma-Aldrich, St. Louis, MO, USA), 50 μM MgCl2 and were boiled for 5 min. Equal amounts of protein extracts were resolved by SDS-polyacrylamide gel electrophoresis (SDS-PAGE) and transferred to a nitrocellulose membrane. After 1 h blocking with 5% non-fat dry milk in 1× PBS, 0.1% Tween20 at room temperature, membranes were incubated with antibodies as follows: anti-DNMT1 (2 μg/mL, Active Motif, Carlsbad, CA, USA), anti-DNMT3A (1:1000, Cell Signaling), anti-H3K36me3 (1:500, Abcam, Cambridge, UK), α-tubulin (1:15,000, Sigma-Aldrich) and anti-histone H3 (1:1000, Abcam). Detection was performed with the appropriate secondary antibodies (Bio-Rad, Hercules, CA, USA) and enhanced luminescence substrate (Pierce ECL, Thermo Fisher Scientific, Waltham, MA, USA). Details of antibodies used are mentioned in Table S6.

4.4. Cell Senescence and Proliferation Assays

Senescent cells were identified by β-galactosidase staining in low-density culture. Caki-2 cells (controls and KOs) were seeded in 6-well plates at 10×10^4 cells/cm^2. In the next day, cells were washed with PBS 1×, fixed for 5 min (RT) in 2% formaldehyde/0.2% glutaraldehyde, washed, and incubated at 37 °C (with no CO_2) with senescence cells histochemical staining kit (Sigma-Aldrich, CS0030) according to manufacturer's recommendations for 12 h. Blue-stained cells and total number of cells was counted under the phase contrast microscope (Leica DM2500, Leica Biosystems, Wetzlar, Germany).

Cellular proliferation for human cancer cell lines (controls and KOs) was measured every 24 h for four days, using AlamarBlue™ (Thermo Fisher Scientific). Briefly, 10×10^4 cells/well were seeded on 96-well plates in a final volume of 100 μL per well. This is a reliable method for measuring cell viability, using the metabolic activity of cells to reduce resazurin (oxidized form: 7-hydroxy-3H-phenoxazin-3-1-10-oxide) to resorufin. The fluorescence of these two forms is measured at 560 nm as excitation wavelength and at 590 nm emission wavelength was measured every 24 h for 72 h, using a microplate reader (Microplate Reader TECAN Infinite M200, Tecan, Mannedorf, Switserland).

4.5. Mitochondria Oxygen Consumption Rate

Mitochondria oxygen consumption rate (OCR) was measured with the XF24 Extracellular Flux Analyzer (Seahorse Bioscience, Agilent, Santa Clara, CA, USA), according to the standard protocol. Briefly, at least 3 months after each knockout, cells were seeded one day prior to the assay in a 24-well XF plates at a density of 2×10^5 cell/well and incubated overnight at 37 °C, 5% CO_2. Twenty-four hours later, cells were incubated with Seahorse XF Base medium supplemented with 10 mM glucose, 2 mM L-glutamine and 1mM sodium pyruvate at pH 7.4 and calibrated for 1 h at 37 °C in the absence of CO_2. Hydration of the sensor cartridge was performed one day prior to the assay at 37 °C in the absence of CO_2. OCR was evaluated in a time course set-up where the following compounds were sequentially injected in the following order: oligomycin (1 µM final concentration), carbonyl cyanide-4-(trifluoromethoxy)phenylhydrazone (FCCP) (0.5 µM final concentration), and rotenone plus antimycin A (0.5 µM final concentration). Rates were normalized to protein concentration measured according to the Bradford method (Bio-Rad, Hercules, CA, USA). Three to five wells from each cell line were measure in a total of $n = 3$ experimental assays. Values for each parameter were calculated as the difference of OCR measures after and before injection:

a. Non-mitochondrial respiration was calculated as the average of OCR measurements after rotenone and antimycin A injection;
b. Basal respiration is calculated as the difference between non-mitochondrial respiration and the third point of baseline cellular oxygen consumption;
c. Maximal respiration corresponds to the difference between the average OCR value after FCCP injection and the non-mitochondria respiration;
d. Spare capacity rate (SCR) is the difference between maximal and basal respiration values.

4.6. Determination of Mitochondrial Morphology

Caki-2 control, Caki-2 DNMT3A and Caki-2 SETD2 cells were seeded on 13 mm coverslips. Twenty-four hours post seeding, cells were washed three times in PBS, fixed in 4% paraformaldehyde for 20 min, washed three times in PBS, permeabilized in 0.1% Triton X-100 in PBS for 10 min, followed by three washes in PBS. Cells were blocked in blocking buffer (0.2% gelatin, 2% fetal bovine serum, 2% BSA, 0.3% bovine serum albumin, 0.3% Triton X-100 in PBS) with 5% goat serum (DAKO) for 1 h. Cells were stained using the primary antibody mouse anti-hsp60 at 1/250 dilution (BD Bioscience) for 2 h. After 3 washes in PBS, cells were incubated with the secondary antibody Alexa Fluor 568 goat anti-mouse at 1/500 dilution (Life Technologies, Carlsbad, CA, USA) for 1 h and with DAPI at 1/10,000 dilution for 10 min. Images were visualized with a confocal laser point-scanning microscope Zeiss LSM 880 with airyscan through an objective of 63× 1.40 oil dipping lens (Zeiss, Oberkochen, Germany). Images were acquired using the ZEN software package (Zeiss) and analyzed in open source Fiji software (https://fiji.sc/).

4.7. Pan-Cancer Data Sets

WES data published in the context of TCGA was downloaded from Broad Institute MAF dashboard https://confluence.broadinstitute.org/display/GDAC/MAF+Dashboard, released (14 April 2017). A total of 2807 patients corresponding to 16 different carcinomas were analyzed: 71 adrenocortical carcinoma (ACC), 270 bladder urothelial carcinoma (BLCA), 228 breast invasive carcinoma (BRCA), 101 cervical squamous cell carcinoma (CESC), 196 head and neck squamous cell carcinoma (HNSC), 167 liver hepatocellular carcinoma (LIHC), 324 lung adenocarcinoma (LUAD),

118 lung squamous cell carcinoma (LUSC), 58 kidney chromophobe (KICH), 274 kidney renal clear cell carcinoma (KIRC), 149 kidney renal papillary cell carcinoma (KIRP), 46 pancreatic adenocarcinoma (PAAD), 349 prostate adenocarcinoma (PRAD), 181 stomach adenocarcinoma (STAD), 163 thyroid carcinoma (THCA), 112 uterine corpus endometrial carcinoma (UCEC). None of the patients were subjected to neoadjuvant therapies (neither chemotherapy or radiotherapy or immunotherapy) before tumor resection. A complete list of samples is given in Table S1. The effect mutations were predicted using cBioportal (Table S3) [42].

4.8. Pan-Cancer Characterization of Genomic Instability and Intratumor Heterogeneity

Genomic instability and ITH were determined using all the somatic point mutations and INDELs downloaded from the Broad Institute MAF dashboard. Genomic instability was calculated as the absolute number of mutations and INDEL observed in each tumor sample. The ITH defined as the genetic heterogeneity was measured considering the same somatic mutations and using the mutant-allele tumor heterogeneity (MATH) approach [24] (see Supplementary Methods for details). Briefly, for each individual tumor we: (1) obtained the mutant-allele fraction (MAF) values of the somatic mutations (the fraction of DNA that shows the mutated allele at a locus), (2) calculated the center (median) and the width of the distribution (median absolute deviation, MAD); (3) multiplied the median by a factor of 1.4826, so that the expected MAD of a normally distributed variable is equal to its standard deviation; (4) calculated the MATH value as the percentage ratio of the MAD to the median distribution of MAFs among the tumor's genomic *loci* (MATH = $100 \times$ MAD/median). Correlation between genomic instability and ITH was determined using Pearson method as implemented in cor.test function of R package [43].

4.9. Pan-Cancer Discovery of Driver-Gene Mutations of ITH

To identify driver-gene mutations, a binary matrix was produced representing the presence/absence of mutations for each gene on each tumor sample, eliminating the bias introduced by hypermutated genes. First, mutated genes were classified according to cancer specific pathways previously defined: epigenetic modifiers, transcription factors/regulators, genome integrity, RTK signaling, cell cycle, MAPK signaling, PI(3)K signaling, TGF-β signaling, Wnt/β-catenin signaling, proteolysis, splicing, HIPPO signaling, metabolism, NFE2L, protein phosphatase, ribosome, TOR [25]. By doing this, we reduced noise from passenger mutations and discover which group of genes is the major contributor of ITH in a wide range of carcinomas. Then, we applied a linear model per cancer type, extracting: explained variance, estimated coefficients, Benjamin-Hochberg adjusted *p*-values for the fitted model and for each estimated coefficient (Table S2). Second, to identify specific gene driver-events we used generalized linear models previously applied to infer association of genetic alterations with other variables [26] (see Supplementary Methods for details). Briefly, ITH for each individual cancer type and all cancers was modelled by Lasso regression as implemented in glmnet R package [44]. Significance of the explained variance by each model was determined for values greater than zero by a margin of more than one standard deviation. Finally, the fitted models were evaluated by comparing the observed and predicted ITH levels based on the tumor mutation profiles and assessing the Pearson correlation.

4.10. Whole-Exome Sequencing from Human Cancer Cell Lines

The genomic DNA from cells was prepared using the QIAamp DNA Mini Kit (Qiagen, Hilden, Germany) following the manufacturer's instructions and the quality and quantity of purified DNA was assessed by NanoDrop™ 2000 (Thermo Fisher Scientific) and gel electrophoresis. Genomic DNA was extracted from control, DNMT3A and SETD2 KOs carcinoma cell lines following 1, 3 and 6 months in culture and then used for WES. Whole-exome capture libraries were constructed using 100 ng of DNA from Caki-2 cells (controls and KOs) sequenced as paired-end 151-bp sequence tags with coverage of $30\times$. Samples were barcoded and prepared for sequencing by GATC Biotech AG (www.gatc-biotech.com) using Illumina protocols. Integrity and quantity of the starting material was determined by appropriate methods (e.g., volume measurement, gel electrophoresis and fluorimeter measurements). Library preparation incorporated adaptor sequences and indexing compatible for Illumina sequencing technology, using proprietary methods of GATC Biotech. Enrichment was performed using Agilents SureSelectXT Human All Exon V6 technology. The quality of the final library was assessed by determination of size distribution and by quantification, following GATC Biotech protocols. Sequencing was carried out on the Illumina HiSeq platform. Delivered raw data is the result of a primary analysis using Illumina CASAVA software (http://cancan.cshl.edu/labmembers/gordon/fastq_illumina_filter/).

4.11. Variant Calling from Whole-Exome Sequencing

Whole-exome sequence data processing and analysis were performed by RubioSeq software (http://rubioseq.bioinfo.cnio.es/) using default parameters for somatic variation analysis [45]. Briefly, sequencing data were first checked by FastQC for quality control checks on raw sequence data and then aligned to the human reference genome (GRCh37/hg19) using Burrows-Wheeler alignment (BWA) [46]. Reads unmapped by BWA were realigned using BFAST [47]. Sequenced samples presented 71% of bases in the targeted exome above $30\times$ coverage (see Supplementary Methods for details and Table S7). For variant calling we used GATK Unified Genotyper v2 [48] applying the "Discovery" genotyping mode and default parameters for filtering. The GATK QUAL field was employed for ranking selected somatic variants. Mutations were filtered to ensure that each variant had at least 5 reads supporting the mutant allele and coverage of $\geq$30. Single-nucleotide variants reported in dbSNP150 were filtered out from VCF output files, unless they were also present in COSMICv85 [49]. Only single nucleotide variants were used for downstream analyses. The filtered variants were annotated with SnpEff (VEP) [50]. Finally, to remove the germinal variants (i.e., present in the original cell population) we filtered out variants present in the earliest replicate (1 month) from each experiment (individual knockouts or control) and with MAF equal to 1.

4.12. Assessing ITH and Subclones Number from Whole-Exome Sequencing

The ITH from control and knockout cell lines was determined using the mutant-allele tumor heterogeneity (MATH) approach [24]. A Bayesian clustering approach was also used to infer clonal population structures present in control and knockout cell lines as implemented in Pyclone [30] (see Supplementary Methods for details). Pyclone analysis was performed jointly on all samples using variants supported at least by 50 reads and with copy number information estimated by RubioSeq and processed using CopyWriteR Bioconductor package [51].

4.13. Statistical Analysis and Graphical Representation

Figures were produced using ggplot R package [52] and default packages from R environment [43] and also Graph Pad Prism5 Software (https://www.graphpad.com/scientific-software/prism/). The statistical significance of differences between groups was evaluated using unpaired Student's *t*-test and Mann-Whitney-Wilcoxon test (* $p < 0.05$; ** $p < 0.01$; *** $p < 0.001$; **** $p < 0.0001$). Results are depicted either as mean $\pm$ standard deviation (SD) or median $\pm$ SD, of minimum 3 independent replicates. Survival was analyzed by Kaplan-Meier curve comparison using a log-rank test and with a multivariate Cox proportional hazards analysis as implemented in the survival R package [53]. Statistical significance was determined using *p*-value < 0.05 as cut-off.

5. Conclusions

Our pan-cancer analyses revealed that mutations in epigenetic modifiers, namely *SETD2* and *DNMT3A*, are major determinants of ITH. These genes are recurrently mutated in several cancer types. For instance, *SETD2* mutations are found in 10% of KIRC [16], 9% of non-small cell lung carcinomas [54], 15% of pediatric high-grade gliomas and 8% of adult high-grade gliomas [55], whereas mutations in

DNMT3A are observed in over 20% acute monocytic leukemias [15]. These numbers illustrate the broad significance of our findings, which provide an unprecedented pan-cancer portrait of the major determinants of ITH. Our experimental validation of the role of specific epigenetic modifier genes in driving ITH reveals novel biomarkers and/or therapeutic targets that may contribute to more effective cancer prognoses and treatment.

Supplementary Materials: The following are available online at http://www.mdpi.com/2072-6694/11/3/391/s1, Method S1: Pan-Cancer Data Sets, Method S2: Intratumor heterogeneity score using mutant-allele tumor heterogeneity (MATH) score, Method S3: Identification of deregulated cancer pathways associated with ITH, Method S4: Pan-cancer discovery of driver-gene mutations of ITH, Method S5: Whole-exome sequencing and variant calling for human cancer cell lines, Method S6: Clonality analyses. This file contains the description of the computational methods used in this study, Table S1: Clinical data and genomic features (genomic instability and MATH values) for samples from 16 different TCGA cancer types, Table S2: Linear models associating mutations in functional groups and ITH for each cancer type, Table S3: Predicted effect of DNMT1, DNMT3A and SETD2 mutations in KIRC samples from cBioportal, Table S4: ITH values (MATH) estimated for control, DNTM3A and SETD2 KO cell lines, Table S5: Mutations generated after SETD2 and DNMT3A knockouts (not present in controls), including the mutations with GO terms associated with mitochondria, Table S6: Material and Methods Table (e.g., plasmids, gRNAs, antibodies, primers and other products), Table S7: Read length, total reads and mapped reads for each condition.

Availability of Data and Material: WES sequencing data that correspond to human cell lines are available in the Sequence Read. Archive (SRA) with the following accession code: SRP153138.

Author Contributions: M.R.d.M., I.P. and A.R.G. analyzed TCGA and WES data. M.R.d.M. established the knockout cell lines. M.R.d.M., A.R.G. and S.F.d.a. designed the study, interpreted data and wrote the manuscript. F.S.C. and V.A.M. measured mitochondria oxygen consumption rates and analyzed mitochondria morphology. All authors read and approved the final manuscript.

Funding: This research was funded by: PTDC/BIM-ONC/0016-2014 and PTDC/BIA-MOL/30438/2017 to S.F.d.A., PTDC/MED-ONC/28660/2017 to A.R.G, EMBO-IG-3309, ERC-StG-679168 and FCT/IF/01693/2014/CP1236/CT0003 to V.A.M.; LISBOA-01-0145-FEDER-016394 project co-funded by FEDER, through POR Lisboa, Portugal 2020-Programa Operacional Regional de Lisboa, PORTUGAL 2020 and Fundação para a Ciência e Tecnologia (FCT); UID/BIM/50005/2019 through Fundação para a Ciência e Tecnologia (FCT)/Ministério da Ciência, Tecnologia e Ensino Superior (MCTES)-Fundos do Orçamento de Estado; the iMM-Laço Fund. A.R.G. is the recipient of an FCT Investigator grant (IF/00510/2014). M.R.d.M. is recipient of a PhD fellowship: SFRH/BD/92208/2013. F.S.C. is the recipient of the fellowship iMM/BPD/122-2016. Funding bodies did not play any role in the design of the study, collection, analysis and interpretation of data or writing the manuscript.

Acknowledgments: We thank Claus Azzalin, João Barata and Afonso Almeida for helpful discussions. We thank all members of the SAlmeida and VMorais labs for their comments and technical assistance. We are also indebted to the IMM Bioimaging facility for excellent technical support.

Conflicts of Interest: The authors declare no conflict of interest.

References

1. Burrell, R.A.; McGranahan, N.; Bartek, J.; Swanton, C. The causes and consequences of genetic heterogeneity in cancer evolution. *Nature* **2013**, 338–345. [CrossRef]

2. Gerlinger, M.; McGranahan, N.; Dewhurst, S.M.; Burrell, R.A.; Tomlinson, I.; Swanton, C. Cancer: Evolution Within a Lifetime. *Annu. Rev. Genet.* **2014**, *48*, 215–236. [CrossRef]

3. McGranahan, N.; Swanton, C. Clonal Heterogeneity and Tumor Evolution: Past, Present, and the Future. *Cell* **2017**, 613–628. [CrossRef] [PubMed]

4. Andor, N.; Graham, T.A.; Jansen, M.; Xia, L.C.; Aktipis, C.A.; Petritsch, C.; Ji, H.P.; Maley, C.C. Pan-cancer analysis of the extent and consequences of intratumor heterogeneity. *Nat. Med.* **2016**, *22*, 105–113. [CrossRef] [PubMed]

5. Waclaw, B.; Bozic, I.; Pittman, M.E.; Hruban, R.H.; Vogelstein, B.; Nowak, M.A. A spatial model predicts that dispersal and cell turnover limit intratumour heterogeneity. *Nature* **2015**, *525*, 261–264. [CrossRef]

6. Cleary, A.S.; Leonard, T.L.; Gestl, S.A.; Gunther, E.J. Tumour cell heterogeneity maintained by cooperating subclones in Wnt-driven mammary cancers. *Nature* **2014**, *508*, 113–117. [CrossRef]

7. Turner, K.M.; Deshpande, V.; Beyter, D.; Koga, T.; Rusert, J.; Lee, C.; Li, B.; Arden, K.; Ren, B.; Nathanson, D.A.; et al. Extrachromosomal oncogene amplification drives tumour evolution and genetic heterogeneity. *Nature* **2017**, *543*, 122–125. [CrossRef] [PubMed]

8. Laughney, A.M.; Elizalde, S.; Genovese, G.; Bakhoum, S.F. Dynamics of Tumor Heterogeneity Derived from Clonal Karyotypic Evolution. *Cell Rep.* **2015**, *12*, 809–820. [CrossRef]

9. Sotillo, R.; Schvartzman, J.M.; Socci, N.D.; Benezra, R. Mad2-induced chromosome instability leads to lung tumour relapse after oncogene withdrawal. *Nature* **2010**, *464*, 436–440. [CrossRef]

10. Hanahan, D.; Weinberg, R.A. Hallmarks of cancer: The next generation. *Cell* **2011**, 646–674. [CrossRef]

11. Berdasco, M.; Esteller, M. Aberrant Epigenetic Landscape in Cancer: How Cellular Identity Goes Awry. *Dev. Cell* **2010**, 698–711. [CrossRef] [PubMed]

12. Kaufman, C.K.; Mosimann, C.; Fan, Z.P.; Yang, S.; Thomas, A.J.; Ablain, J.; Tan, J.L.; Fogley, R.D.; van Rooijen, E.; Hagedorn, E.J.; et al. A zebrafish melanoma model reveals emergence of neural crest identity during melanoma initiation. *Science* **2016**, *351*. [CrossRef] [PubMed]

13. Plass, C.; Pfister, S.M.; Lindroth, A.M.; Bogatyrova, O.; Claus, R.; Lichter, P. Mutations in regulators of the epigenome and their connections to global chromatin patterns in cancer. *Nat. Rev. Genet.* **2013**, 765–780. [CrossRef] [PubMed]

14. Shen, H.; Laird, P.W. Interplay between the cancer genome and epigenome. *Cell* **2013**, 38–55. [CrossRef] [PubMed]

15. Yan, X.J.; Xu, J.; Gu, Z.H.; Pan, C.M.; Lu, G.; Shen, Y.; Shi, J.Y.; Zhu, Y.M.; Tang, L.; Zhang, X.W.; et al. Exome sequencing identifies somatic mutations of DNA methyltransferase gene DNMT3A in acute monocytic leukemia. *Nat. Genet.* **2011**, *43*, 309–315. [CrossRef]

16. Creighton, C.; Morgan, M.; Gunaratne, P.; Wheeler, D.; Gibbs, R.; Robertson, R.; Chu, A.; Beroukhim, R.; Cibulskis, K.; Signoretti, S.; et al. Comprehensive molecular characterization of clear cell renal cell carcinoma. *Nature* **2013**, *499*, 43–49. [CrossRef]

17. Carvalho, S.; Vítor, A.C.; Sridhara, S.C.; Martins, F.B.; Raposo, A.C.; Desterro, J.M.; Ferreira, J.; de Almeida, S.F. SETD2 is required for DNA double-strand break repair and activation of the p53-mediated checkpoint. *Elife* **2014**, *3*, 1–19. [CrossRef]

18. Carvalho, S.; Raposo, A.C.; Martins, F.B.; Grosso, A.R.; Sridhara, S.C.; Rino, J.; Carmo-Fonseca, M.; de Almeida, S.F. Histone methyltransferase SETD2 coordinates FACT recruitment with nucleosome dynamics during transcription. *Nucleic Acids Res.* **2013**, *41*, 2881–2893. [CrossRef] [PubMed]

19. Grosso, A.R.; Leite, A.P.; Carvalho, S.; Matos, M.R.; Martins, F.B.; Vítor, A.C.; Desterro, J.M.; Carmo-Fonseca, M.; de Almeida, S.F. Pervasive transcription read-through promotes aberrant expression of oncogenes and RNA chimeras in renal carcinoma. *Elife* **2015**, *4*. [CrossRef]

20. Dhayalan, A.; Rajavelu, A.; Rathert, P.; Tamas, R.; Jurkowska, R.Z.; Ragozin, S.; Jeltsch, A. The Dnmt3a PWWP domain reads histone 3 lysine 36 trimethylation and guides DNA methylation. *J. Biol. Chem.* **2010**, *285*, 26114–26120. [CrossRef]

21. Timp, W.; Feinberg, A.P. Cancer as a dysregulated epigenome allowing cellular growth advantage at the expense of the host. *Nat. Rev. Cancer.* **2013**, 497–510. [CrossRef] [PubMed]

22. Hao, J.J.; Lin, D.C.; Dinh, H.Q.; Mayakonda, A.; Jiang, Y.Y.; Chang, C.; Jiang, Y.; Lu, C.C.; Shi, Z.Z.; Xu, X.; et al. Spatial intratumoral heterogeneity and temporal clonal evolution in esophageal squamous cell carcinoma. *Nat. Genet.* **2016**, *48*, 1500–1507. [CrossRef]

23. Mazor, T.; Pankov, A.; Johnson, B.E.; Hong, C.; Hamilton, E.G.; Bell, R.J.; Smirnov, I.V.; Reis, G.F.; Phillips, J.J.; Barnes, M.J.; et al. DNA Methylation and Somatic Mutations Converge on the Cell Cycle and Define Similar Evolutionary Histories in Brain Tumors. *Cancer Cell* **2015**, *28*, 307–317. [CrossRef] [PubMed]

24. Mroz, E.A.; Rocco, J.W. MATH, a novel measure of intratumor genetic heterogeneity, is high in poor-outcome classes of head and neck squamous cell carcinoma. *Oral Oncol.* **2013**, *49*, 211–215. [CrossRef] [PubMed]

25. Kandoth, C.; McLellan, M.D.; Vandin, F.; Ye, K.; Niu, B.; Lu, C.; Xie, M.; Zhang, Q.; McMichael, J.F.; Wyczalkowski, M.A.; et al. Mutational landscape and significance across 12 major cancer types. *Nature* **2013**, *502*, 333–339. [CrossRef] [PubMed]

26. Gerstung, M.; Pellagatti, A.; Malcovati, L.; Giagounidis, A.; Della Porta, M.G.; Jädersten, M.; Dolatshad, H.; Verma, A.; Cross, N.C.; Vyas, P.; et al. Combining gene mutation with gene expression data improves outcome prediction in myelodysplastic syndromes. *Nat. Commun.* **2015**, *6*, 5901. [CrossRef]

27. Yang, L.; Fang, J.; Chen, J. Tumor cell senescence response produces aggressive variants. *Cell Death Discov.* **2017**, *3*, 17049. [CrossRef]

28. Coppé, J.-P.; Desprez, P.-Y.; Krtolica, A.; Campisi, J. The Senescence-Associated Secretory Phenotype: The Dark Side of Tumor Suppression. *Annu. Rev. Pathol. Mech. Dis.* **2010**, *5*, 99–118. [CrossRef] [PubMed]

29. Castro-Vega, L.J.; Jouravleva, K.; Ortiz-Montero, P.; Liu, W.Y.; Galeano, J.L.; Romero, M.; Popova, T.; Bacchetti, S.; Vernot, J.P.; Londoño-Vallejo, A. The senescent microenvironment promotes the emergence of heterogeneous cancer stem-like cells. *Carcinogenesis* **2015**, *36*, 1180–1192. [CrossRef] [PubMed]

30. Roth, A.; Khattra, J.; Yap, D.; Wan, A.; Laks, E.; Biele, J.; Ha, G.; Aparicio, S.; Bouchard-Côté, A.; Shah, S.P. PyClone: Statistical inference of clonal population structure in cancer. *Nat. Methods* **2014**, *11*, 396–398. [CrossRef] [PubMed]

31. Porporato, P.E.; Filigheddu, N.; Pedro, J.M.B.-S.; Kroemer, G.; Galluzzi, L. Mitochondrial metabolism and cancer. *Cell Res.* **2017**. [CrossRef] [PubMed]

32. Tan, A.S.; Baty, J.W.; Berridge, M.V. The role of mitochondrial electron transport in tumorigenesis and metastasis. *Biochim. Biophys. Acta* **2014**, *1840*, 1454–1463. [CrossRef] [PubMed]

33. Alam, M.M.; Lal, S.; FitzGerald, K.E.; Zhang, L. A holistic view of cancer bioenergetics: Mitochondrial function and respiration play fundamental roles in the development and progression of diverse tumors. *Clin. Transl. Med.* **2016**, *5*, 3. [CrossRef]

34. Cherry, C.; Thompson, B.; Saptarshi, N.; Wu, J.; Hoh, J. A "Mitochondria" Odyssey. *Trends Mol. Med.* **2016**, 391–403. [CrossRef]

35. Raynaud, F.; Mina, M.; Tavernari, D.; Ciriello, G. Pan-cancer inference of intra-tumor heterogeneity reveals associations with different forms of genomic instability. *PLoS Genet.* **2018**. [CrossRef]

36. De, S.; Michor, F. DNA secondary structures and epigenetic determinants of cancer genome evolution. *Nat. Struct. Mol. Biol.* **2011**, *18*, 950–955. [CrossRef] [PubMed]

37. Schuster-Böckler, B.; Lehner, B. Chromatin organization is a major influence on regional mutation rates in human cancer cells. *Nature* **2012**, *488*, 504–507. [CrossRef] [PubMed]

38. Pfister, S.X.; Ahrabi, S.; Zalmas, L.P.; Sarkar, S.; Aymard, F.; Bachrati, C.Z.; Helleday, T.; Legube, G.; La Thangue, N.B.; Porter, A.C.; et al. SETD2-Dependent Histone H3K36 Trimethylation Is Required for Homologous Recombination Repair and Genome Stability. *Cell Rep.* **2014**, *7*, 2006–2018. [CrossRef]

39. Aymard, F.; Bugler, B.; Schmidt, C.K.; Guillou, E.; Caron, P.; Briois, S.; Iacovoni, J.S.; Daburon, V.; Miller, K.M.; Jackson, S.P.; et al. Transcriptionally active chromatin recruits homologous recombination at DNA double-strand breaks. *Nat. Struct. Mol. Biol.* **2014**, *21*, 366–374. [CrossRef]

40. Gerlinger, M.; Rowan, A.J.; Horswell, S.; Larkin, J.; Endesfelder, D.; Gronroos, E.; Martinez, P.; Matthews, N.; Stewart, A.; Tarpey, P.; et al. Intratumor Heterogeneity and Branched Evolution Revealed by Multiregion Sequencing. *N. Engl. J. Med.* **2012**, *366*, 883–892. [CrossRef] [PubMed]

41. Kanu, N.; Grönroos, E.; Martinez, P.; Burrell, R.A.; Goh, X.Y.; Bartkova, J.; Maya-Mendoza, A.; Mistrík, M.; Rowan, A.J.; Patel, H.; et al. SETD2 loss-of-function promotes renal cancer branched evolution through replication stress and impaired DNA repair. *Oncogene* **2015**, *34*, 5699–5708. [CrossRef] [PubMed]

42. Cerami, E.; Gao, J.; Dogrusoz, U.; Gross, B.E.; Sumer, S.O.; Aksoy, B.A.; Jacobsen, A.; Byrne, C.J.; Heuer, M.L.; Larsson, E.; et al. The cBio Cancer Genomics Portal: An open platform for exploring multidimensional cancer genomics data. *Cancer Discov.* **2012**, *2*, 401–404. [CrossRef] [PubMed]

43. R Core Team. *R: A Language and Environment for Statistical Computing*; R Foundation for Statistical Computing: Vienna, Austria, 2018; Available online: https://www.R-project.org/ (accessed on 19 March 2019).

44. Friedman, J.; Hastie, T.; Tibshirani, R. Regularization Paths for Generalized Linear Models via Coordinate Descent. *J. Stat. Softw.* **2010**, *33*. [CrossRef]

45. Rubio-Camarillo, M.; Gómez-López, G.; Fernández, J.M.; Valencia, A.; Pisano, D.G. RUbioSeq: A suite of parallelized pipelines to automate exome variation and bisulfite-seq analyses. *Bioinformatics* **2013**, *29*, 1687–1689. [CrossRef] [PubMed]

46. Li, H.; Durbin, R. Fast and accurate short read alignment with Burrows-Wheeler transform. *Bioinformatics* **2009**, *25*, 1754–1760. [CrossRef] [PubMed]

47. Homer, N.; Merriman, B.; Nelson, S.F. BFAST: An alignment tool for large scale genome resequencing. *PLoS ONE* **2009**, *4*. [CrossRef] [PubMed]

48. DePristo, M.A.; Banks, E.; Poplin, R.; Garimella, K.V.; Maguire, J.R.; Hartl, C.; Philippakis, A.A.; Del Angel, G.; Rivas, M.A.; Hanna, M.; et al. A framework for variation discovery and genotyping using next-generation DNA sequencing data. *Nat. Genet.* **2011**, *43*, 491–501. [CrossRef] [PubMed]

49. Forbes, S.A.; Beare, D.; Boutselakis, H.; Bamford, S.; Bindal, N.; Tate, J.; Cole, C.G.; Ward, S.; Dawson, E.; Ponting, L.; et al. COSMIC: Somatic cancer genetics at high-resolution. *Nucleic Acids Res.* **2017**, *45*, D777–D783. [CrossRef]

50. Cingolani, P.; Platts, A.; Wang, L.L.; Coon, M.; Nguyen, T.; Wang, L.; Land, S.J.; Lu, X.; Ruden, D.M. A program for annotating and predicting the effects of single nucleotide polymorphisms, SnpEff: SNPs in the genome of Drosophila melanogaster strain w1118; iso-2; iso-3. *Fly* **2012**, *6*, 80–92. [CrossRef] [PubMed]

51. Kuilman, T.; Velds, A.; Kemper, K.; Ranzani, M.; Bombardelli, L.; Hoogstraat, M.; Nevedomskaya, E.; Xu, G.; de Ruiter, J.; Lolkema, M.P.; et al. CopywriteR: DNA copy number detection from off-target sequence data. *Genome Biol.* **2015**, *16*. [CrossRef]

52. Wickham, H. ggplot2: Elegant Graphics for Data Analysis. In *eBook*; Springer: New York, NY, USA, 2016. [CrossRef]

53. Therneau, T.; Grambsch, P. Modeling Survival Data: Extending the Cox Model. *Technometrics* **2002**, *44*, 85–86. [CrossRef]

54. Govindan, R.; Ding, L.; Griffith, M.; Subramanian, J.; Dees, N.D.; Kanchi, K.L.; Maher, C.A.; Fulton, R.; Fulton, L.; Wallis, J.; et al. Genomic landscape of non-small cell lung cancer in smokers and never-smokers. *Cell* **2012**, *150*, 1121–1134. [CrossRef] [PubMed]

55. Fontebasso, A.M.; Schwartzentruber, J.; Khuong-Quang, D.A.; Liu, X.Y.; Sturm, D.; Korshunov, A.; Jones, D.T.; Witt, H.; Kool, M.; Albrecht, S.; et al. Mutations in SETD2 and genes affecting histone H3K36 methylation target hemispheric high-grade gliomas. *Acta Neuropathol.* **2013**, *125*, 659–669. [CrossRef] [PubMed]

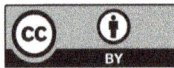

cancers

MDPI

Article

Reverse Engineering Cancer: Inferring Transcriptional Gene Signatures from Copy Number Aberrations with ICAro

Davide Angeli [1], Maurizio Fanciulli [2,†] and Matteo Pallocca [2,*,†]

[1] Department of Paediatric Haematology, IRCCS Ospedale Pediatrico Bambino Gesù, 00146 Rome, Italy; davide.ang@gmail.com
[2] SAFU Unit, IRCCS Regina Elena National Cancer Institute, 00144 Rome, Italy; maurizio.fanciulli@ifo.gov.it
* Correspondence: matteo.pallocca@ifo.gov.it
† These authors contributed equally.

Received: 28 December 2018; Accepted: 13 February 2019; Published: 22 February 2019

Abstract: The characterization of a gene product function is a process that involves multiple laboratory techniques in order to silence the gene itself and to understand the resulting cellular phenotype via several omics profiling. When it comes to tumor cells, usually the translation process from in vitro characterization results to human validation is a difficult journey. Here, we present a simple algorithm to extract mRNA signatures from cancer datasets, where a particular gene has been deleted at the genomic level, ICAro. The process is implemented as a two-step workflow. The first one employs several filters in order to select the two patient subsets: the inactivated one, where the target gene is deleted, and the control one, where large genomic rearrangements should be absent. The second step performs a signature extraction via a Differential Expression analysis and a complementary Random Forest approach to provide an additional gene ranking in terms of information loss. We benchmarked the system robustness on a panel of genes frequently deleted in cancers, where we validated the downregulation of target genes and found a correlation with signatures extracted with the L1000 tool, outperforming random sampling for two out of six L1000 classes. Furthermore, we present a use case correlation with a published transcriptomic experiment. In conclusion, deciphering the complex interactions of the tumor environment is a challenge that requires the integration of several experimental techniques in order to create reproducible results. We implemented a tool which could be of use when trying to find mRNA signatures related to a gene loss event to better understand its function or for a gene-loss associated biomarker research.

Keywords: transcriptional signatures; copy number variation; copy number aberration; TCGA mining; cancer CRISPR; firehose; gene signature extraction; gene loss biomarkers; gene inactivation biomarkers; biomarker discovery

1. Background

Translational research has been hard at work trying to find a way to characterize genes and gene product functions for decades. One successful approach is the study of particular contexts where the gene expression of interest is perturbed. In the past, biologists mostly tried to characterize gene functions by overexpressing its mRNA, whereas more recently, several tools have been introduced in the field of Cellular and Molecular Biology to erase a gene (or its mRNA). Furthermore, a rapid evolution of induced DNA/RNA ablation techniques have emerged from perfectible approaches including siRNA/shRNA to highly specific ones such as TALEN and CRISPRs/Cas9 [1,2].

An induced gene deletion (or mRNA ablation) event brings about a series of phenotypes, both as direct consequences of the gene/protein absence and as epiphenomena mediated by the cellular environment response of such a relevant change.

The granular study of these phenotypes has been accelerated dramatically by the introduction of omic technologies in basic and translational research. For instance, we can easily take a transcriptome-wide picture of the mRNA status or the profile of a large panel of metabolites. All these data can easily help the investigators to apply the "guilt by association" approach in order to better understand a gene function by looking at the correlated omic response [3]. In spite of the elegant workflow (perturbation → omics → understanding), the process is hindered by a series of issues.

In regards to silencing technologies, while CRISPRs have promised to lead much less off-target effects than shRNAs, they still are a challenging technique for several laboratories worldwide and even show little correlation with RNA interference screens, a worrying scenario since thousands of mechanistic papers on cellular and molecular biology are based on these tools [4]. Furthermore, most of these characterizations are conducted in vitro, where the reproducibility of results is being pointed out as a major issue [5–7].

Several efforts have been made towards also automating and standardizing in vitro results to make them reproducible. Among these proposals, the L1000 connectivity map [8,9] is a clear example of a thorough characterization of the mRNA response of thousands of compounds (shRNA, overexpression, and drugs) in several cell lines.

However, when the whole question shifts to a difficult cellular context such as cancer, the situation worsens. The network of intercellular and intracellular interactions of the tumor macroenvironment is extremely complex and inevitably fails to be modeled by a simple mono-population cell line. In relation to this, organoids are an interesting promise [10], but most medium- and small-sized laboratories worldwide still do not have access to these kinds of models.

On the other hand, one resource that is available to any oncology-based research group is access to public cancer datasets. Only The Cancer Genome Atlas (TCGA) contains several molecular profiles from more than 11,000 patients at the time of the writing [11]. We tried to reason whether we could extract huge amounts of data to make the process of elucidating gene functions in cancer contexts easier and more robust. For this reason, we implemented ICAro (gene signature Inference system from Copy number Aberrations), a framework that enables researchers to extract putative gene signatures from publicly available Cancer Genomic datasets.

This overall idea involves treating cancer as a Cas9 model by using Copy Number Variations (CNVs) and inactivating mutations data on a particular gene target to split the patient dataset in control and inactivated groups. Then, we obtained RNA (RNA-seq) expression levels to extract a gene deletion signature. Here, we show that this method can still be a useful resource as an integrated tool for molecular knowledge mining.

2. Implementation

The algorithm is based on the workflow shown in Figure 1: the main inputs of the model are the gene of interest α and the particular tissue context Σ (chosen from the available TCGA cohort codes, e.g., ACC and COAD). Next, the inactivated and control sample sets are built. In the first step, only samples for which both CNV and mRNA-seq data are present in the TCGA database are included.

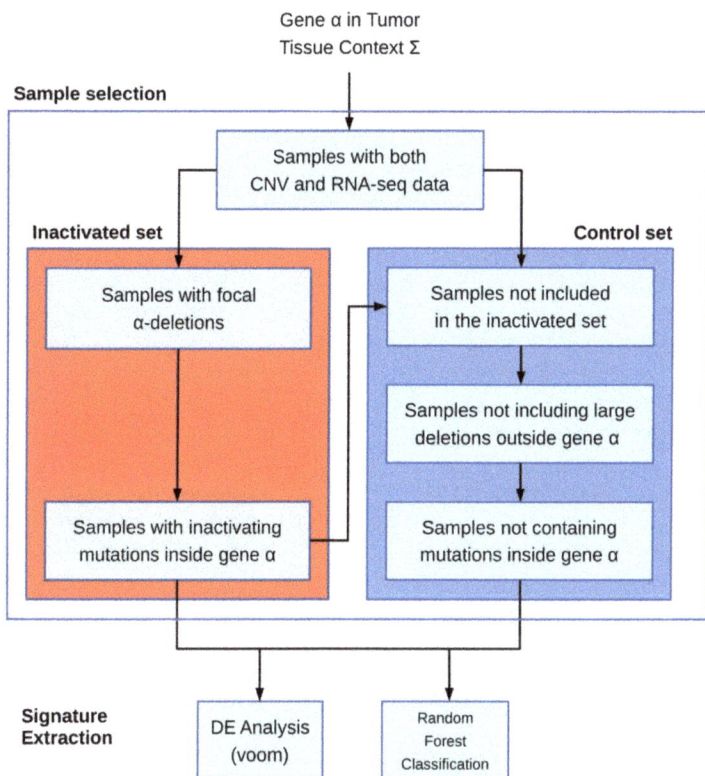

Figure 1. A schematic representation of the ICAro (gene signature Inference system from Copy number Aberrations) workflow. The first part relies on sample filtering based on deletions and inactivating mutations spanning the gene target α in order to build the inactivated and the control sample sets. They are used as input for the signature extraction process, performed via a differential gene expression analysis (the voom function from limma) and a Random Forest classification (randomForest R package).

The inactivated sample selection is performed following two different strategies: in the first one, both deletions and inactivating mutations if provided are used to include samples; in the second one, samples are selected only by inactivating mutations.

The deletion-based filter extracts inactivated samples by selecting CNVs that overlap the gene α location and in which the CNV-GISTIC score [12,13] is lower than -1. An optional filter allows to include only deletions larger than a given threshold. The second filter is based on inactivating mutations and requires an input file containing a list of protein substitution variants in the standard format according to Sequence Variant Nomenclature amino_acid/position/new_amino_acid (e.g., Cys28Ser). Unlike the first filter, it incorporates samples with variations present in the inactivating mutation list. Moreover, the specific format "STOP N" can be added to the list, where N is a number representing the rightmost stop-gain mutation allowing a sample to be included in the set.

The control set is built starting from only samples with both CNV and mRNA-seq data. Other exclusion criteria for the control set include outside the gene α, samples containing CNVs larger than a given threshold (e.g., 1 Mb), or mutations inside the same gene α. With these filters, we tried to minimize the genomic interference of having huge structural rearrangements in the control set.

The downstream analysis is executed only if there are at least five samples in the inactivated set and if the ratio between such a set and the control set is higher than a given threshold (0.05).

RNA-seq raw count data are transformed in count per millions (CPM), and only genes for which CPM is greater than 5 in at least 5 samples are kept.

The second part regarding the signature extraction is performed in two separated methods: the first one is a Differential Expression (DE) strategy in order to fetch up- and downregulated genes with regards to the inactivated set. Secondly, a Random Forest approach (RF) is employed with the aim of building activated and inactivated sets from a binary classifier. From the RF, we extracted a gene ranking list that allows to understand the most discriminatory genes in the classification process and the most likely to be part of our signature.

In the DE approach, the voom function of the limma package is executed on the data and a linear model followed by empirical bayesian statistics are performed in order to find differentially expressed genes between the two sets. On the other hand, Random Forests are built via the randomForest function of the randomForest package which implements the Breiman's random forest algorithm for classification. The preprocessing part is performed via custom Python scripting, whereas the filtered sets are provided as input to an R script that will perform the second step with the voom limma and randomForest [14,15] packages. The data fetch process is automated thanks to the Firebrowse package [16].

The DE output file contains a list of genes with some features, such as the log fold-change and q-value, where the user can observe the putative differentially expressed genes. We appended additional columns to the differential output file in order to give more information on the kind of induction adopted, e.g., two columns with a median expression for each group. The RF output file contains a list of genes ranked by their meanDecreaseGini value, thus having the most important genes in terms of loss of information on top.

The tool is freely available at https://gitlab.com/bioinfo-ire-release/icaro.

3. Results

In order to demonstrate the accuracy of our approach, we extracted 50 pairs of frequently deleted genes (and their matching datasets) from the cBioPortal [17] (Tables S1 and S2) to run the workflow with. Afterwards, from the output signature, we extracted the fold change and the adjusted *p*-value of the target gene to understand whether we are selecting samples in which the target gene is significantly downregulated. Indeed, almost all of the targets are significantly downregulated (94.0%) and have a strong induction (i.e., $\log_2 FC < -0.58$, meaning a 50% regulation, 93.6%) (Figure 2). We performed a similar benchmarking for the RF results on the same genes. When visualizing the meanDecreaseAccuracy (MDA) and meanDecreaseGini (MDG) of such genes, we observed that only 5/50 (10%) gene-dataset pairs had an MDG higher than 1%, while only 2/50 (4%) pairs showed an MDG over 5% (Figure S1).

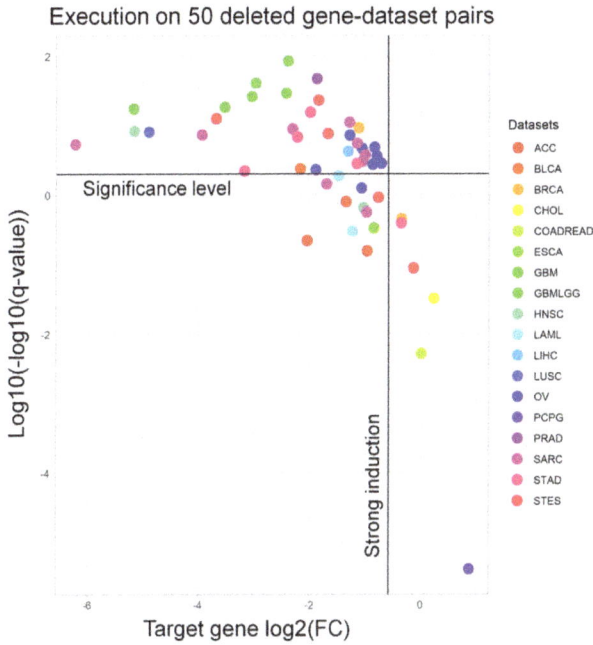

Figure 2. The performance of the ICAro Differential Expression for 50 executions on frequently deleted gene-dataset pairs: Every point represents one ICAro execution on a gene-dataset pair (e.g., TP53 on COADREAD). The different colors represent several TCGA datasets. *X*-axis: log2FC (gene induction), *Y*-axis: transformed *q*-value (statistical significance). Most tests fall in the upper region, meaning that they are significant, and on the center of the *X*-axis, i.e., they are downregulated. The downregulation of deleted genes is a first step towards the in vivo validation of the ICAro process. For a complete key of datasets please refer to Table S1.

We pointed out that inactivated set sizing was the main failure in the workflow. That is, for most datasets, it was difficult to find a high number of patients with focal deletions inside a particular gene. For the RF classification task, it seemed that the deleted gene expression level did not contain a sufficient amount of information in this in vivo setting in order to build a good classifier by itself.

Next, we attempted to demonstrate that the algorithm was able to correlate with other data that were more similar to the typical laboratory approach. The idea involved testing whether the ICAro signature had significant similarities to shRNA knockout perturbations, the routine approach, or other drugs and kinase signatures. To this purpose, we used the aforementioned 50 signatures and we queried L1000 via the Enrichr API [8,9,18] for correlating with the Chemical, Kinase, and Ligand Perturbation. We divided the signatures into up- and downregulated genes; therefore, for each gene-dataset pair, we extracted a L1000 table, 300 in total (Figure 3). On average, every signature correlated with 5 significant terms (adjusted *p*-value < 0.05, median: 5 terms, and mean: 306 terms). When analyzing the particular sub-signatures, up-signatures tended to poorly overlap (median: 0) while down-signatures had better correlation (median from 2 to 660) (Table S3). This difference is to be clearly attributed to the nature of the model that we tested. In fact, our focus is on deletions; therefore a direct gene downregulation trend will overlap better than an in-trans upregulation event.

L1000 significant term count from ICAro signatures

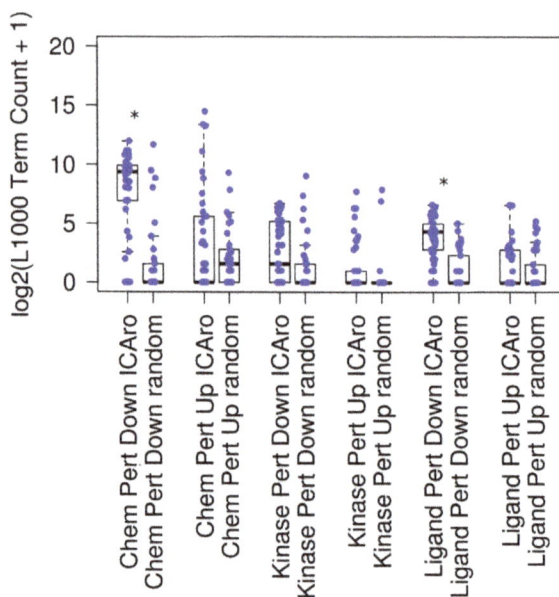

Figure 3. The amount of significant terms for down and up-regulated genes when compared to L1000 signatures: Every point is an ICAro execution with a significant gene set (up or down). Every signature is compared with the amount of significant terms when sampling random gene sets of equal size. Legend: * significant increase between random sampling and ICAro.

In order to show a comparison on the difference between this performance and random distribution, we ran a parallel script, where given N_i, M_i, the number of significant genes from each signature S_i, we extracted N_i, M_i random genes and executed the Enrichr analysis on them. The median number of significant signatures was 0 (adjusted p-value < 0.05, median: 0 terms, and mean: 36 terms), and five out of six classes had a median term number 0 (Figure 3 and Table S3). The mean amount of terms resulted significantly more in 2 out of 6 cases, particularly in the Chemical Perturbation Down and the Ligand Perturbation Down clusters, confirming the aforementioned hypothesis of the ICAro applicability.

As a second validation process, without focusing on frequently deleted genes, we applied the workflow on the genes of interest in tumor genomics, i.e., cancer driver genes. We focused on 459 mutational cancer driver genes (Table S4), deriving from the Integrative Onco Genomics (intOgen) list [19]. Among those, we excluded 23 of them, which were located in sexual chromosomes. Given that we did not separate patients by gender, this would have had a strong bias in the CNV/mRNA separation. The analysis was carried out on 35 datasets (Table S5): only on UCS (Uterine Carcinosarcoma), no results were obtained. For the other datasets, there was a high variability in the number of analyses successfully performed, starting from 2 for CHOL (Cholangiocarcinoma) and DLBC (Diffuse Large B-cell Lymphoma) to 100 for OV (Ovarian serous cystadenocarcinoma), with a mean of 22 successful runs per dataset. From a gene-centered perspective (Table S6), we obtained at least 1 result from 148 genes (34%) and f in which the minimum is 1 for 60 genes and the maximum is 31 for the WNK1 gene, with a mean of 5 analyses for each gene. The main challenge in performing an ICAro analysis is the lack of CNVs on the genes of interest: 59% of analyses failed for this reason. Subsequently, the second main cause for this failure is the absence or the low amount of inactivated mRNA samples: 88% of samples which had passed the previous filters were rejected at this step. Eight analyses were not performed due to a missing control sample. In conclusion, on the whole, only 5% of analyses were successfully performed.

The final step of ICAro modeling features also a Random Forest analysis in addition to the Differential Expression. The aim is to overcome the limitations of linear modeling and to provide a clean gene rank in terms of importance. In order to further describe the relationship among the two analyses, we compared the results of ICAro executions of the aforementioned 50 gene-datasets pairs in terms of the Differential Expression vs. Random Forest results. This profiling presents different scenarios, in which in some cases, the RF approach can massively extend the scope of the DE, that features only a few significant genes (5 out of the top 100 RF genes are significant in DE, Figure 4A). In other cases, the situation is the opposite, and the RF is only an extension of the strong amount of significant DE genes (75 out of the 100 top RF genes are significant in DE, Figure 4B). The full 50 plots are available at the application's webpage.

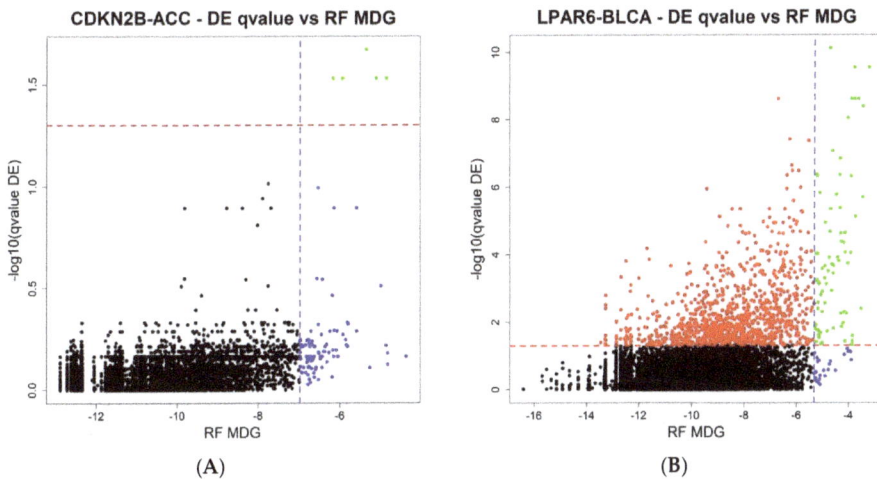

Figure 4. (**A,B**) Two representative plots of the Differential Expression against the Random Forest analysis on the ICAro system. Blue line: the top 100 genes from the Random Forest analysis, ranked by the meanDecreaseGini (MDG). Red line: the adjusted *p*-value significance threshold. Left: only a few genes are significantly regulated in the DE analysis, but more can be studied from the top 100 genes on the RF analysis. Right: the opposite situation where most information lies in the differential expression, and just most of the top 100 RF genes are significant in DE terms.

Finally, in order to present the scope and the possible applications of our system, we produced a use case. We exploited a public transcriptomic dataset (GSE76689), a silencing experiment designed to dissect the role of RB1 in Ovarian carcinoma [20]. We reproduced the DE analysis of the paper. Globally, 2 down- and 8 upregulated genes are confirmed to be significant by the system, thus stressing the importance of these mRNAs to discriminate signatures of RB1 loss in Ovarian carcinoma (Table 1). Furthermore, the Random Forest modeling returned 5/10 of the significant genes to be in the top 100 Gini index ranking.

Table 1. The significant genes validated in the GSE76689 dataset from the ICAro system.

Gene	Log2FC siRB1	Log2FC ICAro	adj PVal siRB1	adj P Val ICAro
RB1	−0.83	−1.12	5.73×10^{-4}	1.81×10^{-6}
SH3BP4	−0.64	−0.63	8.21×10^{-4}	3.35×10^{-2}
NUDT21	0.67	0.29	1.22×10^{-3}	4.46×10^{-2}
SLC27A3	0.64	0.40	5.70×10^{-3}	3.45×10^{-2}
C15orf38	0.77	0.42	1.40×10^{-3}	3.82×10^{-2}
ADCY3	0.76	0.49	7.18×10^{-4}	1.78×10^{-2}
TMEM106C	0.66	0.51	2.69×10^{-3}	2.70×10^{-2}
FANCE	0.47	0.57	2.92×10^{-2}	2.36×10^{-3}
WDR34	0.53	0.59	1.31×10^{-2}	4.94×10^{-4}
TCF19	0.49	0.99	2.68×10^{-2}	1.81×10^{-6}

Taken together, these results highlighted that the algorithm is able to extract a few significantly correlated regulation signatures for genes that are frequently deleted in cancer. The workflow performed better than random sampling and could be used by researchers to extract several "parent" signatures from the target gene in a tumor environment. From the cancer gene driver's point-of-view, a small fraction could be queried for gene signatures thanks to ICAro. Finally, it can be exploited to select a subset of genes of interest in a mRNA profiling experiment.

4. Discussion

The intricate patterns of transcriptional networks are complex to decipher for the biomedical researcher, and in our experience, researchers struggle to find evidence to confirm a regulatory hypothesis. This is one of the main reasons that led us to develop a simple algorithm to help investigators in the field of Cancer Transcriptomics.

The other motivation comes from our experience in handling NGS data and bioinformatic analysis of a medium-sized genomic facility. Translational projects are often designed to start with a whole transcriptomic or a whole epigenomic experiment (e.g., RNA-seq and ChIP-seq), intended to be the hypothesis driver for further investigations. As a matter of fact, the process risks to be interrupted when bioinformaticians present researchers with enormous lists of genes and ontologies. We impute this matter to three main factors: the lack of computational biologists in research groups, the intrinsic difficulty of summarizing large quantity of data, and a slow validation process due to the high number of possible targets as starting points. ICAro comes as an aid for the latter issues, providing hints on mRNA targets that could indeed be validated in vivo.

Many confounding factors are not taken into account in the patient partitioning. These are, for instance, patient stratification by demographic data. This is an issue of many algorithmic signatures of the transcriptomic field that do not seem to care even if they are designed to stratify patients into clinical settings [21,22]. In our case, the scarcity of the inactivated set, usually falling below the count of 5, prevents us in further dividing the patient strata.

In addition, most TCGA mutation datasets do not carry Variant Allele Frequency (VAF) information. For this reason, we may erroneously include a few patients in the inactivation set (that is already suffering from typical smaller size) that carry a stop-gain mutation in only a small fraction of tumor cells (e.g., VAF < 10%). This limitation also applies to CNV data, where the GISTIC threshold output are decided on a sample by sample basis [23]. Furthermore, it should be noted that every sample profiled in the TCGA had a tumor cellularity of at least 80% (recently shifted to 60%) and is not available metadata for which we could correct the CNV/Mutation status.

Our implementation process also lacks some features that we plan to employ in the future. The most obvious one is the lack of a gene amplification study. That is, the possibility to extract a signature when a gene has more copies. This could be a valuable experiment mirroring another frequent laboratory approach such as overexpression models. Another interesting add-on would be appending genomic coordinates of each gene locus to the final output in order to understand whether the differential effect is mostly guided by the CNV itself or by some other regulation pathways. Finally, one more aspect that could be improved in the future is the simple automatization of functional APIs from the result dataset, such as LINCs Cloud and ENRICHR, allowing researchers to better investigate the mechanisms involved.

ICAro testing on a list of mutational cancer driver genes pointed out that the main problem is that less than half of such genes are affected by CNVs, and among the samples with these deletions, only 1 over 12 contains related mRNA experiments, thus preventing us from performing the analysis on a larger set of data.

5. Conclusions

Mining knowledge regarding gene function or seeking inactivation biomarkers is not so trivial tasks. It is for this reason, we developed an automated tool to integrate and mine knowledge from third-level TCGA data. Our testing showed that this workflow is able to extract several transcriptional signatures for a discrete set of genes.

From a biological perspective, the authors are aware that (a) the amount of patients with focal deletions for a given gene will be discrete for the time being, (b) the cancer genomic and transcriptomic background is a disorderly environment very different from engineered cell lines, and (c) it is known that most frequent gene losses have recurrent breakpoints [12]. Nevertheless, we remain confident in the value and feasibility of the presented approach due to the rapid increase in the amount of available high-throughput data and in the vast disappointing failures of in vitro derived models.

We are currently working on an extended version for miRNA signature extraction that will be useful for researchers in the non-coding RNA field. Investigators will fetch via ICAro differential miRNA classes that are up-and downregulated by a particular gene deletion, providing additional insights on miRNA-mRNA interaction.

In a real-life setting, we trust that the ICAro approach would be of value when paired with several other approaches such as in vitro or in vivo knockout models, for instance when understanding biomarkers for the inactivation of a particular gene. In this scenario, it will be useful to implement a novel branch of the workflow to take into account also other emerging large-scale omic approaches such as Reverse-Phase Protein Arrays (RPPA).

Supplementary Materials: The following are available online at http://www.mdpi.com/2072-6694/11/2/256/s1, Figure S1: Performance of ICAro Random Forest classification for 50 executions on frequently deleted gene-dataset pairs. MDA: meanDecreaseAccuracy and MDG: meanDecreaseGini, Table S1: The list of gene-dataset pairs used for benchmarking purposes in Figures 2 and 3, Table S2: A full key of TCGA dataset names from Firebrowse at the time of the writing, Table S3: The average number of significant L1000 signature overlaps from the ICAro output and random sampling. The *cpd, kpd,* etc. stand for classes abbreviations for Chemical Perturbation Down, etc., Table S4: The list of mutational cancer driver autosomal genes used for testing ICAro on each dataset, Table S5: A dataset-centered summary of the ICAro tests using cancer driver genes. The column *total* contains the genes analyzed for each dataset; *no_cnv* is the number of samples without CNVs on the queried gene; *no_or_few_mrna* is the number of samples for which there are no mRNA data, the samples are less than 5, or the ratio between them and the control samples is less than 0.05; *no_control* is the number of samples without mRNA control data; *success* is the number of analysis successfully performed; and *perc_success* is the percentage of succeeded analysis on the total number of analysis attempted for each dataset, Table S6: A gene-centered summary of the ICAro tests using cancer driver genes. The columns follow the same nomenclature as Table S5 but on a gene-centered analysis.

Author Contributions: M.P. conceived the idea, implemented the beta version of the Python algorithm, and wrote the validating script resulting in Figure 3. D.A. tested and extended the first part of the workflow, implemented the whole automated signature extraction in R, and evaluated the algorithm resulting in Figures 1 and 2. M.F. provided the Molecular Biology supervision of the whole process. M.P., D.A., and M.F. wrote the manuscript. All authors read and approved this version of the manuscript.

Funding: Work and publication costs were supported by Ministero della Salute—Ricerca Corrente 2018, Italian Association for Cancer research (AIRC) to M.F. (Grant number 19949) and Alleanza Contro il Cancro-Immunotherapy (ACC-Immuno).

Acknowledgments: We thank Tania Merlino for the editorial assistance. We thank the members of our laboratory for critically reading the manuscript. We thank Eng. Sara Errigo for the critical discussion and data visualization support. We acknowledge the CINECA award under the ISCRA initiative for the availability of the high-performance computing resources and support.

Conflicts of Interest: The authors declare no conflict of interest.

Abbreviations

DE	Differential Expression
RF	Random Forest
CNV	Copy Number Variations
CNA	Copy Number Aberration
siRNA	small interfering RNA
shRNA	short hairpin RNA
CPM	count per million
TALEN	Transcription Activator-Like Effector Nucleases
CRISPR	Clustered Regulatory Interspaced Short Palindromic Repeats
VAF	Variant Allele Frequency

References

1. Boettcher, M.; McManus, M.T. Choosing the Right Tool for the Job: RNAi, TALEN, or CRISPR. *Mol. Cell* **2015**, *58*, 575–585. [CrossRef] [PubMed]

2. Unniyampurath, U.; Pilankatta, R.; Krishnan, M.N. RNA interference in the age of CRISPR: Will CRISPR interfere with RNAi? *Int. J. Mol. Sci.* **2016**, *17*, 291. [CrossRef] [PubMed]

3. Lefever, S.; Anckaert, J.; Volders, P.J.; Luypaert, M.; Vandesompele, J.; Mestdagh, P. decodeRNA- predicting non-coding RNA functions using guilt-by-association. *Database (Oxford)* **2017**, *2017*, 1–8. [CrossRef] [PubMed]

4. Morgens, D.W.; Deans, R.M.; Li, A.; Bassik, M.C. Systematic comparison of CRISPR/Cas9 and RNAi screens for essential genes. *Nat. Biotechnol.* **2016**, *34*, 634–636. [CrossRef] [PubMed]

5. Freedman, L.P. Know thy cells: Improving biomedical research reproducibility. *Sci. Transl. Med.* **2015**, *7*, 2015–2017. [CrossRef] [PubMed]

6. Phillips, P.; Lithgow, G.J.; Driscoll, M. A long journey to reproducible results. *Nature* **2017**, *548*, 387–388.

7. Northcott, P.A. Cancer: Keeping it real to kill glioblastoma. *Nature* **2017**, *547*, 291–292. [CrossRef]

8. Subramanian, A.; Narayan, R.; Corsello, S.M.; Peck, D.D.; Natoli, T.E.; Lu, X.; Gould, J.; Davis, J.F.; Tubelli, A.A.; Asiedu, J.K.; et al. Resource A Next Generation Connectivity Map: L1000 Platform Resource A Next Generation Connectivity Map. *Cell* **2017**, *171*, 1437–1452. [CrossRef]

9. Duan, Q.; Flynn, C.; Niepel, M.; Hafner, M.; Muhlich, J.L.; Fernandez, N.F.; Rouillard, A.D.; Tan, C.M.; Chen, E.Y.; Golub, T.R.; et al. LINCS Canvas Browser: Interactive web app to query, browse and interrogate LINCS L1000 gene expression signatures. *Nucleic Acids Res.* **2014**, *42*, 1–12. [CrossRef] [PubMed]

10. Huch, M.; Knoblich, J.A.; Lutolf, M.P.; Martinez-Arias, A. The hope and the hype of organoid research. *Development* **2017**, *144*, 938–941. [CrossRef] [PubMed]

11. The Cancer Genome Atlas. Available online: https://tcga-data.nci.nih.gov (accessed on 27 November 2017).

12. Zack, T.I.; Schumacher, S.E.; Carter, S.L.; Cherniack, A.D.; Saksena, G.; Tabak, B.; Lawrence, M.S.; Zhang, C.Z.; Wala, J.; Mermel, C.H.; et al. Pan-cancer patterns of somatic copy number alteration. *Nat. Genet.* **2013**, *45*, 1134–1140. [CrossRef] [PubMed]

13. Mermel, C.H.; Schumacher, S.E.; Hill, B.; Meyerson, M.L.; Beroukhim, R.; Getz, G. GISTIC2.0 facilitates sensitive and confident localization of the targets of focal somatic copy-number alteration in human cancers. *Genome Biol.* **2011**, *12*, R41. [CrossRef] [PubMed]

14. Robinson, M.D.; McCarthy, D.J.; Smyth, G.K. edgeR: A Bioconductor package for differential expression analysis of digital gene expression data. *Bioinformatics* **2009**, *26*, 139–140. [CrossRef] [PubMed]

15. Ritchie, M.E.; Phipson, B.; Wu, D.; Hu, Y.; Law, C.W.; Shi, W.; Smyth, G.K. Limma powers differential expression analyses for RNA-sequencing and microarray studies. *Nucleic Acids Res.* **2015**, *43*, e47. [CrossRef] [PubMed]

16. Broad Institute TCGA Genome Data Analysis Center. *Analysis-Ready Standardized TCGA Data from Broad GDAC Firehose 2016_01_28 Run*; Broad Institute of MIT and Harvard: Cambridge, MA, USA, 2016.

17. Gao, J.; Aksoy, B.A.; Dogrusoz, U.; Dresdner, G.; Gross, B.; Sumer, S.O.; Sun, Y.; Jacobsen, A.; Sinha, R.; Larsson, E.; et al. Integrative Analysis of Complex Cancer Genomics and Clinical Profiles Using the cBioPortal Complementary Data Sources and Analysis Options. *Sci. Signal.* **2014**, *6*, 1–20.

18. Kuleshov, M.V.; Jones, M.R.; Rouillard, A.D.; Fernandez, N.F.; Duan, Q.; Wang, Z.; Koplev, S.; Jenkins, S.L.; Jagodnik, K.M.; Lachmann, A.; et al. Enrichr: A comprehensive gene set enrichment analysis web server 2016 update. *Nucleic Acids Res.* **2016**, *44*, 90–97. [CrossRef] [PubMed]

19. cBioPortal for Cancer Genomics::FAQ. Available online: http://www.cbioportal.org/faq.jsp (accessed on 27 November 2017).

20. Comisso, E.; Scarola, M.; Rosso, M.A.; Piazza, S.; Marzinotto, S.; Ciani, Y.; Orsaria, M.; Mariuzzi, L.; Schneider, C.; Schoeftner, S.; et al. OCT4 controls mitotic stability and inactivates the RB tumor suppressor pathway to enhance ovarian cancer aggressiveness. *Oncogene* **2017**, *36*, 4253–4266. [CrossRef] [PubMed]

21. Jiang, P.; Gu, S.; Pan, D.; Fu, J.; Sahu, A.; Hu, X. Signatures of T cell dysfunction and exclusion predict cancer immunotherapy response. *Nat. Med.* **2018**, *24*, 1550–1558. [CrossRef] [PubMed]

22. Charoentong, P.; Finotello, F.; Angelova, M.; Mayer, C.; Efremova, M.; Rieder, D.; Hackl, H.; Trajanoski, Z. Pan-cancer Immunogenomic Analyses Reveal Genotype-Immunophenotype Relationships and Predictors of Response to Checkpoint Blockade Resource Pan-cancer Immunogenomic Analyses Reveal Genotype-Immunophenotype Relationships and Predictors of Response to Checkpoint Blockade. *Cell Rep.* **2017**, *18*, 248–262. [PubMed]

23. Tamborero, D.; Rubio-Perez, C.; Deu-Pons, J.; Schroeder, M.P.; Vivancos, A.; Rovira, A.; Tusquets, I.; Albanell, J.; Rodon, J.; Tabernero, J.; et al. Cancer Genome Interpreter annotates the biological and clinical relevance of tumor alterations. *Genome Med.* **2018**, *10*, 1–8. [CrossRef] [PubMed]

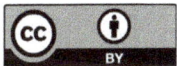

cancers

MDPI

Article

Nucleotide Weight Matrices Reveal Ubiquitous Mutational Footprints of AID/APOBEC Deaminases in Human Cancer Genomes

Igor B. Rogozin [1,*,†], Abiel Roche-Lima [2,†], Artem G. Lada [3,†], Frida Belinky [1], Ivan A. Sidorenko [4], Galina V. Glazko [5], Vladimir N. Babenko [4], David N. Cooper [6] and Youri I. Pavlov [7,8,*]

1   National Center for Biotechnology Information, National Library of Medicine, National Institutes of Health, Bethesda, MD 20894-6075, USA; frida.belinky@gmail.com
2   Center for Collaborative Research in Health Disparities–RCMI Program, Medical Sciences Campus, University of Puerto Rico, San Juan, PR 00936, USA; abiel.roche@upr.edu
3   Department Microbiology and Molecular Genetics, University of California, Davis, CA 95616, USA; alada@ucdavis.edu
4   Institute of Cytology and Genetics, Novosibirsk 630090, Russia; vanyasidorenko22@gmail.com (I.A.S.); babenko@yahoo.com (V.N.B.)
5   Department of Biomedical Informatics, University of Arkansas for Medical Sciences, Little Rock, AR 72205, USA; GVGlazko@uams.edu
6   Institute of Medical Genetics, Cardiff University, Cardiff CF14 4AY, UK; CooperDN@cardiff.ac.uk
7   Departments of Microbiology and Pathology; Biochemistry and Molecular Biology; Genetics, Cell Biology and Anatomy, University of Nebraska Medical Center, Omaha, NE 68198, USA
8   Eppley Institute for Research in Cancer and Allied Diseases, Omaha, NE 68198, USA
*   Correspondence: rogozin@ncbi.nlm.nih.gov (I.B.R.); ypavlov@unmc.edu (Y.I.P.)
†   These authors contributed equally.

Received: 11 January 2019; Accepted: 30 January 2019; Published: 12 February 2019

Abstract: Cancer genomes accumulate nucleotide sequence variations that number in the tens of thousands per genome. A prominent fraction of these mutations is thought to arise as a consequence of the off-target activity of DNA/RNA editing cytosine deaminases. These enzymes, collectively called activation induced deaminase (AID)/APOBECs, deaminate cytosines located within defined DNA sequence contexts. The resulting changes of the original C:G pair in these contexts (mutational signatures) provide indirect evidence for the participation of specific cytosine deaminases in a given cancer type. The conventional method used for the analysis of mutable motifs is the consensus approach. Here, for the first time, we have adopted the frequently used weight matrix (sequence profile) approach for the analysis of mutagenesis and provide evidence for this method being a more precise descriptor of mutations than the sequence consensus approach. We confirm that while mutational footprints of APOBEC1, APOBEC3A, APOBEC3B, and APOBEC3G are prominent in many cancers, mutable motifs characteristic of the action of the humoral immune response somatic hypermutation enzyme, AID, are the most widespread feature of somatic mutation spectra attributable to deaminases in cancer genomes. Overall, the weight matrix approach reveals that somatic mutations are significantly associated with at least one AID/APOBEC mutable motif in all studied cancers.

Keywords: DNA sequence profile; Monte Carlo; mixture of normal distributions; somatic mutation; tumor; mutable motif; activation induced deaminase; AID/APOBEC

1. Introduction

The sequencing of genomes of solid tumors and liquid malignancies associated with different types and stages of cancer has revealed a plethora of genetic changes, from nucleotide substitutions and insertions/deletions to chromosomal rearrangements and chromosome copy number alterations [1–3]. As predicted decades ago by the mutator theory of cancer [4], the elevated mutability in tumors contributes both to their onset and to their further evolution. The underlying causes of this mutagenesis are diverse, from the appearance of mutator mutations to DNA damage by intrinsic or environmental mutagens (e.g., oxidative stress, tobacco smoke, UV light, etc.) [5]. Somatic genome instability leads to the activation of oncogenes and inactivation of tumor suppressors and helps tumor cells to emerge, proliferate, elude immune surveillance, and acquire resistance to anticancer drugs.

In some cancers, the number of single nucleotide variations (SNVs) is in the order of tens of thousands per genome. A few driver mutations [6,7] ultimately lead to cancer, while the role, if any, of the vast majority of mutations, termed "passengers", during tumor development is poorly understood [8,9]. One crucial principle stands out: mutations can be classified into 'families' based upon their flanking DNA sequences [10,11]. Different mutagenic processes generate mutations within different contexts of a neighboring nucleotide sequence (the bases upstream and/or downstream of the mutations, termed "mutation signatures"). Sophisticated approaches have been developed to extract the most prominent signatures from a complex mix of mutational targets resulting from the action of a variety of mutagens, both exogenous and endogenous, operating during tumor evolution [12,13]. Both driver and passenger mutations have been used in the analysis. One of the clearest mutational signatures, found in breast and other cancers [14,15], is characterized by C:G to T:A or C:G to G:C substitutions that are found predominantly in the 5'-TC sequence motif (signatures #2 and 13; listed in the COSMIC database). These signatures have been attributed to the action of nucleic acid-editing enzymes, cytosine deaminases. These enzymes, collectively called APOBECs, deaminate cytosine in single-stranded DNA, yielding uracil. DNA replication past the uracil leads to the insertion of A, thereby giving rise to the C-to-T transition. Also, abasic sites that are produced as intermediates of uracil repair are bypassed by the cytidine transferase activity of REV1 translesion DNA polymerase, leading to C:G to G:C transversions. Cytosine deaminases possess inherent sequence specificity. Thus, for example, activation induced deaminase (AID) prefers to deaminate within 5'-WRC motifs (W = A or T, R = A or G), whereas APOBEC3G acts preferentially on the last cytosine in the 5'-CCC motif, while two other APOBEC3 enzymes, APOBEC3A and APOBEC3B, exhibit a preference for 5'-TC sequences. Another prominent feature of APOBEC enzymes is their ability to act in a processive fashion, i.e., to catalyze multiple deamination events per substrate-binding event [16], thereby inducing kataegis (clustered mutations); however, it should be noted that APOBEC action is only one possible explanation for kataegis in cancer cells [17]. Mutational signatures of cytosine deaminases are detected in many cancers [15]. It is unlikely to be a mere coincidence that the APOBEC3 enzymes are frequently upregulated in tumors [18,19]. It should be noted that if deaminases act on 5-methylcytosine generating "T", a specialized G:T mismatch repair mechanism operates, and the genetic consequences could be different because of the disappearance of an epigenetic mark [20]. There is evidence for the contribution of this process to cancer [21].

Cancer genome studies necessitate working with huge datasets; the obvious problems posed by the analysis of such data are partially solved by the advent of the "mutational signature" technique [12,22,23]. It is not usually possible to define the DNA strand upon which the vast majority of mutations has occurred (but see [24,25]); for example, both a C>T change on one strand and a G>A change on the opposite strand lead to the same CG to TA transition. Therefore, in practice, the analysis may be reduced to the study of only six different types of substitution. Similarly, there are 96 context-dependent mutations (mutation types) that consider two nucleotides in the flanking 5' and 3' positions of the mutated nucleotide [23]. Analysis of the mutational spectra of context-dependent mutations in cancer genomes involves pooling all the mutations from cancer samples into a discrete distribution according to the mutation types, while further analysis involves the so-called non-negative matrix factorization (NMF) method [12,22,23]. There are some variations of this basic technique; indeed, Temiz et al. [26] presented a 32 × 12 mutation matrix, which captures the nucleotide pattern two nucleotides upstream and downstream of each mutation. In this study, a somatic autosomal mutation matrix (SAMM) representing tumor-specific mutations and mechanistic template mutation matrices (MTMMs) representing oxidative DNA damage, ultraviolet-induced DNA damage, (5m)CpG deamination, and APOBEC-mediated cytosine mutation were constructed. MTMMs were mapped to the individual tumor SAMMs to identify mutational mechanisms corresponding to each overall mutational pattern. The method appeared to be sensitive enough to retrospectively allocate the origins of tumors to specific tissues [26].

In an attempt to increase the specificity and sensitivity of the arsenal of techniques available for mutation analysis in whole genomes, we have employed mutable motifs of cytosine deaminases represented in the form of weight matrices (sequence profiles) [27–29]. This approach may be expected to be a more general descriptor of nucleotide sequences as compared to the sequence consensus approach, because it takes into account the variability in the information content ("conservation") across neighboring positions. Control experiments using various constrained samples of randomly selected sequences indicated that the level of false positives obtained using this approach is even lower than the expected false discovery rate (~0.05, see Sections 4.5–4.8 for details). These analyses suggest that the weight matrices method is a powerful tool for the analysis of genomic mutations. Further, we identified prominent mutational footprints of APOBECA and APOBECB in many human cancers. Mutable motifs attributable to AID are less pronounced but are nevertheless present ubiquitously in cancer genomes.

2. Results

2.1. Weight Matrices of AID/APOBEC Mutable Motifs

The information content of AID/APOBEC mutable motifs is shown in Figure 1 (the list and sources of the mutated sequences are shown in Supplementary Table S1). AID/APOBEC cytosine deaminases exhibit substantial variability in terms of their mutable motifs. T in position −1 (number 5 in Figure 1) was the most prominent feature of the APOBEC1, APOBEC3A, and APOBEC3B enzymes, consistent with previous studies (reviewed in [23]). APOBEC3C has a distinct mutable motif with T in position −2. Additionally, APOBEC1 has an excess of T in position −3 (number 3 in Figure 1).

APOBEC3G has a distinct mutation pattern wcCCw (lower case w and c mean substantially lower information content as compared with the upper case, Figure 1), which is a variation of the previously described CCC motif and CCR motif [7,30]. The AID deaminase has the expected context specificity, WRC [16,31].

It is hard to demarcate the mutational signatures of APOBECs using the consensus approach due to the high variability of information content across sites. For example, APOBEC3G has a highly conserved C in positions −4 and −5; however, there is also a less conserved C (and lower information content) in position −3 that may or may not be included in a consensus sequence (Figure 1). We opted to employ the widely used weight matrix technique (see Section 4) in order to avoid uncertainties with the less informative positions.

We compared the nucleotide composition of mutation sites (±5 nucleotides, Supplemental Figure S1) for all the studied AID/APOBEC proteins using the χ^2 test (Table 1). We found that all six AID/APOBEC proteins studied were significantly different with respect to the DNA sequence context of the mutation sites expressed in the form of nucleotide frequency matrices (Table 1). Thus, weight matrices properly represent the DNA sequence context of mutations induced by various AID/APOBEC proteins, as noted in previous studies [5] where a simple consensus approach was used. We aimed to differentiate between the mutable motifs associated with the various AID/APOBEC proteins, although this was not always possible (for example, the sequence contexts of the APOBEC3A, APOBEC3B, and APOBEC3C targets are not as different as other pairwise comparisons, see Table 1).

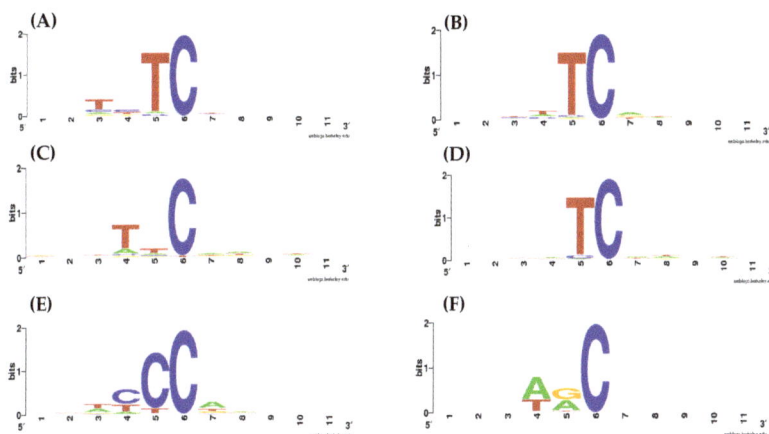

Figure 1. Information content and derived consensus sequences of the DNA context of mutations induced by AID/APOBEC deaminases in yeast genomes (frequencies of nucleotides were used as input). (**A**) APOBEC1, (**B**) APOBEC3A, (**C**) APOBEC3C, (**D**) APOBEC3B, (**E**) APOBEC3G, and (**F**) AID. Position 6 is the position of the somatic mutations. AID/APOBEC weight matrices are shown in Supplementary Figure S1.

Table 1. Pairwise differences between the DNA context (position-specific nucleotide frequencies across ±5 surrounding bases) of the studied AID/APOBEC proteins.

	AID	APOBEC3G	APOBEC3C	APOBEC3B	APOBEC3A
APOBEC1	1986.8	2299.2	203.2	378.6	344.1
APOBEC3A	1674.4	2057.0	138.4	175.7	
APOBEC3B	1764.5	2316.8	175.7		
APOBEC3C	237.2	327.5			
APOBEC3G	2711.8				

The critical χ^2 values = 71.1 (after Bonferroni correction $P = 0.05/15 = 0.0033$, degrees of freedom = 42). The χ^2 test was applied to raw numbers of nucleotides.

We performed four control experiments (for details, see Sections 4.5–4.8): (1) analysis of the sequence context of somatic mutations in mitochondrial DNA as a negative control [32]; (2) analysis of the correlation between the matrices of shuffled sites of mutations and the sites of somatic mutation in cancer cells using the expected false discovery rate approach [33]; (3) analysis of the correlation between matrices of randomly sampled sites from the yeast genome and somatic mutations in cancer cells using the expected false discovery rate approach [33]; and (4) analysis of somatic mutations in human immunoglobulin genes as a positive control [34–36]. The results of all four control experiments (Supplementary Tables S2–S5) strongly support our contention that the weight matrix technique is applicable to the studied AID/APOBECs (for details, see Section 4).

2.2. Analysis of the Correlation between AID/APOBEC Mutable Motifs and Somatic Mutations in Cancer Cells: C:G>T:A Transitions

We examined the correlation of the sites of C:G>T:A mutations in cancers and AID/APOBEC mutable motifs. A correlation between a mutable motif and the DNA context of somatic mutations from the COSMIC database was claimed when the results of two statistical tests (Monte Carlo test and *t*-test, see Section 4) were both significant. A correlation between the mutable motifs of (at least one) deaminase(s) and the sites of somatic C:G>T:A mutations was found for all cancer tissues (Figure 2 and

Supplementary Table S6). AID activity was the most ubiquitous according to the enzyme characteristic signature in various cancer types, whereas the APOBEC1, APOBEC3A, APOBEC3B, and APOBEC3G signatures were detected less frequently, although their signatures were stronger, most notably in breast, lung, cervix, skin, and bladder cancer (Figure 2).

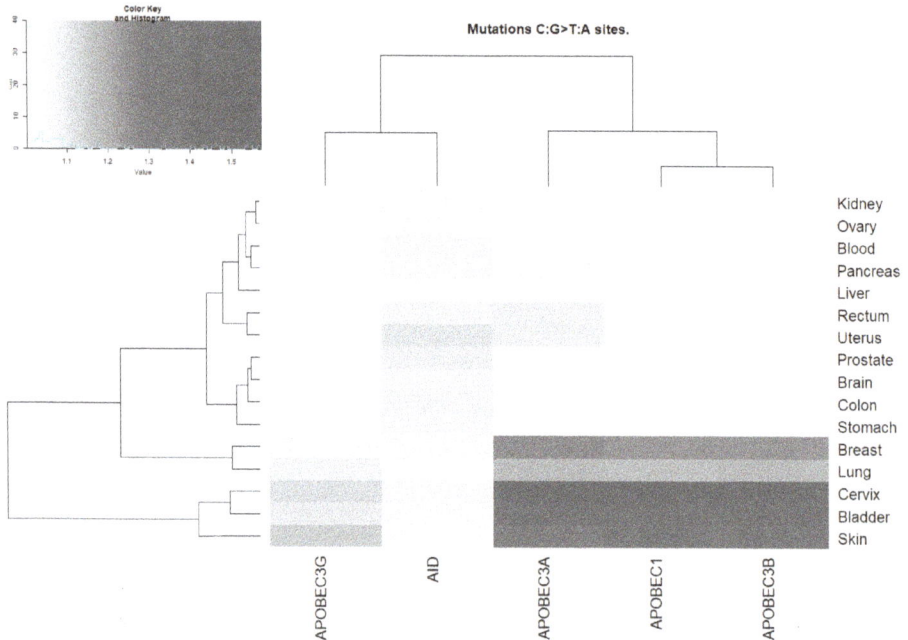

Figure 2. Correlation between AID/APOBEC mutable motifs and the sequence context of somatic C:G>T:A mutations. For the actual data, see Supplementary Table S6. The intensities of the gray color correspond to the ratio values (the ratio being the mean weight of the mutated sites divided by the mean weight of the non-mutated sites). The unweighted pair group method with arithmetic mean (UPGMA) clustering of ratio values for the AID/APOBEC footprints and tissues is shown as dendrograms.

We attempted to estimate the fraction of somatic mutations associated with AID/APOBEC deamination using a mixture of two normal distributions (see Sections 3 and 4 for details). For example, estimated fractions of APOBEC1-associated mutations (0.66, 0.48, 0.74, 0.39, and 0.62) look consistent with the smallest value of 0.39 corresponding to the lowest ratio value (1.064, APOBEC1, lung), although this method sometimes yielded potentially underestimated values (0.17, APOBEC3G, cervix, ratio = 1.113) and overestimated values (0.92, APOBEC3G, bladder, ratio = 1.101) (Supplementary Table S6). The overall distribution of fractions for APOBEC1, APOBEC3A, ABOPECB, and AID deaminases is shown in Supplementary Figure S2. The mean of the fractions in Figure S2 is 0.42 (Supplementary Table S6). This result suggests that a substantial proportion of somatic mutations is associated with AID/APOBEC mutagenesis.

2.3. Analysis of the Correlation between AID/APOBEC Mutable Motifs and Somatic Mutations in Cancer Cells: C:G>G:C and C:G>A:T Transversions

Many C:G > G:C transversions were suggested to be the result of processing abasic sites after the removal of uracils originating via DNA deamination by AID/APOBEC proteins [37]. Consistent with this idea, a significant correlation of these mutations with mutable motifs was found in many cancers (Figure 3 and Supplementary Table S7). The transversions associated with APOBEC1,

APOBEC3A, and APOBEC3B were found to be more abundant in comparison with APOBEC3G and AID, suggesting a role of these three deaminases in generating C:G>G:C somatic mutations in human cancer. The correlation with the three APOBEC motifs was again strongest for breast, bladder, cervix, and lung cancer.

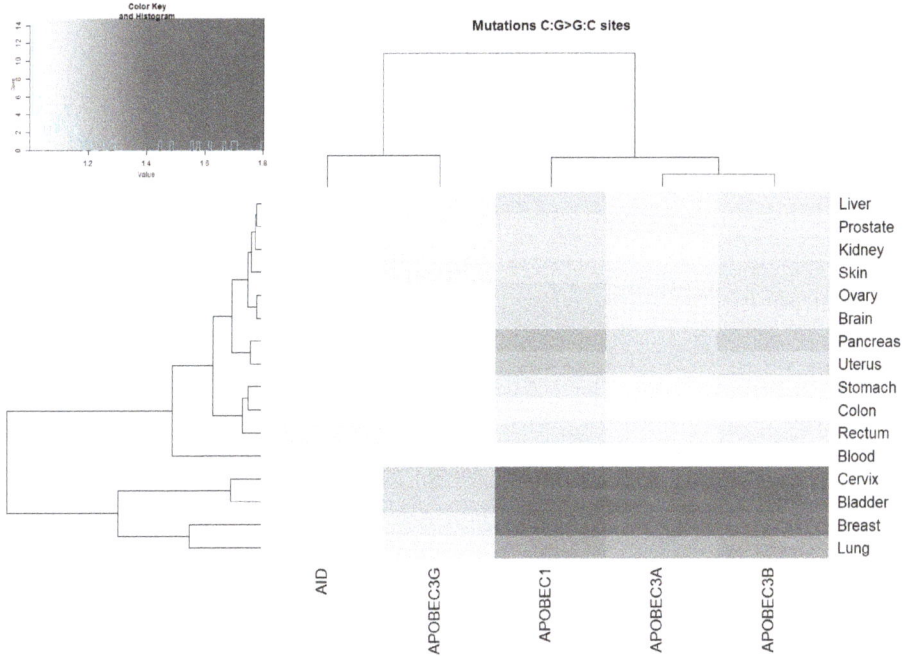

Figure 3. Correlation between AID/APOBEC mutable motifs and the sequence context of somatic C:G>G:C mutations. For actual data, see Supplementary Table S7. The intensities of the gray color correspond to the ratio values (the ratio being the mean weight of the mutated sites divided by the mean weight of the non-mutated sites).

Although it has been proposed that C:G>A:T mutations are a less likely outcome of AID/APOBEC enzymatic action, we found a significant excess of these transversions in many cancers (Figure 4 and Supplementary Table S8), suggesting that a significant portion of C:G>A:T mutations may be caused by processes initiated by deamination by AID/APOBEC enzymes. That the APOBEC3A, APOBEC3B, and APOBEC3G footprints are more abundant in comparison with the APOBEC1 and AID motifs suggests an important role for these three deaminases in generating somatic C:G>A:T mutations in human cancers.

The unweighted pair group method with arithmetic mean (UPGMA) clustering of ratio values for AID/APOBEC footprints and tissues (Figures 2–4) suggests that AID/APOBEC3G form one clade, whereas APOBEC1/3A/3B form another clade according to the distributions of the ratios across tissues (graphs above heatmaps at Figures 2–4). This can be explained by the high similarity of APOBEC1/3A/3B signatures (Figure 1). Breast, bladder, and colon tend to form a separate group according to the distributions of ratios across the AID/APOBEC footprints (graphs above heatmaps at Figures 2–4). In general, these classifications are not consistent, reflecting large variations in transition/transversion ratios (Supplementary Tables S6–S8) and are likely to be a result of variation in the efficiency of DNA repair of such sites in different tissues [5,36,38].

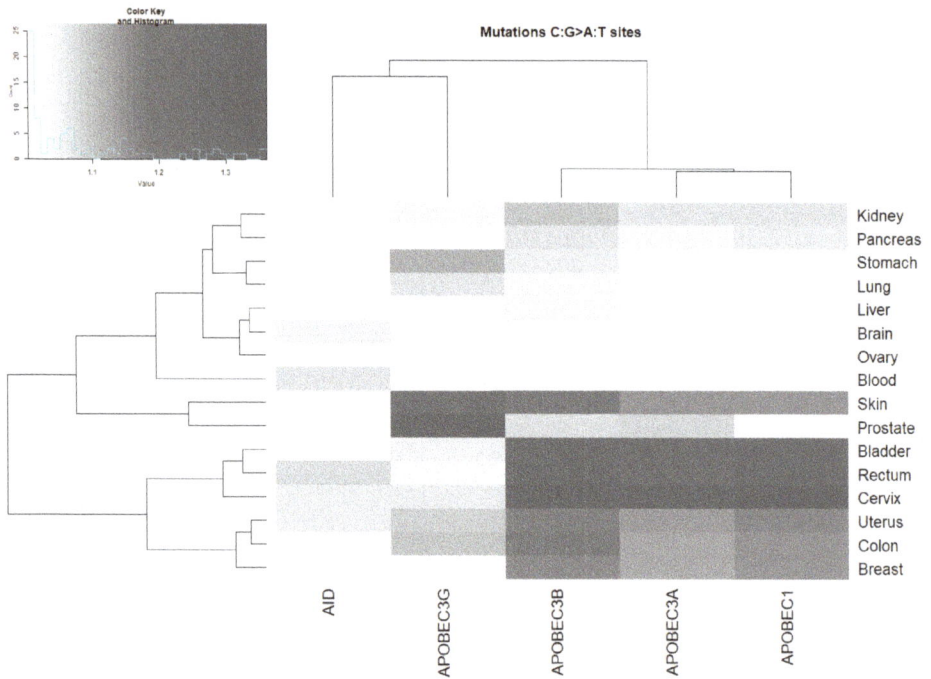

Figure 4. Correlation between AID/APOBEC mutable motifs and the sequence context of somatic C:G>A:T mutations. For actual data, see Supplementary Table S8. The intensities of the gray color correspond to the ratio values (the ratio being the mean weight of the mutated sites divided by the mean weight of the non-mutated sites).

2.4. Analysis of Various Tumor Types in Blood and Skin

Cancers of the blood system were found to be associated with AID and APOBEC3A (Figures 2–4 and Supplementary Tables S6–S8). No other putative associations with APOBEC enzymes were identified. We performed an analysis of two blood cancer subtypes with the highest representation in the COSMIC dataset (see Section 4): acute myeloid leukemia and germinal center B-cell-like (GCB) lymphomas (Table 2). A significant excess of somatic mutations in AID mutable motifs was detected in acute myeloid leukemia (Table 2). In GCB lymphomas, a significant excess of somatic mutations was detected in both AID and APOBEC3A mutable motifs (Table 2). These results suggest that there is variability of mutation context specificity across the same tissue, as seen previously [39].

We also performed an analysis of two skin cancer subtypes with the highest representation in the COSMIC dataset (see Section 4.3) (Table 2): skin cutaneous melanoma and skin adenocarcinoma. Both tumor types yielded somewhat similar results. An overwhelming excess of somatic mutations in APOBEC1 and APOBEC3A/B/G mutable motifs (Table 2) is likely to be due to the known excess of mutations in dipyrimidine dinucleotides (for example, TC) in skin cutaneous melanoma caused by mutagenic UV photoproducts [40]. Accordingly, we interpreted the excess of mutations in the AID/APOBEC3A/B/G contexts (Table 2) to be the result of false positives (as was already suggested by the results of the control experiments; for details, see Section 4.7), but we are also aware of evidence for the direct role of deaminases in skin cancer [41]. We observed a much lower excess of mutations in the mutable motifs observed in skin adenocarcinoma (Table 2). These results are likely to reflect the participation of AID/APOBEC deaminases in mutagenesis, because UV photoproducts do not play any role in the mutagenesis of skin adenocarcinomas [39]. Thus, APOBECs may play a role in a proportion of cases of squamous cell carcinoma [42].

Table 2. Correlation between AID/APOBEC mutable motifs and the context of somatic mutations in C:G sites in various blood and skin tumor types.

Cancer Tissue Type	Number of Mutations	Test	APOBEC1	APOBEC3A	APOBEC3B	APOBEC3G	AID
Blood: acute myeloid leukemia	6844	Ratio	0.920	0.978	0.958	0.977	1.031
		t-test	NSE #	NSE	NSE	NSE	**6.5 ***
		MC test					<0.001
		Fraction					
Blood: GCB lymphomas	2747	Ratio	0.967	1.030	0.979	0.980	1.091
		t-test	NSE	**3.4 ***	NSE	NSE	**12.3 ***
		MC test		<0.001			<0.001
		Fraction		0.208			
Skin: cutaneous melanoma	235043	Ratio	1.388	1.308	1.334	1.138	1.026
		t-test	**321.3 ***	**292.8 ***	**344.6***	**176.2 ***	**35.8 ***
		MC test	<0.001	<0.001	<0.001	<0.001	<0.001
		Fraction	0.608		0.508	0.982	0.687
Skin: adeno-carcinoma	780	Ratio	1.045	1.073	1.088	1.075	1.025
		t-test	NSE	**4.4 ***	**4.8 ***	**4.6 ***	NSE
		MC test		<0.001	<0.001	<0.001	
		Fraction		0.213			

#—NSE (no significant excess) indicates the absence of a significant excess of mutations in the mutable motifs, suggesting that there is no association between mutagenesis and the motifs. The significance of any excess was measured using the Student *t* and Monte Carlo (MC) tests. The bold font and asterisk (*) denote that the corresponding $P < 0.002$ (critical value = 3.1); this is a conservative estimate of the critical overall value of the *t*-test having allowed for multiple testing by means of the Bonferroni correction ($4 \times 6 = 24$). The "Ratio" is the mean weight of the mutated sites divided by the mean weight of the non-mutated sites. The predicted fraction of mutations induced by AID/APOBEC proteins ("Fraction") is shown when a significant excess of somatic mutations in the mutable motif comparisons was detected; all cases where there was a significant difference between the observed and expected distributions ($P > 0.05$) were discarded.

The mixture of two normal distributions yielded fairly predictable results (0.168–0.687, Table 2, see Section 2.2) except for the APOBEC3G mutable motifs in skin cutaneous melanoma samples where the fraction of sites potentially associated with the APOBEC3G mutable motifs is extremely large (0.982, Table 2). The distribution of weights for this case is shown in Figure 5A. A putative component (normal distribution) corresponding to the APOBEC3G mutable motifs (large weights, the rightmost distribution) was less obvious compared with Figure 5B, which can be classified as a reasonable result, because the fraction of sites potentially associated with the APOBEC1 mutable motifs (0.65) is close to the mean of the fractions estimated above (0.42, Supplementary Figure S2). This distorted normal distribution (another problem is a much larger number of sites in the last bin compared with the previous bin) may be a reason why two distributions (Figure 5A) were incorrectly classified (mixed together) yielding an obvious overestimate for the APOBEC3G mutable motifs (see Section 3). This is a known problem in classification analyses of this kind [43,44].

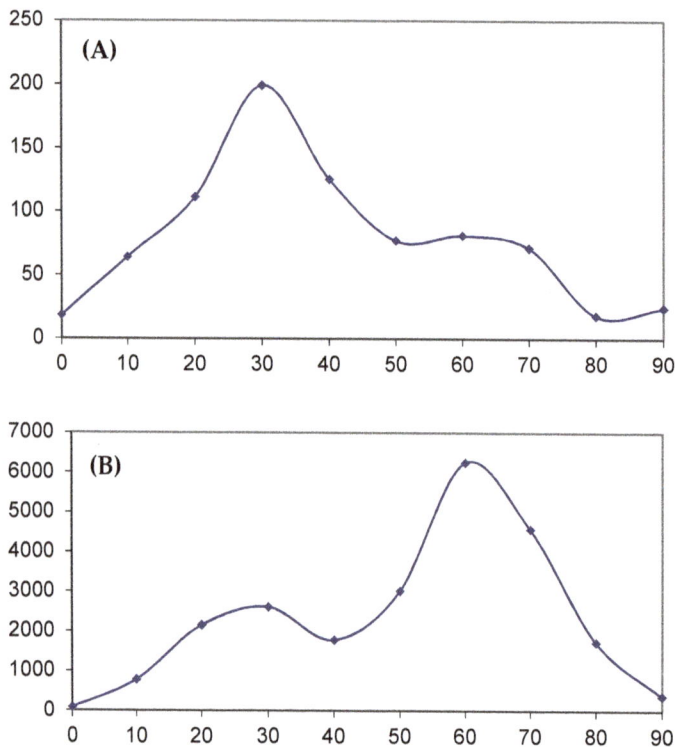

Figure 5. The weight distribution obtained using (**A**) the APOBEC3G weight matrix for skin adenocarcinoma (Table 2) and (**B**) the APOBEC1 weight matrix for bladder tissue (Supplementary Table S6). X axis: 0 stands for 0–9 interval of weights, 1 stands for the 10–19 interval, 2 stands for 20–29, etc.

3. Discussion

The advantage of our approach is that we used a unified computational technique that allowed an objective and accurate comparison of the mutational contribution of various APOBEC enzymes under the same experimental conditions and for the same datasets. We confirm that while the mutational footprints of APOBEC1, APOBEC3A, APOBEC3B, and APOBEC3G are prominent in many cancers, mutable motifs characteristic of the humoral immune response somatic hypermutation machine, AID, are the most widespread feature of the somatic mutation spectra attributed to APOBECs in cancer genomes. It is important to note that the suggested technique does not depend on expert opinion as to the exact consensus sequences and, therefore, objectively represents mutable motifs.

Somatic mutations in all 18 studied cancer types are significantly associated with at least one AID/APOBEC mutable motif. The blood subset of mutations stands apart because only AID mutable motifs are detected (Figures 2–4 and Table 2). Although there are significant differences between the contexts of AID/APOBEC-induced mutations manifested in frequency matrices (Table 1), there are many tissues where mutable sites have been found to be targeted by two or more deaminases (Figures 2–4). In such cases, we cannot reliably differentiate between different deaminases with similar mutable motifs (Figure 1). For example, the frequency matrices of APOBEC1, APOBEC3A, and APOBEC3B are quite similar to each other (Figure 1 and Table 1), and this represents a major problem. To resolve this issue, it may be possible to use additional information, for example, gene expression data. However, the addition of expression data was not particularly informative for the AID and DNA polymerase η mutational footprints [21,39]. The same conclusion was reached in several other studies, because the genomic level of cytosine deamination does not necessarily correlate with the expression of the corresponding AID/APOBEC genes [15,23,45]. For this reason, we did not attempt to compare expression data from different tissue types and relate these data to the results we obtained.

In order to take into account the differences in the base composition between the yeast and human genomes, we used the simplest normalization procedure by taking the frequencies of nucleotides in the non-informative positions −5, −4, +4, and +5 as a null model (Figure 1, see Section 4.7 for details). Although the control experiments suggest that this normalization tends to yield results that are consistent with our expectations (with the exception of bladder, cervix, and skin tumors; see Section 4.7), we cannot exclude the possibility that more sophisticated normalization schemes might be required to generate more accurate results.

In addition, the role of APOBEC3C in mutagenesis remains uncertain and requires further investigation. Another potential methodological problem (at least, for complex computational techniques) is that we have a "positive" set (sites of mutations: sites that contain characteristic features of mutable motifs) and do not have a "negative" set (sites of mutations: sites that do not contain characteristic features of mutable motifs). Randomly sampled sites from yeast chromosomes are far from being a good "negative" set, because distributions of mutations across yeast chromosomes are too sparse and may contain a lot of mutable motifs. This is not a problem for the weight matrix technique, which does not use negative sets as a part of its learning procedures. However, this is the major problem for more sophisticated methods. For example, it is an obstacle for the application of supervised learning methods (e.g., hidden Markov models or support vector machine), because the training of these artificial intelligence (AI) algorithms requires classified or labeled data. However, unsupervised learning methods (such as k-means clustering), which do not need classified data, may be applied to this problem. Another issue is the need to take into account the much higher A:T content of the mutation sites in the yeast genome as compared with the human genome; this should be implemented as a part of a learning procedure.

The results of all the control experiments and somatic mutations in cancers strongly suggest that the weight matrix technique is applicable to various types of mutational signatures. The suggested approach complimented with clustering techniques (Figures 2–4) allows for comparison between the studied enzymes and tissues. The suggested approach can be applied to various exciting questions in cancer genomics, including the underlying causes of the non-uniform distribution of somatic mutations across the human genome and asymmetries of mutagenesis with respect to leading/lagging and non-transcribed/transcribed DNA strands.

We estimated the impact of mutagenesis associated with AID/APOBEC deamination by representing distributions of weights as mixtures of two normal distributions. This approach is based on the method of estimating the protein coding density in a corpus of DNA sequence data, in which a 'protein-coding coding statistic' (which is similar to distributions of weights of somatic mutation contexts) is calculated for a large number of windows for the sequences under study, and the distribution of the statistic is decomposed into two normal distributions, assumed to be the distributions of the coding statistic in the coding and non-coding fractions of the sequence windows [43]. The distribution with the largest mean was assumed to reflect the fraction of protein coding fragments [43]. Similarly, the fraction of sites in a distribution with the largest mean was assumed to be the fraction of mutations induced by the AID/APOBEC enzymes. We noted problems with such an approach for some cases (see Section 2.4). However, the method tends to produce reasonable estimates. Rare deviations from normality caused by the natural boundaries of weight distributions (0 and 100, see the last bin in Figure 5A) is a possible explanation for the problems associated with the use of this classification technique in some cases.

Our analysis suggested that initial deamination events lead to both transitions and transversions. This is already known for somatic mutations initiated by AID in immunoglobulin genes and for APOBEC enzymes in cancer [5,38]. A large variation in transition/transversion ratios (Supplementary Tables S6–S8) is likely to be a result of peculiarities in the relative abundance of proper DNA substrates for deamination and the various efficiency of the DNA repair of such sites [5,36,38]. Overall, our results suggest that AID/APOBEC proteins make a major contribution to several different types of somatic mutations in cancer. The idea that APOBECs can be carcinogenic was originally proposed by Neuberger et al. in early 2000s [46], after the discovery that these proteins can edit DNA [47,48] and, therefore, are by definition mutators. Under normal conditions, deaminases are involved in adaptive (AID) and innate (APOBEC3s) immunity, lipid metabolism (APOBEC1), and possibly even active DNA demethylation [49–51] both in developing and in terminally differentiated cells. Extremely precise, tight, and complex (and therefore, not surprisingly, poorly understood) regulation of AID/APOBEC proteins ensures that in normal cells, they edit cytosines at very specific sites, such as immunoglobulin genes or viral DNA. However, when the regulatory constraints fail, these housekeepers can become much more promiscuous and edit DNA genome-wide.

The overexpression of active APOBECs is highly toxic in human cell lines [18,52], indicating that a precise balance of deaminase production and other factors is required in order to cause non-lethal genome-wide hypermutagenesis and kataegis. This is apparently also true in the case of APOBECs, where only a small fraction of cells with unfettered deaminases and a fine-tuned environment survive and give rise to malignant clones. It is also possible that the sudden overproduction of deaminases in tumor cells with genomes shaped by other mutagenic processes will kill the tumor by extensively damaging its genome, unless the tumor cells can protect themselves against APOBEC.

4. Materials and Methods

4.1. Mutations in Yeast Genomes

Coordinates and types of mutations induced by various APOBEC/AID proteins in yeast were obtained from previously published SNV datasets (see legend to Supplementary Table S1) [37,53–56]. To extract the sequence context of the mutations, we used the getfasta tool from the bedtools package (http://bedtools.readthedocs.org/en/latest/). These datasets are available upon request from I.B.R. The logo description of mutable motifs was constructed using the Weblogo website (http://weblogo.berkeley.edu/logo.cgi).

4.2. Analysis of Mutable Motifs

Several approaches have been developed for the analysis of a set of mutated sequences [27–29]. A mononucleotide weight matrix is a simple and straightforward way to present the structure of a functional signal and to calculate weights for the signal sequence. Each matrix includes information on a normalized frequency of A, T, G, C bases in each of the 10 positions surrounding the detected sites of mutation (5 bases downstream and 5 bases upstream). We calculated the weight matrices for 6f different AID/APOBEC mutational signatures in the yeast genome (Supplementary Table S1).

A simple formula for W(b,j) was used for data analysis: W(b,j) = log2[f(b,j)/e(b)], where f(b,j) is the observed frequency of the nucleotide b in position j and e(b,j) is the expected frequency of the nucleotide b in position j, calculated as the mean nucleotide frequencies of positions $-5, -4, +4, +5$ for sites of mutations in the yeast genome; the resulting W(b,i) matrices are shown in Supplementary Figure S1.

The matching score S(b1, ..., bL) of a sequence b1, ..., bL is as follows:

$$S(b1, ..., bL) = \sum_{j=1}^{L} W(b,j) \tag{1}$$

The matching score between sequence b1, ..., bL and a weight matrix can be further expressed as a percentage:

$$\% \text{ matching score} = 100 \times (S(b1, ..., bL) - Smin)/(Smax - Smin) \tag{2}$$

$$
\begin{array}{cc}
\text{L} & \text{L} \\
\text{Smin} = \Sigma \text{ MIN W(b,j)} \qquad \text{Smax} = \Sigma \text{ MAX W(b,j)} \\
\text{j} = 1 \text{ b} \qquad\qquad\qquad \text{j} = 1 \text{ b}
\end{array} \qquad\qquad (3)
$$

Hereafter, we use the term "weight" instead of "% matching score". We used the positions -3:$+3$ to estimate the weights of the sites.

In addition to the analyses of AID/APOBEC mutational signatures in cancer genomes, we performed a control experiment: we randomly shuffled a dataset of AID/APOBEC contexts in the yeast genome (Supplementary Table S1), keeping position 6 (the position of mutations) intact. Each sequence was shuffled separately; thus, the overall base composition and the base compositions of each sequence were the same. We also performed another control experiment: we randomly extracted sequences from the yeast genome, maintaining the nucleotide composition and the size of sequence sets for each set of mutation sites with AID/APOBEC-induced mutations. Weight matrices were derived from these sampled sites. Where there was a significant difference between an extracted set and the analyzed set (the 2-tailed *t*-test), the sampling procedure was repeated.

4.3. Datasets and Analysis of Somatic Mutations

Somatic mutation data from the ICGC and TCGA cancer genome projects were extracted from the Sanger COSMIC Whole Genome Project v75 (http://cancer.sanger.ac.uk/wgs). The ICGC/TCGA datasets are almost exclusively passenger mutations, and they are unlikely to be subject to selection to promote cellular proliferation. Thus, they are more likely to reflect the original AID/APOBEC mutational spectrum [23]. The tissues and cancer types were defined according to the primary tumor site and the cancer project in question [12,13]. A dataset of somatic mutations in mitochondrial DNA in various cancer types was extracted from [32]. In this set, no excess of mutations in known mutable motifs is to be expected, because the mutation landscape in mitochondrial DNA is shaped by its very specific mode of replication [32]. The mitochondrial mutation set can, therefore, be used as a negative control.

DNA sequences surrounding the mutated nucleotide represent the mutation context. We compared the frequency of known mutable motifs for somatic mutations with the frequency of these motifs in the vicinity of the mutated nucleotide. Specifically, for each base substitution, the 121 bp sequence centered at the mutation was extracted (the DNA neighborhood). We used only the nucleotides immediately flanking the mutations, because the AID/APOBEC enzymes are thought to scan a very limited region of DNA to deaminate (methyl)cytosines in a preferred motif [16,57,58]. This approach does not exclude any specific area of the genome, but rather uses the areas within each sample where mutagenesis has occurred (taking into account the variability in the mutation rates across the human genome) and then evaluates whether the mutagenesis in these samples were enriched for AID/APOBEC motifs [58]. This approach was thoroughly tested, and the high accuracy of the analysis was demonstrated [58]. The mean weight of the mutable motifs (Supplementary Figure S1) in the positions of somatic mutations was compared to the mean weight of the same motifs in the DNA neighborhood using the *t*-test (2-tail test) and Monte Carlo test (MC, 1-tail test) similar to the consensus method, as previously described [58].

4.4. Impact of AID/APOBEC Mutagenesis

In order to estimate the proportion of mutated sites that are likely to be caused by the AID/APOBEC enzymes, we applied a mixture model of two normal distributions [43] to distributions of weights of somatic mutation contexts. An example of such a distribution is shown in Figure 5B. This approach is based on the method of estimating the protein coding density in a corpus of DNA sequence data, in which a 'protein-coding coding statistic' (which is similar to distributions of weights of somatic mutation contexts) is calculated for a large number of windows of the sequence under study. The distribution of the statistic is decomposed into two normal distributions and assumed to be distributions of the coding statistic in the coding and non-coding fractions of the sequence windows [43]. The distribution with the largest mean was assumed to reflect the fraction of protein coding fragments [43]. Similarly, the fraction of sites in a distribution with the largest mean was assumed to be the fraction of mutations induced by the AID/APOBEC enzymes. The results were considered to be reliable only if no significant difference was found between the observed and expected distributions according to the χ^2 test. The suggested classification approach for normal distributions had been tested by Fickett and Guigo and showed good accuracy [43]. All the details of the suggested methodology and underlined statistical Bayesian framework were previously described for analyses of normal and binomial distributions [43,44].

Heatmap visualization analysis for each of the AID/APOBEC pseudo-mutable motifs groups was performed. The R (https://www.R-project.org/) software package heatmap.2 (https://CRAN. R-project.org/package=gplots) was employed to generate the heatmaps for each group. For each group, a specific range of values was established in grayscale representation, from the lowest values to the highest values. For the pseudo-mutable motifs in somatic mutation in the C:G sites group, the range was from 0.01 to 0.84 with intervals between 0.05. Values <0.01 were denoted as white. For the pseudo-mutable motifs in somatic mutation in the C:G>T:A sites group, the range was from 1 to 1.573 with intervals between 0.01. Values <1 were denoted as white. For the pseudo-mutable motifs in somatic mutation in the C:G>C:G sites group, the range was from 1 to 1.802 with intervals between 0.01. Values <1 were denoted as white. For the pseudo-mutable motifs in somatic mutation in the C:G>A:T sites group, the range was from 1 to 1.362 with intervals between 0.02. Values <1 were denoted as white.

4.5. Control Experiment 1: Analysis of Somatic Mutations in Mitochondrial DNA

In the first control experiment, we analyzed the sequence context of somatic mutations in mitochondrial DNA. In this set, no excess of mutations in known mutable motifs was to be expected, because the mutation landscape in mitochondrial DNA is shaped by its very specific mode of replication [32]. Thus, the mitochondrial mutation set can be used as a negative control. No significant excess of AID/APOBEC mutable motifs was found (Supplementary Table S2). This is consistent with a previous study [32]. In all the studied tissues, the ratio of the mean weight of the mutated sites vs. the mean weight of the non-mutated sites was less than or close to 1; this is expected when there is no correlation between mutable motifs and mutation (Supplementary Table S2). We observed only a single case where the Monte Carlo test yielded a significant P-value ($P = 0.031$, APOBEC3B/brain), but this result was not confirmed by use of the t-test and is likely to be an isolated false positive. Thus, the weight matrix appears to be a reliable method for the analysis of somatic mutations.

4.6. Control Experiment 2: Correlation between the Matrices of Shuffled Sites of Mutations and the Sites of Somatic Mutation in Cancer Cells

In order to allow for differences in nucleotide content between the yeast and human genomes, we used normalized weight matrices (see above). To test the robustness of the normalization, a simple control experiment was designed: we randomly shuffled the sequences of the AID/APOBEC mutation sites (Supplementary Table S1). We identified rare cases of a significant deviation from the expected value of the ratio (1.0, the ratio is the mean weight of the mutated sites divided by the mean weight of the non-mutated sites), but those cases constituted only 2.6% of all the studied cases (Supplementary Table S3). This result establishes that the weight matrix technique yields an expected proportion of false positives (the expected false discovery rate should be around 5% according to the standard in the field [33]) and hence is robust with respect to the biased nucleotide composition of mutated sites in the yeast genome. However, the results for colon, skin, and stomach cancers may not be reliable for some APOBECs (the fractions of false positives were found to be large, for example, 0.96 for APOBEC3C/skin; Supplementary Table S3). In general, the APOBEC3C weight matrix tends to yield the largest number of false positives, suggesting that this matrix might be problematic. We conclude that such controls should always be performed when starting work with a new mutation set.

4.7. Control Experiment 3: Correlation between Matrices of Randomly Sampled Sites from the Yeast Genome and Somatic Mutations in Cancer Cells

To check for a potential influence of nucleotide content biases and the extent of a correlation between positions in yeast and human genomes, we randomly extracted sequences from the yeast genome, maintaining the nucleotide composition and size of sequence sets for each set of mutation sites. Weight matrices were derived from these sampled sites. We identified numerous examples of a substantial deviation from the expected values that produced significant results that should be considered to be false positives (Figure 6 and Supplementary Table S4), because we did not expect any meaningful association between randomly sampled sites and somatic mutations. The APOBEC3C weight matrix yielded a large number of significant yet spurious results (false positives) for all the studied tissues (Figure 6 and Supplementary Table S4) and therefore cannot be recommended for the analysis of somatic mutation. This effect may have been due to the much smaller number of mutations in the dataset, a lack of highly informative positions and a high A/T content of sites for APOBEC3C (Figure 1). The results for APOBEC3C are likely to be false positives in this and previous control experiments and were included in the Supplementary Materials only.

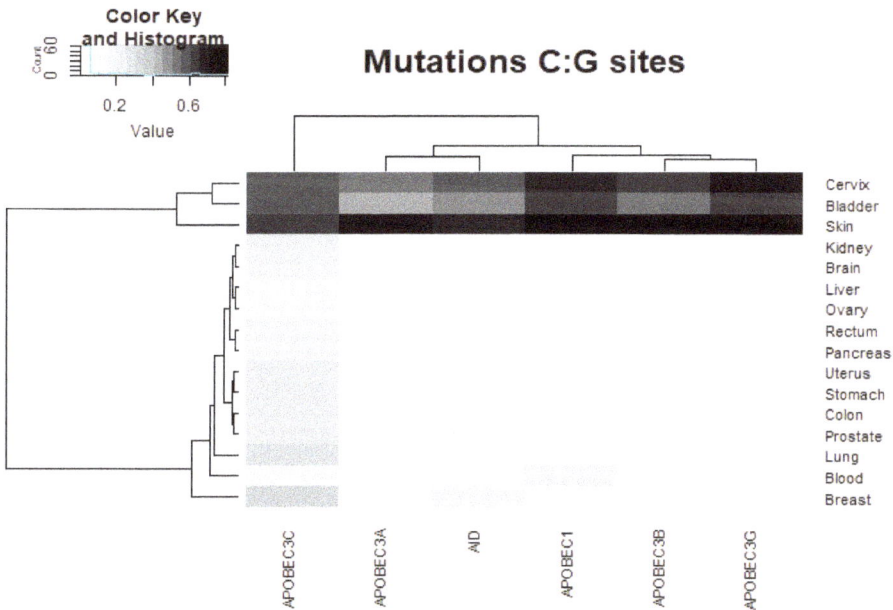

Figure 6. Fraction of random matrices with a significant correlation between AID/APOBEC pseudo-mutable motifs (randomly sampled sites from the yeast genome) and the sequence context of somatic mutations in C:G sites. For the actual data, see Supplementary Table S2. The intensities of the gray color correspond to the fractions of cases with a significant correlation between pseudo-mutable motifs (represented as weight matrices) and the context of somatic mutations in C:G sites.

The analysis of mutations in various tissues suggested that the weight matrix technique may also produce misleading results for bladder, cervix, and skin tumors (Figure 6). The skin tissue consistently produced a high rate of false positives in control experiments 3 and 4; thus, weight matrices should be used with great caution for this tissue. The analysis of nucleotide frequencies for the region ±3 suggested that skin, cervix, and bladder tumors are characterized by a high frequency of T nucleotides around the sites of mutation (Supplementary Table S5), and this is likely to be a reason for the high rate of false positives. It should be noted that other techniques are also likely to produce a high rate of false positives for these tissues, although this type of control experiment has, to our knowledge, never been performed before except for analysis of somatic mutations in normal tissues [21]. The likely reason for high rates of false positives is that APOBEC mutable motifs tend to be A/T-rich (even C-rich APOBEC3G sites contain excessive amounts of A and T nucleotides in positions -3, $+1$, $+2$, and $+3$; Figure 1 and Supplementary Figure S1). We attempted to take this into account by removing sites with a high A/T content ($\geq$50% A+T in the 10-nucleotide region around sites of somatic mutations, Supplementary Table S4). Although there was a substantial improvement in the accuracy of prediction (rates of false positives were much smaller, Supplementary Table S4), problems with the accuracy of prediction for skin tumors persisted (Supplementary Table S4).

4.8. Control Experiment 4: Analysis of Somatic Mutations in Human Immunoglobulin Genes

Somatic mutations in human immunoglobulin genes are known to be associated with AID mutable motifs [35], and these mutations can be used as a positive control set. Indeed, a significant association between the AID mutable motif and mutations was found in all three studied sets of somatic mutations [34,35] (Table 3), suggesting that the AID weight matrix is a reliable descriptor of AID-induced mutagenesis. The APOBEC1/3A/3B/3G weight matrices did not, however, yield significant results for all the studied cases (Table 3). This is consistent with the absence of any traces of APOBEC1/3A/3B/3G-induced mutation in the somatic hypermutation profiles of immunoglobulin genes [36]. The results of all four control experiments suggested that the weight matrix technique is applicable to studied APOBECs.

Table 3. Correlation between the AID/APOBEC mutable motifs and the sequence context of somatic mutations in fragments of human immunoglobulin genes.

Locus	Number of Mutations	Test	APOBEC1	APOBEC3A	APOBEC3B	APOBEC3G	AID
V_H26	708	Ratio	0.931	0.986	0.919	0.908	1.162
		t-test	NSE #	NSE	NSE	NSE	11.1 *
		MC test					<0.001
		Fraction					0.477
J_H4 intron, control individuals	177	Ratio	0.927	0.957	0.887	0.870	1.331
		t-test	NSE	NSE	NSE	NSE	11.9 *
		MC test					<0.001
		Fraction					0.559
J_H4 intron, XP-V patients	235	Ratio	0.981	1.008	0.957	0.930	1.266
		t-test	NSE	NSE	NSE	NSE	9.6 *
		MC test					<0.001
		Fraction					0.366

\#—NSE (no significant excess) indicates the absence of a significant excess of mutations in mutable motifs, suggesting that there is no association between mutagenesis and the motifs. The significance of any excess was measured using the Student *t* and Monte Carlo (MC) tests. The bold font and asterisk (*) denote that the corresponding $P <$ 0.003 (critical value = 3.1); this is a conservative estimate of the critical overall value of the *t*-test having allowed for multiple testing by means of the Bonferroni correction ($3 \times 6 = 18$). The "Ratio" is the mean weight of the mutated sites divided by the mean weight of the non-mutated sites. The predicted fraction of mutations induced by the AID/APOBEC proteins ("Fraction") is shown when a significant excess of somatic mutations in the mutable motif comparisons was detected; all the cases where there was a significant difference between the observed and expected distributions ($P > 0.05$) were discarded.

5. Conclusions

For the first time, we have adopted the weight matrix (sequence profile) approach for the analysis of mutations in cancer genomes, and we provide evidence for this method being a more precise descriptor of mutations than the commonly used sequence consensus approach. Control experiments using shuffled sites and constrained samples of randomly sampled sequences from the yeast genome yielded a low level of false positives.

We confirm that while mutational footprints of APOBEC1, APOBEC3A, APOBEC3B, and APOBEC3G are prominent in many cancers, mutable motifs characteristic of the action of the humoral immune response somatic hypermutation enzyme, AID, are the most widespread feature of the somatic mutation spectra attributed to APOBECs in cancer genomes. The AID and APOBEC3A mutable motifs are the most prominent features of the C:G>T:A transitions that constitute the vast majority of somatic mutations in studied cancers. We also demonstrated an abundance of APOBEC3A/3B/3G mutable motifs in DNA contexts of C:G>A:T transversions. A potential association of AID and APOBEC3A in a certain type of blood cancers is another interesting outcome of our study. Overall, the weight matrix approach revealed that somatic mutations are significantly associated with at least one AID/APOBEC mutable motif in the studied cancer types.

Supplementary Materials: The following are available online at http://www.mdpi.com/2072-6694/11/2/211/s1, Figure S1:AID/APOBEC weight matrices W(b,j).itle; Figure S2: The overall distribution of fraction of somatic C:G>T:A mutations associated with AID/APOBEC deamination (APOBEC1, APOBEC3A, ABOPEC3B, and AID deaminases); Table S1: Datasets of mutations induced by overexpression of AID/APOBEC enzymes in the yeast genome; Table S2: Control study: correlation between AID/APOBEC mutable motifs and the context of somatic mutations in C:G sites in mitochondrial DNA; Table S3: Control study: fractions of random matrices with a significant correlation between AID/APOBEC pseudo-mutable motifs (shuffled sites of mutations) and the context of somatic mutations at C:G sites; Table S4: Control study: fraction of random matrices with a significant correlation between AID/APOBEC pseudo-mutable motifs (randomly sampled sites from the yeast genome) and the context of somatic mutations at C:G sites; Table S5: Nucleotide composition of the DNA context of somatic mutations (±3 nucleotides); Table S6: Correlation between AID/APOBEC mutable motifs and the context of C:G>T:A somatic mutations; Table S7: Correlation between AID/APOBEC mutable motifs and the context of C:G>G:C somatic mutations; and Table S8: Correlation between AID/APOBEC mutable motifs and the context of C:G>A:T somatic mutations.

Author Contributions: Conceptualization, I.B.R. and Y.I.P.; Data curation, I.B.R., A.G.L., F.B., I.A.S., and V.N.B.; Formal analysis, I.B.R., A.R.-L., F.B., I.A.S., and V.N.B.; Investigation, I.B.R., A.R.-L., and Y.I.P.; Methodology, I.B.R., A.R.-L., D.N.C., and Y.I.P.; Resources, I.B.R., A.R.-L, F.B., I.A.S., V.N.B., and Y.I.P.; Software, I.B.R., A.R.-L., A.G.L., I.A.S., G.V.G., and V.N.B.; Validation, I.B.R., A.R.-L., I.A.S., G.V.G., and V.N.B.; Original draft, I.B.R., A.R.-L., D.N.C., and Y.I.P.; and Review and editing of the manuscript, I.B.R., A.R.-L., A.G.L., F.B., I.A.S., G.V.G., V.N.B., D.N.C., and Y.I.P.

Funding: This work was supported by the Intramural Research Program of the National Library of Medicine at the National Institutes of Health (to I.B.R. and F.B.); RCMI grant U54 MD007600 (National Institute on Minority Health and Health Disparities) from the National Institutes of Health (to A.R.-L.), NE DHHS LB506, grant 2017-48 and Fred and Pamela Buffett Pilot Grant 2018-06 (to Y.I.P.); the Fred and Pamela Buffett Cancer Center Support Grant from the National Cancer Institute under award number P30 CA072720 (the content is solely the responsibility of the authors and does not necessarily represent the official views of the National Institutes of Health), and Qiagen Inc through a License Agreement with Cardiff University (to D.N.C.). GVG was supported in part by the NIH IDeA Networks of Biomedical Research Excellence (INBRE) grant P20GM103429 and by the Center for Translational Pediatric Research (CTPR) NIH Center of Biomedical Research Excellence award P20GM121293.

Acknowledgments: We appreciate the help from Elizabeth Moore (Y.I.P. laboratory) during the study and manuscript writing.

References

1. Weinstein, J.N.; Collisson, E.A.; Mills, G.B.; Shaw, K.R.M.; Ozenberger, B.A.; Ellrott, K.; Shmulevich, I.; Sander, C.; Stuart, J.M. The Cancer Genome Atlas Pan-Cancer analysis project. *Nat. Genet.* **2013**, *45*, 1113–1120.

2. Forbes, S.A.; Beare, D.; Gunasekaran, P.; Leung, K.; Bindal, N.; Boutselakis, H.; Ding, M.; Bamford, S.; Cole, C.; Ward, S.; et al. COSMIC: Exploring the world's knowledge of somatic mutations in human cancer. *Nucleic Acids Res.* **2015**, *43*, D805–D811. [CrossRef] [PubMed]

3. Nakagawa, H.; Fujita, M. Whole genome sequencing analysis for cancer genomics and precision medicine. *Cancer Sci.* **2018**, *109*, 513–522. [CrossRef] [PubMed]

4. Loeb, L.A.; Springgate, C.F.; Battula, N. Errors in DNA replication as a basis of malignant changes. *Cancer Res.* **1974**, *34*, 2311–2321. [PubMed]

5. Roberts, S.A.; Gordenin, D.A. Hypermutation in human cancer genomes: Footprints and mechanisms. *Nat. Rev. Cancer* **2014**, *14*, 786–800. [CrossRef] [PubMed]

6. Bailey, M.H.; Tokheim, C.; Porta-Pardo, E.; Sengupta, S.; Bertrand, D.; Weerasinghe, A.; Colaprico, A.; Wendl, M.C.; Kim, J.; Reardon, B.; et al. Comprehensive characterization of cancer driver genes and mutations. *Cell* **2018**, *173*, 371–385. [CrossRef] [PubMed]

7. Bailey, M.H.; Tokheim, C.; Porta-Pardo, E.; Sengupta, S.; Bertrand, D.; Weerasinghe, A.; Colaprico, A.; Wendl, M.C.; Kim, J.; Reardon, B.; et al. Erratum: Comprehensive characterization of cancer driver genes and mutations. *Cell* **2018**, *174*, 1034–1035. [CrossRef]

8. Martincorena, I.; Roshan, A.; Gerstung, M.; Ellis, P.; Van Loo, P.; McLaren, S.; Wedge, D.C.; Fullam, A.; Alexandrov, L.B.; Tubio, J.M.; et al. Tumor evolution. High burden and pervasive positive selection of somatic mutations in normal human skin. *Science* **2015**, *348*, 880–886. [CrossRef]

9. Martincorena, I.; Raine, K.M.; Gerstung, M.; Dawson, K.J.; Haase, K.; Van Loo, P.; Davies, H.; Stratton, M.R.; Campbell, P.J. Universal patterns of selection in cancer and somatic tissues. *Cell* **2017**, *171*, 1029–1041. [CrossRef]

10. Alexandrov, L.B.; Nik-Zainal, S.; Wedge, D.C.; Aparicio, S.A.; Behjati, S.; Biankin, A.V.; Bignell, G.R.; Bolli, N.; Borg, A.; Borresen-Dale, A.L.; et al. Signatures of mutational processes in human cancer. *Nature* **2013**, *500*, 415–421. [CrossRef]

11. Hutchinson, L. Genetics: Signatures of mutational processes in cancer-a big step closer. *Nat. Rev. Clin. Oncol.* **2013**, *10*, 545. [CrossRef] [PubMed]

12. Alexandrov, L.B.; Stratton, M.R. Mutational signatures: The patterns of somatic mutations hidden in cancer genomes. *Curr. Opin. Genet. Dev.* **2014**, *24*, 52–60. [CrossRef] [PubMed]

13. Goncearenco, A.; Rager, S.L.; Li, M.; Sang, Q.X.; Rogozin, I.B.; Panchenko, A.R. Exploring background mutational processes to decipher cancer genetic heterogeneity. *Nucleic Acids Res.* **2017**, *45*, W514–W522. [CrossRef]

14. Burns, M.B.; Temiz, N.A.; Harris, R.S. Evidence for APOBEC3B mutagenesis in multiple human cancers. *Nat. Genet.* **2013**, *45*, 977–983. [CrossRef] [PubMed]

15. Roberts, S.A.; Lawrence, M.S.; Klimczak, L.J.; Grimm, S.A.; Fargo, D.; Stojanov, P.; Kiezun, A.; Kryukov, G.V.; Carter, S.L.; Saksena, G.; et al. An APOBEC cytidine deaminase mutagenesis pattern is widespread in human cancers. *Nat. Genet.* **2013**, *45*, 970–976. [CrossRef] [PubMed]

16. Pham, P.; Bransteitter, R.; Petruska, J.; Goodman, M.F. Processive AID-catalysed cytosine deamination on single-stranded DNA simulates somatic hypermutation. *Nature* **2003**, *424*, 103–107. [CrossRef] [PubMed]

17. Chan, K.; Gordenin, D.A. Clusters of multiple mutations: Incidence and molecular Mechanisms. *Annu. Rev. Genet.* **2015**, *49*, 243–267. [CrossRef]

18. Burns, M.B.; Lackey, L.; Carpenter, M.A.; Rathore, A.; Land, A.M.; Leonard, B.; Refsland, E.W.; Kotandeniya, D.; Tretyakova, N.; Nikas, J.B.; et al. APOBEC3B is an enzymatic source of mutation in breast cancer. *Nature* **2013**, *494*, 366–370. [CrossRef]

19. Kuong, K.J.; Loeb, L.A. APOBEC3B mutagenesis in cancer. *Nat. Genet.* **2013**, *45*, 964–965. [CrossRef]

20. Franchini, D.M.; Schmitz, K.M.; Petersen-Mahrt, S.K. 5-Methylcytosine DNA demethylation: More than losing a methyl group. *Annu. Rev. Genet.* **2012**, *46*, 419–441. [CrossRef]

21. Rogozin, I.B.; Lada, A.G.; Goncearenco, A.; Green, M.R.; De, S.; Nudelman, G.; Panchenko, A.R.; Koonin, E.V.; Pavlov, Y.I. Activation induced deaminase mutational signature overlaps with CpG methylation sites in follicular lymphoma and other cancers. *Sci. Rep.* **2016**, *6*, 38133. [CrossRef] [PubMed]

22. Alexandrov, L.B.; Nik-Zainal, S.; Wedge, D.C.; Campbell, P.J.; Stratton, M.R. Deciphering signatures of mutational processes operative in human cancer. *Cell Rep.* **2013**, *3*, 246–259. [CrossRef] [PubMed]

23. Rogozin, I.B.; Pavlov, Y.I.; Goncearenco, A.; De, S.; Lada, A.G.; Poliakov, E.; Panchenko, A.R.; Cooper, D.N. Mutational signatures and mutable motifs in cancer genomes. *Brief. Bioinform.* **2017**, *19*, 1085–1101. [CrossRef] [PubMed]

24. Seplyarskiy, V.B.; Soldatov, R.A.; Popadin, K.Y.; Antonarakis, S.E.; Bazykin, G.A.; Nikolaev, S.I. APOBEC-induced mutations in human cancers are strongly enriched on the lagging DNA strand during replication. *Genome Res.* **2016**, *26*, 174–182. [CrossRef] [PubMed]

25. Haradhvala, N.J.; Polak, P.; Stojanov, P.; Covington, K.R.; Shinbrot, E.; Hess, J.M.; Rheinbay, E.; Kim, J.; Maruvka, Y.E.; Braunstein, L.Z.; et al. Mutational strand asymmetries in cancer genomes reveal mechanisms of DNA damage and repair. *Cell* **2016**, *164*, 538–549. [CrossRef] [PubMed]

26. Temiz, N.A.; Donohue, D.E.; Bacolla, A.; Vasquez, K.M.; Cooper, D.N.; Mudunuri, U.; Ivanic, J.; Cer, R.Z.; Yi, M.; Stephens, R.M.; et al. The somatic autosomal mutation matrix in cancer genomes. *Hum. Genet.* **2015**, *134*, 851–864. [CrossRef] [PubMed]

27. Staden, R. Computer methods to locate signals in nucleic acid sequences. *Nucleic Acids Res.* **1984**, *12*, 505–519. [CrossRef]

28. Gelfand, M.S. Prediction of function in DNA sequence analysis. *J. Comput. Biol.: J. Comput. Mol. Cell Biol.* **1995**, *2*, 87–115. [CrossRef]

29. Rogozin, I.B.; Milanesi, L. Analysis of donor splice sites in different eukaryotic organisms. *J. Mol. Evol.* **1997**, *45*, 50–59. [CrossRef]

30. Bishop, K.N.; Holmes, R.K.; Sheehy, A.M.; Davidson, N.O.; Cho, S.J.; Malim, M.H. Cytidine deamination of retroviral DNA by diverse APOBEC proteins. *Curr. Biol.* **2004**, *14*, 1392–1396. [CrossRef]

31. Rogozin, I.B.; Pavlov, Y.I. The cytidine deaminase AID exhibits similar functional properties in yeast and mammals. *Mol. Immunol.* **2006**, *43*, 1481–1484. [CrossRef] [PubMed]

32. Ju, Y.S.; Alexandrov, L.B.; Gerstung, M.; Martincorena, I.; Nik-Zainal, S.; Ramakrishna, M.; Davies, H.R.; Papaemmanuil, E.; Gundem, G.; Shlien, A.; et al. Origins and functional consequences of somatic mitochondrial DNA mutations in human cancer. *eLife* **2014**, *3*, e02935. [CrossRef] [PubMed]

33. Benjamini, Y.; Hochberg, Y. Controlling the false discovery rate: A practical and powerful approach to multiple testing. *J. R. Stat. Soc. Ser. B (Methodol.)* **1995**, *57*, 289–300. [CrossRef]

34. Milstein, C.; Neuberger, M.S.; Staden, R. Both DNA strands of antibody genes are hypermutation targets. *Proc. Natl. Acad. Sci. USA* **1998**, *95*, 8791–8794. [CrossRef] [PubMed]

35. Mayorov, V.I.; Rogozin, I.B.; Adkison, L.R.; Frahm, C.R.; Kunkel, T.A.; Pavlov, Y.I. Expression of human AID in yeast induces mutations in context similar to the context of somatic hypermutation at G-C pairs in immunoglobulin genes. *BMC Immunol.* **2005**, *6*, 10. [CrossRef] [PubMed]

36. Zanotti, K.J.; Gearhart, P.J. Antibody diversification caused by disrupted mismatch repair and promiscuous DNA polymerases. *DNA Repair* **2016**, *38*, 110–116. [CrossRef] [PubMed]

37. Taylor, B.J.; Nik-Zainal, S.; Wu, Y.L.; Stebbings, L.A.; Raine, K.; Campbell, P.J.; Rada, C.; Stratton, M.R.; Neuberger, M.S. DNA deaminases induce break-associated mutation showers with implication of APOBEC3B and 3A in breast cancer kataegis. *eLife* **2013**, *2*, e00534. [CrossRef]

38. Neuberger, M.S.; Rada, C. Somatic hypermutation: Activation-induced deaminase for C/G followed by polymerase eta for A/T. *J. Exp. Med.* **2007**, *204*, 7–10. [CrossRef]

39. Rogozin, I.B.; Goncearenco, A.; Lada, A.G.; De, S.; Yurchenko, V.; Nudelman, G.; Panchenko, A.R.; Cooper, D.N.; Pavlov, Y.I. DNA polymerase eta mutational signatures are found in a variety of different types of cancer. *Cell Cycle* **2018**, *17*, 348–355. [CrossRef]

40. Saini, N.; Roberts, S.A.; Klimczak, L.J.; Chan, K.; Grimm, S.A.; Dai, S.; Fargo, D.C.; Boyer, J.C.; Kaufmann, W.K.; Taylor, J.A.; et al. The impact of environmental and endogenous damage on somatic mutation load in human skin fibroblasts. *PLoS Genet.* **2016**, *12*, e1006385. [CrossRef]

41. Pham, P.; Landolph, A.; Mendez, C.; Li, N.; Goodman, M.F. A biochemical analysis linking APOBEC3A to disparate HIV-1 restriction and skin cancer. *J. Biol. Chem.* **2013**, *288*, 29294–29304. [CrossRef] [PubMed]

42. Cho, R.J.; Alexandrov, L.B.; den Breems, N.Y.; Atanasova, V.S.; Farshchian, M.; Purdom, E.; Nguyen, T.N.; Coarfa, C.; Rajapakshe, K.; Prisco, M.; et al. APOBEC mutation drives early-onset squamous cell carcinomas in recessive dystrophic epidermolysis bullosa. *Sci. Transl. Med.* **2018**, *10*, eaas9668. [CrossRef] [PubMed]

43. Fickett, J.W.; Guigo, R. Estimation of protein coding density in a corpus of DNA sequence data. *Nucleic Acid Res.* **1993**, *21*, 2837–2844. [CrossRef] [PubMed]

44. Glazko, G.B.; Milanesi, L.; Rogozin, I.B. The subclass approach for mutational spectrum analysis: Application of the SEM algorithm. *J. Theor. Biol.* **1998**, *192*, 475–487. [CrossRef] [PubMed]

45. Siriwardena, S.U.; Perera, M.L.W.; Senevirathne, V.; Stewart, J.; Bhagwat, A.S. A tumor promoting phorbol ester causes a large increase in APOBEC3A and a moderate increase in APOBEC3B expression in a normal human keratinocyte cell line without increasing genomic uracils. *Mol. Cell. Biol.* **2018**, *39*, e00238-18. [CrossRef] [PubMed]

46. Neuberger, M.S.; Harris, R.S.; Di Noia, J.; Petersen-Mahrt, S.K. Immunity through DNA deamination. *Trends Biochem. Sci.* **2003**, *28*, 305–312. [CrossRef]

47. Harris, R.S.; Petersen-Mahrt, S.K.; Neuberger, M.S. RNA editing enzyme APOBEC1 and some of its homologs can act as DNA mutators. *Mol. Cell* **2002**, *10*, 1247–1253. [CrossRef]

48. Petersen-Mahrt, S.K.; Harris, R.S.; Neuberger, M.S. AID mutates *E. coli* suggesting a DNA deamination mechanism for antibody diversification. *Nature* **2002**, *418*, 99–103. [CrossRef]

49. Bhagwat, A.S. DNA-cytosine deaminases: From antibody maturation to antiviral defense. *DNA Repair* **2004**, *3*, 85–89. [CrossRef]

50. Franchini, D.M.; Petersen-Mahrt, S.K. AID and APOBEC deaminases: Balancing DNA damage in epigenetics and immunity. *Epigenomics* **2014**, *6*, 427–443. [CrossRef]

51. Rebhandl, S.; Huemer, M.; Greil, R.; Geisberger, R. AID/APOBEC deaminases and cancer. *Oncoscience* **2015**, *2*, 320–333. [CrossRef] [PubMed]

52. Landry, S.; Narvaiza, I.; Linfesty, D.C.; Weitzman, M.D. APOBEC3A can activate the DNA damage response and cause cell-cycle arrest. *Embo Rep.* **2011**, *12*, 444–450. [CrossRef] [PubMed]

53. Taylor, B.J.; Wu, Y.L.; Rada, C. Active RNAP pre-initiation sites are highly mutated by cytidine deaminases in yeast, with AID targeting small RNA genes. *eLife* **2014**, *3*, e03553. [CrossRef] [PubMed]

54. Lada, A.G.; Kliver, S.F.; Dhar, A.; Polev, D.E.; Masharsky, A.E.; Rogozin, I.B.; Pavlov, Y.I. Disruption of transcriptional coactivator Sub1 leads to genome-wide re-distribution of clustered mutations induced by APOBEC in active yeast genes. *PLoS Genet.* **2015**, *11*, e1005217. [CrossRef] [PubMed]

55. Lada, A.G.; Krick, C.F.; Kozmin, S.G.; Mayorov, V.I.; Karpova, T.S.; Rogozin, I.B.; Pavlov, Y.I. Mutator effects and mutation signatures of editing deaminases produced in bacteria and yeast. *Biochemistry* **2011**, *76*, 131–146. [CrossRef] [PubMed]

56. Lada, A.G.; Stepchenkova, E.I.; Zhuk, A.S.; Kliver, S.F.; Rogozin, I.B.; Polev, D.E.; Dhar, A.; Pavlov, Y.I. Recombination is responsible for the increased recovery of drug-resistant mutants with hypermutated genomes in resting yeast diploids expressing APOBEC deaminases. *Front. Genet.* **2017**, *8*, 202. [CrossRef] [PubMed]

57. Shi, K.; Carpenter, M.A.; Banerjee, S.; Shaban, N.M.; Kurahashi, K.; Salamango, D.J.; McCann, J.L.; Starrett, G.J.; Duffy, J.V.; Demir, O.; et al. Structural basis for targeted DNA cytosine deamination and mutagenesis by APOBEC3A and APOBEC3B. *Nat. Struct. Mol. Biol.* **2017**, *24*, 131–139. [CrossRef]

58. Nik-Zainal, S.; Wedge, D.C.; Alexandrov, L.B.; Petljak, M.; Butler, A.P.; Bolli, N.; Davies, H.R.; Knappskog, S.; Martin, S.; Papaemmanuil, E.; et al. Association of a germline copy number polymorphism of APOBEC3A and APOBEC3B with burden of putative APOBEC-dependent mutations in breast cancer. *Nat. Genet.* **2014**, *46*, 487–491. [CrossRef]

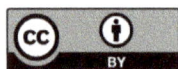

cancers

MDPI

Article

A Toolbox for Functional Analysis and the Systematic Identification of Diagnostic and Prognostic Gene Expression Signatures Combining Meta-Analysis and Machine Learning

**Johannes Vey [1,2,†], Lorenz A. Kapsner [3,†], Maximilian Fuchs [1,4], Philipp Unberath [4],
Giulia Veronesi [5] and Meik Kunz [4,*]**

[1] Functional Genomics and Systems Biology Group, Department of Bioinformatics, University of Würzburg, 97074 Würzburg, Germany; johannes.vey@uni-wuerzburg.de (J.V.); maximilian.fuchs@uni-wuerzburg.de (M.F.)

[2] Institute of Medical Biometry and Informatics, University of Heidelberg, Im Neuenheimer Feld 130.3, 69120 Heidelberg, Germany

[3] Center of Medical Information and Communication Technology, Erlangen University Hospital, 91054 Erlangen, Germany; lorenz.kapsner@uk-erlangen.de

[4] Chair of Medical Informatics, Friedrich-Alexander University of Erlangen-Nürnberg, 91058 Erlangen, Germany; philipp.unberath@fau.de

[5] Unit of Thoracic Surgery, Humanitas Research Hospital, Via Manzoni 56, 20089 Rozzano (Milan), Italy; giuliaveronesi1@gmail.com

* Correspondence: meik.kunz@fau.de; Tel.: +49-9131-85-26767; Fax: +49-9131-85-26754

† These authors contributed equally.

Received: 30 September 2019; Accepted: 15 October 2019; Published: 21 October 2019

Abstract: The identification of biomarker signatures is important for cancer diagnosis and prognosis. However, the detection of clinical reliable signatures is influenced by limited data availability, which may restrict statistical power. Moreover, methods for integration of large sample cohorts and signature identification are limited. We present a step-by-step computational protocol for functional gene expression analysis and the identification of diagnostic and prognostic signatures by combining meta-analysis with machine learning and survival analysis. The novelty of the toolbox lies in its all-in-one functionality, generic design, and modularity. It is exemplified for lung cancer, including a comprehensive evaluation using different validation strategies. However, the protocol is not restricted to specific disease types and can therefore be used by a broad community. The accompanying R package vignette runs in ~1 h and describes the workflow in detail for use by researchers with limited bioinformatics training.

Keywords: Bioinformatics tool; R package; machine learning; meta-analysis; biomarker signature; gene expression analysis; survival analysis; functional analysis

---

1. Introduction

The combination of biomarkers (so-called biomarker signature) allows us to represent the information contained in biological samples and fluids, supporting clinical decisions [1]. Numerous studies demonstrated the clinical usefulness of diagnostic (disease detection) and prognostic (disease outcome) gene-expression signatures derived from microarray analysis [2,3]. For instance, MammaPrint is a 70 gene-expression prognostic signature for powerful disease outcome prediction in breast cancer [4]. The diagnostic miR-Test shows promising results for lung cancer early detection [5].

However, reliable clinical signatures are restricted by dataset availability, which often reduces their statistical power [3,6]. Artificially increasing the number of samples by combining different large cohorts using dataset merging (meta-analysis) is a beneficial solution enabling numerous insights into biological systems [7–10], but methods for biomarker signature identification are currently limited. For instance, the R packages virtualArray [11] and inSilicoMerging [12] allow virtual array merging but are no longer available and are removed from current Bioconductor releases [13]. On the other hand, database tools such as SurvExpress [14] and SurvMicro [3] allow for the assessment of a prognostic signature in cancer. Similarly, the miRpower tool provides survival analysis for miRNA biomarkers using expression data from 2178 breast cancer patients [15] and GOBO based on 1881 breast cancer dataset [16], whereas the Kaplan-Meier Plotter enables outcome analysis for ovarian cancer based on 1287 patients [17]. However, these tools focus on specific diseases and signature types. More importantly, they allow only online analysis, requiring a gene list as input, but not the calculation of signatures from in-house data. These characteristics limit them as stand-alone tools, suggesting new bioinformatics approaches.

Machine learning (ML) approaches have been demonstrated to be useful in medicine. For example, studies report that ML could be used in cancer diagnosis [18] and prognosis [19] as well as prediction of optimal cancer therapies [20]. It can also improve the prediction of heart failure readmissions [21].

Regularized Generalized Linear Models such as L1/L2 regularized and Elastic net regression address overfitting and aim to balance between accuracy and simplicity of a model [22,23]. The Least Absolute Shrinkage and Selection Operator (LASSO) uses L1 regularization, whereas Elastic net implements a mixture of L1 and L2 regularization. Applying these regularization techniques to fit a Generalized Linear Model is widely used for feature selection and is extremely effective when dealing with high dimensional data, which contains a large set of features. The LASSO model allows the shrinkage of the coefficients of the less contributive variables to be exactly zero (the penalty term L1-norm) [22]. Thereby, the tuning parameter lambda controls the strength of the penalization (regularization). The cross-validation calculates the lambda.min value, which reflects the model with the lowest prediction error, whereas the lambda.1se value represents a simpler model but within one standard error of the optimal model. However, the LASSO regression tends to over-regularization and has limited strength in highly correlated data.

The Elastic net balances between LASSO (L1-norm) and ridge penalties (L2-norm) shrinking some coefficients close to zero (like ridge) and some exactly to zero (similar to LASSO) [23]. This model is powerful in datasets with e.g., correlations between variables. For this, the hyper-parameter alpha controls the mixing between the two penalty techniques (alpha = 0 for ridge; alpha = 1 for LASSO) and can be set manually between 0 and 1 to receive a model with the desired size, whereas the parameter lambda fine-tunes the amount of shrinkage [23]. Therefore, the Elastic net is a powerful method for feature selection and can operate with continuous as well as categorical features.

Several statistical methods have been developed for survival data analysis [24,25]. The Cox Proportional Hazard model is the most popular multivariate approach to investigate survival time in medical research [24,26]. It describes the relation between event incidence (hazard function, survival probability) and covariates [24,25].

We previously introduced a sample merging approach that is compatible with current Bioconductor releases [27]. It allows the use of datasets from databases such as Gene Expression Omnibus (GEO), The Cancer Genome Atlas (TCGA), and own experimental data [27], greatly enhancing the number of available datasets for analysis. Starting from this, we developed a protocol for the systematical calculation of diagnostic and prognostic gene signatures that combines (i) meta-analysis (multiple dataset integration) with (ii) functional gene expression analysis and (iii) ML approaches. Our aim was to develop a general framework for functional analysis and signature calculation with high predictive performance that is not restricted to specific disease types and can therefore be used by a broad community.

2. Results

2.1. Meta-Analysis (Dataset Download, Normalization, Merging, Batch Effect Correction)

We demonstrate the workflow of our toolbox by analyzing three lung cancer datasets from microarray profiling downloaded from the GEO database. The datasets GSE18842 (45 non-tumor, 46 tumor samples) and GSE19804 (60 tumor/60 non-tumor samples) were downloaded (getGEO) and are already GCRMA normalized deposited in GEO. For the datasets GSE19188 (91 tumor/ 65 non-tumor samples), we downloaded the raw data (CEL files). The files were imported into the R environment and subsequently GCRMA normalized (resulting "ExpressionSet" object) using the gcrma package version 2.56.0 [28] (Figure S1; datasets from Chip GPL570, Affymetrix Human Genome U133 Plus 2.0). The merged dataset contained 54,675 transcripts and 367 samples (197 tumor/170 non-tumor samples; no gene transcripts were excluded during the merging procedure). The batch effect detection using a gPCA (Top) and the resulting boxplot of the merged dataset after batch effect correction (Bottom) are shown in Figure S2.

2.2. Functional Gene Expression Analysis

The differentially expressed genes (DEG) analysis after batch correction resulted in 699 significantly deregulated transcripts (Table S1; q-value < 0.05, logFC > 2/< −2 as standard criterion for selecting significantly deregulated genes [29]). Figure 1 shows the heatmap of the DEGs, illustrating a clear separation of tumor and non-tumor samples in two expression clusters. Many of them are known key players in lung cancer, for instance G Protein-Coupled Receptor Kinase 5 (GRK5) [30], Solute Carrier Family 46 Member 2 (SLC46A2) [31], and Collagen Type XI Alpha 1 Chain (COL11A1) [32] function as oncogenic factors in lung cancer.

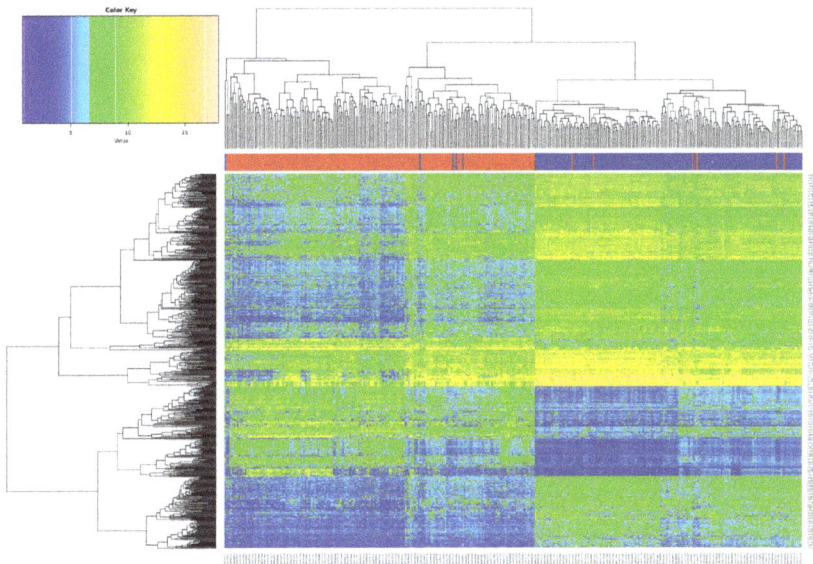

Figure 1. Overview of the differentially expressed genes (DEGs). Heatmap of the 699 DEGs derived from the meta-analysis with the merged datasets GSE18842, GSE19804 and GSE19188 (samples on the x-axis, DEGs on the y-axis; red color represents tumor, blue non-tumor (control) samples).

We further tested the 699 DEGs for enriched Gene Ontology (GO) terms and Kyoto Encyclopedia of Genes and Genomes (KEGG) pathways (Figure 2, enriched GO terms and KEGG pathways after False

Discovery Rate (FDR) control are shown). For instance, the analysis shows enriched functions such as hormone receptor binding and protein serine/threonine kinase activity (Left) and enriched pathways such as Phosphatidylinositol 3-Kinase-Akt (PI3K-Akt) signaling pathway and Mitogen-Activated Protein Kinase (MAPK) signaling pathway (Middle). Moreover, specific pathways depending on the interest of the users can be further investigated. As an example, we show the PI3K-Akt signaling pathway (hsa04151) from the KEGG database including the expression values of the involved DEGs (Figure 2, Right; red: upregulated, green: downregulated).

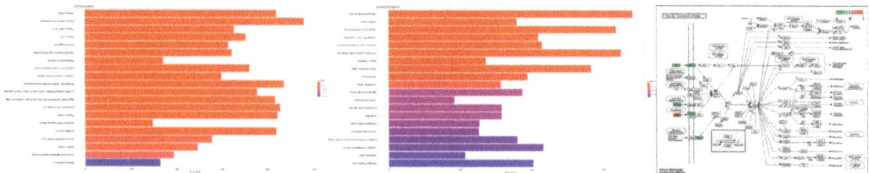

Figure 2. Functional Gene Ontology (GO) term and pathway enrichment analysis. (**Left**) Enriched GO terms including adjusted p-value as color code. (**Middle**) Enriched Kyoto Encyclopedia of Genes and Genomes (KEGG) pathways including adjusted p-value as color code. (**Right**) The phosphatidylinositol 3-kinase (PI3K)-Akt signaling pathway (hsa04151) from the KEGG database including the differentially expressed genes (DEGs) are highlighted considering differential expression.

2.3. Calculation of Diagnostic and Prognostic Signatures

We next analyzed the merged dataset (54,675 transcripts) for a diagnostic signature. We divided the merged dataset into a training dataset (80%; 294 samples) and test dataset (20%, 73 samples). We used a L1/L2 regularized logistic regression to fit a Generalized Linear Model in order to perform a feature selection to include only the potentially most predictive variables (here genes) in the model. The 10-fold cross-validation results in a lambda of 0.009260 and 0.059521 (Figure 3; alpha = 1). The lambda.min identifies a selection of 64 transcript variables (55 unique gene symbols) whose coefficients were not forced to be zero, whereas the lambda.1se identifies a 26 gene transcript signature (24 unique gene symbols) (Table S2). Figure 3 shows the cross-validation error (Left) and the confusion matrix (Right) for the calculated LASSO signatures predicting the test data samples.

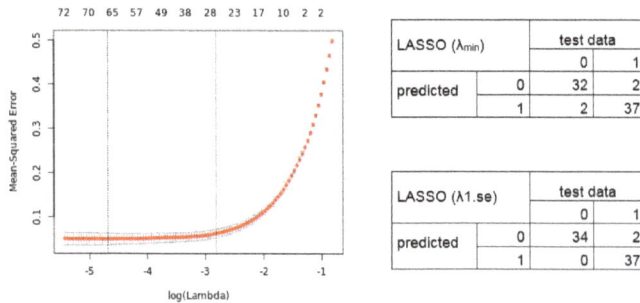

Figure 3. Mean-Squared error for 10-fold cross-validation according to the log of lambda on the training lung cancer dataset. (**Left**) The cross-validation errors and the upper and lower standard deviation along the lambda values of the Least Absolute Shrinkage and Selection Operator (LASSO) regression model are shown. The vertical dotted lines represent the two selected lambdas. The lambda.min value (left line) minimizes the prediction error (MSE), whereas lambda.1se (right line) gives the most regularized model (most simple model within one standard deviation of the optimal model). Values above the plot show the number of variables included in the model. (**Right**) Confusion matrix depicting the diagnostic potential of the signatures validated on the test dataset (0 = healthy, 1 = tumor).

We further applied the Elastic net regression. The 10-fold cross-validation shows a lambda of 0.010288 and 0.063129 (alpha = 0.9). Notably, we manually set alpha = 0.9 as the grid search for lambda (0 to 0.0001 with 100 intervals) calculates an alpha = 0.1 (lambda = 0.521401), resulting in a signature without an improved predictive performance. The Elastic net regression model identified, for lambda.min, an 80 gene transcript signature (69 unique gene symbols), and for lambda.1se, a 41 transcript signature (36 unique gene symbols) (Table S2). The calculated cross-validation error (Left) and resulting confusion matrix (Right) of the predicted test data samples by the Elastic net model are shown in Figure 4.

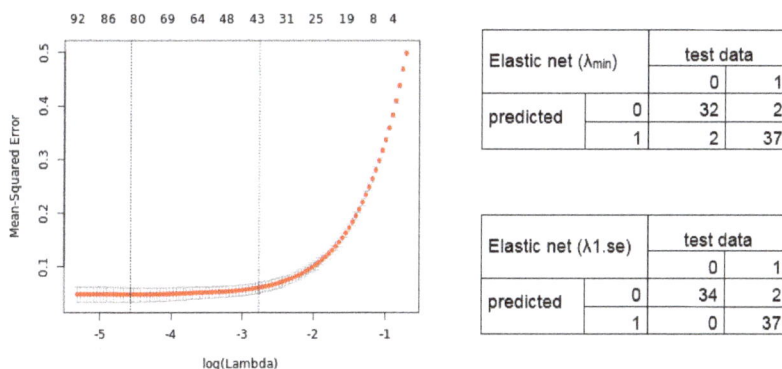

Elastic net (λ_{min})		test data	
		0	1
predicted	0	32	2
	1	2	37

Elastic net (λ1.se)		test data	
		0	1
predicted	0	34	2
	1	0	37

Figure 4. Elastic net regression model. (**Left**) The plot displays the 10-fold cross-validation errors and the upper and lower standard deviation along to the lambda values of the Elastic net regression model. The vertical dotted lines represent the two selected lambdas. The lambda.min value (left line) minimizes the prediction error (MSE), whereas lambda.1se (right line) gives the most regularized model (most simple model within one standard deviation of the optimal model). Values above the plot show the number of variables included in the model. (**Right**) Confusion matrix depicting the diagnostic potential of the signatures validated on the test dataset (0 = healthy, 1 = tumor).

To address overfitting and reduce model instability, the framework allows to include further datasets for validation. We validated the gene signatures in three independent datasets (GSE30219, 293 lung/14 non lung cancer samples; GSE102287, 32 lung/34 non lung cancer samples; GSE33356, 60 lung/60 non lung cancer samples; 54,675 genes). The GSE30219 contains <5% non-cancerous samples, whereas the GSE102287 and GSE33356 are more balanced validation datasets. The results of the validation are depicted in Figure 5 (confusion matrices) and Supplementary Table S3 (diagnostic values), showing a high diagnostic power to classify between lung cancer and non-lung cancer samples.

After determining the diagnostic signature, we tested for a relevant prognostic signature. For this, we analyzed the significant influence of the 699 DEGs on the patient survival outcome using a Univariate Cox Proportional Hazard Model (82 patient survival outcome data from GSE19188). The Cox regression analysis revealed 22 DEGs that have a significant influence (effect size) on the patient survival (Table S4; *p*-value < 0.05). We found known lung cancer drivers such as Lipoprotein Lipase (LPL) [33] and CC Chemokine Receptor 2 (CCL2) [34].

A: Confusion matrix Independent dataset GSE30219   B: Confusion matrix Independent dataset GSE102287   C: Confusion matrix Independent dataset GSE33356

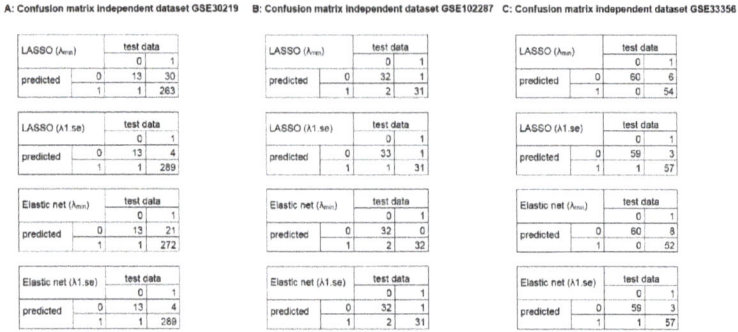

Figure 5. Confusion matrices of the identified diagnostic signatures in independent datasets. The plots illustrate the diagnostic classification using the identified signatures in the independent validation dataset (54,675 genes; 0 = healthy, 1 = tumor). (**A**) GSE30219, 293 lung cancer samples, 14 non lung cancer samples. (**B**) GSE102287, 32 lung cancer samples, 34 non lung cancer samples. (**C**) GSE33356, 60 lung cancer samples, 60 non lung cancer samples.

Next, we trained the prognostic 22 gene classifier using an algorithm comparing the expression profiles between tumor and healthy samples of the merged datasets GSE18842 and GSE19804 (we excluded GSE19188 for classification to avoid selection bias, as it is the dataset for the identification of survival correlated genes). We additionally validated the identified 22 prognostic gene signature in two independent datasets (GSE30219: 278 from 293 patients with survival data, GSE50081: 181 patients with survival data) to evaluate its impact on the patient outcome. Here, we tested whether the 22 gene signature can classify patients with high and low mortality risk. Therefore, we classified the patient samples into high risk and low risk groups using the trained classifier.

The Kaplan-Meier estimators in Figure 6 demonstrate the significant patient classification achieved regarding high and low risk groups for the 22 genes in the validation dataset GSE30219 (Left: p-value = 0.0002166) and GSE50081 (Right: p-value = 0.02919). This indicates that the identified 22 gene classifier reflects a common prognostic signature of dominant tumor factors that can differentiate between high and low risk tumor disease.

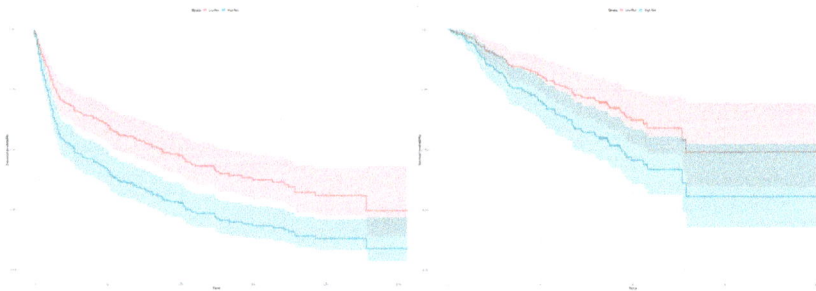

Figure 6. Kaplan-Meier estimators with computed 95% confidence interval to evaluate the patient classification in high and low risk groups deploying the 22 gene signature on two independent datasets. The classification in high and low risk groups is based on the expression profiles between tumor and healthy samples of the merged datasets (GSE18842, GSE19804). (Left) The plot shows a classification in high and low risk groups for the 293 patients from the validation dataset GSE30219 based on the 22 survival correlated genes (p-value = 0.0002166; low risk: 121 samples, high risk: 172 samples, number of events/deaths: 188). (Right) The 22 gene signature can classify the 181 patients in the validation dataset GSE50081 in high and low risk groups (p-value = 0.02919; low risk: 88 samples, high risk: 93 samples, number of events/deaths: 75).

3. Discussion

Our intention was to develop a general and easy to use toolbox that identifies reliable diagnostic and prognostic signatures including the important steps of data augmentation and validation, especially for users with limited bioinformatics resources. It is therefore a step-by-step protocol rather than an improved algorithm or ML method approach.

The tool applies a comparison between the two ML models LASSO and Elastic net, which aim to balance between accuracy and simplicity of a model. LASSO and Elastic net regularization are well-established methods for gene expression analysis, allowing to construct predictive models from datasets with non-linear and large dimensional variable numbers [21]. Especially for generalization of data with additive variable and outcome dimensions or a low number of training datasets they generate predictive results similar to complex ML algorithms [19]. Complex ML approaches such as support vector machines, neural networks, random forest, and gradient boosting algorithms allow unbiased predictive models using complex variable selection and huge datasets but tend to overfitting in the identification of large biomarker combinations [1,19,35]. However, the combinations of biomarkers show better discriminatory power for clinical decision support rather than a single biomarker [1].

The use of ML implies the need for a substantial amount of data in order to train the model, in which the integration of different datasets might be required. However, gene expression analysis often suffers from selection bias, poor sample quality, and poor sample size estimation, influencing the statistical power and validity of downstream analysis [1,36,37]. Combing different gene expression datasets using meta-analysis has been shown to increase statistical power and overcome selection biases including the identification of diagnostic and prognostic biomarkers [7–10,38–40]. However, differentially gene expression selection using meta-analysis is mostly based on univariate p-value statistics which introduces the problem to identify sets of genes with non-redundant information and to find the correct number of genes that describe the data [8]. This limits application for diagnostic and prognostic signatures that integrate several feature selections and covariates such as patient characteristics (e.g., survival) and histology [8]. We overcome this by implementing a meta-analysis for the integration of multiple gene expression datasets into a merging array and then applied ML methods to identify biomarker signatures from datasets with non-linear and large dimensional variable numbers.

Several studies calculate signatures using ML approaches, but often fail during independent validation stages [36]. To overcome overfitting and reduce model instability, we identified a classifier in the training dataset and applied a comprehensive evaluation using different validation strategies—in particular, a split sample, internal validation (cross-validation) and testing in independent datasets. Moreover, we applied a multiple-testing correction using the Benjamini and Hochberg method and set a stringent q-value of 0.05. We recommend using a stringent q-value (can be set by the user) to reduce the false positives and find real biologically deregulated genes but also considering sample size and power estimation approaches based on statistical and clinical significance [1,41]. This strengthens the robustness for the biomarker signature identification capability and validity for clinical usefulness.

In our example, the identified gene signatures from two different ML models show a high diagnostic power and might be promising for the clinic to classify between lung cancer and non-cancer samples. The confusion matrix for the LASSO and Elastic net regression models are similar. Comparing the calculated signatures shows a common set of 12 transcripts (12 unique gene symbols), and similar accuracy and predictive performance. However, this is of course not always the case. For example, studies in breast cancer reported two independent prognostic signatures identified with similar approaches showing only few common genes, which were experimentally validated [42]. This illustrates that different mathematical models should be applied to find the most reliable signature rather than using only one method. Hence, using several methods reduces false positive results even for challenging datasets and avoids misclassification in experimental and clinical testing. This strengthens the validity and clinical usefulness of signatures extracted from large gene expression datasets.

The common gene set contains known cancer markers. For instance, TMEM106B has been shown to be a valuable marker of lung cancer metastasis [43], whereas COL10A1 [44] plays a diagnostic role of circulating extracellular matrix-related proteins. However, LGR4 [45] is known as a diagnostic marker in prostate cancer. This highlights that our analysis approach allows the identification of reliable diagnostic signatures. The next step is then to validate and iteratively refine the marker signature derived from our tool in prospective clinical studies to find an optimal biomarker signature, with the help of more complex ML models.

The significance and novelty of the toolbox lies in its functionality as an „all-in-one tool": it offers an analysis path combining meta-analysis with functional gene expression analysis and robust diagnostic and prognostic signature calculation. The code is implemented in an R package. The four main functions—*sigidentDEG*, *sigidentEnrichment*, *sigidentDiagnostic*, and *sigidentPrognostic*—are wrapper functions around all included smaller functions to execute the analysis steps. However, these can also be run separately, depending on the interests of the users.

The toolbox benefits from its generic design and modularity. We designed it for Affymetrix as a widely used microarray profiling platform [46] and illustrate the generality of the approach using lung cancer gene expression datasets (tumor/healthy) downloaded from the GEO database. The generic design of the tool allows the analysis of different types of gene expression signatures, e.g., mRNA, lncRNA, and miRNA. Furthermore, it supports analysis in front of the high biological complexity of tumors, for instance analysis of tumor subtypes and heterogeneity.

We demonstrated the method's power to be applied to datasets containing a large number of gene probes using the Affymetrix HG-U133 Plus 2.0 platform. However, the merging algorithm is not restricted to this platform, allowing the potential integration of other popular microarray profiling platforms such as HG-U133A, HG-U133B, and HG-U133A 2.0. Moreover, the modularity of the framework allows the future incorporation of additional platforms, such as Illumina, but also other high-throughput data such as genomic, proteomic, metabolomic, and radiomic data. For instance, the Elastic net model shows applicability to genome-scale data such as the identification of genomic markers of drug sensitivity [8,47]. Indeed, the implementation of this complex data requires programming skills and is therefore recommended only for experienced users. Such a broad applicability is in principle possible but was not the intention of the current version of the framework and should be the focus of future work. Further efforts should also focus on the integration of the toolbox into a web application to provide its functionality to users without R programming skills.

Existing tools such as SurvMicro [3] and SurvExpress [14] allow for the online validation of prognostic signatures, but are restricted to datasets from TCGA and limited to cancer. Our toolbox has the advantage to be disease independent and allows the integration of data from TCGA and GEO, but also from in-house experiments.

The framework from Hughey et al. 2015 identifies a diagnostic signature combining meta-analysis with an Elastic net regression [8]. This approach is similar to our method, but our tool calculates prognostic signatures as a further relevant biomarker signature for clinical application. Additionally, the regularization methods LASSO and Elastic net can be applied for the aim of feature selection to identify variables correlated to the desired response variable. The toolbox also integrates an automated method to identify DEGs, including a summary table with gene annotations and functional enrichment analysis. In this way, our method can also be used to perform a functional DEG analysis from merged datasets without the calculation of signatures. In conclusion, the user-friendly R package, the all-in-one functionality, and modularity make the framework useful to a broad community.

4. Materials and Methods

Figure 7 illustrates the workflow of our toolbox. It has been developed and tested on R version 3.6.1 (R Bioconductor version 3.9). We implemented the code into the R package "sigident" (https://gitlab.miracum.org/clearly/sigident), which provides the four main functions—*sigidentDEG*, *sigidentEnrichment*, *sigidentDiagnostic*, and *sigidentPrognostic*. The whole workflow is documented in detail in the R package vignette.

Supplementary Table S5 lists the used R packages. The newly created "sigident" R package integrates a (i) meta-analysis (multiple dataset integration), (ii) functional gene expression analysis, and (iii) the calculation of statistically robust multi-gene signature combinations. As an application example, we used lung cancer datasets from the GEO database (GSE18842, GSE19804, and GSE19188). After merging, we divided the dataset into a training (80%) and test (20%) dataset for the calculation of the diagnostic signature. Moreover, we validated the diagnostic signature in three independent datasets (GSE30219, GSE102287, GSE33356). For the prognostic signature, we performed a survival analysis using the GSE19188 which includes survival information and validated the signature in two independent datasets (GSE30219, GSE50081).

For the meta-analysis (dataset download, normalization, merging) and the functional gene expression analysis (analysis for DEGs, heatmap), we used our previously published sample merging approach, which is based on a modified code of the inSilicoMerging package combined with the limma package [27]. This approach has been developed further in order to integrate it into the "sigident" R package framework. In detail, it uses the R package GEOquery version 2.52.0 for dataset downloading [48], gcrma package version 2.56.0 for CEL file loading, background correction, quantile normalization, and log2-transformation [28], Biobase package version 2.44.0 for integration of standardized data structures [13], gplots package version 3.0.1.1 for graphical representation [49], and the limma package version 3.40.6 for the DEG analysis [50]. We extended the code by detecting batch effects using a guided principal component analysis from the gPCA package version 1.0 [51]. For batch effect correction, we used empirical Bayes framework applying the ComBat function from the sva package version 3.32.1 [52] considering different groups (tumor, ctrl). As a DEG analysis is known to generate false positive results [36], we applied a multiple-testing correction using the Benjamini and Hochberg approach to control the FDR [53]. We used a stringent q-value (adjusted FDR value) of 0.05.

Furthermore, for the DEGs we added a functional gene ontology (GO) and KEGG pathway enrichment analysis using the goana and kegga functions from the limma package (Entrez IDs as input). A further GO and pathway over-representation test is implemented using the clusterProfiler package version 3.12.0 [54] (including FDR control, DEGs are mapped to their Entrez-IDs as input), whereas specific pathways can be further investigated using the pathview package version 1.24.0 [55].

The calculation of statistically robust multi-gene signature combinations focuses on diagnostic and prognostic signatures. For diagnostic signatures, we used the LASSO and Elastic net penalty as implemented in the R package glmnet version 2.0.18 [56]. The hyper-parameter alpha can manually be set to a value between 0 and 1 or can automatically be calculated in combination with the tuning parameter lambda based on cross-validation and a grid search applying the wrapper function train as implemented in the caret package version 6.0.84 [57]. In the case of a fixed value for alpha, lambda is determined by 10-fold cross-validation, and a leave-one-out cross-validation is also possible. For calculation of the Receiver Operating Characteristics (ROC) and the Area Under the Curve (AUC) value of the ML models we used the pROC package version 1.15.3 [58].

For the prognostic signature detection we applied a survival and risk assessment analysis using a Cox Proportional Hazard Model as implemented in the survival R package version 2.44.1.1 [59]. The Cox Proportional Hazard regression analysis identifies genes that have a significant effect size on the survival outcome. To generate a prognostic signature, we applied a classification algorithm that assigns patients in high and low risk groups based on the expression profiles of the identified survival correlated genes between tumor and non-tumor samples. Survival curves were plotted using the survminer package version 0.4.5 [60].

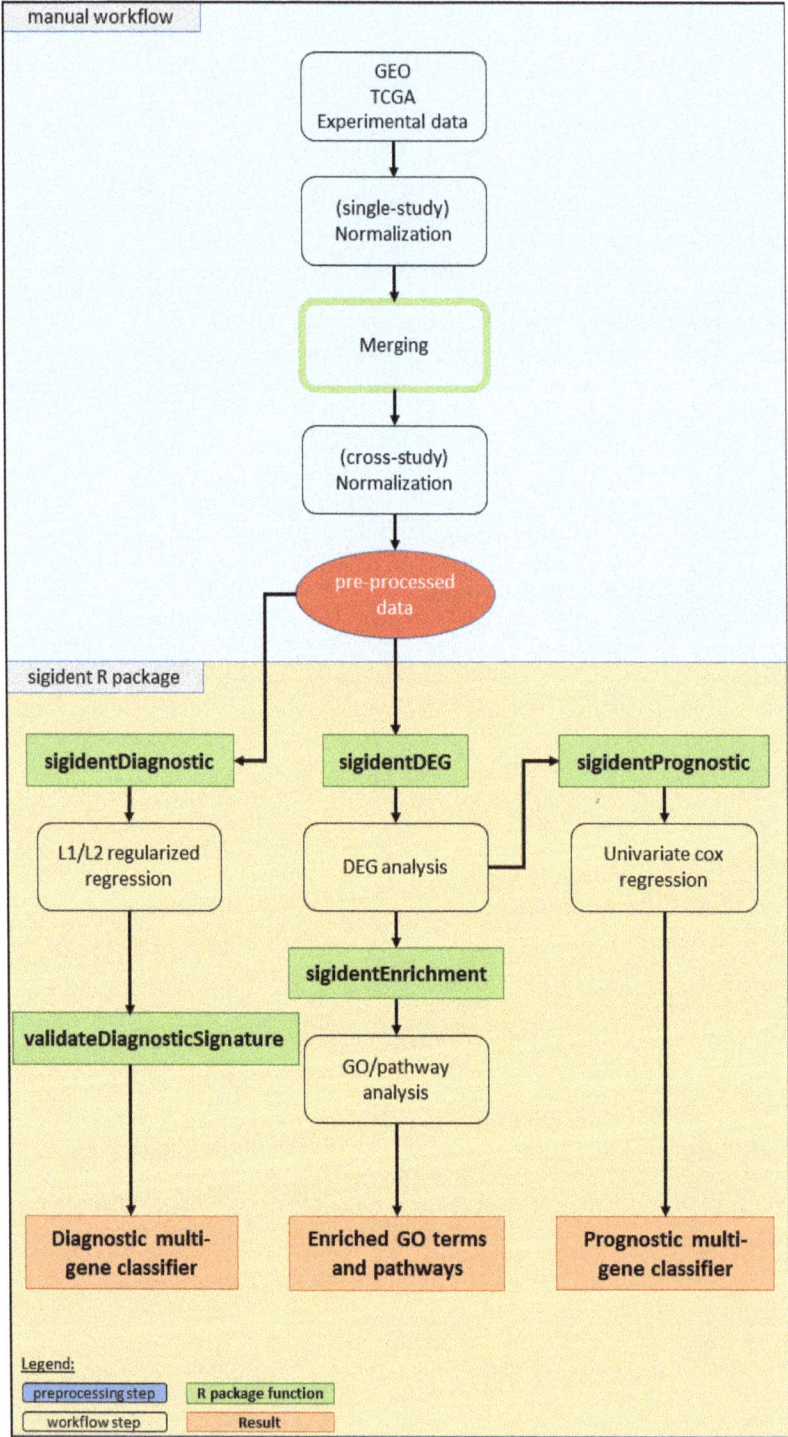

Figure 7. Overview of the workflow of our toolbox. The boxes show the analysis steps, colored rectangles represent the R package functions and results (see legend).

5. Conclusions

We developed an efficient toolbox for the identification of diagnostic and prognostic gene signatures. It is the first R package tool that combines meta-analysis with gene expression analysis and ML approaches for the systematical calculation of statistically robust gene signatures. This helps to reduce study biases and improves the statistical power for the identification of reliable signatures from large sample cohorts. Importantly, the tool is not restricted to a specific disease. We believe that our toolbox will be useful for the research community and opens new windows for an effective analysis of data and a better clinical management of diseases.

Supplementary Materials: The following are available online at http://www.mdpi.com/2072-6694/11/10/1606/s1, Figure S1. Boxplots of the GCRMA normalized expression data (training and test dataset). The dataset GSE18842 contains 45 non-tumor and 46 tumor samples (Left), the GSE19804 dataset 60 non-tumor and 60 tumor samples (Middle) and the GSE19188 dataset 65 non-tumor and 91 tumor samples (Right). (GCRMA normalized; datasets from Chip GPL570, Affymetrix Human Genome U133 Plus 2.0); Figure S2. Plots for the batch effect detection using the gPCA (training and test dataset). (Top) The merged dataset contains 54,675 transcripts and 367 samples (170 non-tumor (control), 197 tumor samples; no gene transcript were excluded during the merging process). The plots show the gPCA before (Left) and after (Right) batch correction. (Bottom) Boxplots of the merged datasets before (left) and after (right) batch effect removal; Table S1. List of the 699 DEGs. The table lists the 699 DEGs (q-value < 0.05, logFC > 2/< −2) in the merged dataset after batch effect correction (517 unique gene symbols of total 699 ID transcripts); Table S2. Overview of the calculated signatures from the LASSO and Elastic net regression models; Table S3. Predictive parameters of the identified diagnostic signatures in the independent dataset. (A) GSE30219, 293 lung cancer samples, 14 non lung cancer samples. (B) GSE102287, 32 lung cancer samples, 34 non lung cancer samples. (C) GSE33356, 60 lung cancer samples, 60 non lung cancer samples. total: 54,675 genes; Table S4. List of the 22 DEGs. The table lists the 22 DEGs that are significantly associated with the survival outcome (affy gene ID according to affy_hg_u133_plus_2; p-value < 0.05; 20 unique genes of total 22 transcripts, two variants of each DLC1 and LPL; HR > 1: poor prognosis, HR < 1: good prognosis, HR = 1: no effect); Table S5. Overview of the used R packages (for details see https://gitlab.miracum.org/clearly/sigident).

Data Availability: The toolbox is publicly available as R package under the URL https://gitlab.miracum.org/clearly/sigident.

Author Contributions: J.V. and L.A.K., design of software, data analysis, interpretation of data, and manuscript writing; G.V., corrections and advice on cancer signature; M.F. and P.U., expert analysis and corrections. M.K., conceptualization, methodology, design of the study and software, data analysis, interpretation of data, and manuscript writing. All authors approved the submitted manuscript version.

Funding: This research was supported by the Federal Ministry of Education and Research (BMBF), grant FKZ 031L0129B to M.K., Era-Net grant 01KT1801 to M.K., M.F., and J.V., 01ZZ1801A to P.U and L.A.K., 031L0073A to P.U.

Acknowledgments: We thank Oisin Roche-Lancaster for native speaker and language corrections. Andreas Pittroff is acknowledged for programming input.

Conflicts of Interest: The authors declare no conflict of interest. The funders had no role in the design of the study; in the collection, analyses, or interpretation of data; in the writing of the manuscript, or in the decision to publish the results.

References

1. Borrebaeck, C.A.K. Precision diagnostics: Moving towards protein biomarker signatures of clinical utility in cancer. *Nat. Rev. Cancer* **2017**, *17*, 199–204. [CrossRef] [PubMed]
2. Kunz, M.; Wolf, B.; Schulze, H.; Atlan, D.; Walles, T.; Walles, H.; Dandekar, T. Non-coding rnas in lung cancer: Contribution of bioinformatics analysis to the development of non-invasive diagnostic tools. *Genes* **2016**, *8*, 8. [CrossRef] [PubMed]
3. Aguirre-Gamboa, R.; Trevino, V. Survmicro: Assessment of miRNA-based prognostic signatures for cancer clinical outcomes by multivariate survival analysis. *Bioinformatics* **2014**, *30*, 1630–1632. [CrossRef] [PubMed]
4. Cusumano, P.G.; Generali, D.; Ciruelos, E.; Manso, L.; Ghanem, I.; Lifrange, E.; Jerusalem, G.; Klaase, J.; de Snoo, F.; Stork-Sloots, L.; et al. European inter-institutional impact study of mammaprint. *Breast* **2014**, *23*, 423–428. [CrossRef]
5. Montani, F.; Marzi, M.J.; Dezi, F.; Dama, E.; Carletti, R.M.; Bonizzi, G.; Bertolotti, R.; Bellomi, M.; Rampinelli, C.; Maisonneuve, P.; et al. miR-test: A blood test for lung cancer early detection. *J. Natl. Cancer Inst.* **2015**, *107*. [CrossRef]

6. Taminau, J.; Lazar, C.; Meganck, S.; Nowé, A. Comparison of merging and meta-analysis as alternative approaches for integrative gene expression analysis. *ISRN Bioinform.* **2014**, *2014*, 345601. [CrossRef]

7. Xu, L.; Tan, A.C.; Winslow, R.L.; Geman, D. Merging microarray data from separate breast cancer studies provides a robust prognostic test. *BMC Bioinform.* **2008**, *9*, 125. [CrossRef]

8. Hughey, J.J.; Butte, A.J. Robust meta-analysis of gene expression using the elastic net. *Nucleic Acids Res.* **2015**, *43*, e79. [CrossRef]

9. Ramasamy, A.; Mondry, A.; Holmes, C.C.; Altman, D.G. Key issues in conducting a meta-analysis of gene expression microarray datasets. *PLoS Med.* **2008**, *5*, e184. [CrossRef]

10. Tseng, G.C.; Ghosh, D.; Feingold, E. Comprehensive literature review and statistical considerations for microarray meta-analysis. *Nucleic Acids Res.* **2012**, *40*, 3785–3799. [CrossRef]

11. Heider, A.; Alt, R. virtuAlarray: A R/Bioconductor package to merge raw data from different microarray platforms. *BMC Bioinform.* **2013**, *14*, 75. [CrossRef] [PubMed]

12. Taminau, J.; Meganck, S.; Lazar, C.; Steenhoff, D.; Coletta, A.; Molter, C.; Duque, R.; de Schaetzen, V.; Weiss Solis, D.Y.; Bersini, H.; et al. Unlocking the potential of publicly available microarray data using inSilicoDb and inSilicoMerging R/Bioconductor packages. *BMC Bioinform.* **2012**, *13*, 335. [CrossRef] [PubMed]

13. Huber, W.; Carey, V.J.; Gentleman, R.; Anders, S.; Carlson, M.; Carvalho, B.S.; Bravo, H.C.; Davis, S.; Gatto, L.; Girke, T.; et al. Orchestrating high-throughput genomic analysis with bioconductor. *Nat. Methods* **2015**, *12*, 115–121. [CrossRef] [PubMed]

14. Aguirre-Gamboa, R.; Gomez-Rueda, H.; Martínez-Ledesma, E.; Martínez-Torteya, A.; Chacolla-Huaringa, R.; Rodriguez-Barrientos, A.; Tamez-Peña, J.G.; Treviño, V. Survexpress: An online biomarker validation tool and database for cancer gene expression data using survival analysis. *PLoS ONE* **2013**, *8*, e74250. [CrossRef] [PubMed]

15. Lanczky, A.; Nagy, A.; Bottai, G.; Munkacsy, G.; Szabo, A.; Santarpia, L.; Gyorffy, B. miRpower: A web-tool to validate survival-associated miRNAs utilizing expression data from 2178 breast cancer patients. *Breast Cancer Res. Treat.* **2016**, *160*, 439–446. [CrossRef]

16. Ringner, M.; Fredlund, E.; Hakkinen, J.; Borg, A.; Staaf, J. Gobo: Gene expression-based outcome for breast cancer online. *PLoS ONE* **2011**, *6*, e17911. [CrossRef]

17. Gyorffy, B.; Lanczky, A.; Szallasi, Z. Implementing an online tool for genome-wide validation of survival-associated biomarkers in ovarian-cancer using microarray data from 1287 patients. *Endocr. Relat. Cancer* **2012**, *19*, 197–208. [CrossRef]

18. Schweitzer, S.; Kunz, M.; Kurlbaum, M.; Vey, J.; Kendl, S.; Deutschbein, T.; Hahner, S.; Fassnacht, M.; Dandekar, T.; Kroiss, M. Plasma steroid metabolome profiling for the diagnosis of adrenocortical carcinoma. *Eur. J. Endocrinol.* **2019**, *180*, 117–125. [CrossRef]

19. Beck, A.H.; Sangoi, A.R.; Leung, S.; Marinelli, R.J.; Nielsen, T.O.; van de Vijver, M.J.; West, R.B.; van de Rijn, M.; Koller, D. Systematic analysis of breast cancer morphology uncovers stromal features associated with survival. *Sci. Transl. Med.* **2011**, *3*, 108ra113. [CrossRef]

20. Huang, C.; Mezencev, R.; McDonald, J.F.; Vannberg, F. Open source machine-learning algorithms for the prediction of optimal cancer drug therapies. *PLoS ONE* **2017**, *12*, e0186906. [CrossRef]

21. Mortazavi, B.J.; Downing, N.S.; Bucholz, E.M.; Dharmarajan, K.; Manhapra, A.; Li, S.X.; Negahban, S.N.; Krumholz, H.M. Analysis of machine learning techniques for heart failure readmissions. *Circulation. Cardiovasc. Qual. Outcomes* **2016**, *9*, 629–640. [CrossRef] [PubMed]

22. Tibshirani, R. Regression shrinkage and selection via the lasso. *J. R. Stat. Soc. Ser. B* **1996**, *58*, 267–288. [CrossRef]

23. Zou, H.; Hastie, T. Regularization and variable selection via the elastic net. *J. R. Statist. Soc. B* **2005**, *67*, 301–320. [CrossRef]

24. Bradburn, M.J.; Clark, T.G.; Love, S.B.; Altman, D.G. Survival analysis part II: Multivariate data analysis—An introduction to concepts and methods. *Br. J. Cancer* **2003**, *89*, 431–436. [CrossRef] [PubMed]

25. Clark, T.G.; Bradburn, M.J.; Love, S.B.; Altman, D.G. Survival analysis part I: Basic concepts and first analyses. *Br. J. Cancer* **2003**, *89*, 232–238. [CrossRef]

26. Cox, D.R. Regression models and life-tables. *J. R. Stat. Society. Ser. B* **1972**, *34*, 187–220. [CrossRef]

27. Kunz, M.; Pittroff, A.; Dandekar, T. Systems biology analysis to understand regulatory miRNA networks in lung cancer. In *Computational Cell Biology*; Humana Press: New York, NY, USA, 2018; pp. 235–247.

28. Wu, J.; Gentry, R. Gcrma: Background Adjustment Using Sequence Information. Available online: https://bioc.ism.ac.jp/packages/3.7/bioc/html/gcrma.html (accessed on 27 September 2019).

29. Conesa, A.; Madrigal, P.; Tarazona, S.; Gomez-Cabrero, D.; Cervera, A.; McPherson, A.; Szcześniak, M.W.; Gaffney, D.J.; Elo, L.L.; Zhang, X.; et al. A survey of best practices for RNA-seq data analysis. *Genome Biol.* **2016**, *17*, 13. [CrossRef]

30. Jiang, L.-P.; Fan, S.-Q.; Xiong, Q.-X.; Zhou, Y.-C.; Yang, Z.-Z.; Li, G.-F.; Huang, Y.-C.; Wu, M.-G.; Shen, Q.-S.; Liu, K.; et al. Grk5 functions as an oncogenic factor in non-small-cell lung cancer. *Cell Death Dis.* **2018**, *9*, 295. [CrossRef]

31. Kim, K.Y.; Lee, G.; Yoon, M.; Cho, E.H.; Park, C.-S.; Kim, M.G. Expression analyses revealed thymic stromal co-transporter/Slc46A2 is in stem cell populations and is a putative tumor suppressor. *Mol. Cells* **2015**, *38*, 548–561. [CrossRef]

32. Shen, L.; Yang, M.; Lin, Q.; Zhang, Z.; Zhu, B.; Miao, C. COL11A1 is overexpressed in recurrent non-small cell lung cancer and promotes cell proliferation, migration, invasion and drug resistance. *Oncol. Rep.* **2016**, *36*, 877–885. [CrossRef]

33. Trost, Z.; Sok, M.; Marc, J.; Cerne, D. Increased lipoprotein lipase activity in non-small cell lung cancer tissue predicts shorter patient survival. *Arch. Med Res.* **2009**, *40*, 364–368. [CrossRef] [PubMed]

34. Li, L.; Liu, Y.D.; Zhan, Y.T.; Zhu, Y.H.; Li, Y.; Xie, D.; Guan, X.Y. High levels of CCL2 or CCL4 in the tumor microenvironment predict unfavorable survival in lung adenocarcinoma. *Thorac. Cancer* **2018**, *9*, 775–784. [CrossRef] [PubMed]

35. Chen, T.; Guestrin, C. Xgboost: A scalable tree boosting system. In Proceedings of the 22nd Acm Sigkdd International Conference on Knowledge Discovery and Data Mining, San Francisco, CA, USA, 13–17 August 2016; pp. 785–794.

36. Chibon, F. Cancer gene expression signatures—The rise and fall? *Eur. J. Cancer* **2013**, *49*, 2000–2009. [CrossRef] [PubMed]

37. Ching, T.; Huang, S.; Garmire, L.X. Power analysis and sample size estimation for RNA-seq differential expression. *Rna* **2014**, *20*, 1684–1696. [CrossRef]

38. Wirapati, P.; Sotiriou, C.; Kunkel, S.; Farmer, P.; Pradervand, S.; Haibe-Kains, B.; Desmedt, C.; Ignatiadis, M.; Sengstag, T.; Schutz, F.; et al. Meta-analysis of gene expression profiles in breast cancer: Toward a unified understanding of breast cancer subtyping and prognosis signatures. *Breast Cancer Res.* **2008**, *10*, R65. [CrossRef]

39. Chen, R.; Khatri, P.; Mazur, P.K.; Polin, M.; Zheng, Y.; Vaka, D.; Hoang, C.D.; Shrager, J.; Xu, Y.; Vicent, S.; et al. A meta-analysis of lung cancer gene expression identifies PTK7 as a survival gene in lung adenocarcinoma. *Cancer Res.* **2014**, *74*, 2892–2902. [CrossRef]

40. Sorlie, T.; Tibshirani, R.; Parker, J.; Hastie, T.; Marron, J.S.; Nobel, A.; Deng, S.; Johnsen, H.; Pesich, R.; Geisler, S.; et al. Repeated observation of breast tumor subtypes in independent gene expression data sets. *Proc. Natl. Acad. Sci. USA* **2003**, *100*, 8418–8423. [CrossRef]

41. Jia, B.; Lynn, H.S. A sample size planning approach that considers both statistical significance and clinical significance. *Trials* **2015**, *16*, 213. [CrossRef]

42. Van't Veer, L.J.; Dai, H.; van de Vijver, M.J.; He, Y.D.; Hart, A.A.; Mao, M.; Peterse, H.L.; van der Kooy, K.; Marton, M.J.; Witteveen, A.T.; et al. Gene expression profiling predicts clinical outcome of breast cancer. *Nature* **2002**, *415*, 530–536. [CrossRef]

43. Kundu, S.T.; Grzeskowiak, C.L.; Fradette, J.J.; Gibson, L.A.; Rodriguez, L.B.; Creighton, C.J.; Scott, K.L.; Gibbons, D.L. TMEM106B drives lung cancer metastasis by inducing TFEB-dependent lysosome synthesis and secretion of cathepsins. *Nat. Commun.* **2018**, *9*, 2731. [CrossRef]

44. Andriani, F.; Landoni, E.; Mensah, M.; Facchinetti, F.; Miceli, R.; Tagliabue, E.; Giussani, M.; Callari, M.; de Cecco, L.; Colombo, M.P.; et al. Diagnostic role of circulating extracellular matrix-related proteins in non-small cell lung cancer. *BMC Cancer* **2018**, *18*, 899. [CrossRef] [PubMed]

45. Liang, F.; Yue, J.; Wang, J.; Zhang, L.; Fan, R.; Zhang, H.; Zhang, Q. GPCR48/LGR4 promotes tumorigenesis of prostate cancer via PI3K/Akt signaling pathway. *Med Oncol.* **2015**, *32*, 49. [CrossRef]

46. Zhou, W.; Han, L.; Altman, R.B. Imputing gene expression to maximize platform compatibility. *Bioinformatics* **2016**, *33*, 522–528. [CrossRef] [PubMed]

47. Garnett, M.J.; Edelman, E.J.; Heidorn, S.J.; Greenman, C.D.; Dastur, A.; Lau, K.W.; Greninger, P.; Thompson, I.R.; Luo, X.; Soares, J.; et al. Systematic identification of genomic markers of drug sensitivity in cancer cells. *Nature* **2012**, *483*, 570–575. [CrossRef] [PubMed]

48. Davis, S.; Meltzer, P.S. GEOquery: A bridge between the Gene Expression Omnibus (GEO) and bioconductor. *Bioinformatics* **2007**, *23*, 1846–1847. [CrossRef] [PubMed]

49. Warnes, G.; Bolker, B.; Bonebakker, L.; Gentleman, R.; Liaw, W.; Lumley, T.; Maechler, M.; Magnusson, A.; Moeller, S.; Schwartz, M.; et al. *Gplots: Various R Programming Tools for Plotting Data*; R package version 3.0.1. Available online: https://cran.r-project.org/web/packages/gPCA/index.html (accessed on 27 September 2019).

50. Ritchie, M.E.; Phipson, B.; Wu, D.; Hu, Y.; Law, C.W.; Shi, W.; Smyth, G.K. Limma powers differential expression analyses for RNA-sequencing and microarray studies. *Nucleic Acids Res.* **2015**, *43*, e47. [CrossRef] [PubMed]

51. Reese, S. *Batch Effect Detection via Guided Principal Components Analysis*, R package version 1.0; Available online: https://rdrr.io/cran/gPCA/man/gPCA-package.html (accessed on 27 September 2019).

52. Leek, J.T.; Johnson, W.E.; Parker, H.S.; Jaffe, A.E.; Storey, J.D. The sva package for removing batch effects and other unwanted variation in high-throughput experiments. *Bioinformatics* **2012**, *28*, 882–883. [CrossRef]

53. Benjamini, Y.; Hochberg, Y. Controlling the false discovery rate: A practical and powerful approach to multiple testing. *J. R. Stat. Society. Ser. B* **1995**, *57*, 289–300. [CrossRef]

54. Yu, G.; Wang, L.G.; Han, Y.; He, Q.Y. clusterProfiler: An R package for comparing biological themes among gene clusters. *Omics A J. Integr. Biol.* **2012**, *16*, 284–287. [CrossRef]

55. Luo, W.; Brouwer, C. Pathview: An R/Bioconductor package for pathway-based data integration and visualization. *Bioinformatics* **2013**, *29*, 1830–1831. [CrossRef]

56. Friedman, J.; Hastie, T.; Tibshirani, R. Regularization paths for generalized linear models via coordinate descent. *J. Stat. Softw.* **2010**, *33*, 1–22. [CrossRef] [PubMed]

57. Kuhn, M. *Classification and Regression Training*, R package version 6.0-80; Available online: https://cran.r-project.org/web/packages/caret/index.html (accessed on 27 September 2019).

58. Robin, X.; Turck, N.; Hainard, A.; Tiberti, N.; Lisacek, F.; Sanchez, J.-C.; Müller, M. pROC: An open-source package for R and S+ to analyze and compare ROC curves. *BMC Bioinform.* **2011**, *12*, 77. [CrossRef] [PubMed]

59. Therneau, T. *A Package for Survival Analysis in S*, R package version 2.38; Available online: https://CRAN.R-Proj..Org/Package=Surviv (accessed on 27 September 2019).

60. Alboukadel, K.; Marcin, K. *Survminer: "Drawing Survival Curves Using 'Ggplot2'"*, R package version 0.3.1; Available online: https://cran.r-project.org/web/packages/survminer/index.html (accessed on 27 September 2019).

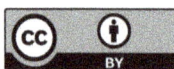

cancers

MDPI

Article

Association Analysis of Deep Genomic Features Extracted by Denoising Autoencoders in Breast Cancer

Qian Liu [1] and Pingzhao Hu [1,2,3,*]

[1]   Department of Biochemistry and Medical Genetics, College of Medicine, Faculty of Health Sciences, University of Manitoba, Winnipeg, MB R3E 0J9, Canada; qianl@myumanitoba.ca
[2]   Research Institute in Oncology and Hematology, CancerCare Manitoba, Winnipeg, MB R3E 0V9, Canada
[3]   Department of Computer Science, University of Manitoba, Winnipeg, MB R3T 2N2, Canada
*   Correspondence: pingzhao.hu@umanitoba.ca; Tel.: +1-204-789-3229

Received: 17 March 2019; Accepted: 4 April 2019; Published: 7 April 2019

Abstract: Artificial intelligence-based unsupervised deep learning (DL) is widely used to mine multimodal big data. However, there are few applications of this technology to cancer genomics. We aim to develop DL models to extract deep features from the breast cancer gene expression data and copy number alteration (CNA) data separately and jointly. We hypothesize that the deep features are associated with patients' clinical characteristics and outcomes. Two unsupervised denoising autoencoders (DAs) were developed to extract deep features from TCGA (The Cancer Genome Atlas) breast cancer gene expression and CNA data separately and jointly. A heat map was used to view and cluster patients into subgroups based on these DL features. Fisher's exact test and Pearson' Chi-square test were applied to test the associations of patients' groups and clinical information. Survival differences between the groups were evaluated by Kaplan–Meier (KM) curves. Associations between each of the features and patient's overall survival were assessed using Cox's proportional hazards (COX-PH) model and a risk score for each feature set from the different omics data sets was generated from the survival regression coefficients. The risk scores for each feature set were binarized into high- and low-risk patient groups to evaluate survival differences using KM curves. Furthermore, the risk scores were traced back to their gene level DAs weights so that the three gene lists for each of the genomic data points were generated to perform gene set enrichment analysis. Patients were clustered into two groups based on concatenated features from the gene expression and CNA data and these two groups showed different overall survival rates (p-value = 0.049) and different ER (Estrogen receptor) statuses (p-value = 0.002, OR (odds ratio) = 0.626). All the risk scores from the gene expression and CNA data and their concatenated one were significantly associated with breast cancer survival. The patients with the high-risk group were significantly associated with patients' worse outcomes (p-values $\leq$ 0.0023). The concatenated risk score was enriched by the AMP-activated protein kinase (AMPK) signaling pathway, the regulation of DNA-templated transcription, the regulation of nucleic acid-templated transcription, the regulation of apoptotic process, the positive regulation of gene expression, the positive regulation of cell proliferation, heart morphogenesis, the regulation of cellular macromolecule biosynthetic process, with FDR (false discovery rate) less than 0.05. We confirmed DAs can effectively extract meaningful genomic features from genomic data and concatenating multiple data sources can improve the significance of the features associated with breast cancer patients' clinical characteristics and outcomes.

Keywords: denoising autoencoders; breast cancer; feature extraction and interpretation; concatenated deep feature

1. Introduction

Advanced hardware technologies have highly increased computational power, which makes the implementation of computation-consuming algorithms possible. At the same time, the development of biological technologies has greatly reduced the cost of genomic sequencing, which produced a huge amount of high-dimensional genomic data. Under these circumstances, bioinformatics becomes an exciting research field for researchers to explore the possibility to interpret genomic data using advanced computational technologies [1].

Different types of high-dimensional genomic data have been associated with cancer clinical characteristics and outcomes. The most commonly used ones are gene expression data and copy number alteration (CNA) data [2]. The activity of gene expression in tumor tissues is quite different from that in normal tissues [3] and has been established to have the ability to distinguish the characteristics of cancers [4]. There are some repeated segments in normal DNA, and during the process of cancer development, the repeated number of the segments may be changed due to abnormal DNA replication in tumor cells. This phenomenon is called copy number alteration [5]. CNA may result in chromosome structure changes in the forms of duplication or deletion in DNA segments. It has been shown that CNA plays an important role in the development of many types of cancers including breast cancer [6]. Therefore, it is highly necessary to mine the prognostic and diagnostic significance of the genome-wide cancer genomic data. From a clinical point of view, the prognosis of the genomic factors is always a necessary consideration because of its importance in making treatment plans [7]. In previous studies, prognosis significance was evaluated mainly based on clinical features, such as tumor grades and tumor subtypes [7] and molecular features, such as expression related gene signatures (e.g., PAM50 subtypes) [8,9]. Results from these studies showed that the gene signatures tend to have better prognosis significance than traditional pathological assessment [7]. This might be due to the integration ability of these gene signatures. For instance, PAM50 can combine the information from the tumor stage, tumor grade and tumor subtype together [9]. However, the known gene signatures are only based on single genomic data source such as gene expression. This might be not adequate since other types of genomic data such as copy number alterations should also include important cancer prognosis information [9]. Advanced algorithms now give us new tools to explore the possibility of integrating different data sources together. For example, Chi, et al. identified several genes and pathways with a high prognostic significance for young breast cancer patients based on their gene expression and copy number alteration data using a graph-based machine learning (ML) method [9].

Traditional ML methods such as artificial neural networks (ANN) and support vector machines (SVM) may suffer some problems in dealing with the high-dimensional, noisy and massive genomic data [10]. Recently, a special case of ANN with more nodes and layers has emerged as an efficient method to handle these high-dimensional and noisy data. The idea of ANN was originated from the information processing and communication patterns in a human nervous system [11]. As the new development of the traditional ANN, deep learning (DL) presents a large group of interconnected artificial neurons with many more layers. Like other learning methods, DL could be implemented in a supervised or unsupervised way, which depends on whether the input data is labeled or not. Although both supervised and unsupervised DL algorithms have been successfully applied to the analysis of genomic data, they could be used to solve different biology problems. Supervised learning algorithms are often used to predict gene functions and gene-gene interactions or to identify new driver genes [12], while unsupervised learning algorithms are often used to cluster the strong signals in the data [13,14]. Among the unsupervised learning algorithms, autoencoder is a new technology that uses the data itself as the learning objective or label. Therefore, it is also known as self-labeled or self-supervised deep learning. Traditional autoencoders may face the invalid learning problem when the number of hidden nodes is larger than the input size. To avoid this potential risk, denoising autoencoders (DAs) came up with the solution of adding some noise into the input data on purpose.

Vincent, et al. brought the concept of DAs into DL and built a specialized feature extraction DL architecture [15]. The key idea of DAs as mentioned above is to add random noise into the raw data before it is input into the network. After the encode and decode processes, the raw data would be reconstructed from the noisy data, while the compact and efficient representations from the raw data could be learned as well [15]. These representations are the DAs-based genomic features.

DL as a special case of ML and ANN has been applied to mine deep information from complex genomic data and has generated interesting results [16]. Its high integration and reconstruction abilities give us large flexibility to combine different types of genomic data to extract valuable information from them. It has been expected that deep features extracted by DL models would perform better in clinical association and prognosis prediction than standard gene or pathway signatures [17]. For example, Tan, et al. reported a deep feature representing ER status and a deep feature with high prognosis significance based on breast cancer gene expression data [13]. These deep features were constructed by a DAs and performed better in the downstream analyses [13]. However, these studies were based on only a single genomic source.

This study aims to extract the integrated features from both the gene expression and CNA data by a concatenated DAs model. As a comparison, we also built a standard DAs model to extract deep features from gene expression and CNA data separately. The comparisons were made in terms of the performance in association analysis as well as prognosis analysis. The study design and analysis procedures are shown in Figure 1.

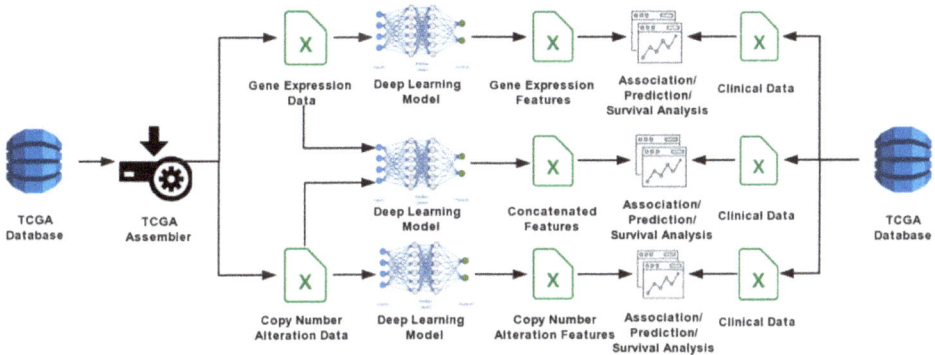

Figure 1. A flowchart illustrating the analysis procedures in this study.

2. Materials and Methods

2.1. Data Sources

Datasets used in this study came from The Cancer Genome Atlas (TCGA) [18], which is one of the most comprehensive genomic databases. TCGA provides 1098 breast cancer patients' clinical data along with their genomic data. These genomic data include gene expressions, CNA, protein expressions, micro RNA (miRNA) expressions, and somatic mutations.

For gene expression data, the sequencing, alignment, quality control and quantification were performed previously [18]. Using the TCGA-Assembler tool [19], we downloaded the gene expression raw count, then filtered out unexpressed genes and those genes with a count per million (CPM) less than 1 in 3 patients. We performed normalization of the data using Upper Quartile Fragments per Kilobase of transcript per Million mapped reads (FPKM-UQ) [20]. FPKM-UQ is a modified FPKM algorithm in which the total read count is replaced by the 75th percentile read count for a given sample.

Similar to the gene expression data, upstream processes of CNA data were done previously as well [18]. Using the downloaded chromosome-region specific log2 copy number data, we calculated the gene-level CNA values using the TCGA-Assembler tool. Several data cleaning procedures such as removing all-NAs were also performed to avoid potential format issues in the follow-up analysis.

After normalization and preprocessing, there were 18,163 genes from each of the 1095 patients left for gene expression data and 23,563 genes from the 1098 patients left for CNA data. To keep the gene dimension and scale matched in the two data sources, both of them were linearly transformed into a range between 0 and 1, resulting in the decreasing of the data dimension to 16,197 (genes) × 1085 (patients) for both data sources.

2.2. DA Models

Two DAs models were developed using Keras [21] with Tensorflow [22] as the backend to extract deep genomic features. One model was for feature extraction from a single genomic source, named as one-input DAs model (Figure 2). The other, named as the two-input DAs model (Figure 3), was for concatenated feature extraction from the integrated genomic sources.

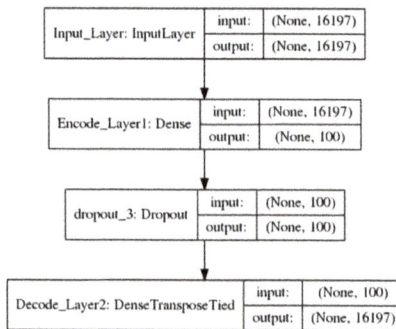

Figure 2. The one-input denoising autoencoders model. There are two hidden layers in the encode phase and two decode layers. The input can be either gene expression data or copy number alteration data.

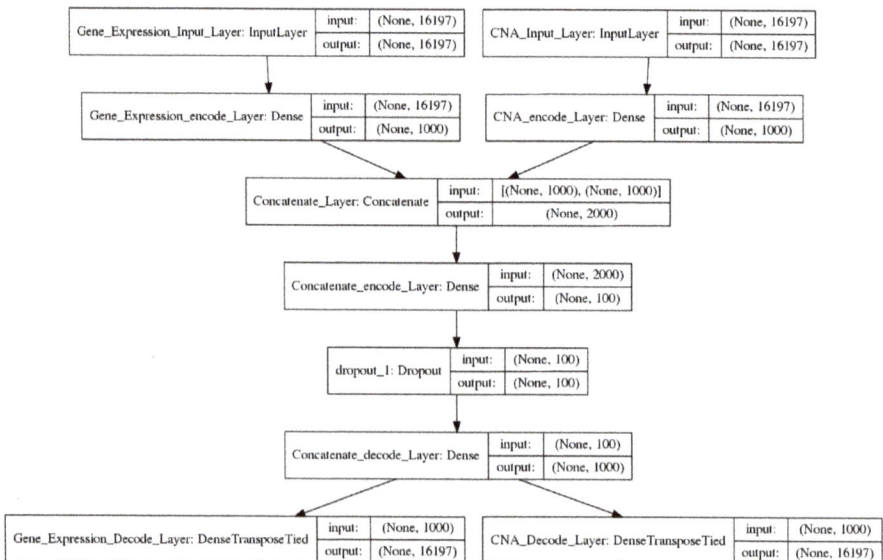

Figure 3. The two-input DAs model. There are two hidden layers in the encode phase and one decode layer. Concatenation was performed between the two encode layers.

2.2.1. One-Input DAs Model

This architecture was composed of one input layer, one fully connected encode hidden layer with 100 nodes which were chosen to be the deep features used in this study and one decode layer which uses the transpose of encoding layer' weights. This procedure can be formulated as below:

$$
\begin{aligned}
\text{encode} &= \text{sigmoid} \ (W \times \text{input} + b) \\
\text{decode} &= \text{sigmoid} \ (W' \times \text{encode} + b')
\end{aligned}
\tag{1}
$$

where W is the weight metrics between the layers with the size of $16{,}197 \times 100$, b is the bias for each node, and the sigmoid function is sigmoid $(x) = 1 \ / \ (1 + e^{-x})$. The counterparts with the superscript refer to the transpose metrics. A dropout layer was added after the encode layer, which randomly set 50% of the output of encode layer to 0 to prevent overfitting. The encode item was chosen to be the activity values of the deep features in this model.

2.2.2. Two-Input DAs Model

Literally, the two-input DAs model contained two input layers, followed by one encode layer with 1000 nodes for each input layer, then followed by a concatenated layer, and another encode layer with 100 nodes which were chosen to be the deep concatenated features. Finally, there were two decode layers. The procedure can be formulated as follow:

$$
\begin{aligned}
\text{input}_1\_\text{encode}_1 &= \text{sigmoid} \ (\text{input}_1\_W_1 \times \text{input}_1 + \text{input}_1\_b_1) \\
\text{input}_2\_\text{encode}_1 &= \text{sigmoid} \ (\text{input}_2\_W_1 \times \text{input}_2 + \text{input}_2\_b_1) \\
\text{concate}\_\text{encode}_1 &= \text{concatenate} \ (\text{input}_1\_\text{encode}_1, \text{input}_2\_\text{encode}_1) \\
\text{concate}\_\text{encode}_2 &= \text{sigmoid} \ (\text{concate}\_W_2 \times \text{concate}\_\text{encode}_1 + \text{concate}\_b_2) \\
\text{output}_1 &= \text{sigmoid} \ (\text{input}_1\_W_1' \times \text{concate}\_\text{encode}_2 + \text{input}_1\_b_1') \\
\text{output}_2 &= \text{sigmoid} \ (\text{input}_2\_W_1' \times \text{concate}\_\text{encode}_2 + \text{input}_2\_b_1')
\end{aligned}
\tag{2}
$$

where $\text{input}_1\_W_1$, $\text{input}_2\_W_1$, and concate_W_2 are the weight metrics between the layers with the size of $16{,}197 \times 1000$, $16{,}197 \times 1000$, 2000×100 respectively. The $\text{input}_1\_b_1$, $\text{input}_2\_b_1$, and concate_b_2 are the biases for each node. The counterparts with superscript refer to the transpose metrics. A dropout layer was added after $\text{concate}\_\text{encode}_2$ layer, which randomly set 50% of the output of that layer to 0. The $\text{concate}\_\text{encode}_2$ was chosen to be the activity values of the deep features in this model.

2.3. Train the Models

Before the training process, the input data sets were disrupted by a noise factor of 0.25, which is the proportion of the number of genes in the data sources. These genes were selected randomly and their values were set to 0. The binary cross-entropy function shown below was used to measure the difference between the input layer and the output layer:

$$
L \ (input, output) = -(1/N) \ \Sigma \ (input_k \times log(output_k) + (1 - input_k) \times log(1 - output_k))
\tag{3}
$$

where $L \ (input, output)$ is the binary cross-entropy, K is the index of batches, N is the total number of batches. Thus, the training task is to minimize the $L \ (input, output)$.

For the optimizer, e.g., the strategy to update the weights and bias so that the minima could be found, we selected stochastic gradient descent (SGD), which has several arguments to be set freely. After having different trials, the learning rate was finally set to 0.1; the batch size and epoch were set to 64 and 100 respectively. The models were finally trained under the parameters mentioned above. The activity values and weight metrics related to deep features were read out.

2.4. Visualization and Clustering

Heatmap3 [23] was used to visualize the activity values of these deep feature sets. We used the complete linkage function in the hierarchical clustering process and visual-guided criteria by analysis of the dendrogram to decide the number of clusters. First, the clinical data downloaded from TCGA were carefully scanned and the most clinical-relevant characteristics such as pathological status (T, N, M), tumor stage, estrogen receptor (ER) status, progesterone receptor (PR) status, human epidermal growth factor receptor 2 (HER2) status, triple negative status, and PAM50 subtypes (i.e., Luminal A, Luminal B, Basal-like, HER2-enriched, and Normal-like) were extracted. These clinical characteristics were shown as the sidebar of the heat map.

2.5. Association Analysis

To test whether the identified patient clusters are associated with known clinical and molecular characteristics, we applied both Fisher's exact test and Pearson' Chi-square test.

Survival differences between the identified patients groups were evaluated by Kaplan–Meier (KM) curves. Furthermore, associations between each deep feature in the three feature sets (gene expression, CNA, the concatenated one) and patient's overall survival was assessed using Cox's proportional hazards (COX-PH) model [24]. The hazard function is

$$h(t) = h_0(t) \times exp(bx) \tag{4}$$

where t represents the survival time. b is the coefficient which measures the impact of the covariate x. Later, a risk score for each feature set was generated from the COX-PH coefficients:

$$r = \Sigma (b_i \times a_i) \tag{5}$$

where r is the risk score, b_i is the coefficient from the COX-PH model and a_i is the related activity value of the given feature. Afterward, the risk scores were binarized into high-risk and low-risk groups using R package xtile function with a *prob* parameter set to 0.55, which means we use the 55% quantile as the cutoff to bin the patients into the high-risk and low-risk groups. Finally, the survival differences between these two groups were evaluated by the KM curve.

2.6. Gene Sets Enrichment Analysis

For each of the three DAs models for gene expression, CNA and their concatenated one, we traced back their gene-level weights based on

$$W_g = W \times B \tag{6}$$

where W is the 16,197 $\times$ 100 dimensional weights that were extracted from a given DAs model previously. B is the vector of COX-PH coefficients. The gene-specific weights W_g were filtered by a cutoff 0.01, which resulted in the three selected gene lists with 6954, 5381 and 6297 genes, respectively. Finally, the three gene lists were used to perform gene set enrichment analysis (GSEA) by the Enricr tool [25] to identify the up-regulated and down-regulated pathways. Kyoto Encyclopedia of Genes and Genomes (KEGG) [26] and Gene Ontology (GO) [27] Biological Process 2018 version were chosen to be the reference gene sets.

3. Results

Based on the normalized and processed breast cancer genomic data, our models were trained and the activity values of the 100 deep features for each of the three data sets as well as the weights matrices were extracted (Table 1). Then we clustered these activity values for each of the three data sets. Overall, there were no clear patterns shown in the deep features from a single genomic source (gene expression or CNA data). However, patients were roughly clustered into 2 groups according to the activity values of the concatenated deep features (Figure 4).

Table 1. The size and organization of deep features obtained from the models. The size and structure of the deep features extracted from gene expression data and copy number alteration data by the two denoising autoencoders (DAs) models.

Model	Data Source	Deep Features (Noise Factors = 0.25)	
One-input DAs	Gene expressions	Activity values	1085×100
		weights	$16{,}197 \times 100$
	Copy number alterations	Activity values	1085×100
		weights	$16{,}197 \times 100$
Two-input DAs	Gene expressions Copy number alterations	Activity values	1085×100
		weights	$16{,}197 \times 100$

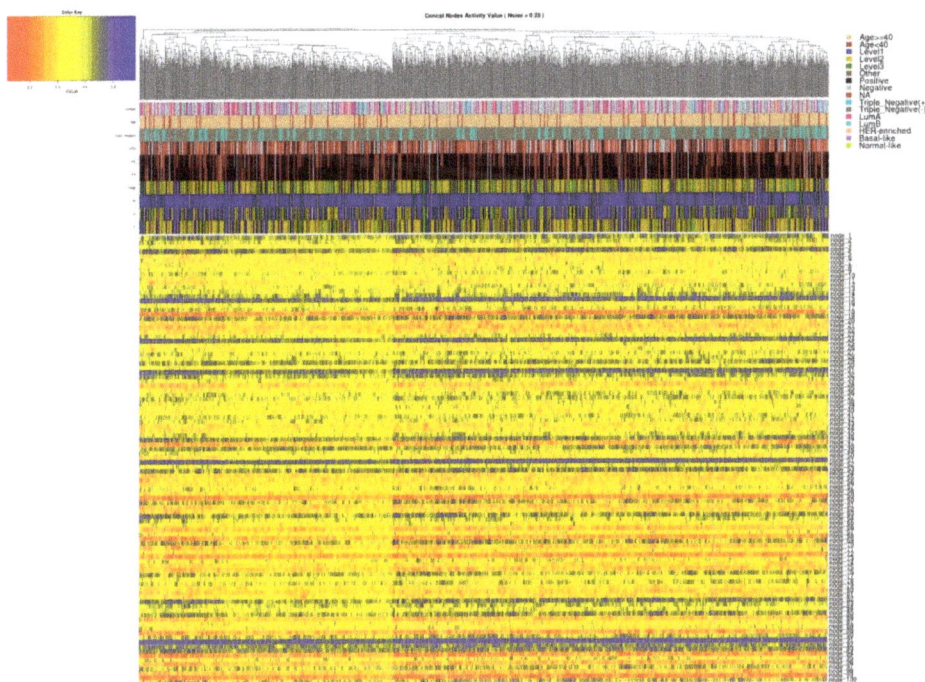

Figure 4. The clustering of activity values of concatenated deep features extracted under the noise factor of 0.25. The columns are the 1085 patients and the rows are the 100 deep features. The sidebar contains the corresponding clinical information of the patients. Values are clustered by both columns and rows.

Results from the association tests between the two patient groups and their clinical characteristics are shown in Table 2. The two patient groups showed significant survival (Figure 5) and ER status difference (Table 2) with *p*-values 0.049 and 0.002, respectively, which mean that the concatenated features have learned the ER information and performed well in predicting patient's prognosis. The odds ratio of ER status is 0.626, indicating that the second group tends to be associated with ER-negative patients. From the KM plot (Figure 5), we can see that the patients in Group 2 suffered from a poor prognosis, which happens to be associated with ER-negative status. It has been shown that ER-negative breast cancer patients usually have a poor prognosis.

Table 2. The results of clinical association analysis. * patients were classified as young (age < 40) and old (age $\geq$ 40) groups.

Clinical Characteristics	Fisher's Exact p-Value	Chi-Square Test p-Value
Pathological T	0.69	0.69
Pathological N	0.95	0.96
Pathological M	0.95	0.94
Tumor Stage	0.93	0.93
ER Status	0.002	0.002
PR Status	1.00	0.99
HER Status	0.43	0.44
Age *	0.58	0.67
Triple Negative Status	0.15	0.17
Tumor Subtype	0.35	0.36

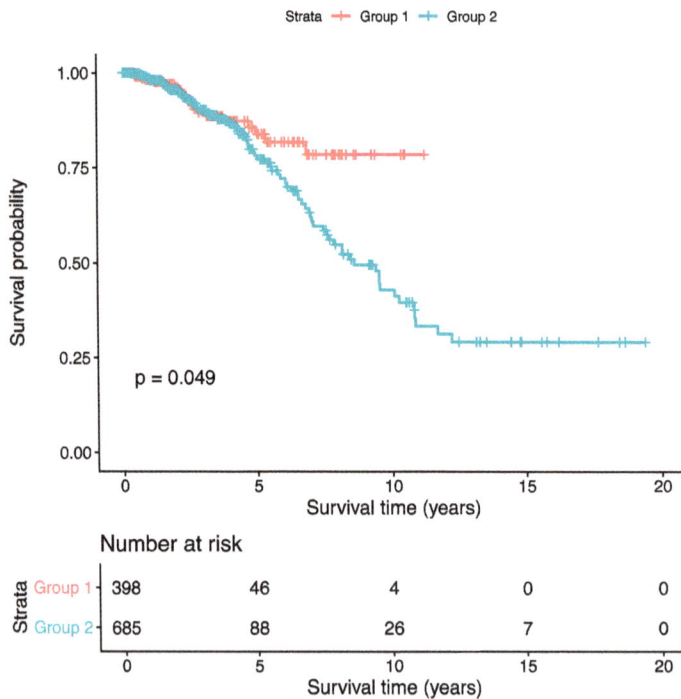

Figure 5. The Kaplan–Meier (KM) plot of the two patient groups clustered by the concatenated features.

According to the results of COX-PH models, the high-risk scores generated from each of the three deep feature sets are all significantly associated with a poor overall survival with p-values less than 1×10^{-5} (Table 3). The concatenated features showed a higher hazard ratio (HR) with 95% confidence interval (CI) (1.27, 1.16–1.40) than gene expression features (1.009, 1.005–1.013) and CNA features (1.23, 1.15–1.32). These results indicated that the risk scores from the deep features, especially the concatenated risk score, predict patient's poor prognosis. The similar patterns were observed in KM plots (Figure 6), where the patient group with high-risk scores always suffered from a poor prognosis.

Table 3. Cox's proportional hazards (COX-PH) results for risk scores.

Risk Score	HR	Lower.95_HR	Upper.95_HR	*p*-Value
Gene expression	1.009	1.005	1.013	1.06×10^{-5}
CNA	1.23	1.15	1.32	7.86×10^{-9}
Concatenated	1.27	1.16	1.40	5.62×10^{-7}

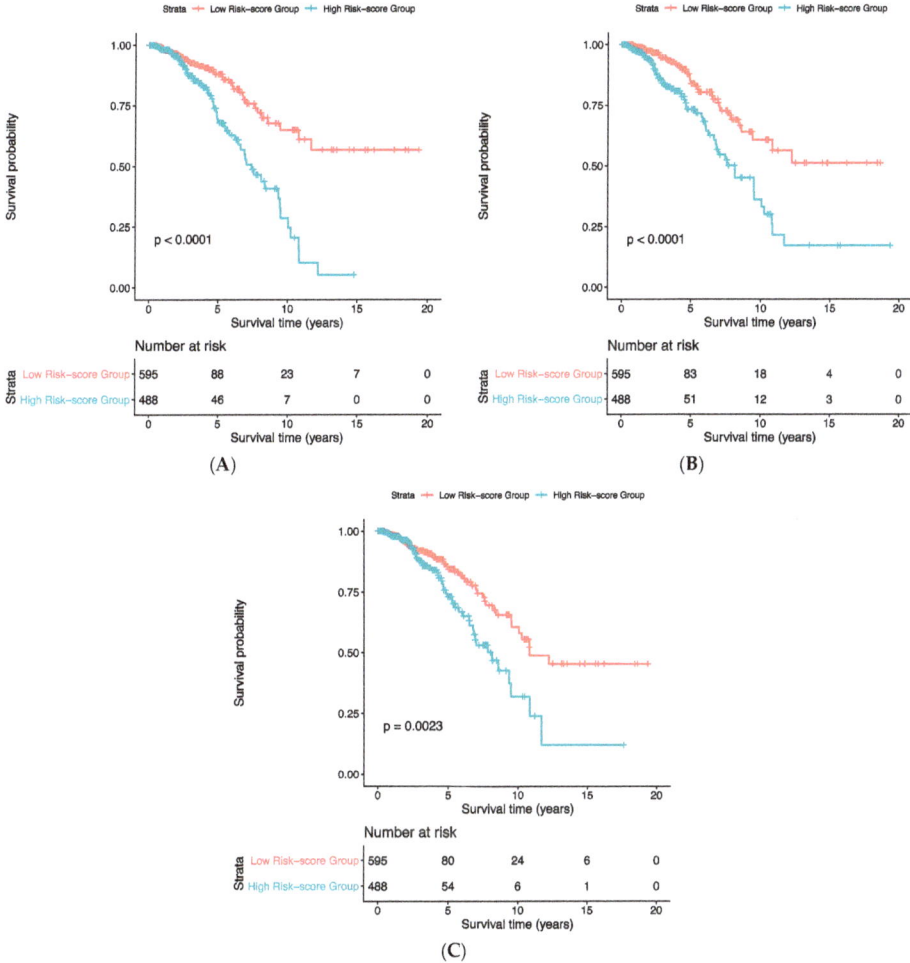

(A)

(B)

(C)

Figure 6. The KM-plots for risk scores based on the deep feature sets. (**A**) Gene expression data; (**B**) copy number alteration data; (**C**) the concatenated data.

GSEA using the 6,297 genes selected based on the concatenated deep feature set showed that the AMP-activated protein kinase (AMPK) signaling pathway in the KEGG family was significantly down-regulated with a false discovery rate (FDR) less than 0.05, and several GO-based regulation processes, such as the regulation of DNA-templated transcription, the regulation of nucleic acid-templated transcription, the regulation of apoptotic process, the positive regulation of gene expression, the positive regulation of cell proliferation, and the regulation of cellular macromolecule biosynthetic process were significantly enriched as well, with an FDR less than 0.05 (Table 4).

Table 4. The gene set enrichment analysis using Enricr.

Gene Sets	*p*-Value	Adjusted *p*-Value
regulation of transcription, DNA-templated	2.25×10^{-7}	0.001
regulation of nucleic acid-templated transcription	6.03×10^{-5}	0.04
regulation of apoptotic process	6.19×10^{-5}	0.04
positive regulation of gene expression	5.89×10^{-5}	0.04
positive regulation of cell proliferation	4.78×10^{-5}	0.04
AMPK signaling pathway_Homo sapiens_hsa04152	6.08×10^{-5}	0.018

AMPK is an important cellular metabolism and energy homeostasis regulator in mammalian tissues. It is situated in the center of a signaling network which contains tumor suppressors such as LKB1, TSC2 and p53 [25]. Some evidence has been reported that AMPK plays an anti-tumorigenic role and a lot of work are ongoing to involve agonists of AMPK for cancer treatment [28]. Furthermore, all those enriched GO regulation processes are critical as hallmarks in cancer occurrence and progression [29].

4. Discussion

In building the DA model, one of the key parameters we need to set up is the noise level used to partially destroy the inputs. We tried to add different levels of noise (e.g., 0%, 10%, 25% and 50%) into the DA model. Similar to the observations made by Vincent et al. [15], we also found that the more noise was added the better the network learns dependencies between the features. With low noise levels, the learned features do not stand out. As we set the noise level at 0.25, denoising training can capture more distinctive deep features.

Comparing with conventional breast cancer biomarkers, such as CA15-3 for measuring how breast cancer treatment is working and looking for cancer that has come back or recurred, after treatment [30], and NCC-ST-439 for measuring breast cancer progression [31], the explanation of the deep genomic features or biomarkers from the DA model for breast cancers is more complicated. Each of the extracted deep features is a high-level summary of the raw features or conventional biomarkers. These high-level features or biomarkers can be more robust against noise in the conventional biomarkers. Furthermore, these high-level features can potentially significantly improve the breast cancer outcome prediction by integrating information from both breast cancer histology images and genomic biomarkers [32]. The extracted features based on the proposed deep learning model can be also used to predict the statuses of malignancy, relapse, and reactivity for anticancer if the related data sources are available. We will explore the method in other large data sets and cancer types in the future. This can further validate the usefulness of the method for risk stratification of cancer patients.

In order to extract robust deep features using the proposed DA model, we took a strategy to add noise into the input genomic data by the partial corruption of the input pattern. It is expected that the learned deep features from the partially destroyed inputs can yield almost the same representation of the raw genomic data. In order to further boost the performance of using the learned deep features to predict breast cancer outcome or traits, another interesting strategy is to incorporate the prior knowledge about breast cancer hallmarks, which can be represented by a few molecular or signaling networks [33], into the deep learning procedure. This can be potentially implemented in different ways. For example, the interaction information among different genes or mutations collected in the molecular or signaling network databases can be used to assign the weights in different layers of the network among different neurons. We will explore the interesting strategy in future studies.

5. Conclusions

In this study, we showed that unsupervised DAs as an effective model to extract meaningful deep genomic features from either single- or multi- genomic sources from breast cancer patients. These features were significantly associated with the breast cancer ER status and had the prognosis significance. We also showed that the concatenated deep features were enriched by breast cancer relevant pathways.

This study can be improved in two potential ways. The first one is to develop new DAs model structures such as stacking more layers into DAs or adding a regression layer to make it supervised [34]. The second one is to combine all types of possible data sources together, such as somatic mutation data, protein expressions, miRNA expressions, etc. We will explore these ideas in future analyses.

Author Contributions: Q.L. and P.H. were involved in the conceptualization, development of methodologies and manuscript writing; P.H. was involved in supervision, project administration and funding acquisition.

Funding: This research was supported in part by Canadian Breast Cancer Foundation, Natural Sciences and Engineering Research Council of Canada, Manitoba Health Research Council and University of Manitoba.

Conflicts of Interest: The authors declare no conflict of interest.

Abbreviations

DL	Deep learning
CNA	Copy number alteration
DAs	Denoising autoencoders
TCGA	The Cancer Genome Atlas
KM	Kaplan-Meier
COX-PH	Cox's proportion hazard
OR	Odds ratio
AMPK	AMP-activated protein kinase
FDR	False discovery rate
GSEA	Gene sets enrichment analysis
ML	Machine learning
ANN	Artificial neural network
SVM	Support vector machine
ER	Estrogen receptor
miRNA	Micro RNA
CPM	Count per million
FPKM-UQ	Upper quartile fragments per kilobase of transcript per Million mapped reads
SGD	Stochastic gradient descent
KEGG	Kyoto Encyclopedia of Genes and Genomes
GO	Gene Ontology

References

1. Lesk, A.M. *Introduction to Bioinformatics*, 3rd ed.; Oxford University Press: Oxford, UK, 2008.
2. Bergamaschi, A.; Kim, Y.H.; Wang, P.; Sørlie, T.; Hernandez-Boussard, T.; Lonning, P.E.; Tibshirani, R.; Borresen-Dale, A.L.; Pollack, J.R. Distinct patterns of DNA copy number alteration are associated with different clinicopathological features and gene-expression subtypes of breast cancer. *Genes Chromosomes Cancer* **2006**, *45*, 1033–1040. [CrossRef]
3. Ramaswamy, S.; Tamayo, P.; Rifkin, R.; Mukherjee, S.; Yeang, C.H.; Angelo, M.; Ladd, C.; Reich, M.; Latulippe, E.; Mesirov, J.P.; et al. Multiclass cancer diagnosis using tumor gene expression signatures. *Proc. Natl. Acad. Sci. USA* **2001**, *98*, 15149–15154. [CrossRef]

4. Sorlie, T.; Tibshirani, R.; Parker, J.; Hastie, T.; Marron, J.S.; Nobel, A.; Deng, S.; Johnsen, H.; Pesich, R.; Geisler, S.; et al. Repeated observation of breast tumor subtypes in independent gene expression data sets. *Proc. Natl. Acad. Sci. USA* **2003**, *100*, 8418–8423. [CrossRef] [PubMed]

5. Wu, H.T.; Hajirasouliha, I.; Raphael, B.J. Detecting independent and recurrent copy number aberrations using interval graphs. *Bioinformatics* **2014**, *30*, i195–i203. [CrossRef]

6. Beroukhim, R.; Mermel, C.H.; Porter, D.; Wei, G.; Raychaudhuri, S.; Donovan, J.; Barretina, J.; Boehm, J.S.; Dobson, J.; Urashima, M.; et al. The landscape of somatic copy-number alteration across human cancers. *Nature* **2010**, *463*, 899–905. [CrossRef]

7. Boughorbel, S.; Al-Ali, R.; Elkum, N. Model Comparison for Breast Cancer Prognosis Based on Clinical Data. *PLoS ONE* **2016**, *11*, e0146413. [CrossRef] [PubMed]

8. Nielsen, T.O.; Parker, J.S.; Leung, S.; Voduc, D.; Ebbert, M.; Vickery, T.; Davies, S.R.; Snider, J.; Stijleman, I.J.; Reed, J.; et al. A comparison of PAM50 intrinsic subtyping with immunohistochemistry and clinical prognostic factors in tamoxifen-treated estrogen receptor-positive breast cancer. *Clin. Cancer Res.* **2010**, *16*, 5222–5232. [CrossRef] [PubMed]

9. Chi, C.; Murphy, L.C.; Hu, P. Recurrent copy number alterations in young women with breast cancer. *Oncotarget* **2018**, *9*, 11541–11558. [CrossRef] [PubMed]

10. Auria, L.; Moro, R.A. *Support Vector Machines (SVM) as a Technique for Solvency Analysis*; DIW Discussion Papers 811; DIW Berlin, German Institute for Economic Research: Berlin, Germany, 2008.

11. Olshen, A.B.; Venkatraman, E.S.; Lucito, R.; Wigler, M. Circular binary segmentation for the analysis of array-based DNA copy number data. *Biostatistics* **2004**, *5*, 557–572. [CrossRef]

12. Schadt, E.E.; Lamb, J.; Yang, X.; Zhu, J.; Edwards, S.; Guhathakurta, D.; Sieberts, S.K.; Monks, S.; Reitman, M.; Zhang, C.; et al. An integrative genomics approach to infer causal associations between gene expression and disease. *Nat. Genet.* **2005**, *37*, 710–717. [CrossRef]

13. Tan, J.; Ung, M.; Cheng, C.; Greene, C.S. Unsupervised feature construction and knowledge extraction from genome-wide assays of breast cancer with denoising autoencoders. *Pac. Symp. Biocomput.* **2014**, *20*, 132–143.

14. Guyon, I.; Elisseeff, A. Feature Extraction, Foundations and Applications: An introduction to feature extraction. *Stud. Fuzziness Soft Comput.* **2006**, *207*, 1–25.

15. Vincent, P.; Larochelle, H.; Bengio, Y.; Manzagol, P.A. Extracting and composing robust features with denoising autoencoders. In Proceedings of the 25th International Conference on Machine Learning, Helsinki, Finland, 5–9 July 2008; ACM: New York, NY, USA, 2008; pp. 1096–1103.

16. Khan, J.; Wei, J.S.; Ringnér, M.; Saal, L.H.; Ladanyi, M.; Westermann, F.; Berthold, F.; Schwab, M.; Antonescu, C.R.; Peterson, C.; et al. Classification and diagnostic prediction of cancers using gene expression profiling and artificial neural networks. *Nat. Med.* **2001**, *7*, 673–679. [CrossRef] [PubMed]

17. Angermueller, C.; Pärnamaa, T.; Parts, L.; Oliver, S. Deep Learning for Computational Biology. *Mol. Syst. Biol.* **2016**, *12*, 878. [CrossRef] [PubMed]

18. Tomczak, K.; Czerwińska, P.; Wiznerowicz, M. The Cancer Genome Atlas (TCGA): An immeasurable source of knowledge. *Wspolczesna Onkol.* **2015**, *19*, A68–A77. [CrossRef] [PubMed]

19. Zhu, Y.; Qiu, P.; Ji, Y. TCGA-assembler: Open-source software for retrieving and processing TCGA data. *Nat. Methods* **2014**, *11*, 599–600. [CrossRef]

20. Bullard, J.H.; Purdom, E.; Hansen, K.D.; Dudoit, S. Evaluation of statistical methods for normalization and differential expression in mRNA-Seq experiments. *BMC Bioinform.* **2010**, *11*, 94. [CrossRef] [PubMed]

21. Chollet, F. Building Autoencoders in Keras. *The Keras Blog*, 2016. Available online: https://blog.keras.io/building-autoencoders-in-keras.html (accessed on 20 January 2019).

22. Abadi, M.; Barham, P.; Chen, J.; Chen, Z.; Davis, A.; Dean, J.; Devin, M.; Ghemawat, S.; Irving, G.; Isard, M.; et al. TensorFlow: A System for Large-Scale Machine Learning. In Proceedings of the 12th USENIX Symposium on Operating Systems Design and Implementation (OSDI'16), Savannah, GA, USA, 2–4 November 2016; pp. 265–284.

23. Wu, G.; Xing, M.; Mambo, E.; Huang, X.; Liu, J.; Guo, Z.; Chatterjee, A.; Goldenberg, D.; Gollin, S.M.; Sukumar, S.; et al. Somatic mutation and gain of copy number of PIK3CA in human breast cancer. *Breast Cancer Res.* **2005**, *7*, R609–R616. [CrossRef]

24. Ching, T.; Zhu, X.; Garmire, L.X. Cox—Nnet: An artificial neural network method for prognosis prediction on high—Throughput omics data. *PLoS Comput. Biol.* **2016**, *14*, e1006076. [CrossRef]

25. Chen, E.Y.; Tan, C.M.; Kou, Y.; Duan, Q.; Wang, Z.; Meirelles, G.V.; Clark, N.R.; Ma'ayan, A. Enrichr: Interactive and collaborative HTML5 gene list enrichment analysis tool. *BMC Bioinform.* **2013**, *14*, 128. [CrossRef]

26. Ogata, H.; Goto, S.; Sato, K.; Fujibuchi, W.; Bono, H.; Kanehisa, M. KEGG: Kyoto encyclopedia of genes and genomes. *Nucleic Acids Res.* **1999**, *27*, 29–34. [CrossRef]

27. Ashburner, M.; Ball, C.A.; Blake, J.A.; Botstein, D.; Butler, H.; Cherry, J.M.; Davis, A.P.; Dolinski, K.; Dwight, S.S.; Eppig, J.T.; et al. Gene ontology: Tool for the unification of biology. *Nat. Genet.* **2000**, *25*, 25–29. [CrossRef]

28. Giordanetto, F.; Karis, D. Direct AMP-activated protein kinase activators: A review of evidence from the patent literature. *Expert Opin. Ther. Pat.* **2012**, *22*, 1467–1477. [CrossRef]

29. Hanahan, D.; Weinberg, R.A. Hallmarks of cancer: The next generation. *Cell* **2011**, *144*, 646–674. [CrossRef]

30. Harris, L.; Fritsche, H.; Mennel, R.; Norton, L.; Ravdin, P.; Taube, S.; Somerfield, M.R.; Hayes, D.F.; Bast, R.C., Jr. American Society of Clinical Oncology 2007 update of recommendations for the use of tumor markers in breast cancer. *J. Clin. Oncol.* **2007**, *25*, 5287–5312. [CrossRef]

31. Miyahara, E.; Toi, M.; Wada, T.; Yamada, H.; Osaki, A.; Yanagawa, E.; Toge, T. The expression of NCC-ST-439, a tumor marker, in human breast cancer patients. *Gan No Rinsho* **1990**, *36*, 2023–2026.

32. Mobadersany, P.; Yousefi, S.; Amgad, M.; Gutman, D.A.; Barnholtz-Sloan, J.S.; Vega, J.E.V.; Brat, D.J.; Cooper, L.A.D. Predicting cancer outcomes from histology and genomics using convolutional networks. *Proc. Natl. Acad. Sci. USA* **2018**, *115*, E2970–E2979. [CrossRef]

33. Wang, E.; Zaman, N.; Mcgee, S.; Milanese, J.S.; Masoudi-Nejad, A.; O'Connor-McCourt, M. Predictive genomics: A cancer hallmark network framework for predicting tumor clinical phenotypes using genome sequencing data. *Semin. Cancer Biol.* **2015**, *30*, 4–12. [CrossRef]

34. Vincent, P.; Larochelle, H.; Lajoie, I.; Bengio, Y.; Manzagol, P.A. Stacked denoising autoencoders: Learning useful representations in a deep network with a local denoising criterion. *J. Mach. Learn. Res.* **2010**, *11*, 3371–3408.

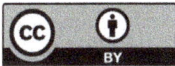

cancers

MDPI

Article

Potential Applications of DNA, RNA and Protein Biomarkers in Diagnosis, Therapy and Prognosis for Colorectal Cancer: A Study from Databases to AI-Assisted Verification

Xueli Zhang [1,2], Xiao-Feng Sun [3,*], Bairong Shen [2,*] and Hong Zhang [1,*]

[1] School of Medicine, Institute of Medical Sciences, Örebro University, SE-70182 Örebro, Sweden;
    zhang.xueli@oru.se
[2] Centre for Systems Biology, Soochow University, Suzhou 215006, China
[3] Department of Oncology and Clinical and Experimental Medicine, Linköping University,
    SE-58183 Linköping, Sweden
* Correspondence: xiao-feng.sun@liu.se (X.-F.S.); bairong.shen@suda.edu.cn (B.S.); hong.zhang@oru.se (H.Z.);
    Tel.: +46-101-032-066 (X.-F.S.); +86-521-6511-0951 (B.S.); +46-193-013-02 (H.Z.)

Received: 11 December 2018; Accepted: 29 January 2019; Published: 1 February 2019

Abstract: In order to find out the most valuable biomarkers and pathways for diagnosis, therapy and prognosis in colorectal cancer (CRC) we have collected the published CRC biomarkers and established a CRC biomarker database (CBD: http://sysbio.suda.edu.cn/CBD/index.html). In this study, we analysed the single and multiple DNA, RNA and protein biomarkers as well as their positions in cancer related pathways and protein-protein interaction (PPI) networks to describe their potential applications in diagnosis, therapy and prognosis. CRC biomarkers were collected from the CBD. The RNA and protein biomarkers were matched to their corresponding DNAs by the miRDB database and the PubMed Gene database, respectively. The PPI networks were used to investigate the relationships between protein biomarkers and further detect the multiple biomarkers. The Kyoto Encyclopaedia of Genes and Genomes (KEGG) pathway enrichment analysis and Gene Ontology (GO) annotation were used to analyse biological functions of the biomarkers. AI classification techniques were utilized to further verify the significances of the multiple biomarkers in diagnosis and prognosis for CRC. We showed that a large number of the DNA, RNA and protein biomarkers were associated with the diagnosis, therapy and prognosis in various degrees in the CRC biomarker networks. The CRC biomarkers were closely related to the CRC initiation and progression. Moreover, the biomarkers played critical roles in cellular proliferation, apoptosis and angiogenesis and they were involved in Ras, p53 and PI3K pathways. There were overlaps among the DNA, RNA and protein biomarkers. AI classification verifications showed that the combined multiple protein biomarkers played important roles to accurate early diagnosis and predict outcome for CRC. There were several single and multiple CRC protein biomarkers which were associated with diagnosis, therapy and prognosis in CRC. Further, AI-assisted analysis revealed that multiple biomarkers had potential applications for diagnosis and prognosis in CRC.

Keywords: DNA; RNA; protein; single-biomarkers; multiple-biomarkers; cancer-related pathways; colorectal cancer

---

1. Introduction

Colorectal cancer (CRC) is one of the most common types of malignancies and third leading cause of cancer-related death [1]. In 2017, there were 135 430 individuals who were diagnosed for CRC and 50 260 dead from CRC only in the United States of the America [2]. Accumulating evidence has shown that the outcome of CRC is clearly dependent on the cancer stage [2,3] and follows the strict rule: early diagnosis with better survival and later diagnosis with worse prognosis [4]. If the CRC patients are diagnosed at stage I cancer the 5-year survival rate is more than 90%, while for the stage IV patients the 5-year survival is around 10% [5]. However, more than 50% of CRC patients are already in stage III + IV at diagnosis [2]. This means that they have already passed the golden diagnostic time: early diagnosis. The rule for better cancer therapy is that it is always more complicated to treat the later stages of the cancers than to treat the early cancer patients [5]. Therefore, we lose the best therapy opportunity for the CRC patients when the golden diagnosis has been missed. Although advanced cancer therapeutic techniques have improved the outcome of cancer patients, the individuals with the same types of cancer respond remarkably differently to the same therapies. A group of cancer may respond very well to the therapy, another group may not respond to the same therapy at all and even some patients will die due to the side effects of the therapy.

Studies have shown that there is great variation among patients concerning cancer therapy and patient survival [6]. During the last decades, the publications concerning genomics, proteomics and molecular pathology have reported a large amount of cancer biomarkers from a plenty of studies from various laboratories. However, there are still huge gaps between the results from the research benches to clinical bedsides. In order to understand how and when the biomarkers can be integrated into clinical practice it is crucial to translate the laboratory results into reality. More accurate early diagnosis and individual therapy will lead us to the better cancer therapy and further improve cancer patient survival [7,8].

Recently, numerous CRC-related biomarkers have been identified and hundreds of these biomarkers have been found to be associated with early diagnosis, therapy and survival of CRC [9]. The knowledge concerning applications of the biomarkers has been considered as one of the most optimal alternative way to improve the diagnosis, therapy and prognosis for CRC [10]. The development of bioinformatics, computer science and computer-assisted biomarker analysis techniques have proven very useful tools for further biomarker investigations [11]. Consequently, several biomarker databases concerning various diseases have been created which provide a large amount of valuable data to further study the functions, interactions and even applications of biomarkers in various diseases [12–15]. However, there is no such public database focusing only on CRC biomarkers and providing comprehensive information and overview of the CRC biomarkers for both basic and clinic studies. With this question in our minds, we have recently established a CRC biomarker database (CBD: http://sysbio.suda.edu.cn/CBD/index.html) [9].

In this study, we used the biomarker data from our CBD database and other public databases to analyse the aspects of the potential applications of DNA, RNA and protein biomarkers focusing in diagnosis, therapy and prognosis for CRC. AI-assisted classification techniques were used to verify the diagnostic and prognostic significances of the single and multiple biomarkers for CRC. We attempted to further clarify the important single and multiple biomarkers as well as biomarker pathways from the laboratory benches to the clinical bedside and to provide more precise criteria in diagnosis, therapy and prognosis and to benefit the CRC patients.

2. Results

2.1. Applications of CRC Biomarkers and Their Interactions in Cancer Diagnosis, Therapy and Prognosis

Applications of CRC biomarkers and their interactions in diagnosis, therapy and prognosis and relationships of the biomarkers to the diagnosis, therapy and prognosis were analysed. As shown in Figure 1A, there were 157 biomarkers which were associated with CRC diagnosis, 152 biomarkers were related to cancer therapy and 707 with cancer prognosis. According to frequency of CRC biomarkers from our database, the sub networks were reconstructed by biomarkers in the high frequency research articles. According to Figure 1B, among the 157 diagnostic biomarkers the most common biomarkers were carcinoembryonic antigen (CEA) and cyclooxygenase-2 (COX-2). For the therapy biomarkers, thymidylate synthase (TS), leucine-rich repeat-containing G protein-coupled receptor 5 (LGR5) and vascular endothelial growth factor (VEGF) were the common ones. CEA most frequently prognostic biomarkers. Interactions among the diagnostic biomarkers, therapeutic biomarkers and prognostic biomarkers were further analysed and the interactions of the multiple functional biomarkers were presented in Figure 1C.

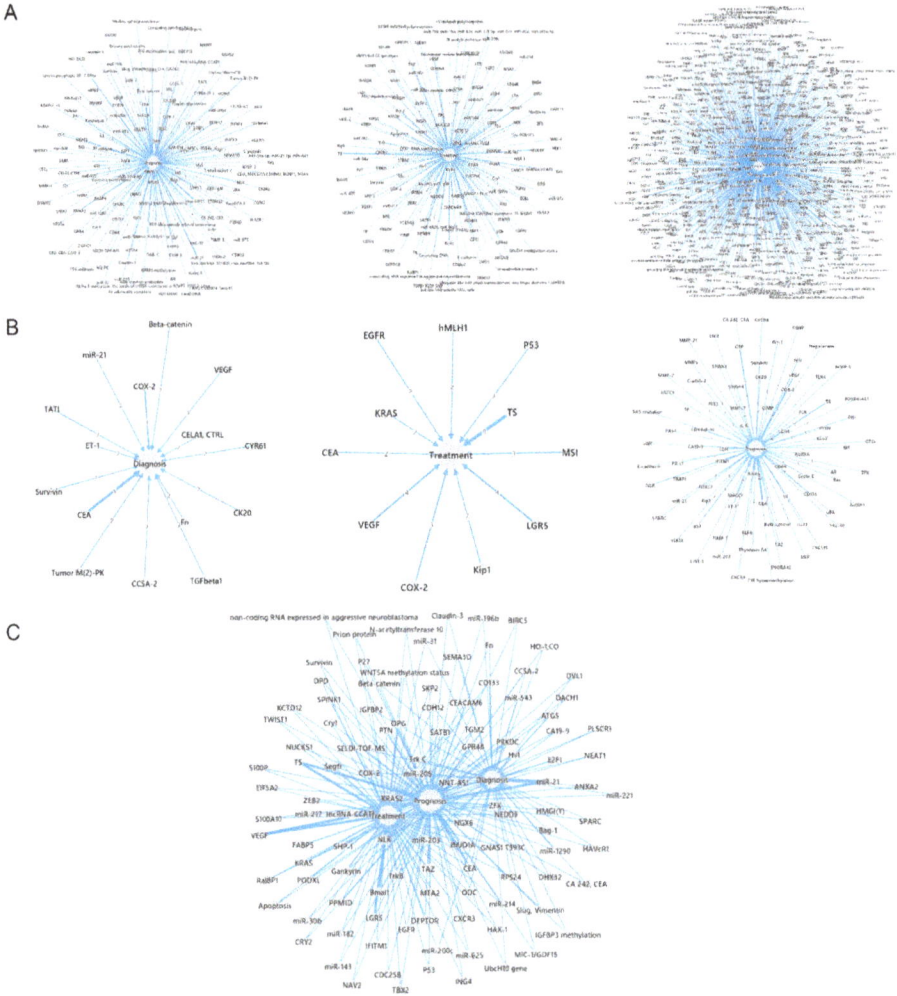

Figure 1. Distributions and interactions of CRC diagnosis, therapy and prognosis biomarkers from the CBD. The numbers mentioned on the lines means the amounts of articles for the correlated biomarkers. (**A**) The CRC biomarkers were classified according to their functions of diagnosis, therapy and prognosis. (**B**) The biomarkers reported by more than 2 articles are presented. (**C**) The interactions of diagnosis, therapy and prognosis biomarkers.

2.2. Applications of PPI Networks for CRC Diagnostic, Therapeutic and Prognostic Protein Biomarkers

As shown in Figure 2, the CRC protein biomarkers were further analysed in the PPI networks for CRC diagnosis, therapy and prognosis. The biomarkers with the highest degree for the diagnosis were TP53, VEGF, IGF1 and CD44 (Figure 2A), for therapy were TP53, PCNA, CDH1 and so forth,

(Figure 2B) and for prognosis were TP53, EGFR, MYC and so forth, (Figure 2C). TP53 was found as the biomarker with highest degree for all CRC diagnosis, therapy and prognosis. EGFR, Ras, CDH1 and BCL2 have been related to both CRC therapy and prognosis. (KRAS protein with therapy and HRAS protein with prognosis) CD44 is associated with both CRC diagnosis and prognosis. Most of the protein biomarkers were associated with CRC prognosis. The top 10 high degree protein biomarkers in each PPI network are selected and presented in Figure 2.

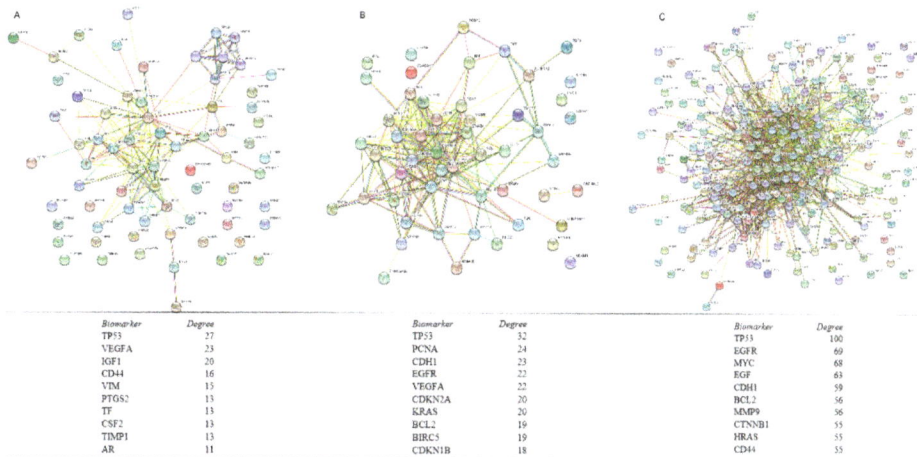

Biomarker	Degree		Biomarker	Degree		Biomarker	Degree
TP53	27		TP53	32		TP53	100
VEGFA	23		PCNA	24		EGFR	69
IGF1	20		CDH1	23		MYC	68
CD44	16		EGFR	22		EGF	63
VIM	15		VEGFA	22		CDH1	59
PTGS2	13		CDKN2A	20		BCL2	56
TF	13		KRAS	20		MMP9	56
CSF2	13		BCL2	19		CTNNB1	55
TIMP1	13		BIRC5	19		HRAS	55
AR	11		CDKN1B	18		CD44	55

Figure 2. PPI networks of CRC protein biomarkers in diagnosis, therapy and prognosis. Distributions of protein biomarkers in diagnosis (**A**), therapy (**B**) and prognosis (**C**) of CRC are displayed. Top 10 most frequent protein biomarkers in related to the diagnosis, therapy and prognosis of the CRC are listed.

We utilized KEGG pathway enrichment to further analyse the top 10 pathways in related to diagnosis, therapy and prognosis in CRC, respectively. Results are shown in Table 1. The top enriched pathways for CRC diagnosis were Ribosome, Pathway in cancer, HIF-1 signalling pathway, Wnt signalling pathway and MicroRNAs in cancer (Table 1A). The pathways for CRC therapy were Pathways in cancer, Bladder cancer, MicroRNAs in cancer, Hepatitis B and Colorectal cancer (Table 1B). Moreover, the pathways for CRC prognosis were MicroRNAs in cancer, bladder cancer, Pathway in cancer, p53 signalling pathway and HTL V-I infection (Table 1C). Pathways in cancer and microRNAs in cancer shared essential roles in CRC diagnosis, therapy and prognosis.

The CRC biomarkers in functional pathways were further analysed by GO analysis and the results showed GO annotation in biological process for diagnosis, therapy and prognosis biomarkers (Table 2). In the CRC diagnosis, phosphorylation was an important functional pathway, such as Positive regulation of phosphorylation, Positive regulation of phosphate metabolic process, Positive regulation of protein phosphorylation and Protein complex subunit organization (Table 2A). For CRC therapy, Negative regulation of cell death, Regulation of apoptotic processes, Response to abiotic stimulus, Regulation of cell death and Negative regulation of apoptotic processes (Table 2B). Regulation of cell proliferation, Response to stress, System development, Positive regulation of cellular processes and Negative regulation of cellular processes seemed playing important roles (Table 2C). Phosphorylation was essential for CRC diagnosis. Regulation of cellular death was critical for CRC therapy. Regulations for cell proliferation and cellular processes were important for CRC prognosis. It seems that different groups of cellular functional pathways play their unique roles for CRC diagnosis, therapy and prognosis, respectively.

Table 1. KEGG pathway enrichment results for CRC protein biomarkers.

Pathway ID	Pathway Description	Counts	FDR
A. KEGG pathway enrichment for diagnosis biomarkers			
03010	Ribosome	6	0.00157
05200	Pathways in cancer	8	0.00213
04066	HIF-1 signalling pathway	5	0.00281
04310	Wnt signalling pathway	5	0.00765
05206	MicroRNAs in cancer	5	0.00803
05131	Shigellosis	3	0.049
B. KEGG pathway enrichment for treatment biomarkers			
05200	Pathways in cancer	15	4.52×10^{-13}
05219	Bladder cancer	7	6.28×10^{-10}
05206	MicroRNAs in cancer	9	8.43×10^{-9}
05161	Hepatitis B	8	1.56×10^{-7}
05210	Colorectal cancer	6	3.78×10^{-7}
04110	Cell cycle	7	9.35×10^{-7}
05218	Melanoma	6	9.35×10^{-7}
05215	Prostate cancer	6	2.7×10^{-6}
05212	Pancreatic cancer	5	1.48×10^{-5}
05220	Chronic myeloid leukaemia	5	2.48×10^{-5}
C. KEGG pathway enrichment for prognosis biomarkers			
05206	MicroRNAs in cancer	23	1.16×10^{-17}
05219	Bladder cancer	13	1.47×10^{-14}
05200	Pathways in cancer	26	3.98×10^{-13}
04115	p53 signalling pathway	12	7.01×10^{-10}
05166	HTLV-I infection	18	3.39×10^{-8}
04060	Cytokine-cytokine receptor interaction	18	5.3×10^{-8}
04151	PI3K-Akt signalling pathway	20	7.36×10^{-8}
05215	Prostate cancer	11	1.15×10^{-7}
05205	Proteoglycans in cancer	16	1.28×10^{-7}

Table 2. GO analysis results in biological process level for CRC protein biomarkers.

Pathway ID	Pathway Description	Counts	FDR
A. GO analysis in biological process level for diagnosis biomarkers			
Go:0042327	Positive regulation of phosphorylation	20	6.22×10^{-9}
Go:0045937	Positive regulation of phosphate metabolic process	21	6.22×10^{-9}
Go:0001934	Positive regulation of protein phosphorylation	19	1.42×10^{-8}
Go:0071822	Protein complex subunit organization	24	1.42×10^{-8}
Go:0042127	Regulation of cell proliferation	24	2.08×10^{-8}
Go:0042981	Regulation of apoptotic process	23	3.65×10^{-8}
Go:0048583	Regulation of response to stimulus	34	4.31×10^{-8}
Go:0043933	Macromolecular complex subunit organization	27	9.8×10^{-8}
Go:0043066	Negative regulation of apoptotic process	18	1.39×10^{-7}
Go:0008284	Positive regulation of cell proliferation	17	4.33×10^{-7}
B. GO analysis in biological process level for treatment biomarkers			
GO:0060548	Negative regulation of cell death	20	7.29×10^{-11}
GO:0042981	Regulation of apoptotic process	21	5.27×10^{-9}
GO:0009628	Response to abiotic stimulus	19	8.77×10^{-9}
GO:0010941	Regulation of cell death	21	8.77×10^{-9}
GO:0043066	Negative regulation of apoptotic process	17	8.77×10^{-9}
GO:0031325	Positive regulation of cellular metabolic process	26	8.79×10^{-8}
GO:0010604	Positive regulation of macromolecule metabolic process	25	1.34×10^{-7}
GO:0009893	Positive regulation of metabolic process	28	1.89×10^{-7}

Table 2. *Cont.*

Pathway ID	Pathway Description	Counts	FDR
GO:0009605	Response to external stimulus	21	3.8×10^{-7}
GO:0048523	Negative regulation of cellular process	29	4.12×10^{-7}
C. GO analysis in biological process level for prognosis biomarkers			
GO:0042127	Regulation of cell proliferation	76	3.63×10^{-29}
GO:0006950	Response to stress	100	4.56×10^{-21}
GO:0048731	System development	101	1.33×10^{-20}
GO:0048522	Positive regulation of cellular process	111	5.31×10^{-20}
GO:0048523	Negative regulation of cellular process	105	5.31×10^{-20}
GO:0031325	Positive regulation of cellular metabolic process	88	6.82×10^{-20}
GO:0048518	Positive regulation of biological process	119	8.49×10^{-20}
GO:0010604	Positive regulation of macromolecule metabolic process	84	2.55×10^{-19}
GO:0048519	Negative regulation of biological process	107	7.7×10^{-19}
GO:0051247	Positive regulation of protein metabolic process	60	1.19×10^{-18}

However, when we further estimated molecular functions of the CRC biomarkers and their pathways associated with CRC diagnosis, therapy and prognosis with GO analysis the results (Table 3) showed that protein binding, identical protein binding, binding and enzyme binding are the four pathways shared in CRC diagnosis (Table 3A), therapy (Table 3B) and diagnosis (Table 3C). Cellular Component GO analysis for the CRC biomarkers and pathways revealed in Table 4 that CRC diagnosis and prognosis biomarkers shared extracellular space, vesicle, extracellular region and extracellular region part pathways.

Table 3. GO analysis results in molecular function level for CRC protein biomarkers.

Pathway ID	Pathway Description	Counts	FDR
A. GO Analysis in molecular function level for diagnosis biomarkers			
GO:0005515	Protein binding	44	2.81×10^{-10}
GO:0005102	Receptor binding	20	4.2×10^{-7}
GO:0042802	Identical protein binding	15	0.000526
GO:0005488	Binding	53	0.00127
GO:0001968	Fibronectin binding	3	0.0307
GO:0005539	Glycosaminoglycan binding	6	0.0353
GO:0003735	Structural constituent of ribosome	5	0.0358
GO:0005126	Cytokine receptor binding	6	0.0358
GO:0032403	Protein complex binding	9	0.0358
GO:0019899	Enzyme binding	14	0.0365
B. GO Analysis in molecular function level for treatment biomarkers			
GO:0005515	Protein binding	36	3.52×10^{-10}
GO:0042802	Identical protein binding	16	8.85×10^{-7}
GO:0046983	Protein dimerization activity	13	1.15×10^{-5}
GO:0005488	Binding	42	0.000317
GO:0019899	Enzyme binding	15	0.000317
GO:0042803	Protein homodimerization activity	10	0.000445
GO:0043566	Structure-specific DNA binding	7	0.00061
GO:0046982	Protein heterodimerization activity	7	0.00061
GO:0030983	Mismatched DNA binding	3	0.000839
GO:0004861	Cyclin-dependent protein serine/threonine kinase inhibitor activity	3	0.00138
C. GO Analysis in molecular function level for prognosis biomarkers			
GO:0005515	Protein binding	131	4.67×10^{-29}
GO:0005102	Receptor binding	45	1.18×10^{-11}
GO:0044877	Macromolecular complex binding	44	1.98×10^{-11}
GO:0005488	Binding	160	2.91×10^{-9}
GO:0042802	Identical protein binding	35	1.63×10^{-7}
GO:0019899	Enzyme binding	41	5.39×10^{-7}
GO:0032403	Protein complex binding	25	6.42×10^{-7}
GO:0003684	Damaged DNA binding	9	8.98×10^{-6}
GO:0043566	Structure-specific DNA binding	15	1.09×10^{-5}
GO:0019900	Kinase binding	19	9.05×10^{-5}

Table 4. GO analysis results in cellular component level for CRC protein biomarkers.

Pathway ID	Pathway Description	Counts	FDR
A. GO analysis in cellular component level for diagnosis biomarkers			
GO:0005615	Extracellular space	20	1.49×10^{-6}
GO:0022627	Cytosolic small ribosomal subunit	6	1.49×10^{-6}
GO:0031982	Vesicle	33	1.49×10^{-6}
GO:0031988	Membrane-bounded vesicle	32	2.34×10^{-6}
GO:0005576	Extracellular region	36	2.74×10^{-6}
GO:0044421	Extracellular region part	32	7.96×10^{-6}
GO:0034774	Secretory granule lumen	6	1.67×10^{-5}
GO:0022626	Cytosolic ribosome	6	8.62×10^{-5}
GO:0030141	Secretory granule	9	8.62×10^{-5}
GO:0031093	Platelet alpha granule lumen	5	8.62×10^{-5}
B. GO analysis in cellular component level for treatment biomarkers			
GO:0005829	Cytosol	24	4.63×10^{-5}
GO:0044428	Nuclear part	26	4.63×10^{-5}
GO:0032991	Macromolecular complex	27	0.000117
GO:0043233	Organelle lumen	26	0.000117
GO:0043234	Protein complex	25	0.000117
GO:0044427	Chromosomal part	11	0.000117
GO:0031981	Nuclear lumen	23	0.000149
GO:0005654	Nucleoplasm	21	0.000153
GO:0005694	Chromosome	11	0.000164
GO:0070013	Intracellular organelle lumen	24	0.000662
C. GO analysis in cellular component level for prognosis biomarkers			
GO:0005576	Extracellular region	96	1.33×10^{-10}
GO:0005615	Extracellular space	46	1.62×10^{-10}
GO:0044421	Extracellular region part	85	1.96×10^{-10}
GO:0005829	Cytosol	72	6.05×10^{-8}
GO:0005912	Adherens junction	23	1.13×10^{-7}
GO:0005924	Cell-substrate adherens junction	21	2.33×10^{-7}
GO:0043227	Membrane-bounded organelle	163	3.07×10^{-7}
GO:0009986	Cell surface	28	3.94×10^{-7}
GO:0005925	Focal adhesion	20	6.84×10^{-7}
GO:0031982	Vesicle	73	1.04×10^{-6}

2.3. CRC Biomarkers in Pathway in Cancer and miRNAs in Cancer Pathway

CRC biomarkers were analysed in association with Pathways in cancer (Figure 3). There were many biomarkers and pathways which are found in the Pathways in cancer which were associated with CRC. However, the most common and important pathways were p53, Ras and PI3K and apoptosis, cell proliferation and angiogenesis pathways.

CRC miRNA biomarkers in the miRNAs in cancer pathway have been closely associated with the Vogelstein's CRC developing model. Different miRNAs and interactions among the miRNAs and a variety of genes, such as APC and K-ras have been involved in CRC initiation and progression process. MiR-135 inhibits APC at CRC initiating level; Let-7, miR-18a and miR-143 inhibit K-ras at CRC progression level; miR-21 and miR-200 involve in the CRC metastasis (Figure 4).

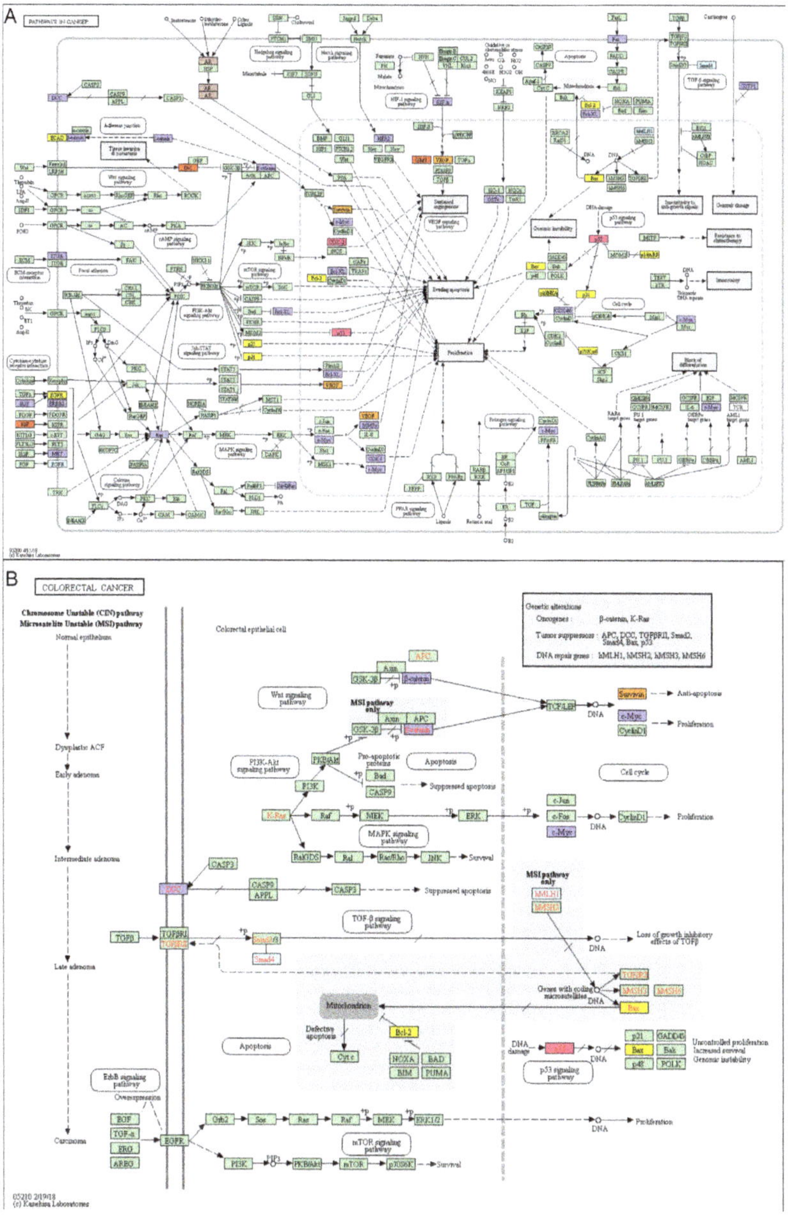

Figure 3. Biomarkers in the Pathways in cancer. (**A**) Various cancer pathways involve in different cancer initiation and progression. (**B**) CRC biomarkers for diagnosis, therapy and prognosis biomarkers in the CBD were mapped in different colours in Pathways in cancer. The CRC biomarkers have been associated with apoptosis, cell proliferation, VEGF signalling pathway and Ras signalling pathway in the Pathways in cancer. Red: diagnosis biomarker; Blue: treatment biomarker; Purple: prognosis biomarker; Orange: diagnosis & treatment biomarker; Yellow: treatment & prognosis biomarker; Pink: diagnosis & treatment & prognosis biomarker.

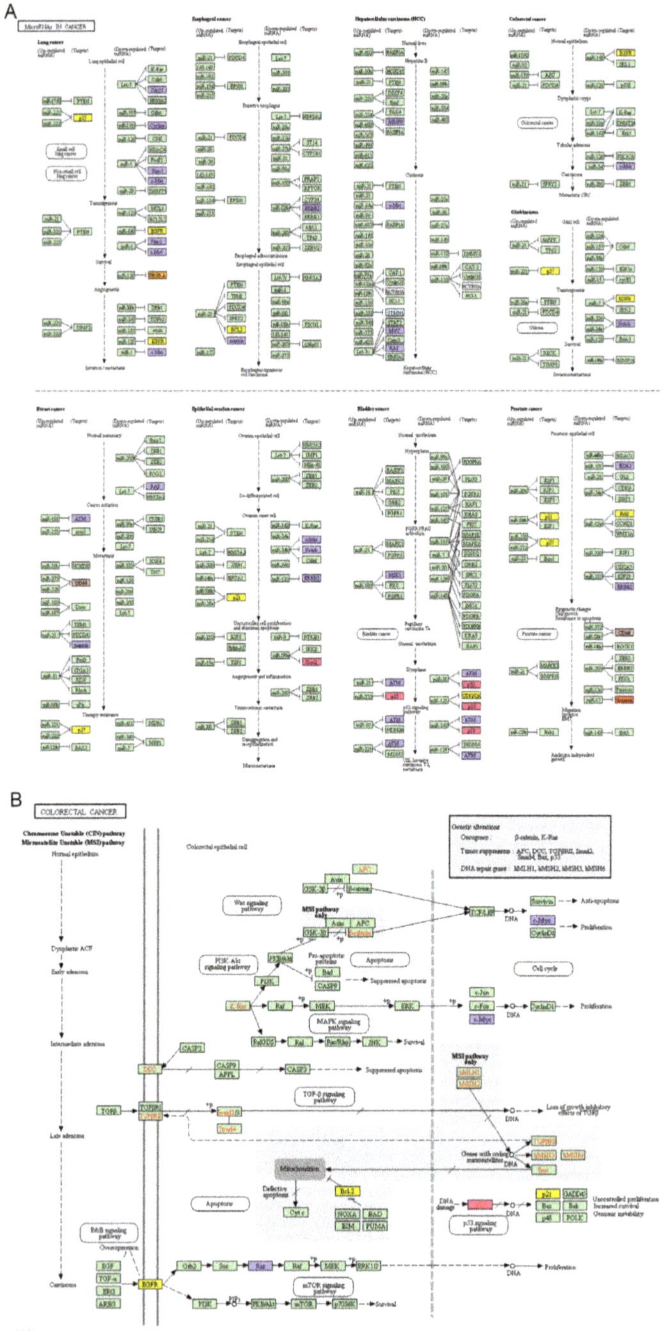

Figure 4. MiRNA in cancers. (**A**) MiRNAs involve in different types of cancers. (**B**) CRC Biomarkers in the miRNAs in cancer pathway. Different miRNAs and interactions among the miRNAs and a variety of genes, such as APC and K-ras have been involved in CRC initiation and progression process.

2.4. miRNAs and Proteins Biomarkers for CRC Diagnosis, Therapy and Prognosis

As shown in Figure 5, we analysed miRNA and protein biomarkers concerning CRC diagnosis, therapy and prognosis in our CBD database and found that there are 16 miRNA and 71 protein biomarkers for diagnosis in the CBD database. After standardization through miRBase (http://www.mirbase.org/) and NCBI protein database (https://www.ncbi.nlm.nih.gov/protein), the miRNAs and proteins were converted to their corresponding target DNAs in the miRDB database and NCBI Gene database. 1041 target genes in the miRDB were found for their 18 diagnosis miRNA biomarkers in our CBD and 71 corresponding genes in the NCBI Gene database were found for the 71 diagnostic protein biomarkers in the CBD. The converted DNAs for diagnostic miRNA and protein biomarkers were overlapped in the check points IGFBP3 and PTPRG. For the CRC therapy biomarkers, there were 16 miRNAs and 61 proteins. After the standardization and converting to DNAs, MYA6 was found as the check point for both miRNAs and proteins for CRC therapy. There were 61 miRNAs and 421 proteins were found as the CRC prognostic biomarkers in our CBD database. After the standardization and converting to their corresponding DNAs, 24 check points were found to associate with CRC prognosis between 1187 for miRNAs and 421 for proteins.

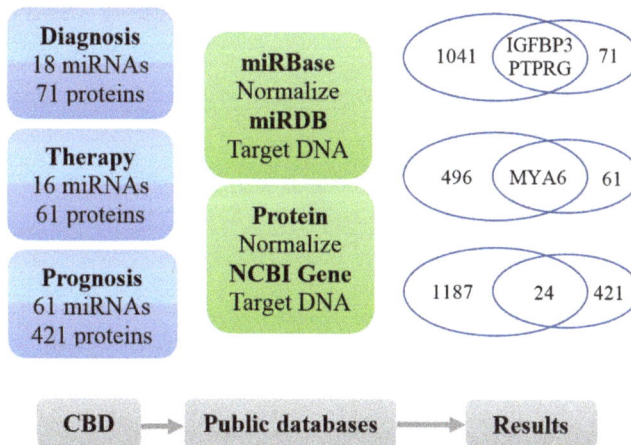

Figure 5. Associations of DNA, RNA and protein biomarkers in diagnosis, therapy and prognosis of CRC. The RNA and protein biomarkers from our CBD were converted to their corresponding genes and the relationships between the overlapping genes were further analysed. There were two genes (IGFBP1 and PTPRG) from both RNA and protein biomarkers which were associated to CRC diagnosis and one gene (MYA6) was related to therapy. However, there were 24 genes which were associated with prognosis.

2.5. Prognostic DNA Biomarkers in CRC

For prognosis biomarkers, the protein-miRNA biomarkers overlapping genes are as follows: ATP11A, CASK, CD44, DEK, DUSP5, DYRK2, EIF5A2, EPAS1, HOXB7, KRAS, MACC1, NRCAM, PRRX1, PTEN, RALBP1, S1PR1, SATB1, SLIT2, STAT3, TAGLN2, TBL1XR1, ZEB1, ZEB2, ZFX. After searching in the CBD we find that KRAS gene has been reported as DNA biomarker in CRC [16]. The biological analysis results for these overlapped DNA are shown in Table 5.

Table 5. Biological functional analysis for overlapping DNA transferred by prognosis biomarkers.

Pathway ID	Pathway Description	Counts	FDR
A. KEGG pathway enrichment for overlapping DNA transferred by prognosis biomarkers			
05206	MicroRNAs in cancer	5	0.000171
04068	FoxO signalling pathway	3	0.0466
05200	Pathways in cancer	4	0.0466
B. GO analysis result in biological process level for overlapping DNA transferred by prognosis biomarkers			
GO:0009887	Organ morphogenesis	9	0.00107
GO:0010468	Regulation of gene expression	16	0.00107
GO:0010557	Positive regulation of macromolecule biosynthetic process	11	0.00107
GO:0010628	Positive regulation of gene expression	11	0.00107
GO:2000112	Regulation of cellular macromolecule biosynthetic process	15	0.00107
GO:0031328	Positive regulation of cellular biosynthetic process	11	0.00118
GO:0048514	Blood vessel morphogenesis	6	0.00514
GO:0010556	Regulation of macromolecule biosynthetic process	14	0.00588
GO:0010604	Positive regulation of macromolecule metabolic process	12	0.00608
GO:0001568	Blood vessel development	6	0.00631

In order to find the relationship of the CRC prognostic biomarkers and the prognostic DNA biomarkers in CRC were mapped in PPI network (Figure 6). There were many single genes which were confirmed to be associated in the PPI networks. We showed also 15 significant gene interactions such as KRAS/PTEN and ZEB1/ZEB2 in the PPI networks, which may serve as combined biomarkers.

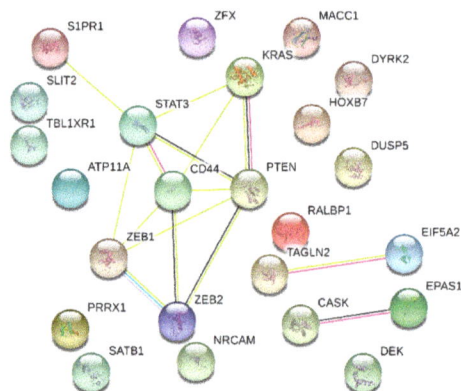

Figure 6. PPI network for the 24 overlapping prognosis genes. There were 13 genes which can been used to predict patients survival. The remaining genes worked in pairs or in groups to predict the prognosis.

2.6. Verifications of Protein Biomarkers in Diagnosis and Prognosis

AI-assisted classification techniques were utilized to further verify the significance of the 15 commonly combined multiple biomarkers predicted from PPI networks in diagnosis and prognosis for CRC. In Figure 2 we showed that many biomarkers can be applied in more than one ways along diagnosis, treatment and prognosis. So the diagnostic value for these 15 multiple biomarkers were further analysed. Figure 7 revealed the diagnostic ROC curves and distributions of AUC across biosignatures of the combined multiple protein biomarkers in CRC. The combined multiple protein biomarker of KRAS-PTEN-STAT3-CD44-ZEB1-ZEB2-S1PR1 had the most significant value amount the 15 combined biomarkers and it played the most significant role in CRC diagnosis.

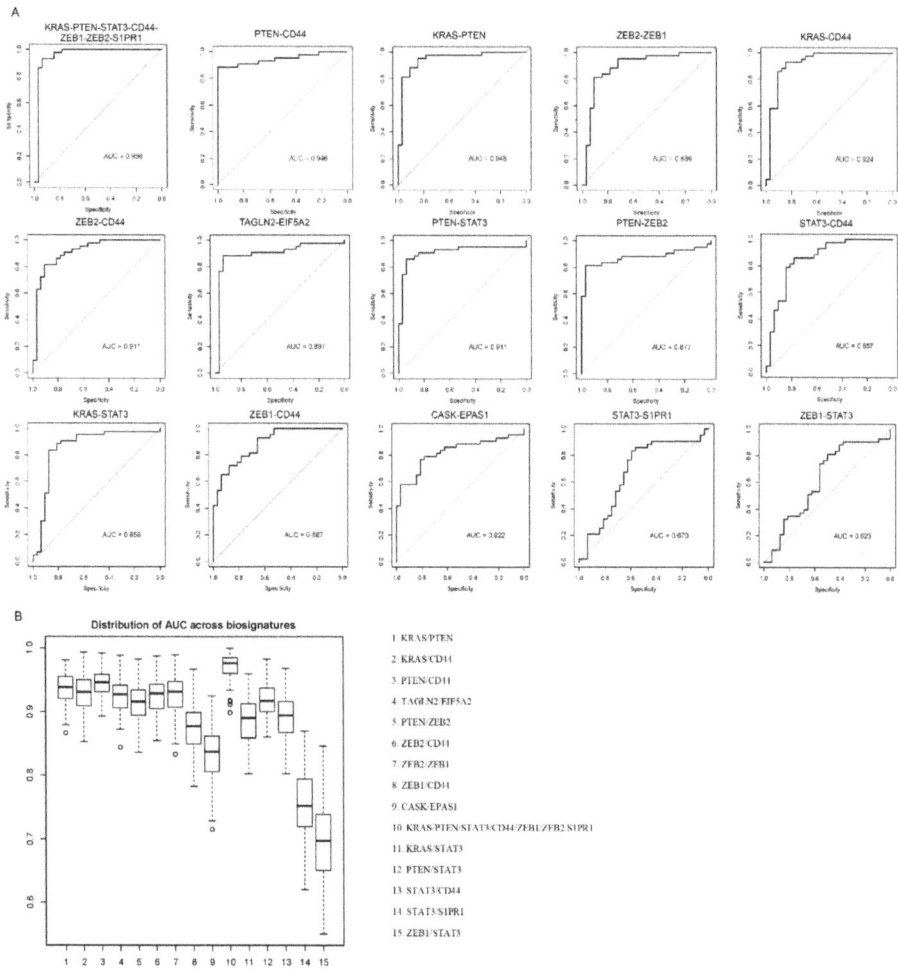

Figure 7. Diagnostic performance of multiple biomarkers for CRC. (**A**) The receiver operating (ROC) curves of all the 15 multiple biomarkers. (**B**) Distributions of AUC across biosignatures. The area under curve (AUC) statistics from 100 random training/testing divisions. The 15 multiple biomarkers were ranked.

AI-assisted prognosis analysis showed that five of the 15 combined had statistical significance to predict CRC prognosis. Of these, 5 biosignatures were significant at a level of 0.05 using the log-rank test. After multiplicity correction using the Holm FWER correction, a single biosignature was significant, the PTEN-ZEB2 pair. Its corresponding Log rank Score is 9.31. Further analyses revealed that the CRC patients with lower S1PR1 levels had better prognosis and those with higher S1PR1 levels had worse prognosis, independent of PTEN and STAT3 (Figure 8).

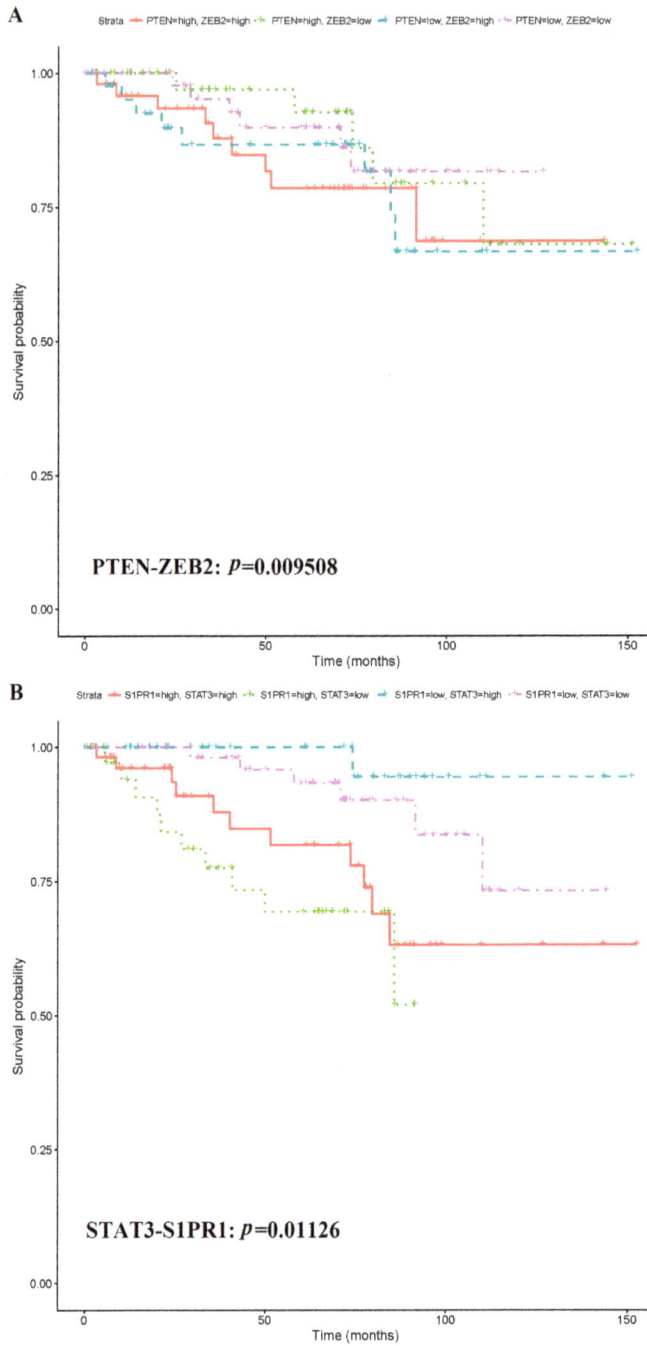

A

B

Figure 8. *Cont.*

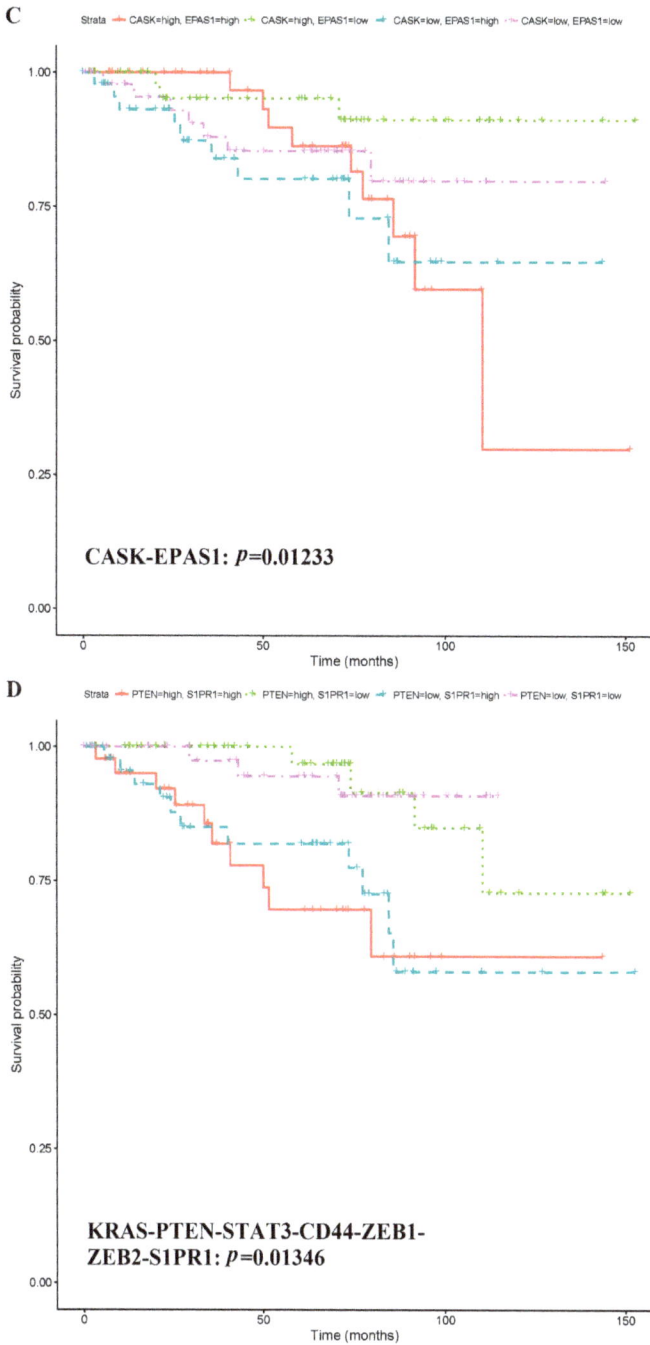

C

CASK-EPAS1: *p*=0.01233

D

KRAS-PTEN-STAT3-CD44-ZEB1-
ZEB2-S1PR1: *p*=0.01346

Figure 8. *Cont.*

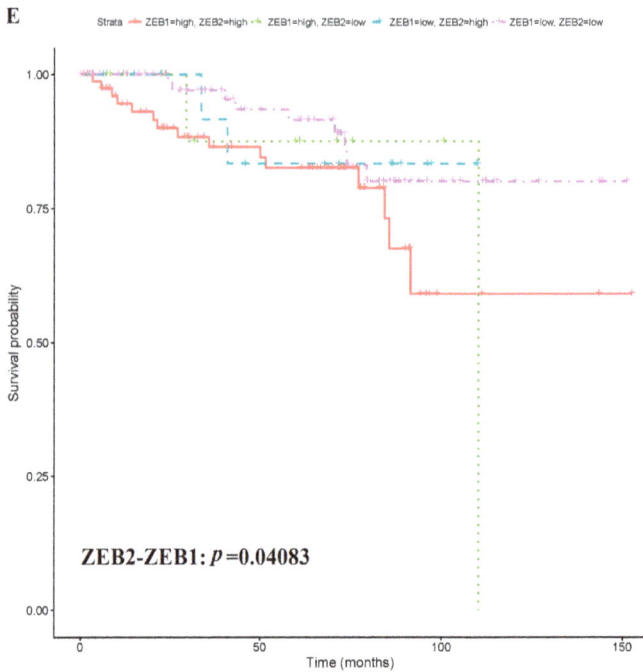

Figure 8. Kaplan-Meier survival curves of five multiple biomarkers with significant prognosis value. (A) Kaplan-Meier survival curves of multiple biomarker combined by PTEN and ZEB2. (B) Kaplan-Meier survival curves of multiple biomarker combined by STAT3 and S1PR1. (C) Kaplan-Meier survival curves of multiple biomarker combined by CASK and EPAS1. (D) Kaplan-Meier survival curves of multiple biomarker combined by KRAS, PTEN, STAT3, CD44, ZEB1, ZEB2 and S1PR1. (E) Kaplan-Meier survival curves of multiple biomarker combined by ZEB2 and ZEB1.

3. Discussion

In the CBD database [9] we have collected all the reported CRC biomarkers from the PubMed, which has provided a useful platform for CRC researchers to further investigate the effects of the biomarkers in early diagnosis, beneficial therapy and improved prediction for CRC patient survival. In this study, the potential applications of CRC biomarkers and their interactions in cancer diagnosis, therapy and prognosis and relationships of the biomarkers among the diagnosis and prognosis were further analysed and verified by AI-assisted techniques. We found there were several single and multiple functional biomarkers which are important in diagnosis, therapy and prognosis for CRC.

Although accumulating evidence concerning studies of biomarkers in cancers have been focused on cancer diagnosis, therapy and prognosis there are only few biomarkers which have been clinically utilized for early diagnosis, selecting the suitable cancer patients for better therapy and predicting prognosis. In this study, the applications of the CRC biomarkers in diagnosis, therapy and prognosis were investigated at cellular, molecular and pathway levels to further understand the biological and molecular process of the biomarkers. GO analysis showed that various biological processes, such as molecular functions and cellular composition of the protein biomarkers are involved in CRC diagnosis, therapy and prognosis. Protein phosphorylation and cell proliferation have been associated with the CRC diagnosis. Cell death and apoptosis are related to the CRC therapy and cell proliferation and biological process to the CRC prognosis. We provided clear evidence from molecular pathways and cell biology levels that the CRC biomarkers can be utilized to early diagnosis, better therapy and predicting patients outcome.

CRC biomarkers in various molecule networks and biological pathways are important for CRC. In this study, we showed the top enriched pathways in diagnosis, therapy and prognosis with the KEGG enrichment analysis. The Pathways in cancer and miRNA in cancer pathway are the most common pathways for the CRC biomarkers. As expected, the CRC biomarkers have been mainly working for the molecular binding and there are the similar pathways for the molecular binding function of CRC protein biomarkers. In the biological processes, most of annotated pathways are positive regulators for diagnosis and prognosis biomarkers and negative regulators for therapy biomarkers, indicating that protein biomarkers play different roles in CRC diagnosis, therapy and prognosis.

Proteins are the major consistency of CRC biomarkers and biological functions are always implemented by several different proteins. In this study, we collected all the protein biomarkers from our CBD [9] and drew PPI networks concerning diagnosis, therapy and prognosis, respectively. Most of the protein biomarkers were connected to the PPI networks. There were several protein biomarkers which acted as essential hubs in all the three PPI networks, such as TP53, EGFR, CDH11 and BCL2. GO analysis showed that these proteins played an important role in positive regulation of intracellular transportation, cellular protein localization and cell-cell adhesion, which provided the evidence that our future study should focus on such hub proteins as the biomarkers for CRC.

Potential applications of the CRC protein biomarkers in PPI networks for diagnostic, therapeutic and prognostic biomarkers were further analysed and we found that the most frequent protein biomarkers were associated with CRC prognosis. However, the roles of CRC protein biomarkers for diagnosis, therapy and prognosis can be overlapped with multiple functions, such as TP53 in CRC therapy and prognosis [17–19], Ras [20], BCL2 [21], CD44 [22], CEA [23] in CRC prognosis. The similar results from gene expression and PPI data analysis for accurate prediction have been found in leukaemia [24]. The molecular functions in protein networks of the protein biomarkers decided whether the protein biomarkers play a single or multiple roles in CRC. High degree protein biomarkers from our CRC database [9] were found to associate with p53, Ras, PI3K, apoptosis, proliferation and angiogenesis, which are the essential pathways in CRC formation, diagnosis, therapy and prognosis. We further analysed the CRC protein biomarkers from our database by KEGG pathway enrichment concerning diagnosis, therapy and prognosis, respectively. The diagnosis, therapy and prognosis protein biomarkers have been found to share the same pathways, such as pathway in cancer and microRNAs in cancer. Moreover, the CRC diagnosis protein biomarkers were enriched in the Wnt signalling pathway. The therapy-associated protein biomarkers were found in the colorectal cancer pathway and prognosis protein biomarkers in p53 signalling pathway, indicating that there are single and multiple cancer pathways which may play various role in CRC diagnosis, therapy and prognosis.

Various miRNAs and their interactions with different genes, such as APC and KRAS, have been involved in CRC initiation, development and progression processes. The miRNAs have been considered as important players in the tumorigenesis. A number of miRNAs have been identified with miRNA microarrays as potential biomarkers for cancers [25–27]. Different miRNAs and genes are involved in various CRC progression, such as miR-135 with APC and miR-21 with PDCD4 in the CRC initiation (Figure 4). In addition, miRNAs in cancer pathway has been related to cancer initiation, development and progression of several cancer types (Figure 4). In this study, we showed that different miRNAs played different roles in the CRC development and progression by suing NCBI, miRBase, miRDB, KEGG, GO Consortium and STRING databases which contain a huge amount of genomics and proteomics data. Systematic and integrated analyses of the CRC biomarkers in the miRNAs in cancer pathway provided an evidence the multiple miRNA biomarkers should play more critical roles in diagnosis, therapy and prognosis of CRC. Under CRC progression from the normal epithelial cells to primary and metastatic cancer cells, there are up-regulated and down-regulated miRNAs which are involved in this molecular process, such as the up-regulated miRNA-135 inhibiting expression of APC gene to block the process from the normal cells to dysplastic cells. EGFR as a therapy and prognosis biomarker and c-Met as a prognosis biomarker have both down-regulated under the CRC progression. EGFR is regulated by miR-145, which has been reported as a biomarker for acute pulmonary embolism [28], bipolar mania [29], temporal lobe epilepsy [30], breast cancer [31] and lung cancer [32]. C-Met is regulated by miR-34, which is a known biomarker in CRC, [33] indicating that different miRNAs may involve in a variety of cancer types and cancer progression in various cancer types may be regulated by the same miRNAs.

There were many protein biomarkers which were regulated by various miRNAs that identified as biomarkers for CRC. Moreover, further analyses of the relationship between protein and miRNA biomarkers showed that DNA was considered as the connection between protein miRNA biomarkers. Multiple biomarkers played better roles in the diagnosis [34–36], therapy [37,38] and prognosis [39–41] for CRC although there was disagreement concerning combination of two biomarkers [35].

In this study, we utilized AI-assisted classification techniques to further verify the significance of both the single and multiple protein biomarkers in diagnosis and prognosis for CRC. The multiple biomarkers revealed strongly statistical significance to precise diagnosis and predict prognosis in CRC and a more optimal and precise tool to investigate cancer biomarkers.

4. Materials and Methods

4.1. Data Collection and Construction of the CRC Biomarker Application Networks

870 CRC biomarkers were collected from the published articles indexed in PubMed to construct a CBD database [8]. In this study, we selected the CRC biomarkers concerning diagnosis, therapy and prognosis to produce the CRC biomarker application networks and further analyse significant importance of the biomarkers from our CBD in the diagnosis, therapy and prognosis biomarkers for CRC. The gene expression data collected from Gene Expression Omnibus (GEO) database: Series GSE87211, Platform GPL13497 were used to test the prognosis and diagnosis value of multiple biomarkers, which contains 203 rectal tumour samples and 160 control samples and was obtained from Affymetrix Human Genome arrays [42].

4.2. Systematic Analysis for the CRC Protein Biomarkers

In order to perform a systematic analysis for protein biomarkers, all the 583 CRC protein biomarkers from the CBD were collected to construct the protein-protein interaction (PPI) networks using the STRING database (https://string-db.org/). The relationship between the biomarkers and diagnosis, therapy and prognosis were further investigated. The pathway enrichment analysis was conducted with the Kyoto Encyclopaedia of Genes and Genomes (KEGG) database (http://www.genome.jp/kegg/) to further cluster these protein biomarkers at pathway levels. The Gene Ontology Consortium database (GO: http://www.geneontology.org/) was used to annotate the CRC protein biomarkers into corresponding pathways at three levels: biological process, cellular component and molecular function. The enriched pathways were ranked according to the false discovery rate (FDR) and gene counts.

4.3. Overlapping Analysis of miRNA and Protein Biomarkers

In order to make comprehensive overlapping analysis of the CRC biomarker, both miRNA and protein biomarkers were matched to their corresponding genes. The miRDB database (http://www.mirdb.org/) was utilized to assign the miRNA biomarkers to their gene targets (the genes with more than 95 target prediction score were selected). The algorithm for the prediction score (S) of each gene is as following:

$$S = 100 \times (1 - \prod_{ni=1} Pi)$$

where n represents the number of predicted target gene sites number and Pi is statistical significance of gene sites calculated by support vector machines (SVMs) [43]. For each target gene, higher predicted score represents greater statistical confidence.

The NCBI Gene database (https://www.ncbi.nlm.nih.gov/gene) was used to match the protein biomarkers to their coding genes. The biological functions of the overlap between the genes matching the miRNA and protein biomarkers were further investigated. The STRING PPI network was utilized to analyse the relationships among the overlapping genes and to search for multiple biomarkers. The biological functions of the biomarkers were studied with KEGG pathway enrichment analysis and GO annotation.

4.4. AI-assisted Verification

Tissue samples were classified as cancerous according to a binary classification model. The tissue classes were normal mucosa (0) and tumour (1) tissues. The tissue class Y was modelled according to logistic regression,

$$\log\left(\frac{E(Y)}{1 - E(Y)}\right) = \beta_0 + \sum_{j=1}^{J} \beta_j x_j$$

where $p = E(Y)$ is the expected proportion belonging to the tumour class and parameter β_j corresponds to biomarker j.

Altogether, 15 models (multiple biomarkers found in PPI network) were considered, one for each of the candidate biosignatures. For each candidate, we randomly divided the data set into a training and testing set according to an 80/20 division. We then fit the model to the training set and evaluated the predictive performance on the testing set according to the area under the curve (AUC), a measure of a model's ability to discriminate between classes. To evaluate the stability of each model, we replicated the above procedure 100 times to generate 100 AUC statistics for each model.

Associated with these samples were censored survival times, with the event death due to tumour being recorded. We modelled time of death due to tumour according to a Cox Proportional Hazards Model using the list of 15 biosignatures. The corresponding Kaplan-Meier survival curve test were used to estimate the statistical significances of the multiple biomarkers in CRC prognosis. When the p-values < 0.05, the results were considered as statistically significant.

The statistical package R (3.4.3) was used to analyses gene expression data. R-package GEOquery (2.46.15) was used to access data from the GEO repository. R-package pROC (1.10.0) was used to calculate AUCs. R-package survival was used to fit proportional hazards models. R-packages ggplot2 (2.2.1) and survminer (0.4.2) were used to produce Kaplan-Meier curves.

5. Conclusions

In this study, we showed the potential applications of the CRC biomarkers in diagnosis, therapy and prognosis for CRC. We reported that there were many single biomarkers which were associated with the early diagnosis, better therapy and predict prognosis in CRC. However, the combinations of multiple biomarkers and pathways might play more critical roles in diagnosis, therapy and prognosis for CRC than the single biomarkers. Therefore, the applications of multiple biomarkers and pathways could provide more precise criteria as valuable tools for early diagnosis, benefiting therapy and predicting prognosis for CRC patients.

Author Contributions: X.Z. executed and drafted the manuscript. X.-F.S., B.S. and H.Z. supervised the study and edited the manuscript. All authors read and approved the final manuscript.

Funding: This study was financially supported by the Swedish Cancer Foundation and the Swedish Research Council.

Acknowledgments: The authors are grateful to the staff in our research groups who involved in the study for their valuable contributions and discussions. The authors also thank Stephen T.A. Rush for his help in the bioinformatics AI-assisted analysis and linguistics revision.

Conflicts of Interest: The authors declare no conflict of interest.

References

1. Siegel, R.L.; Miller, K.D.; Jemal, A. Cancer statistics, 2018. *CA Cancer J. Clin.* **2018**, *68*, 7–30. [CrossRef] [PubMed]
2. Siegel, R.L.; Miller, K.D.; Fedewa, S.A.; Ahnen, D.J.; Meester, R.G.S.; Barzi, A. Colorectal cancer statistics, 2017. *CA Cancer J. Clin.* **2017**, *67*, 177–193. [CrossRef] [PubMed]

3. Shah, R.; Jones, E.; Vidart, V.; Kuppen, P.J.; Conti, J.A.; Francis, N.K. Biomarkers for early detection of colorectal cancer and polyps: Systematic review. *Cancer Epidemiol. Biomark. Prev.* **2014**, *23*, 1712–1728. [CrossRef] [PubMed]

4. SEER. Available online: http://seer.cancer.gov/statfacts/html/colorect.html (accessed on 31 January 2019).

5. Brenner, H.; Kloor, M.; Pox, C.P. Colorectal cancer. *Lancet* **2014**, *383*, 1490–1502. [CrossRef]

6. Center, M.M.; Jemal, A.; Smith, R.A.; Ward, E. Worldwide variations in colorectal cancer. *CA Cancer J. Clin.* **2009**, *59*, 366–378. [CrossRef] [PubMed]

7. Shin, S.H.; Bode, A.M.; Dong, Z. Precision medicine: The foundation of future cancer therapeutics. *NPJ Precis. Oncol.* **2017**, *1*, 12. [CrossRef] [PubMed]

8. Henry, N.L.; Hayes, D.F. Cancer biomarkers. *Mol. Oncol.* **2012**, *6*, 140–146. [CrossRef] [PubMed]

9. Zhang, X.; Sun, X.F.; Cao, Y.; Ye, B.; Peng, Q.; Liu, X.; Shen, B.; Zhang, H. CBD: A biomarker database for colorectal cancer. *Database* **2018**. [CrossRef]

10. Schirripa, M.; Lenz, H.J. Biomarker in Colorectal Cancer. *Cancer J.* **2016**, *22*, 156–164. [CrossRef]

11. Lin, Y.; Qian, F.; Shen, L.; Chen, F.; Chen, J.; Shen, B. Computer-aided biomarker discovery for precision medicine: Data resources, models and applications. *Brief. Bioinform.* **2017**. [CrossRef]

12. Lobdell, D.T.; Mendola, P. Development of a biomarkers database for the National Children's Study. *Toxicol. Appl. Pharmacol.* **2005**, *206*, 269–273. [CrossRef] [PubMed]

13. Yerlikaya, S.; Broger, T.; MacLean, E.; Pai, M.; Denkinger, C.M. A tuberculosis biomarker database: The key to novel TB diagnostics. *Int. J. Infect. Dis.* **2017**, *56*, 253–257. [CrossRef] [PubMed]

14. Yang, I.S.; Ryu, C.; Cho, K.J.; Kim, J.K.; Ong, S.H.; Mitchell, W.P.; Kim, B.S.; Oh, H.B.; Kim, K.H. IDBD: Infectious disease biomarker database. *Nucleic Acids Res.* **2008**, *36*, D455–D460. [CrossRef]

15. Dai, H.J.; Wu, J.C.; Lin, W.S.; Reyes, A.J.; Dela Rosa, M.A.; Syed-Abdul, S.; Tsai, R.T.; Hsu, W.L. LiverCancerMarkerRIF: A liver cancer biomarker interactive curation system combining text mining and expert annotations. *Database* **2014**. [CrossRef] [PubMed]

16. Osumi, H.; Shinozaki, E.; Suenaga, M.; Matsusaka, S.; Konishi, T.; Akiyoshi, T.; Fujimoto, Y.; Nagayama, S.; Fukunaga, Y.; Ueno, M.; et al. RAS mutation is a prognostic biomarker in colorectal cancer patients with metastasectomy. *Int. J. Cancer* **2016**, *139*, 803–811. [CrossRef] [PubMed]

17. Sun, X.F.; Carstensen, J.M.; Zhang, H.; Stal, O.; Wingren, S.; Hatschek, T.; Nordenskjold, B. Prognostic significance of cytoplasmic p53 oncoprotein in colorectal adenocarcinoma. *Lancet* **1992**, *340*, 1369–1373. [CrossRef]

18. Wang, M.J.; Ping, J.; Li, Y.; Adell, G.; Arbman, G.; Nodin, B.; Meng, W.J.; Zhang, H.; Yu, Y.Y.; Wang, C.; et al. The prognostic factors and multiple biomarkers in young patients with colorectal cancer. *Sci Rep.* **2015**, *5*, 10645. [CrossRef] [PubMed]

19. Pathak, S.; Meng, W.J.; Nandy, S.K.; Ping, J.; Bisgin, A.; Helmfors, L.; Waldmann, P.; Sun, X.F. Radiation and SN38 treatments modulate the expression of microRNAs, cytokines and chemokines in colon cancer cells in a p53-directed manner. *Oncotarget* **2015**, *6*, 44758–44780. [CrossRef]

20. Sun, X.F.; Ekberg, H.; Zhang, H.; Carstensen, J.M.; Nordenskjold, B. Overexpression of ras is an independent prognostic factor in colorectal adenocarcinoma. *APMIS* **1998**, *106*, 657–664. [CrossRef]

21. Sun, X.F.; Bartik, Z.; Zhang, H. Bcl-2 expression is a prognostic factor in the subgroups of patients with colorectal cancer. *Int. J. Oncol.* **2003**, *23*, 1439–1443. [CrossRef]

22. Iseki, Y.; Shibutani, M.; Maeda, K.; Nagahara, H.; Ikeya, T.; Hirakawa, K. Significance of E-cadherin and CD44 expression in patients with unresectable metastatic colorectal cancer. *Oncol. Lett.* **2017**, *14*, 1025–1034. [CrossRef] [PubMed]

23. Ning, S.; Wei, W.; Li, J.; Hou, B.; Zhong, J.; Xie, Y.; Liu, H.; Mo, X.; Chen, J.; Zhang, L. Clinical significance and diagnostic capacity of serum TK1, CEA, CA 19-9 and CA 72-4 levels in gastric and colorectal cancer patients. *J. Cancer* **2018**, *9*, 494–501. [CrossRef] [PubMed]

24. Yuan, X.; Chen, J.; Lin, Y.; Li, Y.; Xu, L.; Chen, L.; Hua, H.; Shen, B. Network Biomarkers Constructed from Gene Expression and Protein-Protein Interaction Data for Accurate Prediction of Leukemia. *J. Cancer* **2017**, *8*, 278–286. [CrossRef]

25. McGuire, A.; Brown, J.A.; Kerin, M.J. Metastatic breast cancer: The potential of miRNA for diagnosis and treatment monitoring. *Cancer Metastasis. Rev.* **2015**, *34*, 145–155. [CrossRef] [PubMed]

26. Shin, V.Y.; Chu, K.M. MiRNA as potential biomarkers and therapeutic targets for gastric cancer. *World J. Gastroenterol.* **2014**, *20*, 10432–10439. [CrossRef] [PubMed]

27. De Robertis, M.; Poeta, M.L.; Signori, E.; Fazio, V.M. Current understanding and clinical utility of miRNAs regulation of colon cancer stem cells. *Semin. Cancer Biol.* **2018**. [CrossRef] [PubMed]

28. Xiao, J.; Jing, Z.C.; Ellinor, P.T.; Liang, D.; Zhang, H.; Liu, Y.; Chen, X.; Pan, L.; Lyon, R.; Liu, Y.; et al. MicroRNA-134 as a potential plasma biomarker for the diagnosis of acute pulmonary embolism. *J. Transl. Med.* **2011**, *9*, 159. [CrossRef]

29. Rong, H.; Liu, T.B.; Yang, K.J.; Yang, H.C.; Wu, D.H.; Liao, C.P.; Hong, F.; Yang, H.Z.; Wan, F.; Ye, X.Y.; et al. MicroRNA-134 plasma levels before and after treatment for bipolar mania. *J. Psychiatr. Res.* **2011**, *45*, 92–95. [CrossRef]

30. Wang, X.; Luo, Y.; Liu, S.; Tan, L.; Wang, S.; Man, R. MicroRNA-134 plasma levels before and after treatment with valproic acid for epilepsy patients. *Oncotarget* **2017**, *8*, 72748–72754. [CrossRef]

31. O'Brien, K.; Lowry, M.C.; Corcoran, C.; Martinez, V.G.; Daly, M.; Rani, S.; Gallagher, W.M.; Radomski, M.W.; MacLeod, R.A.; O'Driscoll, L. miR-134 in extracellular vesicles reduces triple-negative breast cancer aggression and increases drug sensitivity. *Oncotarget* **2015**, *6*, 32774–32789. [CrossRef]

32. Wang, T.; Lv, M.; Shen, S.; Zhou, S.; Wang, P.; Chen, Y.; Liu, B.; Yu, L.; Hou, Y. Cell-free microRNA expression profiles in malignant effusion associated with patient survival in non-small cell lung cancer. *PLoS ONE* **2012**, *7*, e43268. [CrossRef]

33. Lu, G.; Sun, Y.; An, S.; Xin, S.; Ren, X.; Zhang, D.; Wu, P.; Liao, W.; Ding, Y.; Liang, L. MicroRNA-34a targets FMNL2 and E2F5 and suppresses the progression of colorectal cancer. *Exp. Mol. Pathol.* **2015**, *99*, 173–179. [CrossRef] [PubMed]

34. Zhu, M.; Huang, Z.; Zhu, D.; Zhou, X.; Shan, X.; Qi, L.W.; Wu, L.; Cheng, W.; Zhu, J.; Zhang, L.; et al. A panel of microRNA signature in serum for colorectal cancer diagnosis. *Oncotarget* **2017**, *8*, 17081–17091. [CrossRef] [PubMed]

35. Carpelan-Holmstrom, M.A.; Haglund, C.H.; Roberts, P.J. Differences in serum tumor markers between colon and rectal cancer. Comparison of CA 242 and carcinoembryonic antigen. *Dis. Colon Rectum.* **1996**, *39*, 799–805. [CrossRef] [PubMed]

36. Han, M.; Liew, C.T.; Zhang, H.W.; Chao, S.; Zheng, R.; Yip, K.T.; Song, Z.Y.; Li, H.M.; Geng, X.P.; Zhu, L.X.; et al. Novel blood-based, five-gene biomarker set for the detection of colorectal cancer. *Clin. Cancer Res.* **2008**, *14*, 455–460. [CrossRef] [PubMed]

37. Komuro, Y.; Watanabe, T.; Tsurita, G.; Muto, T.; Nagawa, H. Evaluating the combination of molecular prognostic factors in tumor radiosensitivity in rectal cancer. *Hepatogastroenterology* **2005**, *52*, 666–671.

38. Nakajima, T.E.; Yamada, Y.; Shimoda, T.; Matsubara, J.; Kato, K.; Hamaguchi, T.; Shimada, Y.; Okayama, Y.; Oka, T.; Shirao, K. Combination of O6-methylguanine-DNA methyltransferase and thymidylate synthase for the prediction of fluoropyrimidine efficacy. *Eur. J. Cancer* **2008**, *44*, 400–407. [CrossRef]

39. Chen, H.; Sun, X.; Ge, W.; Qian, Y.; Bai, R.; Zheng, S. A seven-gene signature predicts overall survival of patients with colorectal cancer. *Oncotarget* **2017**, *8*, 95054–95065. [CrossRef]

40. Ge, J.; Chen, Z.; Li, R.; Lu, T.; Xiao, G. Upregulation of microRNA-196a and microRNA-196b cooperatively correlate with aggressive progression and unfavorable prognosis in patients with colorectal cancer. *Cancer Cell Int.* **2014**, *14*, 128. [CrossRef]

41. Tatsuta, S.; Tanaka, S.; Haruma, K.; Yoshihara, M.; Sumii, K.; Kajiyama, G.; Shimamoto, F. Combined expression of urokinase-type plasminogen activator and proliferating cell nuclear antigen at the deepest invasive portion correlates with colorectal cancer prognosis. *Int. J. Oncol.* **1997**, *10*, 125–129. [CrossRef]

42. Hu, Y.; Gaedcke, J.; Emons, G.; Beissbarth, T.; Grade, M.; Jo, P.; Yeager, M.; Chanock, S.J.; Wolff, H.; Camps, J.; et al. Colorectal cancer susceptibility loci as predictive markers of rectal cancer prognosis after surgery. *Genes Chromosomes Cancer* **2018**, *57*, 140–149. [CrossRef] [PubMed]

43. Wang, X. Improving microRNA target prediction by modeling with unambiguously identified microRNA-target pairs from CLIP-ligation studies. *Bioinformatics* **2016**, *32*, 1316–1322. [CrossRef] [PubMed]

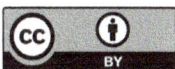

cancers

MDPI

Article

Predicting 90-Day Mortality in Locoregionally Advanced Head and Neck Squamous Cell Carcinoma after Curative Surgery

Lei Qin [1,†], Tsung-Ming Chen [2,†], Yi-Wei Kao [3], Kuan-Chou Lin [4], Kevin Sheng-Po Yuan [5], Alexander T. H. Wu [6], Ben-Chang Shia [7,*] and Szu-Yuan Wu [8,9,*]

[1] School of Statistics, University of International Business and Economics, Beijing 100029, China; qinlei@uibe.edu.cn
[2] Department of Otorhinolaryngology, Shuang-Ho Hospital, Taipei Medical University, New Taipei City 23561, Taiwan; 09326@s.tmu.edu.tw
[3] Graduate Institute of Business Administration, Fu Jen Catholic University, Taipei 116, Taiwan; kyw498762030@gmail.com
[4] Department of Oral and Maxillofacial Surgery, Wanfang Hospital, Taipei Medical University, Taipei 116, Taiwan; kclin0628@hotmail.com
[5] Department of Otorhinolaryngology, Wanfang Hospital, Taipei Medical University, Taipei 116, Taiwan; dryuank@gmail.com
[6] Ph.D. Program for Translational Medicine, Taipei Medical University, Taipei 116, Taiwan; chaw1211@tmu.edu.tw
[7] College of Management, Taipei Medical University, Taipei 106, Taiwan
[8] Department of Radiation Oncology, Wanfang Hospital, Taipei Medical University, Taipei 116, Taiwan
[9] Department of Internal Medicine, School of Medicine, College of Medicine, Taipei Medical University, Taipei 110, Taiwan
* Correspondence: stat1001@tmu.edu.tw (B.-C.S.); szuyuanwu5399@gmail.com (S.-Y.W.)
† These authors have contributed equally to this study (joint primary authors).

Received: 4 September 2018; Accepted: 18 October 2018; Published: 22 October 2018

Abstract: *Purpose:* To propose a risk classification scheme for locoregionally advanced (Stages III and IV) head and neck squamous cell carcinoma (LA-HNSCC) by using the Wu comorbidity score (WCS) to quantify the risk of curative surgeries, including tumor resection and radical neck dissection. *Methods:* This study included 55,080 patients with LA-HNSCC receiving curative surgery between 2006 and 2015 who were identified from the Taiwan Cancer Registry database; the patients were classified into two groups, mortality (n = 1287, mortality rate = 2.34%) and survival (n = 53,793, survival rate = 97.66%), according to the event of mortality within 90 days of surgery. Significant risk factors for mortality were identified using a stepwise multivariate Cox proportional hazards model. The WCS was calculated using the relative risk of each risk factor. The accuracy of the WCS was assessed using mortality rates in different risk strata. *Results:* Fifteen comorbidities significantly increased mortality risk after curative surgery. The patients were divided into low-risk (WCS, 0–6; 90-day mortality rate, 0–1.57%), intermediate-risk (7–11; 2.71–9.99%), high-risk (12–16; 17.30–20.00%), and very-high-risk (17–18 and >18; 46.15–50.00%) strata. The 90-day survival rates were 98.97, 95.85, 81.20, and 53.13% in the low-, intermediate-, high-, and very-high-risk patients, respectively (log-rank p < 0.0001). The five-year overall survival rates after surgery were 70.86, 48.62, 22.99, and 18.75% in the low-, intermediate-, high-, and very-high-risk patients, respectively (log-rank p < 0.0001). *Conclusion:* The WCS is an accurate tool for assessing curative-surgery-related 90-day mortality risk and overall survival in patients with LA-HNSCC.

Keywords: comorbidity score; mortality; locoregionally advanced; HNSCC; curative surgery

1. Introduction

The incidence of head and neck squamous cell carcinoma (HNSCC) in Taiwan is different from that in Western countries. Betel nut chewing is endemic to Taiwan and is observed in >90% patients with HNSCC in Taiwan [1–5]. Betel nut chewing results in a high risk of local recurrence and second primary HNSCC in patients with HNSCC in Taiwan [1–5]. Due to betel nut chewing, the proportion of oral cavity and nonoral cavity cancers in patients with HNSCC in Taiwan is approximately 66 and 34%, respectively [1–6]. The proportion of oral cavity cancers in patients with HNSCC is higher in Taiwan than in other countries [1–6]. Treatments for Taiwanese patients with HNSCC might be complicated, and the frequency of reirradiation is higher in Taiwan than in areas where betel nut chewing is not endemic [1–5]. Therefore, comprehensive curative surgery is the main treatment (accounting for 64.09% of all HNSCC treatments) for patients with HNSCC in Taiwan [1–6]. In addition, in Taiwan, at initial diagnosis, >50% of HNSCC cases are locoregionally advanced (Stages III and IV) HNSCC (LA-HNSCC) [6]. Instead of RT or chemotherapy, the initial treatment for LA-HNSCC is surgical resection of the primary tumor and neck dissection, followed by postoperative radiotherapy (RT) or concurrent chemoradiotherapy (CCRT).

Curative head and neck surgery, including radical neck dissection, is associated with a mortality rate of 1.5–8.5% [7–11]; however, the time interval between curative surgery and mortality has not been specified in the literature. Most studies on curative surgery for HNSCC were published in the 1970s to 1980s [7–11]; however, surgical techniques have improved considerably in the past 20 years [12,13]. Definitive data on mortality rates after curative surgery for LA-HNSCC in the past 20 years, particularly in Asia, are not available. In this study, we estimated mortality rates after curative surgery in patients with LA-HNSCC between 2006 and 2015. A new comorbidity score to predict mortality rates in patients with LA-HNSCC receiving curative surgery was also proposed because modern RT techniques, chemotherapy regimens, induction chemotherapy, and immune therapy might be more suitable alternative curative-intent treatments than curative surgery for high-mortality risk patients with LA-HNSCC [2–4,14–21].

The mean age of patients with HNSCC in Taiwan has been reported to be 55 years; consequently, the patients are generally individuals who provide the main economic support to their families [1–6]. We hope to reduce mortality rates after aggressive treatments in LA-HNSCC and propose a new comorbidity score to preoperatively predict 90-day mortality and overall survival in patients with LA-HNSCC who will receive curative surgery. The new comorbidity score can be used to determine whether curative surgery or other curative-intent aggressive treatments are the optimal treatment [2,4,14–21].

2. Patients and Methods

Ethics approval and consent: Our protocols were reviewed and approved by the Institutional Review Board of Taipei Medical University (TMU-JIRB No. 201712019).

2.1. Database

The study population was identified from the Taiwan Cancer Registry database (TCRD). The TCRD is a crucial research resource for epidemiological studies, and the results obtained using the database can be used as a reference when developing medical and health policies. The Cancer Registry database of Collaboration Center of Health Information Application contains detailed cancer-related information on clinical stages, RT doses, habits (smoking, betel nut chewing, and drinking), surgical procedures, techniques, and chemotherapy regimens [2,4,22,23]. The Institutional Review Board of Taipei Medical University approved this study (TMU-No. 201712019). The TCRD is released to the public for research purposes after identification numbers are scrambled and personal information is de-identified.

2.2. Selection of Patients and Controls

This study included 55,080 patients with LA-HNSCC who had received curative surgeries, including tumor resection and ipsilateral radical neck dissection, between 1 January 2006 and 31 December 2015. In the patients with HNSCC, clinical staging was performed according to the American Joint Committee on Cancer (AJCC), Seventh Edition. Squamous cell carcinoma was confirmed in all study patients identified from the TCRD. Patients with the following contraindications for curative surgery were excluded from the study: An Eastern Cooperative Oncology Group performance status of ≥ 2, a fixed neck mass in the deep cervical fascia, skull base involvement, circumferential or near circumferential involvement, and invasion of the carotid vessels if the patient could not tolerate a balloon occlusion test. All head and neck surgeons in Taiwan are head and neck oncology specialists certified by the Taiwan Ministry of Health and Welfare. We only included patients aged >18 years to restrict our study population to adults. Patients with metastatic HNSCC were excluded. The included patients were classified into two groups, namely mortality (*n* = 1287, mortality rate = 2.34%) and survival (*n* = 53,793, survival rate = 97.66%) groups, according to the event of mortality within 90 days after curative surgery. For each patient, the index date was designated as the date of curative surgery.

2.3. Statistical Analysis

All statistical analyses were performed using SAS statistical software (SAS for Windows, version 9.2, SAS Institute, Cary, NC, USA). Statistical significance was set at $p \leq 0.05$.

For demographic characteristics, age group (18–29, 30–39, 40–49, 50–59, 60–69, and ≥ 70) and sex were selected as the basic information of the patients. Age was calculated as the time interval between the index date and birth date, and data on sex were extracted from the database. Comorbidities were evaluated using the Charlson comorbidity index (CCI), and before surgery, physical status was determined according to the American Society of Anesthesiologists (ASA) Physical Status Classification System [2,4,24–26]. Patients with recent (within 6 months before the index date) myocardial infarction (MI), cerebral vascular accident (CVA), transient ischemic attack (TIA), or coronal arterial disease (CADs) with stents, ongoing cardiac ischemia or severe valve dysfunction, severe reduction of ejection fraction, sepsis, disseminated intravascular coagulation (DIC), adult respiratory distress syndrome (ARDS), or end-stage renal disease (ESRD) were excluded from the study. Only comorbidities observed 6 months before the index date were included in the analysis; comorbidities were identified and included according to the main International Classification of Diseases, Ninth Revision, Clinical Modification (ICD-9-CM) diagnostic codes for the first admission or 3 or more repeated main diagnosis codes for visits to outpatient departments. The comorbidities of interest were diabetes mellitus (DM), hypertension (HTN), pneumonia, chronic obstructive pulmonary disease (COPD), hepatitis B (HBV) infection, hepatitis C (HCV) infection, implanted pacemaker, MI, CVA, TIA, CADs, angina, heart valve dysfunction, ESRD, sepsis, chronic kidney disease (CKD), heart failure, DIC, ARDS, aortic aneurysm, peripheral vascular disease (PVD), peptic ulcer disease (PUD), dementia, chronic pulmonary disease, connective tissue disease, mild liver disease, hemiplegia, moderate or severe renal disease, any non-HNSCC solid cancer, leukemia, lymphoma, moderate or severe liver disease, metastatic non-HNSCC solid cancer, previous thoracic surgery, smoking, obesity, asthma, and bowel obstruction. The chi-square test was used to compare demographic characteristics and comorbidities between the mortality and survival groups.

In this study, we aimed to identify significant risk factors for mortality within 90 days after curative surgery and proposed the Wu comorbidity score (WCS) to assess mortality risk associated with curative surgery in patients with HNSCC. Univariate and multivariate Cox proportional hazard models were constructed to calculate the hazard ratios (HRs) of the variables and corresponding 95% confidence intervals (CIs). A stepwise selection method was used to select all the variables that exerted significant effects on the survival duration in the patients. Variables with coefficients of >0 or HRs of >1 were selected as risk factors to construct the WCS by adding points according to the HRs. We divided all the patients into different strata according to the WCS and confirmed that the patients with high scores had high mortality risk after curative surgery. The cumulative mortality rate was estimated using the Kaplan–Meier method, and differences among the risk strata were determined using the log-rank test. Two-tailed $p < 0.05$ was considered statistically significant.

3. Results

Table 1 shows a comparison of demographic characteristics and mortality rates within 90 days after curative surgery between the mortality and survival groups. Significant differences were observed between the groups in the age ($p < 0.0001$), sex ($p < 0.0001$), and comorbidities, such as DM, HTN, and pneumonia.

Table 1. Demographic characteristics between death within 90 days and survival groups receiving curative surgery in locoregionally advanced head and neck squamous cell carcinoma patients.

Factor	Death No.	Death Rate	Survival No.	Survival Rate	*p* Value
Number of patients	1287		53,793		
Age (years)					<0.0001
18–29	2	0.16%	696	1.29%	
30–39	40	3.11%	4978	9.25%	
40–49	231	17.95%	14,379	26.73%	
50–59	352	27.35%	16,611	30.88%	
60–69	263	20.44%	10,046	18.68%	
≥70	399	31.00%	7083	13.17%	
Sex					<0.0001
Female	195	7.38%	5697	10.59%	
Male	1192	92.62%	48,096	89.41%	
Comorbidity					
DM	80	6.22%	1804	3.35%	<0.0001
HTN	477	37.06%	16,260	30.23%	<0.0001
Pneumonia	250	19.43%	2665	4.95%	<0.0001
COPD	240	18.65%	4517	8.40%	<0.0001
Hepatitis B	8	0.62%	425	0.79%	0.4989
Hepatitis C	32	2.49%	1003	1.86%	0.1045
Implanted pacemaker	2	0.16%	22	0.04%	0.0518
MI, CVA, TIA, angina, or CAD	280	21.76%	6957	12.93%	<0.0001
Heart valve dysfunction	35	2.72%	659	1.23%	<0.0001
ESRD	0	0.00%	0	0.00%	
Sepsis	172	13.36%	882	1.64%	<0.0001
CKD	165	12.82%	1754	3.26%	<0.0001
Heart failure	92	7.15%	1000	1.86%	<0.0001
DIC	5	0.39%	5	0.01%	<0.0001
ARDS	4	0.31%	18	0.03%	<0.0001
Aortic aneurysm	4	0.31%	58	0.11%	0.0319
PVD	33	2.56%	707	1.31%	0.0001
PUD	268	20.82%	7394	13.75%	<0.0001
Dementia	71	5.52%	1100	2.04%	<0.0001
Chronic pulmonary disease	222	17.25%	4810	8.94%	<0.0001
Connective tissue disease	23	1.79%	614	1.14%	0.0323
Mild liver disease	255	19.81%	7733	14.38%	<0.0001
Hemiplegia	107	8.31%	1970	3.66%	<0.0001
Moderate or severe renal disease	166	12.90%	1757	3.27%	<0.0001
Any non-HNSCC Solid Cancer	659	51.20%	14,591	27.12%	<0.0001
Leukemia	2	0.16%	33	0.06%	0.1858
Lymphoma	22	1.71%	647	1.20%	0.101
Moderate or severe liver disease	89	6.92%	2487	4.62%	0.0001
Metastatic non-HNSCC solid cancer	548	42.58%	13,390	24.89%	<0.0001
Smoking	1158	89.98%	48,413	90.00%	0.8989
Previous thoracic surgery	6	0.47%	268	0.50%	0.6767
Obesity	11	1.24%	699	1.30%	0.7756
Asthma	10	0.78%	429	0.80%	0.9573
Bowel obstruction	3	0.23%	123	0.23%	0.8457

Diabetes mellitus: DM; hypertension: HTN; Chronic Obstructive Pulmonary Disease: COPD; Hepatitis B: HBV; Hepatitis C: HCV; myocardial infarction: MI; cerebral vascular accident: CVA; transient ischemic attack: TIA; coronal arterial disease: CAD; end stage renal disease: ESRD; Chronic kidney disease: CKD; disseminated intravascular coagulation: DIC; adult respiratory distress syndrome: ARDS; peripheral vascular disease: PVD; peptic ulcer disease: PUD.

Tables 2 and 3 present the relative risk for each variable estimated using univariate and multivariate Cox proportional hazard models. Fewer variables were significant in the multivariate model than in the univariate model, indicating strong collinearity between the variables. Therefore, we used a stepwise method in the multivariate model for variable selection (Table 4). Among comorbidities, significant variables were HTN, pneumonia, COPD, sepsis, heart failure, DIC, ARDS, dementia, mild to severe liver disease, hemiplegia, moderate or severe renal disease, any tumor, and metastatic solid tumor.

Table 2. Mortality risk assessment through univariate Cox proportional hazard model in locoregionally advanced head and neck squamous cell carcinoma patients receiving curative surgery.

Factor	HR	95% CI	*p* Value
Age (years)			
18–29	1	(Reference)	
≥30	1.277	2.077, 32.989	0.0027
≥40	1.463	2.546, 4.709	<0.0001
≥50	2.19	1.916, 2.503	<0.0001
≥60	2.245	2.012, 2.504	<0.0001
≥70	2.915	2.59, 3.28	<0.0001
Sex			
Female	1	(Reference)	
Male	1.48	1.201, 1.824	0.0002
Comorbidities			
DM	1.894	1.51, 2.374	<0.0001
HTN	1.356	1.211, 1.518	<0.0001
Pneumonia	4.476	3.898, 5.138	<0.0001
COPD	2.466	2.143, 2.838	<0.0001
Hepatitis B	0.787	0.393, 1.576	0.4986
Hepatitis C	1.342	0.945, 1.905	0.1004
Implanted pacemaker	3.716	0.928, 14.874	0.0636
MI, CVA, TIA, angina, or CAD	1.857	1.627, 2.12	<0.0001
Heart valve dysfunction	2.224	1.589, 3.111	<0.0001
Sepsis	8.647	7.364, 10.153	<0.0001
CKD	4.245	3.605, 4.999	<0.0001
Heart failure	3.965	3.207, 4.902	<0.0001
DIC	32.834	13.643, 79.019	<0.0001
ARDS	9.058	3.395, 24.166	<0.0001
Aortic aneurysm	2.818	1.056, 7.519	0.0385
PAD	1.962	1.389, 2.772	0.0001
PUD	1.64	1.433, 1.876	<0.0001
Dementia	2.735	2.153, 3.475	<0.0001
Chronic pulmonary disease	2.1	1.817, 2.427	<0.0001
Connective tissue disease	1.567	1.037, 2.367	0.0328
Mild liver disease	1.465	1.277, 1.68	<0.0001
Hemiplegia	2.35	1.928, 2.865	<0.0001
Moderate or severe renal disease	4.272	3.629, 5.028	<0.0001
Any non-HNSCC Solid Cancer	2.753	1.917, 3.953	<0.0001
Leukemia	2.506	0.626, 10.032	0.1941
Lymphoma	1.423	0.934, 2.168	0.1008
Moderate or severe liver disease	1.525	1.229, 1.891	0.0001
Metastatic non-HNSCC solid cancer	2.21	1.979, 2.468	<0.0001
Smoking	0.964	0.405, 1.459	0.3571
Previous thoracic surgery	1.168	0.778, 2.589	0.6734
Obesity	1.473	0.746, 1.896	0.8197
Asthma	1.384	0.804, 8.09	0.7592
Bowel obstruction	1.132	0.494, 2.873	0.8112

Diabetes mellitus: DM; hypertension: HTN; Chronic Obstructive Pulmonary Disease: COPD; Hepatitis B: HBV; Hepatitis C: HCV; myocardial infarction: MI; cerebral vascular accident: CVA; transient ischemic attack: TIA; coronal arterial disease: CAD; end stage renal disease: ESRD; Chronic kidney disease: CKD; disseminated intravascular coagulation: DIC; adult respiratory distress syndrome: ARDS; peripheral vascular disease: PVD; peptic ulcer disease: PUD.

Table 3. Mortality risk assessment through multivariate Cox proportional hazard model in locoregionally advanced head and neck squamous cell carcinoma patients receiving curative surgery.

Factor	HR	95% CI	*p* Value
Age (years)			
18–29	1	(Reference)	
≥30	1.012	0.486, 3.336	0.3348
≥40	1.125	1.304, 2.555	0.0004
≥50	1.309	1.107, 1.547	0.0016
≥60	1.218	1.037, 1.432	0.0166
≥70	1.902	1.618, 2.236	<0.0001
Sex			
Female	1	(Reference)	
Male	1.439	1.163, 1.78	0.0008
Comorbidities			
DM	1.188	0.942, 1.5	0.1463
HTN	0.811	0.713, 0.922	0.0014
Pneumonia	2.093	1.79, 2.447	<0.0001
COPD	1.262	1.007, 1.581	0.0431
Hepatitis B	0.864	0.429, 1.741	0.6823
Hepatitis C	0.746	0.488, 1.142	0.1772
Implanted pacemaker	1.453	0.36, 5.873	0.6001
MI, CVA, TIA, angina, or CAD	0.891	0.745, 1.066	0.2072
Heart valve dysfunction	1.215	0.858, 1.721	0.2716
Sepsis	4.079	3.418, 4.869	<0.0001
CKD	1.117	0.658, 1.897	0.6818
Heart failure	2.037	1.617, 2.567	<0.0001
DIC	7.585	3.105, 18.53	<0.0001
ARDS	4.04	1.494, 10.923	0.0059
Aortic aneurysm	1.059	0.394, 2.845	0.9093
PAD	1.107	0.777, 1.578	0.5733
PUD	1.063	0.923, 1.225	0.3953
Dementia	1.583	1.234, 2.029	0.0003
Chronic pulmonary disease	0.97	0.774, 1.216	0.7916
Connective tissue disease	1.173	0.772, 1.781	0.4551
Mild liver disease	1.211	1.043, 1.407	0.0121
Hemiplegia	1.426	1.117, 1.821	0.0044
Moderate or severe renal disease	2.092	1.235, 3.544	0.0061
Any non-HNSCC solid cancer	2.306	1.599, 3.325	<0.0001
Leukemia	1.989	0.496, 7.981	0.332
Lymphoma	1.455	0.952, 2.225	0.0832
Moderate or severe liver disease	1.212	1.104, 1.519	0.0025
Metastatic non-HNSCC solid Cancer	2.144	1.916, 2.399	<0.0001
Smoking	0.846	0.618, 1.126	0.5753
Previous thoracic surgery	0.957	0.901, 1.976	0.8251
Obesity	1.015	0.879, 1.705	0.9088
Asthma	1.203	0.798, 1.511	0.8603
Bowel obstruction	1.047	0.505, 1.984	0.9221

Diabetes mellitus: DM; hypertension: HTN; Chronic Obstructive Pulmonary Disease: COPD; Hepatitis B: HBV; Hepatitis C: HCV; myocardial infarction: MI; cerebral vascular accident: CVA; transient ischemic attack: TIA; coronal arterial disease: CAD; end stage renal disease: ESRD; Chronic kidney disease: CKD; disseminated intravascular coagulation: DIC; adult respiratory distress syndrome: ARDS; peripheral vascular disease: PVD; peptic ulcer disease: PUD.

Table 4. Stepwise selection results and comorbidity score for multivariate Cox proportional hazard model in locoregionally advanced head and neck squamous cell carcinoma patients receiving curative surgery.

Factor	HR	95% CI	*p* Value	Points
Age (years)				
≥40	1.913	1.376, 2.659	0.0001	1
≥50	1.309	1.107, 1.547	0.0016	1
≥60	1.221	1.039, 1.435	0.0154	1
≥70	1.894	1.613, 2.225	<0.0001	1
Sex				
Female	1	(Reference)		
Male	1.425	1.153, 1.76	0.001	1
Comorbidities				
HTN	0.803	0.708, 1.11	0.1006	0
Pneumonia	2.092	1.79, 2.446	<0.0001	2
COPD	1.227	1.052, 1.431	0.0093	1
Sepsis	4.161	3.492, 4.958	<0.0001	4
Heart failure	2.056	1.646, 2.566	<0.0001	2
DIC	7.683	3.152, 18.728	<0.0001	7
ARDS	3.897	1.444, 10.52	0.0073	3
Dementia	1.598	1.247, 2.048	0.0002	1
Mild liver disease	1.251	1.087, 1.439	0.0018	1
Hemiplegia	1.342	1.089, 1.654	0.0059	1
Moderate or severe renal disease	2.361	1.983, 2.81	<0.0001	2
Any non-HNSCC solid cancer	2.289	1.588, 3.3	<0.0001	2
Moderate or severe liver disease	1.284	1.034, 1.473	0.0083	1
Metastatic non-HNSCC solid cancer	2.142	1.915, 2.397	<0.0001	2

Diabetes mellitus: DM; hypertension: HTN; Chronic Obstructive Pulmonary Disease: COPD; Hepatitis B: HBV; Hepatitis C: HCV; myocardial infarction: MI; cerebral vascular accident: CVA; transient ischemic attack: TIA; coronal arterial disease: CAD; end stage renal disease: ESRD; Chronic kidney disease: CKD; disseminated intravascular coagulation: DIC; adult respiratory distress syndrome: ARDS; peripheral vascular disease: PVD; peptic ulcer disease: PUD.

The WCS was calculated using significant variables other than HTN because the HR of HTN was <1. Although HTN increased the risk of outcomes, which can be observed from univariate analysis (Table 2, HR = 1.356, CI: 1.211–1.518), collinearity in multivariate model may have reduced the HR to <1 (Table 4, HR = 0.803, CI: 0.708–0.91), which is a common statistical phenomenon. We calculated the WCS by adding points according to the HR of each risk factor. The points of each risk factor were assigned as the largest integer less than or equal to its HR (last column in Table 4); for example, 2 points for pneumonia with an HR of 2.092 and 3 points for ARDS with an HR of 3.897. In the WSC, a high number of points were assigned to risk factors with high relative mortality risk within 90 days. In our study, the minimum and maximum values of the WCS were 0 and 18+, respectively. We collapsed the range of the WCS into 4 strata, namely the low-risk (WCS, 0–6; 90-day mortality rate, 0–1.57%), intermediate-risk (7–11; 2.71–9.99%), high-risk (12–16, 17.30–20.00%), and very-high-risk (17 to 18+; 46.15–50.00%) strata (Table 4). We used the CCI for scoring to predict 90-day mortality compared with the current scoring system (Figures S1 and S2), the risk groups of CCI were not feasible for predicting 90-day mortality in LA-HNSCC patients receiving curative surgery and could not reach statistical significance. In addition, there were scarcely LA-HNSCC patients with ASA classifications I and IV–V receiving curative surgery in our database. Therefore, we cannot use ASA classifications I–V to predict 90-day mortality in LA-HNSCC patients receiving curative surgery. The 90-day mortality rate tended to increase as the WCS increased, indicating the accuracy of the WCS. The 90-day mortality rate and five-year survival in the patients were estimated using the Kaplan–Meier method to analyze the risk of mortality associated with the 4 risk strata (Figures 1 and 2). The 90-day survival rates were 98.97, 95.85, 81.20, and 53.13% in the low-, intermediate-, high-, and very-high-risk strata, respectively (log-rank test $p < 0.0001$; Figure 1). The five-year overall survival rates were 70.86, 48.62, 22.99, and 18.75% in the low-, intermediate-, high-, and very-high-risk strata, respectively (log-rank $p < 0.0001$; Figure 2).

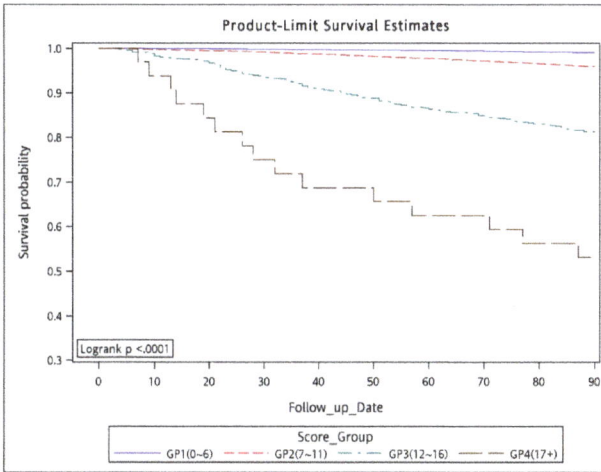

Figure 1. Kaplan–Meier curves for 90-day survival in patients with locoregionally advanced head and neck squamous cell carcinoma receiving curative surgery associated with the four risk groups. Note: *p*-value of Log Rank Test is <0.0001.

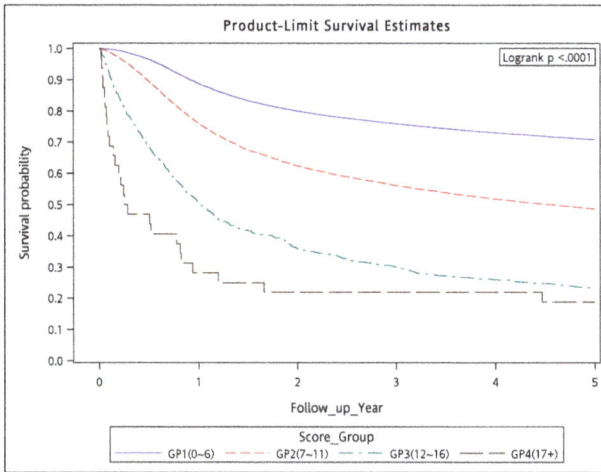

Figure 2. Kaplan–Meier curves for five years overall survival in patients with locoregionally advanced head and neck squamous cell carcinoma receiving curative surgery associated with the four risk groups. Note: *p*-value of Log Rank Test is <0.0001.

4. Discussion

According to the Taiwan Cancer Registry report, 2017 edition [6], >90% of curative surgery procedures for LA-HNSCC are conducted in top-ranking medical centers. The ranking is based on accreditation of hospitals in Taiwan into 4 levels since 1988 (medical center, regional hospitals, local hospital, clinics); the accreditation grade affects the service quality and specific patient volume of the hospital [6]. Most curative surgery procedures were performed in hospitals with sufficient patient volume (>100 newly diagnosed patients with LA-HNSCC per year), thus leading to consistent patient outcomes for LA-HNSCC in Taiwan [6,27–30]. Therefore, in Taiwan, the overall mortality rate within 90 days after curative surgery in the patients with LA-HNSCC was only 2.34% (Table 5) after consultation with a professional head and neck surgeon and anesthesia consultation. In Table 1, <3% of the patients with LA-HNSCC and heart valve dysfunctions and <5% of the patients with LA-HNSCC and moderate or severe liver disease received curative surgery. Surgeons were unwilling to perform curative surgery on the patients with LA-HNSCC and ESRD. However, the 90-day mortality remained 2.34%. Therefore, we wanted to develop a highly accurate predictor score to estimate mortality rates after curative surgery because CCRT or induction chemotherapy, followed by CCRT, might be an alternative treatment for patients with LA-HNSCC [3,4]. The proportion of the patients with LA-HNSCC with smoking habit (approximately 90%) in Table 1 was consistent with that reported in previous studies in Taiwan [1–5]. The 90-day mortality rate was proportional to age, particularly in the patients aged >70 years. This is the first study to show that age is a predictor of 90-day mortality in the patients with LA-HNSCC after curative surgery (Tables 1–3).

Table 5. Mortality (%) by different cumulative comorbidity scores among locoregionally advanced head and neck squamous cell carcinoma patients receiving curative surgery.

Score	No of Patient	No of Death	Death Rate
0	107	0	0.00%
1	277	0	0.00%
2	1104	5	0.45%
3	4289	16	0.37%
4	8948	67	0.75%
5	11,317	124	1.10%
6	10,621	167	1.57%
7	8423	228	2.71%
8	4621	168	3.64%
9	2514	154	6.13%
10	1263	109	8.63%
11	681	68	9.99%
12	393	68	17.30%
13	236	44	18.64%
14	149	32	21.48%
15	70	15	21.43%
16	35	7	20.00%
17	26	12	46.15%
18+	6	3	50.00%
Total	55,080	1287	2.34%

Univariate and multivariate analyses revealed that age is an independent predictor of 90-day mortality after curative surgery in patients (Tables 2 and 3). The male patients had higher 90-day mortality risk than did the female patients after curative surgery. These findings are consistent with those of previous studies, which reported endpoints different from those in our study [31,32]. From Table 3, the patients with LA-HNSCC and pneumonia or COPD exhibited high mortality rates. These findings are consistent with those of previous studies [33,34]. However, this is the first study to demonstrate that preoperative pneumonia increases mortality rates in the patients with LA-HNSCC who received curative surgery. Notably, although heart valve dysfunction, MI, CVA, TIA, angina, or CADs were listed as risk factors in the ASA Physical Status Classification System before surgery [24,26], these factors were not risk factors for 90-day mortality in our study. This discrepancy can be explained by our inclusion of comorbidities observed >6 months before the index date and exclusion of the comorbidities observed within 6 months of the index date. The mortality rates of these acute vascular diseases might decrease considerably after 6 months of having these diseases [35–38]. This is the first study to show the absence of correlations between heart valve dysfunction, MI, CVA,

TIA, angina, or CADs and 90-day mortality rates associated with curative surgery in the patients with LA-HNSCC. These findings are reliable references for head and neck surgeons in the future.

Notably, HF, DIC, and ARDS were independent risk factors for 90-day mortality, even when comorbidities observed 6 months before the index date were included. This is because HF, DIC, and ARDS are chronic diseases [39–42] and not acute vascular diseases. In addition, HF, DIC, and ARDS were also listed in the ASA Physical Status Classification System before surgery [24,26]. Dementia and hemiplegia might affect self-care by patients who receive surgery and might result in an increased mortality rate after surgery [31,43]. Our study is the first to demonstrate that dementia and hemiplegia were independent risk factors for mortality in the patients with LA-HNSCC who had received head and neck curative surgery. Head and neck surgeons should carefully consider curative surgery for patients with LA-HNSCC and dementia or hemiplegia. Furthermore, in our study, liver disease or renal disease were independent risk factors for 90-day mortality. Moreover, Cramer et al. showed that liver disease increases the risk of perioperative mortality in patients with HNSCC, and this risk should be carefully considered during surgical decision-making and postoperative care [44]. ESRD was also an independent 90-day mortality risk factor in our study; this finding is consistent with the results of a previous study, which reported a slightly different endpoint from ours [45]. However, leukemia and lymphoma were not risk factors for 90-day mortality in our study (Table 3). Most patients with leukemia or lymphoma have long survival durations of >1 year [46,47]; this long survival duration might explain why leukemia and lymphoma did not affect 90-day mortality in our study. By contrast, non-HNSCC cancer with or without metastasis was an independent risk factor for 90-day mortality (Table 3). This result may be attributable to the weakening of overall physical health, immunity, and the hematological system owing to previous cancer treatments, such as systemic chemotherapy, major surgical procedures, or RT, which increase 90-day mortality rates because of systemic infection complications, hospitalizations, and uncontrolled coagulation or hematological problems [48–50]. For patients with LA-HNSCC and non-HNSCC cancer with or without metastasis, alternative curative-intent aggressive treatments might be considered [4].

In our analysis, the WCS corresponded with not only the 90-day mortality rates but also with the overall survival rates (Figure 2). Developing a new comorbidity score for predicting 90-day mortality in patients with LA-HNSCC who will receive curative surgery is currently valuable because of the evolution of contemporary chemotherapy, RT techniques, target therapy, or immunotherapy, particularly in the past 10 years [14–21]. An increasing number of alternative curative-intent aggressive treatments are available for patients with LA-HNSCC [14–21].

Because the development of new surgical procedures has minimized surgical morbidity and mortality, the contraindications to curative surgery for LA-HNSCC remain controversial [12,13]. However, patients with LA-HNSCC who have a high surgical risk because of comorbidities and whose condition cannot be optimized preoperatively should not be considered for new surgical procedures. Even after treatment by a professional head and neck surgeon and careful anesthesia consultation, the 90-day mortality in Taiwan remained at 2.34% from 2006 to 2015 (Table 5). The WCS can serve as a valuable tool for preoperative prediction of the risk associated with curative surgery in patients with LA-HNSCC. After predicting the risk, other alternative curative-intent aggressive treatments can be considered in LA-HNSCC patients [4,14–21].

To the best of our knowledge, our study is the first to use a comorbidity score to predict the 90-day mortality in the patients with LA-HNSCC who had received curative surgery. Figures revealed significant differences between low-, intermediate-, high-, and very-high-risk strata. These findings suggest that the WCS is a valid and specific tool for predicting 90-day and overall mortality in patients with LA-HNSCC who will receive curative surgery. Our literature review also revealed that our study also had the largest sample size among the studies that have proposed new comorbidity scores in the past 10 years.

This study has some limitations. First, the morbidity of curative surgery could not be determined because of differences in the levels of experience among surgeons and across hospitals; therefore, head and neck curative-surgery-related mortality estimates may have been biased. However, the Taiwan Cancer Registry report, 2017 edition, revealed that curative surgery for LA-HNSCC in Taiwan are mostly performed in hospitals with high patient volumes and large medical centers [6]. Therefore, the outcomes of head and neck curative surgery would be consistent in Taiwan. Second, because all the patients with LA-HNSCC were enrolled from an Asian population and all the surgical procedures were performed by Taiwanese surgeons, the corresponding ethnic and regional susceptibility to this disease remain unclear; hence, our results should be cautiously extrapolated to non-Asian populations. Third, the diagnoses of all comorbid conditions were based on ICD-9-CM codes. However, the Taiwan Cancer Registry administration randomly reviews charts and interviews patients to verify the accuracy of the diagnoses. Hospitals with outlier chargers or practices may be audited and be subsequently heavily penalized if malpractice or discrepancies are identified. In addition, the quality and precision of ICD-9-CM codes in Taiwan have been verified and proven by previous studies [51,52]. Therefore, to obtain accurate information on population specificity and disease occurrence, large-scale randomized trials that compare carefully selected patients who had received suitable treatments are required. Fourth, we have scarcely very-high WCS patients (32/55,080 = 0.05%) and scarcely high WCS patients (<1000/55,080 = 1.60%). For remaining more than 98 percent of the patients only two risk strata groups are left and this is the same problem what we have with the ASA II and ASA III patients. Nevertheless, the individual 90-day mortality can be predicted upon the findings of this study because a big cancer registry supports this data. Finally, the TCRD does not contain information on dietary habits, socioeconomic status, or body mass index, which may all be risk factors for mortality. However, considering the magnitude and statistical significance of the effects observed in this study, these limitations are unlikely to have affected the conclusions.

5. Conclusions

The WCS is a valid tool for predicting 90-day mortality and overall survival in patients with LA-HNSCC who will receive curative surgery. Other alternative curative-intent aggressive treatments can be considered for patients with LA-HNSCC in the high- to very-high-risk strata instead of curative surgery.

Supplementary Materials: The following are available online at http://www.mdpi.com/2072-6694/10/10/392/s1. Figure S1: Kaplan–Meier curves for 90-day survival in patients with locoregionally advanced head and neck squamous cell carcinoma receiving curative surgery associated with the four risk groups from Charlson Comorbidity Index, Figure S2: Kaplan–Meier curves for 90-day survival in patients with locoregionally advanced head and neck squamous cell carcinoma receiving curative surgery associated with the four risk groups from Wu comorbidity score.

Author Contributions: Study concept and design, S.-Y.W. and L.Q.; financial support, Taipei Medical University (TMU105-AE1-B26); collection and organization of data, Y.-W.K.; data analysis and interpretation, all authors; administrative Support, S.-Y.W.; manuscript writing, all authors; final approval of manuscript, all authors.

Funding: Lei Qin's work was supported by Beijing Natural Science Foundation (No. 4164100) and the National Natural Science Foundation of China (Grant No. 61603092). Szu-Yuan Wu's work was supported by Taipei Medical University (TMU105-AE1-B26) and by Wanfang Hospital (107-wf-swf-08).

Acknowledgments: We thank National Natural Science Foundation of China (Grant No. 61603092), National Statistical Science Research Key Project (2016LZ35), University of International Business and Economics Huiyuan outstanding young scholars research funding (17YQ15) for the financial support provided to Lei Qin. We also thank Taipei Medical University (TMU105-AE1-B26) and Wanfang Hospital (funding 107-wf-swf-08) for the financial support provided to Szu-Yuan Wu.

Conflicts of Interest: The authors declare no potential conflict of interest.

Abbreviations

AJCC	American Joint Committee on Cancer
ARDS	Adult Respiratory Distress Syndrome
ASA	American Society of Anesthesiologists
CAD	Coronal Arterial Disease
CCI	Charlson Comorbidity Index
CCRT	Concurrent Chemoradiotherapy
CI	Confidence Interval
CKD	Chronic Kidney Disease
COPD	Chronic Obstructive Pulmonary Disease
CVA	Cerebral Vascular Accident
DIC	Disseminated Intravascular Coagulation
ESRD	End-Stage Renal Disease
HBV	Hepatitis B
HCV	Hepatitis C
HNSCC	Head and Neck Squamous Cell Carcinoma
HR	Hazard Ratio
HTN	Diabetes Mellitus DM Hypertension
ICD-9-CM	International Classification of Diseases Ninth Revision Clinical Modification
LA-HNSCC	Locoregionally Advanced Head and Neck Squamous Cell Carcinoma
MI	Myocardial Infarction
PUD	Peptic Ulcer Disease
PVD	Peripheral Vascular Disease
RT	Radiotherapy
TCRD	Taiwan Cancer Registry Database
TIA	Transient Ischemic Attack

References

1. Chen, J.H.; Yen, Y.C.; Chen, T.M.; Yuan, K.S.; Lee, F.P.; Lin, K.C.; Lai, M.T.; Wu, C.C.; Chang, C.L.; Wu, S.Y. Survival prognostic factors for metachronous second primary head and neck squamous cell carcinoma. *Cancer Med.* **2017**, *6*, 142–153. [CrossRef] [PubMed]
2. Chang, C.L.; Yuan, K.S.; Wu, S.Y. High-dose or low-dose cisplatin concurrent with radiotherapy in locally advanced head and neck squamous cell cancer. *Head Neck* **2017**, *39*, 1364–1370. [CrossRef] [PubMed]
3. Chen, J.H.; Yen, Y.C.; Liu, S.H.; Yuan, S.P.; Wu, L.L.; Lee, F.P.; Lin, K.C.; Lai, M.T.; Wu, C.C.; Chen, T.M.; et al. Outcomes of Induction Chemotherapy for Head and Neck Cancer Patients: A Combined Study of Two National Cohorts in Taiwan. *Medicine (Baltimore)* **2016**, *95*, e2845. [CrossRef] [PubMed]
4. Chen, J.H.; Yen, Y.C.; Yang, H.C.; Liu, S.H.; Yuan, S.P.; Wu, L.L.; Lee, F.P.; Lin, K.C.; Lai, M.T.; Wu, C.C.; et al. Curative-intent aggressive treatment improves survival in elderly patients with locally advanced head and neck squamous cell carcinoma and high comorbidity index. *Medicine (Baltimore)* **2016**, *95*, e3268. [CrossRef] [PubMed]
5. Chang, J.H.; Wu, C.C.; Yuan, K.S.; Wu, A.T.H.; Wu, S.Y. Locoregionally recurrent head and neck squamous cell carcinoma: Incidence, survival, prognostic factors, and treatment outcomes. *Oncotarget* **2017**, *8*, 55600–55612. [CrossRef] [PubMed]
6. Health Promotion Administration, M.o.H.a.W. Taiwan Cancer Registry Report, 2017 Edition. Available online: http://www.hpa.gov.tw/BHPNet/Web/Stat/StatisticsShow.aspx?No=201404160001 (accessed on 28 December 2017).
7. McGuirt, W.F.; Loevy, S.; McCabe, B.F.; Krause, C.J. The risks of major head and neck surgery in the aged population. *Laryngoscope* **1977**, *87*, 1378–1382. [CrossRef] [PubMed]
8. Gueret, G.; Bourgain, J.L.; Luboinski, B. Sudden death after major head and neck surgery. *Curr. Opin. Otolaryngol. Head Neck Surg.* **2006**, *14*, 89–94. [CrossRef] [PubMed]
9. Krause, L.G.; Moreno-Torres, A.; Campos, R. Radical neck dissection. Evaluation of 230 consecutive cases. *Arch. Otolaryngol.* **1971**, *94*, 153–157. [CrossRef] [PubMed]

10. Yarington, C.T., Jr.; Yonkers, A.J.; Beddoe, G.M. Radical neck dissection. Mortality and morbidity. *Arch. Otolaryngol.* **1973**, *97*, 306–308. [CrossRef] [PubMed]

11. MacComb, W.S. Mortality from radical neck dissection. *Am. J. Surg.* **1968**, *115*, 352–354. [CrossRef]

12. Shaha, A.R. Neck dissection: An operation in evolution. *World J. Surg. Oncol.* **2005**, *3*, 22. [CrossRef] [PubMed]

13. Myers, E.N.; Gastman, B.R. Neck dissection: An operation in evolution: Hayes Martin lecture. *Arch. Otolaryngol. Head Neck Surg.* **2003**, *129*, 14–25. [CrossRef] [PubMed]

14. Seiwert, T.Y.; Salama, J.K.; Vokes, E.E. The concurrent chemoradiation paradigm—General principles. *Nat. Clin. Pract. Oncol.* **2007**, *4*, 86–100. [CrossRef] [PubMed]

15. Ang, K.K.; Zhang, Q.; Rosenthal, D.I.; Nguyen-Tan, P.F.; Sherman, E.J.; Weber, R.S.; Galvin, J.M.; Bonner, J.A.; Harris, J.; El-Naggar, A.K.; et al. Randomized phase III trial of concurrent accelerated radiation plus cisplatin with or without cetuximab for stage III to IV head and neck carcinoma: RTOG 0522. *J. Clin. Oncol.* **2014**, *32*, 2940–2950. [CrossRef] [PubMed]

16. Seiwert, T.Y.; Burtness, B.; Mehra, R.; Weiss, J.; Berger, R.; Eder, J.P.; Heath, K.; McClanahan, T.; Lunceford, J.; Gause, C.; et al. Safety and clinical activity of pembrolizumab for treatment of recurrent or metastatic squamous cell carcinoma of the head and neck (KEYNOTE-012): An open-label, multicentre, phase 1b trial. *Lancet Oncol.* **2016**, *17*, 956–965. [CrossRef]

17. Chow, L.Q.M.; Haddad, R.; Gupta, S.; Mahipal, A.; Mehra, R.; Tahara, M.; Berger, R.; Eder, J.P.; Burtness, B.; Lee, S.H.; et al. Antitumor activity of pembrolizumab in biomarker-unselected patients with recurrent and/or metastatic head and neck squamous cell carcinoma: Results from the phase IB KEYNOTE-012 expansion cohort. *J. Clin. Oncol.* **2016**, *34*, 3838–3845. [CrossRef] [PubMed]

18. Bauml, J.; Seiwert, T.Y.; Pfister, D.G.; Worden, F.; Liu, S.V.; Gilbert, J.; Saba, N.F.; Weiss, J.; Wirth, L.; Sukari, A.; et al. Pembrolizumab for Platinum-and Cetuximab-Refractory Head and Neck Cancer: Results from a Single-Arm, Phase II Study. *J. Clin. Oncol.* **2017**, *35*, 1542–1549. [CrossRef] [PubMed]

19. Owen, D.; Iqbal, F.; Pollock, B.E.; Link, M.J.; Stien, K.; Garces, Y.I.; Brown, P.D.; Foote, R.L. Long-term follow-up of stereotactic radiosurgery for head and neck malignancies. *Head Neck* **2015**, *37*, 1557–1562. [CrossRef] [PubMed]

20. Mageras, G.S.; Mechalakos, J. Planning in the IGRT context: Closing the loop. *Semin. Radiat. Oncol.* **2007**, *17*, 268–277. [CrossRef] [PubMed]

21. Lee, N.; Puri, D.R.; Blanco, A.I.; Chao, K.S. Intensity-modulated radiation therapy in head and neck cancers: An update. *Head Neck* **2007**, *29*, 387–400. [CrossRef] [PubMed]

22. Yen, Y.C.; Chang, J.H.; Lin, W.C.; Chiou, J.F.; Chang, Y.C.; Chang, C.L.; Hsu, H.L.; Chow, J.M.; Yuan, K.S.; Wu, A.T.; et al. Effectiveness of esophagectomy in patients with thoracic esophageal squamous cell carcinoma receiving definitive radiotherapy or concurrent chemoradiotherapy through intensity-modulated radiation therapy techniques. *Cancer* **2017**. [CrossRef] [PubMed]

23. Chang, C.L.; Tsai, H.C.; Lin, W.C.; Chang, J.H.; Hsu, H.L.; Chow, J.M.; Yuan, K.S.; Wu, A.T.H.; Wu, S.Y. Dose escalation intensity-modulated radiotherapy-based concurrent chemoradiotherapy is effective for advanced-stage thoracic esophageal squamous cell carcinoma. *Radiother. Oncol.* **2017**. [CrossRef] [PubMed]

24. Wijeysundera, D.N.; Austin, P.C.; Beattie, W.S.; Hux, J.E.; Laupacis, A. A population-based study of anesthesia consultation before major noncardiac surgery. *Arch. Intern. Med.* **2009**, *169*, 595–602. [CrossRef] [PubMed]

25. Lin, W.C.; Ding, Y.F.; Hsu, H.L.; Chang, J.H.; Yuan, K.S.; Wu, A.T.H.; Chow, J.M.; Chang, C.L.; Chen, S.U.; Wu, S.Y. Value and application of trimodality therapy or definitive concurrent chemoradiotherapy in thoracic esophageal squamous cell carcinoma. *Cancer* **2017**, *123*, 3904–3915. [CrossRef] [PubMed]

26. Cohen, M.M.; Duncan, P.G.; Tate, R.B. Does anesthesia contribute to operative mortality? *JAMA* **1988**, *260*, 2859–2863. [CrossRef] [PubMed]

27. Chowdhury, M.M.; Dagash, H.; Pierro, A. A systematic review of the impact of volume of surgery and specialization on patient outcome. *Br. J. Surg.* **2007**, *94*, 145–161. [CrossRef] [PubMed]

28. Lau, R.L.; Perruccio, A.V.; Gandhi, R.; Mahomed, N.N. The role of surgeon volume on patient outcome in total knee arthroplasty: A systematic review of the literature. *BMC Musculoskelet. Disord.* **2012**, *13*, 250. [CrossRef] [PubMed]

29. Wen, H.C.; Tang, C.H.; Lin, H.C.; Tsai, C.S.; Chen, C.S.; Li, C.Y. Association between surgeon and hospital volume in coronary artery bypass graft surgery outcomes: A population-based study. *Ann. Thorac. Surg.* **2006**, *81*, 835–842. [CrossRef] [PubMed]

30. Birkmeyer, J.D.; Siewers, A.E.; Finlayson, E.V.; Stukel, T.A.; Lucas, F.L.; Batista, I.; Welch, H.G.; Wennberg, D.E. Hospital volume and surgical mortality in the United States. *N. Engl. J. Med.* **2002**, *346*, 1128–1137. [CrossRef] [PubMed]

31. Turrentine, F.E.; Wang, H.; Simpson, V.B.; Jones, R.S. Surgical risk factors, morbidity, and mortality in elderly patients. *J. Am. Coll. Surg.* **2006**, *203*, 865–877. [CrossRef] [PubMed]

32. Van Bokhorst-de van der, S.; van Leeuwen, P.A.; Kuik, D.J.; Klop, W.M.; Sauerwein, H.P.; Snow, G.B.; Quak, J.J. The impact of nutritional status on the prognoses of patients with advanced head and neck cancer. *Cancer* **1999**, *86*, 519–527. [CrossRef]

33. Sylvester, M.J.; Marchiano, E.; Park, R.C.; Baredes, S.; Eloy, J.A. Impact of chronic obstructive pulmonary disease on patients undergoing laryngectomy for laryngeal cancer. *Laryngoscope* **2017**, *127*, 417–423. [CrossRef] [PubMed]

34. Patterson, J.T.; Bohl, D.D.; Basques, B.A.; Arzeno, A.H.; Grauer, J.N. Does Preoperative Pneumonia Affect Complications of Geriatric Hip Fracture Surgery? *Am. J. Orthop. (Belle Mead NJ)* **2017**, *46*, E177–E185. [PubMed]

35. Volpi, A.; De Vita, C.; Franzosi, M.G.; Geraci, E.; Maggioni, A.P.; Mauri, F.; Negri, E.; Santoro, E.; Tavazzi, L.; Tognoni, G. Determinants of 6-month mortality in survivors of myocardial infarction after thrombolysis. Results of the GISSI-2 data base. The Ad hoc Working Group of the Gruppo Italiano per lo Studio della Sopravvivenza nell'Infarto Miocardico (GISSI)-2 Data Base. *Circulation* **1993**, *88*, 416–429. [CrossRef] [PubMed]

36. Johansson, S.; Rosengren, A.; Young, K.; Jennings, E. Mortality and morbidity trends after the first year in survivors of acute myocardial infarction: A systematic review. *BMC Cardiovasc. Disord.* **2017**, *17*, 53. [CrossRef] [PubMed]

37. Kwiatkowski, T.G.; Libman, R.B.; Frankel, M.; Tilley, B.C.; Morgenstern, L.B.; Lu, M.; Broderick, J.P.; Lewandowski, C.A.; Marler, J.R.; Levine, S.R.; et al. Effects of tissue plasminogen activator for acute ischemic stroke at one year. National Institute of Neurological Disorders and Stroke Recombinant Tissue Plasminogen Activator Stroke Study Group. *N. Engl. J. Med.* **1999**, *340*, 1781–1787. [CrossRef] [PubMed]

38. Wang, Y.; Zhao, X.; Liu, L.; Wang, D.; Wang, C.; Li, H.; Meng, X.; Cui, L.; Jia, J.; Dong, Q.; et al. Clopidogrel with aspirin in acute minor stroke or transient ischemic attack. *N. Engl. J. Med.* **2013**, *369*, 11–19. [CrossRef] [PubMed]

39. Marwick, T.H. The viable myocardium: Epidemiology, detection, and clinical implications. *Lancet* **1998**, *351*, 815–819. [CrossRef]

40. Allman, K.C.; Shaw, L.J.; Hachamovitch, R.; Udelson, J.E. Myocardial viability testing and impact of revascularization on prognosis in patients with coronary artery disease and left ventricular dysfunction: A meta-analysis. *J. Am. Coll. Cardiol.* **2002**, *39*, 1151–1158. [CrossRef]

41. Sack, G.H., Jr.; Levin, J.; Bell, W.R. Trousseau's syndrome and other manifestations of chronic disseminated coagulopathy in patients with neoplasms: Clinical, pathophysiologic, and therapeutic features. *Medicine (Baltimore)* **1977**, *56*, 1–37. [CrossRef] [PubMed]

42. Katzenstein, A.L.; Myers, J.L.; Mazur, M.T. Acute interstitial pneumonia. A clinicopathologic, ultrastructural, and cell kinetic study. *Am. J. Surg. Pathol.* **1986**, *10*, 256–267. [CrossRef] [PubMed]

43. Kassahun, W.T. The effects of pre-existing dementia on surgical outcomes in emergent and nonemergent general surgical procedures: Assessing differences in surgical risk with dementia. *BMC Geriatr.* **2018**, *18*, 153. [CrossRef] [PubMed]

44. Cramer, J.D.; Patel, U.A.; Samant, S.; Yang, A.; Smith, S.S. Liver disease in patients undergoing head and neck surgery: Incidence and risk for postoperative complications. *Laryngoscope* **2017**, *127*, 102–109. [CrossRef] [PubMed]

45. Piccirillo, J.F.; Lacy, P.D.; Basu, A.; Spitznagel, E.L. Development of a new head and neck cancer-specific comorbidity index. *Arch. Otolaryngol. Head Neck Surg.* **2002**, *128*, 1172–1179. [CrossRef] [PubMed]

46. Siegel, R.; Ward, E.; Brawley, O.; Jemal, A. Cancer statistics, 2011: The impact of eliminating socioeconomic and racial disparities on premature cancer deaths. *CA Cancer J. Clin.* **2011**, *61*, 212–236. [CrossRef] [PubMed]

47. Ward, E.; DeSantis, C.; Robbins, A.; Kohler, B.; Jemal, A. Childhood and adolescent cancer statistics, 2014. *CA Cancer J. Clin.* **2014**, *64*, 83–103. [CrossRef] [PubMed]

48. Dees, E.C.; O'Reilly, S.; Goodman, S.N.; Sartorius, S.; Levine, M.A.; Jones, R.J.; Grochow, L.B.; Donehower, R.C.; Fetting, J.H. A prospective pharmacologic evaluation of age-related toxicity of adjuvant chemotherapy in women with breast cancer. *Cancer Investig.* **2000**, *18*, 521–529. [CrossRef]

49. Gomez, H.; Mas, L.; Casanova, L.; Pen, D.L.; Santillana, S.; Valdivia, S.; Otero, J.; Rodriguez, W.; Carracedo, C.; Vallejos, C. Elderly patients with aggressive non-Hodgkin's lymphoma treated with CHOP chemotherapy plus granulocyte-macrophage colony-stimulating factor: Identification of two age subgroups with differing hematologic toxicity. *J. Clin. Oncol.* **1998**, *16*, 2352–2358. [CrossRef] [PubMed]

50. Schild, S.E.; Stella, P.J.; Geyer, S.M.; Bonner, J.A.; McGinnis, W.L.; Mailliard, J.A.; Brindle, J.; Jatoi, A.; Jett, J.R. The outcome of combined-modality therapy for stage III non-small-cell lung cancer in the elderly. *J. Clin. Oncol.* **2003**, *21*, 3201–3206. [CrossRef] [PubMed]

51. Cheng, C.L.; Lee, C.H.; Chen, P.S.; Li, Y.H.; Lin, S.J.; Yang, Y.H. Validation of acute myocardial infarction cases in the national health insurance research database in Taiwan. *J. Epidemiol.* **2014**, *24*, 500–507. [CrossRef] [PubMed]

52. Hsing, A.W.; Ioannidis, J.P. Nationwide Population Science: Lessons from the Taiwan National Health Insurance Research Database. *JAMA Intern. Med.* **2015**, *175*, 1527–1529. [CrossRef] [PubMed]

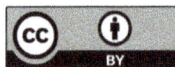

Brief Report

Breast Cancer Prognosis Using a Machine Learning Approach

Patrizia Ferroni [1,2,*], **Fabio M. Zanzotto** [3], **Silvia Riondino** [1,4], **Noemi Scarpato** [2], **Fiorella Guadagni** [1,2] **and Mario Roselli** [4]

1   BioBIM (InterInstitutional Multidisciplinary Biobank), IRCCS San Raffaele Pisana, Via di Val Cannuta 247, 00166 Rome, Italy; silvia.riondino@sanraffaele.it (S.R.); fiorella.guadagni@sanraffaele.it (F.G.)

2   Department of Human Sciences & Quality of Life Promotion, San Raffaele Roma Open University, Via di Val Cannuta 247, 00166 Rome, Italy; noemi.scarpato@unisanraffaele.gov.it

3   Department of Enterprise Engineering, University of Rome "Tor Vergata", Viale Oxford 81, 00133 Rome, Italy; fabio.massimo.zanzotto@uniroma2.it

4   Department of Systems Medicine, Medical Oncology, Tor Vergata Clinical Center, University of Rome "Tor Vergata", Viale Oxford 81, 00133 Rome, Italy; mario.roselli@uniroma2.it

*   Correspondence: patrizia.ferroni@sanraffaele.it or ferronipatrizia@gmail.com; Tel.: +39-06-52253733; Fax: +39-(06)-52255668

Received: 18 December 2018; Accepted: 4 March 2019; Published: 7 March 2019

Abstract: Machine learning (ML) has been recently introduced to develop prognostic classification models that can be used to predict outcomes in individual cancer patients. Here, we report the significance of an ML-based decision support system (DSS), combined with random optimization (RO), to extract prognostic information from routinely collected demographic, clinical and biochemical data of breast cancer (BC) patients. A DSS model was developed in a training set ($n = 318$), whose performance analysis in the testing set ($n = 136$) resulted in a C-index for progression-free survival of 0.84, with an accuracy of 86%. Furthermore, the model was capable of stratifying the testing set into two groups of patients with low- or high-risk of progression with a hazard ratio (HR) of 10.9 ($p < 0.0001$). Validation in multicenter prospective studies and appropriate management of privacy issues in relation to digital electronic health records (EHR) data are presently needed. Nonetheless, we may conclude that the implementation of ML algorithms and RO models into EHR data might help to achieve prognostic information, and has the potential to revolutionize the practice of personalized medicine.

Keywords: breast cancer prognosis; artificial intelligence; machine learning; decision support systems

1. Introduction

The breast cancer (BC) death rate has declined steadily over the past two decades, progress that can be attributed to the deployment of innovative management pathways, from early detection to treatment. Nevertheless, BC still represents the leading cause of cancer death among females worldwide [1]. Accordingly, BC survivability prediction represents a challenging task that could strongly benefit from the development of personalized predictive models. In this context, contemporary oncology has witnessed a growing interest in digital technologies, whose integration with big healthcare data has raised new hopes for personalized medicine.

Artificial intelligence (AI) and machine learning (ML) have been used to diagnose and classify cancer for nearly 20 years, but only a few studies have investigated their relevance in cancer prognosis [2]. In particular, ML or semi-supervised learning techniques have been recently applied to develop models for BC progression and survivability. Most of them, however, were built on datasets from the SEER (Surveillance Program, Epidemiology, and End Results), not including important prognostic parameters such as the St. Gallen criteria (hormones receptor status, HER2/Neu expression or Ki67 proliferation index) [3–5], while other studies were performed on hybrid models containing microarray data [6] or on mammographic images [7,8]. Lately, an unsupervised ML approach that can admit any number of prognostic factors, was used to build prognostic systems for cancer patients [9]. Also, in this case, the SEER dataset used did not include information on HER2/Neu expression, whose prognostic significance has been emphasized in the 8th edition TNM staging system for BC [10]. Thus, the unmet need to develop prognostic classification models that embody the newest AI technologies and can be used to predict outcomes in individual cancer patients for personalized patient care has been highlighted [11].

In this context, we have recently demonstrated the potential of a semi-explainable decision support system (DSS), based on multiple kernel learning (MKL) [12], that can be adapted to different medical problems [13,14] and gives the possibility to inspect the learned model. The model combines a support vector machine (SVM) [15] algorithm and random optimization (RO) [16]. Hence, it can offer an explanation on how routinely collected demographic, clinical and biochemical data are important in predictions. This MKL model, originally developed for cancer-associated thrombosis risk assessment [13], has been here adapted to estimate the risk of disease progression in an oncology setting of BC patients. To achieve this objective, a proof-of-concept study was specifically designed to assess whether a customized MKL-based DSS could be a useful prognostic tool in the clinical management of BC patients.

2. Results

A set of predictors (named ML-RO) was identified using a 3-fold cross-validation technique on a training set (n = 318). A testing set (n = 136) was used to compute the final performance of risk predictors. To devise the DSS, we selected ML-RO-4 as the best performing out of a range of ten runs, in terms of the area under the curve (AUC), on the training set (Table 1).

Table 1. Analytical performance of machine learning with random optimization in the training set.

ML Predictor	AUC (SE)	95% CI	Sensitivity (95% CI)	Specificity (95% CI)	+LR	−LR
ML-RO-4	0.778 (0.0290)	0.728–0.822	67.1 (55.4–77.5)	88.4 (83.7–92.2)	5.80	0.37
ML-RO-1	0.769 (0.0293)	0.719–0.814	65.8 (54.0–76.3)	88.0 (83.2–91.8)	5.49	0.39
ML-RO-7	0.767 (0.0293)	0.717–0.813	67.1 (55.4–77.5)	86.4 (81.4–90.4)	4.92	0.38
ML-RO-3	0.759 (0.0296)	0.708–0.805	65.8 (54.0–76.3)	86.0 (80.9–90.1)	4.68	0.40
ML-RO-6	0.759 (0.0296)	0.708–0.805	65.8 (54.0–76.3)	86.0 (80.9–90.1)	4.68	0.40
ML-RO-8	0.755 (0.0297)	0.703–0.801	65.8 (54.0–76.3)	85.1 (80.0–89.4)	4.42	0.40
ML-RO-0	0.753 (0.0297)	0.701–0.799	65.8 (54.0–76.3)	84.7 (79.5–89.0)	4.30	0.40
ML-RO-2	0.748 (0.0299)	0.697–0.795	64.5 (52.7–75.1)	85.1 (80.0–89.4)	4.33	0.42
ML-RO-9	0.739 (0.0302)	0.687–0.786	61.8 (50.0–72.8)	86.0 (80.9–90.1)	4.40	0.44
ML-RO-5	0.722 (0.0306)	0.669–0.770	59.2 (47.3–70.4)	85.1 (80.0–89.4)	3.98	0.48

AUC: Area under the curve; CI: Confidence interval; LR: Likelihood ratio; ML: Machine learning; RO: Random optimization.

As shown in Table 1, most predictors had a receiver operating characteristic (ROC) curve with an AUC $\geq$0.75 (the threshold generally accepted as clinically useful) [17]. Among these, ML-RO-0 was further selected as it provided a major relative importance to the group of features linked to glucose metabolism (Group 5) (Table 2), which is currently considered an important contributor to BC progression [18,19], at the point that metformin—an anti-diabetic drug with insulin-lowering effects—has been proposed in combination with chemotherapy [20,21] and is currently being considered vs. placebo in a phase-III randomized trial in early stage BC (ClinicalTrials.gov Identifier: NCT01101438).

Table 2. Weights of attribute groups in the training set.

Method	Group					Sum of the Weights	Normalized Group Weights				
	1	2	3	4	5		1	2	3	4	5
ML+RO-4	0.41890	1.04551	0.60311	0.33909	0.58969	2.996321	0.13980	0.34893	0.20128	0.11316	0.19680
ML+RO-0	0.77299	1.86062	1.39445	0.90456	1.00740	5.940053	0.13013	0.31323	0.23475	0.15228	0.16959
ML+RO-6	0.42756	0.91373	1.16514	0.39297	0.58755	3.486968	0.12261	0.26204	0.33414	0.11269	0.16849
ML+RO-8	0.44878	1.28224	0.63075	0.44350	0.53398	3.339267	0.13439	0.38399	0.18888	0.13281	0.15991
ML+RO-1	0.46149	1.17742	0.55782	0.34141	0.47660	3.014770	0.15307	0.39055	0.18503	0.11324	0.15809
ML+RO-7	0.54682	1.40025	0.79264	0.59119	0.61023	3.941154	0.13874	0.35529	0.20112	0.15000	0.15483
ML+RO-3	0.64274	1.13249	0.36078	0.39482	0.45241	2.983255	0.21545	0.37961	0.12093	0.13234	0.15165

Data are absolute numbers for group weights. ML: Machine Learning; RO: Random Optimization.

When both predictors were incorporated into a DSS model for BC progression, their combined use (both positive, either positive, both negative) in the testing set translated in a c-statistic = 0.84 (95% CI: 0.76–0.90). The level with the best Youden index at ROC analysis (>1, i.e., risk estimate achieved by both predictors, according to voting on the positive class) was then selected as the cutoff value for further evaluation of the combined DSS. A comparison of the analytical performance of the trained models and derived DSS on the testing set is reported in Table 3.

Table 3. Analytical performance of machine learning with random optimization in the testing set.

Performance Parameter	ML-RO-0	ML-RO-4	DSS Model [a]
F-measure [b]	0.696	0.677	0.698
Accuracy	0.853	0.838	0.860
Area under the curve (AUC)	0.822	0.813	0.815
(+)LR (95% CI)	9.1 (4.3–20.8)	8.5 (3.9–19.6)	8.6 (4.2–18.0)
(−)LR (95% CI)	0.4 (0.3–0.6)	0.4 (0.3–0.6)	0.4 (0.2–0.5)
HR (95% CI)	10.7 (4.6–24.8)	10.3 (4.5–23.7)	10.9 (4.5–26.6)

LR: Likelihood ratio; C.I.: Confidence interval; HR: Hazard ratio; [a] Analytical performance was evaluated after categorization 0/1 based on risk estimate achieved by both predictors; [b] F-measure represents a harmonic mean of precision [(P) positive predictive value in machine learning] and recall [(R) sensitivity in machine learning] and is calculated as: $2PR/(P+R)$.

At a criterion >1, the DSS model was capable of stratifying primary BC patients into two groups with a low- or high-risk of progression, either in the training (n = 279; log-rank = 3.23, p = 0.001) or in the testing set (n = 118; log-rank = 3.42, p < 0.001). Figure 1 reports the Kaplan–Meier curves of progression-free survival (PFS) in the 136 BC women included in the testing set and followed-up for a mean time of 3.5 years (ranging from 0.3–9.7 years). As shown, patients estimated at high risk (>1) of progression by the combined DSS model had a 5-year progression-free survival probability significantly lower than that observed in BC patients estimated at low-risk (≤1) (26% vs. 85%, respectively; log-rank = 6.82, p < 0.0001).

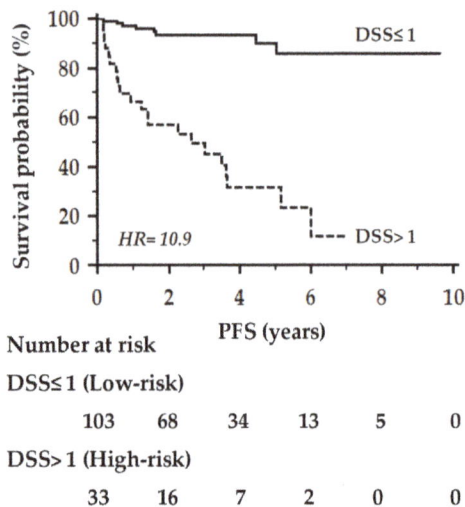

Number at risk

DSS≤1 (Low-risk)

	103	68	34	13	5	0

DSS>1 (High-risk)

	33	16	7	2	0	0

Figure 1. Kaplan–Meier curves of progression-free survival (PFS) of the 136 BC women included in the testing set. Comparison between patients at high (>1) or low-risk (≤1) of progression by the combined decision support system (DSS) model.

3. Discussion

Treatment decisions are particularly challenging in early-stage BC patients with conflicting prognostic features, especially node-negative ones, in which the question of whether to pursue an adjuvant treatment with chemotherapy or endocrine therapies is still unclear. Putative biomarkers, so far, have not demonstrated sufficient predictive ability to be clinically useful. Ki67 itself lacks reproducibility and its use, if not part of an AI model, has been largely re-dimensioned [22].

Identification of predictive tools of tumor responsiveness, risk of recurrence, and mortality, providing the possibility to avoid unnecessary toxicities are thus very appealing. As reported above, ML has started to take hold across the oncology community to develop prognostic classifications models of BC progression and survivability [9]. In this regard, the possibility to perform an automated survival prediction in metastatic cancer patients using high-dimensional electronic health records (EHR) data has been recently highlighted [23]. By using an ML approach on EHR-derived predictor variables (clustered into categories), Gensheimer et al., in fact, devised an AI system, with a better c-statistic than previously reported prognostic models, which could be deployed in a DSS to help improve quality of care in the metastatic setting [23]. More recently, four major nonlinear ML methods (integrating multiple clinicopathological features and genomic data) were used to compare survival predictions in a large cohort of BC patients [24]. Although no model significantly outperformed others, the Nottingham Prognostic Index, age, tumor stage and size, ER/PR/HER2 and breast surgery status strongly influenced survival across repeated runs and models, while the gene expression cluster was a moderately influential factor [24].

The results here reported confirm and extend the findings by Zhao et al., as the use of an SVM has proven effective in devising an AI-based DSS for the prognostic assessment of non-metastatic BC patients. In particular, the combined use of ML and RO techniques, allowed the construction of a set of prognostic discriminators from routinely collected clinicopathological features and biochemical data of BC patients, which showed a better performance than the predictors developed by Zhao et al. (c-statistic 0.82 vs. 0.66 and an accuracy of 86% vs. 73%, respectively) [24]. In our opinion, this combined approach might hold potential for improving model precision through weighting the relative importance of attributes. Moreover, with respect to models based on neural networks [7], the combination of ML and RO techniques offers a model that can be learned with small datasets and that is more interpretable, as were Bayesian networks applied to BC [25]. Furthermore, the devised DSS included a number of prognostic and metabolic parameters, not previously analyzed, that could be easily extracted by EHR, meaning that ML may add significant and sustained benefits to personalized medicine at no additional cost to the health system.

Of course, there are limitations to acknowledge. First, the study was mono-institutional. Second, the sample size was relatively small, which may have lowered the power of ML. Nonetheless, we believe that implementation of ML algorithms and RO models into high-dimensional EHR data might help to achieve prognostic information, and has the potential to revolutionize the practice of personalized medicine.

4. Patients and Methods

Starting from January 2007, the PTV Bio.Ca.Re. (Policlinico Tor Vergata Biospecimen Cancer Repository) and the SR-BioBIM (Interinstitutional Multidisciplinary Biobank, IRCCS San Raffaele Pisana, Rome, Italy) are actively involved in the recruitment of ambulatory patients with primary or metastatic cancer, who are prospectively followed under the appropriate institutional ethics approval, as part of a Clinical Database and Biobank project. Among these, a cohort of 454 consecutive BC patients in whom prognostic and pre-treatment biochemical factors were available, were selected for the present analysis. The study was performed in accordance with the principles embodied in the Declaration of Helsinki. All patients gave written informed consent, previously approved by our Institutional Ethics Committee (ISR/DMLBA/405, 15 November 2006). BC was pathologically staged according to the latest prognostic TNM staging system [8]. Three hundred and ninety-seven women (87%) had primary BC and underwent radical surgery followed by radiation and/or adjuvant treatment as per current guidelines. The remaining 57 (13%) patients presented with metastatic disease. Prognostic routinely-collected factors such as BC stage, menopausal status, pathological grading as well as the St. Gallen criteria (e.g., estrogen and progesterone receptors, HER2/neu expression and the proliferation index Ki67) were available for each patient. In particular, grading was assessed according to the Nottingham grading system (Elston–Ellis modification of the Scarff–Bloom–Richardson grading system) for BC [8]. The immunohistochemical analyses were performed on formalin-fixed, paraffin-embedded tumor sections for hormone receptor presence [26], HER2/neu expression [27] and proliferation index (Ki67) [28]. HER2/neu positivity was defined according to the American Society of Clinical Oncology-College of American Pathologists (ASCO-CAP) guidelines as an immunohistochemical staining of 3+ or 2+ with evidence of gene amplification by fluorescence in situ hybridization (FISH) [27]. The Ki67 proliferative index in surgical specimens was assigned by the pathologist based on the percentage of positivity on at least 500 neoplastic cells counted in the peripheral area of the nodule. A cut–off value of $\geq$20% was used in all association analyses, according to the recommendations of the St. Gallen International Expert Consensus on the primary therapy of early BC 2013 [28].

Furthermore, given the increasing awareness that metabolic features might represent an important contributor to BC progression, Type 2 diabetes, glycemic parameters and the body mass index (BMI) were introduced in the model [18,19]. Routine biochemical analyses were performed on fresh blood samples taken in the morning after an overnight fast at the time of enrolment and prior to any treatment (surgery, adjuvant, either chemotherapy or endocrine, or metastatic). The demographic and clinical characteristics of the recruited population are summarized in Table 4.

Table 4. Clinical-pathological characteristics of breast cancer (BC) patients. Comparison between training and testing set.

Clinical-Pathological Characteristics	Training Set (*n* = 318)	Testing Set (*n* = 136)
Age (years), Mean ± SD	56 ± 13	57 ± 12
Menopausal status, N (%)		
Pre	141 (44)	51 (38)
Post	177 (56)	85 (63)
Body Mass Index, Mean ± SD	25.2 ± 4.5	25.7 ± 5.2
Histological diagnosis, N (%)		
Ductal	263 (83)	121 (89)
Lobular	37 (12)	9 (7)
Others	18 (5)	6 (4)
Molecular Type [a], N (%)		
Triple-negative	39 (12)	17 (12)
Luminal-like A	97 (31)	37 (27)
Luminal-like B	172 (54)	77 (57)
HER2 pos	10 (3)	5 (4)
Grading, N (%) [b]		
1	20 (7)	15 (13)
2	108 (39)	45 (38)
3	151 (54)	58 (49)
Tumor, N (%) [b]		
T1	141 (50)	59 (50)
T2	91 (33)	42 (36)
T3	28 (10)	5 (4)
T4	19 (7)	12 (10)
Node, N (%) [b]		
N0	134 (48)	54 (46)
N+	145 (52)	64 (54)
Prognostic stage, N (%)		
I	177 (56)	70 (50)
II	53 (17)	20 (15)
III	45 (14)	26 (19)
IV	4 (1)	2 (1)
Metastatic	39 (12)	18 (13)
Receptor status, N (%) [c]		
ER+/PR+	235 (74)	94 (69)
ER+/PR−	29 (9)	19 (14)
ER-/PR+	5 (2)	1 (1)
ER-/PR−	49 (15)	22 (16)
HER2/neu+, N (%) [c]	66 (21)	34 (25)
Ki67 proliferation index ≥20%, N (%) [c]	204 (67)	93 (71)
Type 2 Diabetes, N (%)	39 (12)	11 (8%)
Glucose metabolic asset [d]		
Fasting blood glucose (mg/dl), Mean ± SD	105 ± 31	102 ± 32
Fasting insulin (μIU/ml), Median (IQR)	11.9 (6.4–27.0)	10.6 (5.6–19.6)
HbA$_{1c}$ (%), Mean ± SD	5.8 ± 0.8	5.8 ± 0.7
HOMA Index, Mean ± SD	3.0 (1.4–8.3)	2.9 (1.2–6.3)
Follow-up (years)		
Mean (range)	3.4 (0.29–10.5)	3.5 (0.26–9.65)

[a] According to St. Gallen Consensus Conference. [b] Evaluated at time of diagnosis. [c] Evaluated in a population of 397 primary breast cancer patients. [d] Evaluated at time of enrollment and prior to any treatment. ER/PR: estrogen/progesterone receptors; HER2: Human epidermal growth factor receptor 2; IQR: Interquartile range; HbA$_{1c}$: Glycosylated hemoglobin; HOMA Index: Homeostasis model assessment index.

The machine learning used for the primary analysis was run using the kernel-based learning platform (KeLP) [29], as previously reported [13]. Multiple kernel learning (MKL), based on support vector machines (SVM) and random optimization (RO) models, were used to produce prognostic discriminators (referred as machine-learning (ML)-RO) yielding the best classification performance over a training (3-fold cross-validation) and testing set. The training set consisted of 318 BC patients (70% of the dataset); the remaining 136 patients were allocated to the testing set (30% of the cases). No significant difference was observed for demographic, clinical and biochemical characteristics between the training and testing set (Table 4). The numerical attributes were analyzed as continuous values. Missing clinical attribute values were treated according to the predictive value imputation (PVI) method by replacing missing values with the average of the attribute observed in the training set. The variables were clustered into five groups according to clinical significance. A detailed list of all the features applied to construct the predictor is reported in Table 5. RO was used to devise their relative weights in the final prediction. In RO, relative weights are initialized with a random number and estimated by maximizing performance in the 3-fold cross-validation. These weights can be used to interpret the importance of the groups of features within the model. Thus, the final DSS is interpretable.

Table 5. Features included in the model.

Patient-Related	Tumor-Related	Biochemical
Group 1: Age Menopausal status Body Mass Index	**Group 2:** Molecular type Histological diagnosis Grading TNM stage	**Group 4:** Total BilirubinCreatinine
	Group 3: Estrogen receptors Progesterone receptors HER2/NEU Ki67 proliferation index	**Group 5:** Fasting glycemia Fasting insulinemia Glycosylated hemoglobin HOMA index (insulin resistance) Type 2 diabetes

Statistical analysis

The receiver operating characteristic (ROC) curve and univariate Cox proportional hazards analyses were performed by MedCalc Statistical Software version 13.1.2 (MedCalc Software bvba, Ostend, Belgium). The area under the curve (AUC) was calculated on a three-level risk: 2 (if both predictors estimated the risk), 1 (if only one predictor estimated the risk) or 0 (if both predictors did not estimate the risk) to investigate whether the combined DSS could distinguish between recurrent and non-recurrent patients. The level with the best Youden index (>1, i.e., risk estimate achieved by both predictors) was selected as the cutoff value for the combined DSS. Bayesian analysis was performed, and positive (+LR) and negative (−LR) likelihood ratios were used to estimate the probability of BC progression. The survival curves were calculated by the Kaplan–Meier and log-rank methods using computer software packages (MedCalc Software bvba, Ostend, Belgium and Statistica 8.0, StatSoft Inc., Tulsa, OK, USA). The PFS represented the study endpoint and was calculated from the date of enrollment until disease progression. The patients who had no disease progression were censored at the time of the last follow-up. For administrative censoring, the follow-up ended on 31 December, 2017. All tests were two-tailed and only *p*-values lower than 0.05 were regarded as statistically significant.

5. Conclusions

ML has recently started to take hold across the oncology community to develop prognostic classifications models of cancer progression and survivability. In our opinion, a combined approach of ML algorithms and RO models might hold potential for improving model precision through weighting the relative importance of attributes. In line with the actual trend, in fact, the proposed model seeks not only decision, but also interpretability of the model itself, which, together with the use of a real-world BC dataset, represents the novel aspect of our research. Validation in multicenter prospective studies and appropriate management of privacy issues in relation to digital EHR data are required before making any ML approach into the clinical practice available.

Author Contributions: P.F. and M.R. designed the study, analyzed and interpreted the clinical data, and wrote the manuscript; F.M.Z. and N.S. designed the algorithm, performed the machine learning experiments, and wrote the manuscript; S.R. collected clinical and laboratory data, interpreted the data and wrote the manuscript; F.G. designed the study, analyzed and interpreted the data, and critically revised the manuscript. All authors revised and approved the final version of the manuscript.

Funding: This work was partially supported by the European Social Fund, under the Italian Ministries of Education, University and Research (PNR 2015-2020 ARS01_01163 PerMedNet—CUP B66G18000220005) and Economic Development ("HORIZON 2020" PON I&C 2014-2020—F/050383/01-03/X32).

Conflicts of Interest: The authors declare no conflict of interest.

References

1. Torre, L.A.; Bray, F.; Siegel, R.L.; Ferlay, J.; Lortet-Tieulent, J.; Jemal, A. Global cancer statistics, 2012. *CA Cancer J. Clin.* **2015**, *65*, 87–108. [CrossRef] [PubMed]

2. Kourou, K.; Exarchos, T.P.; Exarchos, K.P.; Karamouzis, M.V.; Fotiadis, D.I. Machine learning applications in cancer prognosis and prediction. *Comput. Struct. Biotechnol. J.* **2014**, *13*, 8–17. [CrossRef] [PubMed]

3. Delen, D.; Walker, G.; Kadam, A. Predicting breast cancer survivability: A comparison of three data mining methods. *Artif. Intell. Med.* **2005**, *34*, 113–127. [CrossRef] [PubMed]

4. Kim, J.; Shin, H. Breast cancer survivability prediction using labeled, unlabeled, and pseudo-labeled patient data. *J. Am. Med. Inform. Assoc.* **2013**, *20*, 613–618. [CrossRef] [PubMed]

5. Park, K.; Ali, A.; Kim, D.; An, Y.; Kim, M.; Shin, H. Robust predictive model for evaluating breast cancer survivability. *Eng. Appl. Artif. Intell.* **2013**, *26*, 2194–2205. [CrossRef]

6. Sun, Y.; Goodison, S.; Li, J.; Liu, L.; Farmerie, W. Improved breast cancer prognosis through the combination of clinical and genetic markers. *Bioinformatics* **2007**, *23*, 30–37. [CrossRef] [PubMed]

7. Burt, J.R.; Torosdagli, N.; Khosravan, N.; RaviPrakash, H.; Mortazi, A.; Tissavirasingham, F.; Hussein, S.; Bagci, U. Deep learning beyond cats and dogs: Recent advances in diagnosing breast cancer with deep neural networks. *Br. J. Radiol.* **2018**, *91*, 20170545. [CrossRef] [PubMed]

8. Yousefi, B.; Ting, H.N.; Mirhassani, S.M.; Hosseini, M. Development of computer-aided detection of breast lesion using gabor-wavelet BASED features in mammographic images. In Proceedings of the 2013 IEEE International Conference on Control System, Computing and Engineering (ICCSCE), Penang, Malaysia, 29 November–1 December 2013; pp. 127–131.

9. Hueman, M.T.; Wang, H.; Yang, C.Q.; Sheng, L.; Henson, D.E.; Schwartz, A.M.; Chen, D. Creating prognostic systems for cancer patients: A demonstration using breast cancer. *Cancer Med.* **2018**, *7*, 3611–3621. [CrossRef] [PubMed]

10. Amin, M.B.; Edge, S.; Greene, F.; Byrd, D.R.; Brookland, R.K.; Washington, M.K.; Gershenwald, J.E.; Compton, C.C.; Hess, K.R.; Sullivan, D.C.; et al. (Eds.) *AJCC Cancer Staging Manual*, 8th ed.; Springer: New York, NY, USA, 2017.

11. O'Sullivan, B.; Brierley, J.; Byrd, D.; Bosman, F.; Kehoe, S.; Kossary, C.; Piñeros, M.; Van Eycken, E.; Weir, H.K.; Gospodarowicz, M. The TNM classification of malignant tumours-towards common understanding and reasonable expectations. *Lancet Oncol.* **2017**, *18*, 849–851. [CrossRef]

12. Gönen, M.; Alpaydın, E. Multiple kernel learning algorithms. *J. Mach. Learn. Res.* **2011**, *12*, 2211–2268.

13. Ferroni, P.; Zanzotto, F.M.; Scarpato, N.; Riondino, S.; Nanni, U.; Roselli, M.; Guadagni, F. Risk assessment for venous thromboembolism in chemotherapy treated ambulatory cancer patients: A precision medicine approach. *Med. Dec. Mak.* **2017**, *37*, 234–242. [CrossRef] [PubMed]

14. Ferroni, P.; Roselli, M.; Zanzotto, F.M.; Guadagni, F. Artificial Intelligence for cancer-associated thrombosis risk assessment. *Lancet Haematol.* **2018**, *5*, e391. [CrossRef]

15. Cristianini, N.; Shawe-Taylor, J. An Introduction to Support Vector Machines and other kernel based learning methods. *Ai Magazine* **2000**, *22*, 190.

16. Matyas, J. Random optimization. *Automat. Rem. Control* **1965**, *26*, 246–253.

17. Fan, J.; Upadhye, S.; Worster, A. Understanding receiver operating characteristic (ROC) curves. *Can. J. Emerg. Med.* **2006**, *8*, 19–20. [CrossRef]

18. Zhu, Q.L.; Xu, W.H.; Tao, M.H. Biomarkers of the Metabolic Syndrome and Breast Cancer Prognosis. *Cancers* **2010**, *2*, 721–739. [CrossRef] [PubMed]

19. Ferroni, P.; Riondino, S.; Laudisi, A.; Portarena, I.; Formica, V.; Alessandroni, J.; D'Alessandro, R.; Orlandi, A.; Costarelli, L.; Cavaliere, F.; et al. Pre-treatment insulin levels as a prognostic factor for breast cancer progression. *Oncologist* **2016**, *21*, 1041–1049. [CrossRef] [PubMed]

20. Yam, C.; Esteva, F.J.; Patel, M.M.; Raghavendra, A.S.; Ueno, N.T.; Moulder, S.L.; Hess, K.R.; Shroff, G.S.; Hodge, S.; Koenig, K.H.; et al. Efficacy and safety of the combination of metformin, everolimus and exemestane in overweight and obese postmenopausal patients with metastatic, hormone receptor-positive, HER2-negative breast cancer: A phase II study. *Investig. New Drugs* **2019**. [CrossRef] [PubMed]

21. Martin-Castillo, B.; Pernas, S.; Dorca, J.; Álvarez, I.; Martínez, S.; Pérez-Garcia, J.M.; Batista-López, N.; Rodríguez-Sánchez, C.A.; Amillano, K.; Domínguez, S.; et al. A phase 2 trial of neoadjuvant metformin in combination with trastuzumab and chemotherapy in women with early HER2-positive breast cancer: The METTEN study. *Oncotarget* **2018**, *9*, 35687–35704. [CrossRef] [PubMed]

22. Thakur, S.S.; Li, H.; Chan, A.M.Y.; Tudor, R.; Bigras, G.; Morris, D.; Enwere, E.K.; Yang, H. The use of automated Ki67 analysis to predict Oncotype DX risk-of-recurrence categories in early-stage breast cancer. *PLoS ONE* **2018**, *13*, e0188983. [CrossRef] [PubMed]

23. Gensheimer, M.F.; Henry, A.S.; Wood, D.J.; Hastie, T.J.; Aggarwal, S.; Dudley, S.A.; Pradhan, P.; Banerjee, I.; Cho, E.; Ramchandran, K.; et al. Automated survival prediction in metastatic cancer patients using high-dimensional electronic medical record data. *J. Natl. Cancer Inst.* **2019**, *111*, djy178. [CrossRef] [PubMed]

24. Zhao, M.; Tang, Y.; Kim, H.; Hasegawa, K. Machine learning with k-means dimensional reduction for predicting survival outcomes in patients with breast cancer. *Cancer Inf.* **2018**, *17*, 1–7. [CrossRef] [PubMed]

25. Cruz-Ramírez, N.; Acosta-Mesa, H.G.; Carrillo-Calvet, H.; Nava-Fernández, L.A.; Barrientos-Martínez, R.E. Diagnosis of breast cancer using Bayesian networks: A case study. *Comput. Biol. Med.* **2007**, *37*, 1553–1564. [CrossRef] [PubMed]

26. Hammond, M.E.; Hayes, D.F.; Dowsett, M.; Allred, D.C.; Hagerty, K.L.; Badve, S.; Fitzgibbons, P.L.; Francis, G.; Goldstein, N.S.; Hayes, M.; et al. American Society of Clinical Oncology/College of American Pathologists guideline recommendations for immunohistochemical testing of estrogen and progesterone receptors in breast cancer. *J. Clin. Oncol.* **2010**, *28*, 2784–2795. [CrossRef] [PubMed]

27. Wolff, A.C.; Hammond, M.E.; Schwartz, J.N.; Hagerty, K.L.; Allred, D.C.; Cote, R.J.; Dowsett, M.; Fitzgibbons, P.L.; Hanna, W.M.; Langer, A.; et al. American Society of Clinical Oncology/College of American Pathologists. American Society of Clinical Oncology/College of American Pathologists guideline recommendations for human epidermal growth factor receptor 2 testing in breast cancer. *Arch. Pathol. Lab. Med.* **2007**, *131*, 18–43. [PubMed]

28. Goldhirsch, A.; Winer, E.P.; Coates, A.S.; Gelber, R.D.; Piccart-Gebhart, M.; Thürlimann, B.; Senn, H.J.; Panel Members. Personalizing the treatment of women with early breast cancer: Highlights of the St Gallen International Expert Consensus on the Primary Therapy of Early Breast Cancer 2013. *Ann. Oncol.* **2013**, *24*, 2206–2223. [CrossRef] [PubMed]

29. Filice, S.; Castellucci, G.; Croce, D.; Basili, R. KeLP: A Kernel-based Learning Platform for Natural Language Processing. In Proceedings of the ACL-IJCNLP 2015 System Demonstrations, Beijing, China, 26–31 July 2015; pp. 19–24.

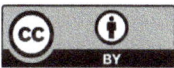

cancers

MDPI

Article

Mining of Self-Organizing Map Gene-Expression Portraits Reveals Prognostic Stratification of HPV-Positive Head and Neck Squamous Cell Carcinoma

Laura D. Locati [1,†], Mara S. Serafini [2,†], Maria F. Iannò [2], Andrea Carenzo [2], Ester Orlandi [3], Carlo Resteghini [1], Stefano Cavalieri [1], Paolo Bossi [1], Silvana Canevari [2], Lisa Licitra [1,4] and Loris De Cecco [2,*]

[1] Head and Neck Medical Oncology Department, Fondazione IRCCS Istituto Nazionale dei Tumori di Milano, 20133 Milan, Italy
[2] Integrated Biology Platform, Department of Applied Research and Technology Development, Fondazione IRCCS Istituto Nazionale dei Tumori di Milano, 20133 Milan, Italy
[3] Radiation Oncology Department, Fondazione IRCCS Istituto Nazionale dei Tumori di Milano, 20133 Milan, Italy
[4] Department of Oncology, University of Milan, 20122 Milan, Italy
*   Correspondence: loris.dececco@istitutotumori.mi.it
†   Authors contributed equally to this paper.

Received: 10 July 2019; Accepted: 24 July 2019; Published: 26 July 2019

Abstract: Patients (pts) with head and neck squamous cell carcinoma (HNSCC) have different epidemiologic, clinical, and outcome behaviors in relation to human papillomavirus (HPV) infection status, with HPV-positive patients having a 70% reduction in their risk of death. Little is known about the molecular heterogeneity in HPV-related cases. In the present study, we aim to disclose the molecular subtypes with potential biological and clinical relevance. Through a literature review, 11 studies were retrieved with a total of 346 gene-expression data points from HPV-positive HNSCC pts. Meta-analysis and self-organizing map (SOM) approaches were used to disclose relevant meta-gene portraits. Unsupervised consensus clustering provided evidence of three biological subtypes in HPV-positive HNSCC: Cl1, immune-related; Cl2, epithelial–mesenchymal transition-related; Cl3, proliferation-related. This stratification has a prognostic relevance, with Cl1 having the best outcome, Cl2 the worst, and Cl3 an intermediate survival rate. Compared to recent literature, which identified immune and keratinocyte subtypes in HPV-related HNSCC, we confirmed the former and we separated the latter into two clusters with different biological and prognostic characteristics. At present, this paper reports the largest meta-analysis of HPV-positive HNSCC studies and offers a promising molecular subtype classification. Upon further validation, this stratification could improve patient selection and pave the way for the development of a precision medicine therapeutic approach.

Keywords: self-organizing map; head and neck cancer; treatment de-escalation; HP; molecular subtypes; tumor microenvironment

1. Introduction

Worldwide, head and neck squamous cell carcinoma (HNSCC) affects more than 550,000 patient cases/year with around 380,000 deaths annually [1]. Traditionally, alcohol exposure and tobacco smoking are identified as exogenous risk factors. However, human papillomavirus (HPV) infection, caused predominantly by HPV type 16, is currently recognized as an independent causal factor for the development of HNSCC. Since the 1990s, there was a significant increase in HPV-related HNSCC in western countries, whilst the incidence of HPV-negative HNSCC is globally declining [2,3], in parallel with the decline in tobacco smoking rates. This high incidence of HPV-positive cases establishes HNSCC as one of the most common HPV-related cancers, second only to cervical cancer [4]. Moreover, it is estimated that the annual incidence could increase and eventually surpass the annual incidence of cervical cancer by 2020. Previous epidemiological studies showed that around 25% of all HNSCCs are related to HPV infection, with a tendency for the oropharynx (OPSCC) to be the specific site, compared to infection in other sites (oral cavity, larynx, and hypopharynx) [5]. It is known that HPV-related HNSCC patients have different epidemiologic and clinical behaviors in comparison with HPV-negative HNSCC patients, allowing the identification of HPV-positive HNSCC as a specific distinct disease with peculiar prognostic characteristics [6]. In fact, HPV-positive HNSCC is diagnosed at a younger age than HPV-negative HNSCC, and the five-year survival rate for HPV-positive HNSCC is 60–90% as compared with 20–70% for HPV-negative HNSCC [7], conferring a more favorable prognosis for HPV-positive HNSCC patients. The differences in outcomes between HPV-positive and HPV-negative tumors were already provided, and a multitude of molecular differences comparing HPV-negative and HPV-positive HNSCC patients were reported [8–10]. However, a clear biological picture behind their broad diversity is not yet elucidated. Moreover, considering the better prognosis of HPV-positive HNSCC patients compared with their HPV-negative HNSCC counterparts and the median younger age of patients at diagnosis, the question about how to treat HPV-positive patients requires an answer. De-escalation of treatment protocols, for this subgroup of patients, is currently ongoing [11], with the final aim being to reduce the intensity of treatments (both chemoradiation and surgery) and the burden of treatment-related toxicities over the next few years. A further investigation on HPV-related HNSCC is needed. As already reported in the literature, in addition to the diversity of HPV-positive HNSCC compared with HPV-negative HNSCC, it is possible to also observe an intrinsic biological heterogeneity in the HPV-positive HNSCC. In particular, we refer to Keck et al. [12], who identified two different clusters on the basis of their gene expression, and to Zhang et al. [13], who classified these two groups as HPV-positive immune-related (HPV-IMU) and HPV-positive with keratinocyte differentiation (HPV-KRT) HNSCC. Both of these studies had the ability to explore the biology related to HPV infection, unfortunately without showing a significant survival difference.

High-throughput technologies allow the assessment of thousands of features, posing challenges to data analysis. To deal with increased data complexity, researchers apply machine learning approaches to improve biological knowledge via intuitive visualization, even at single-sample resolution. This allows questions, such as biomarker discovery and functional biological information mining, to be addressed. A particular method, self-organizing maps (SOM), provides important benefits including dimension reduction, multidimensional scaling, visualization capabilities over alternative methods such as non-negative matrix factorization, and hierarchical clustering [14]. SOM gained immediate attention in the bioinformatics field, and early microarray studies reported its application [15,16]. Since then, a number of studies on different cancer types proved its robustness [17,18].

In the present analysis, we focused our attention on HPV-positive HNSCC with annotated gene expression data and clinical annotations by exploiting a meta-analysis approach. We applied the SOM machine learning method on a total of 346 HPV-positive tumor samples. This allowed us to dissect the molecular heterogeneity of the disease and to make suggestions for de-escalation treatment.

2. Results

2.1. Case Material

In order to dissect the molecular heterogeneity in HPV-positive HNSCC, 11 eligible published studies reporting gene expression data were selected for a systematic survey (Table S1, Supplementary Materials). Of these studies, all but one utilized microarray technology for gene expression analysis, and, in the majority of cases, HPV status was assessed with qPCR or HPV genotyping. The resulting meta-analysis dataset, containing 346 samples and 8254 EntrezID genes, was used for the genomic analysis. HPV infection was assessed by p16 immunohistochemistry (IHC) (13 cases, 4%) or DNA or RNA from HPV testing (333, 96%) (Table S1, Supplementary Materials). All the methods used are recognized and utilized in clinical practice [19].

According to the clinical information (Table 1), a male preponderance (83%) and median age of 58.7 years (range, 35–87) were observed, in line with the epidemiological data reported in the literature. The main subsite of origin was the oropharynx (68%), followed by the oral cavity (17%), larynx (6%), and hypopharynx (3%). Stages, assessed following malignant tumor classification system (TNM edition 7, American Joint Committee on Cancer, AJCC), were divided into stages I–II (35), stages III–IV (229), and information not available (82). Locally advanced stages (III–IV) were the most represented (66%), followed by not available (24%) and early stages (I–II; 10%). Survival data were available for 197 cases (57%) and not present for 149 cases (43%). Smoking habits were reported for 245 patients (169 smokers, 76 never smokers), and were unknown for 101 patients (Table 1).

Table 1. Demographic and clinical data of the head and neck squamous cell carcinoma (HNSCC) human papillomavirus (HPV)-positive patients entered in the meta-analysis.

Characteristics	No.	%
Age, years		
(median; range)	57 (35–87)	77%
Not available	78	23%
Gender (male:female ratio)	287/59	83%/17%
Subsite		
Oropharynx	235	68%
Oral cavity	59	17%
Larynx	20	6%
Hypopharynx	10	3%
Not available	22	6%
Stage according to TNM edition 7		
Stage I–II	35	10%
Stage III–IV	229	66%
Not available	82	24%
Smoking		
Smoker	169	49%
Not smoker	76	22%
Not available	101	29%
Availability of follow-up data		
Yes	197	57%
No	149	43%
Total	**346**	100%

2.2. HPV-Positive HNSCC Tumor Clusters: First-Level Self-Organizing Map (SOM) and Unsupervised Clustering Analysis

We applied the SOM machine learning algorithm to convert the meta-analysis dataset into a matrix of meta-gene expression data. Starting from the 8254 genes, we imposed the log-intensity variation p-value < 0.01, and a data matrix of 3498 genes was yielded. These 3498 genes were aggregated in meta-genes (average 10 genes each), resulting in a matrix of 18 × 18 meta-genes. Consensus unsupervised clustering was applied on the meta-gene data, revealing three clusters of samples.

The cluster had well-defined boundaries, as shown by the consensus heatmap (Figure 1a). To exclude the existence of under-represented clusters, the consistency of sample assignment was evaluated by silhouette plot analysis. The resulting clustering configuration was appropriate (Figure 1b), since most samples in each cluster had a positive value (average $< s >$: Cluster 1, Cl1 = 0.68; Cluster 2, Cl2 = 0.53; Cluster 3, Cl3 = 0.48). Only seven samples (two belonging to Cl2 and five belonging to Cl3), corresponding to 2% of the entire case material, had negative values but were in the range between -0.01 and -0.04. These seven samples were assigned by silhouette analysis, as follows: two Cl2 samples to Cl1, three Cl3 samples to Cl2, and three Cl3 samples to Cl1. We assessed the sample size adequacy by estimating the power for the detection of the three clusters; the robustness of the classification was ensured since at least 87% of genes had a power level of 0.9 (Figure S1, Supplementary Materials). By training the SOM algorithm, each sample was portrayed by displaying its molecular fingerprint. The generated subtype SOM images revealed a series of adjacent mosaic tiles coherently over- or under-expressed, and the resulting gallery of SOM portraits was used to intuitively visualize the coherent cluster patterns. In this way, we highlighted cluster-specific tiles in the SOM portraits, independent of the patient's individuality (Figure 1c).

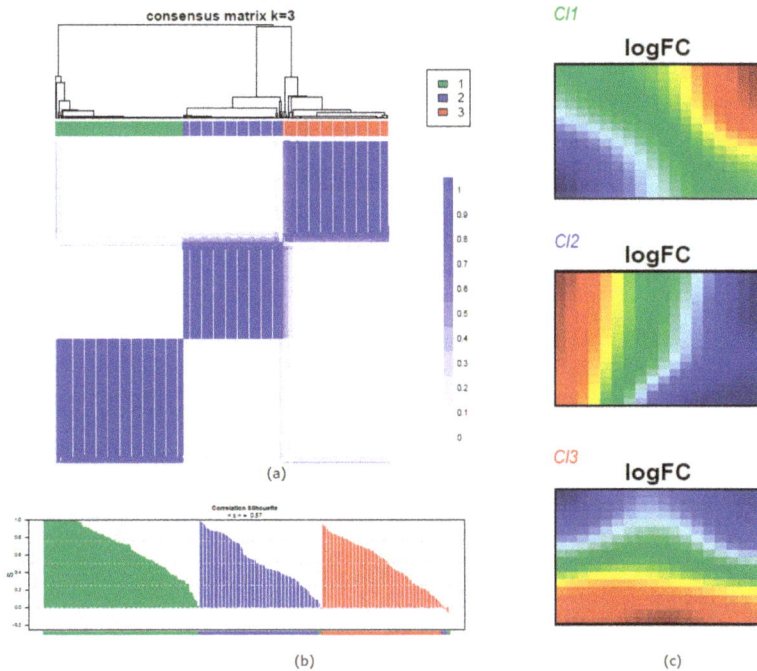

Figure 1. Human papillomavirus (HPV)-positive head and neck squamous cell carcinoma (HNSCC) tumor clusters: first-level self-organizing map (SOM) and unsupervised clustering analysis. (**a**) Consensus matrix heatmap imposing three clusters: Cl1 ($n = 134$; 39%), Cl2 ($n = 104$; 30%), and Cl3 ($n = 108$; 31%). The consensus values are reported in a range from 0 (white, samples that never cluster together) to 1 (blue, samples showing the highest clustering affinity). (**b**) Silhouette plot analysis. The samples are ranked based on silhouette values (S) in each cluster. The heights indicate a strong similarity of the samples within their clusters compared with the samples belonging to other clusters. The colors in the lower bar show the predicted membership by silhouette analysis; the colors correspond to the consensus clustering assignment for all samples with the exception of the seven samples with a negative number but close to 0. (**c**) First level of the SOM gallery of the three clusters with cluster-specific tiles highlighted. The expression patterns are translated into a color code indicating over- and under-expression in a range from red to blue spots, respectively.

We also investigated the influence related to technical sources of variability on our findings. An alluvial diagram was used to show the three-cluster membership, based on the study of origin and the platform used for the expression profiling (Figure 2). The percentage of variation, explained by these variables, was investigated compared with the variation associated with the present cluster stratification, and this is summarized in the violin plots (Figure S2, Supplementary Materials). Our findings supported the biological value behind our three-subtype stratification, with a negligible influence of technical covariates.

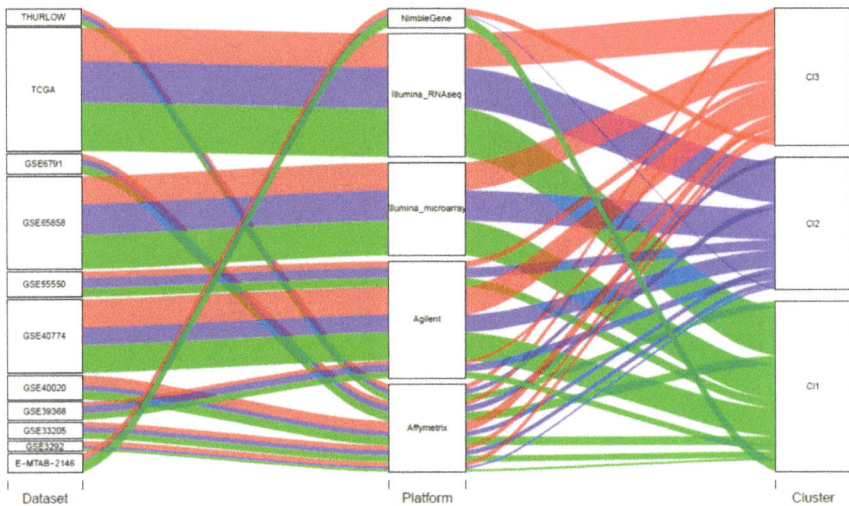

Figure 2. Alluvial diagram. In the diagram, each of the blocks corresponds to the number of features, and the stream fields between the blocks represent changes in the composition of the different blocks. The sizes of the blocks are proportional to the number of samples. We explored the cluster membership taking into account (i) the study of origin of each sample (11 strata); (ii) the different technology platforms used for expression profiling (five strata). Study of the origin: χ^2 test = 12.08, *p*-value = 0.913; Platform χ^2 test = 5.93, *p*-value = 0.655.

2.3. HPV-Positive HNSCC Cluster Similarity Relationships: Second-Level SOM

The second-level SOM analysis investigated the similarity relationships among the first-level sample SOM portraits.

We applied three different sample similarity approaches to estimate the mutual distances among samples, based on metagene expression data and using different metrics and algorithms. The first approach, independent component analysis (ICA), displayed three clusters supporting the identified stratification, although the boundaries between them were not strictly defined (Figure 3a, left panel). Additional information could be retrieved from the three independent components (component 1, component 2, and component 3): the projections onto the component 1/component two axes (Figure 3a, right lower panel) segregated Cluster 1 (Cl1, green spots) from Cl2 and Cl3 (blue and red spots, respectively); however, regions of high density Cl2 and Cl3 showed distinct behavior without clear separation. On the contrary, when the component 1/component three axes were considered, Cl2 and Cl3 were more clearly divided (Figure 3a, right upper panel).

As a second alternative metric, we investigated a correlation network approach: the resulting structure was visualized into a graph to highlight the correlation network (Figure 3b), and it confirmed the presence of a main cluster including Cl1 with few connections to Cl2 and Cl3.

The third approach exploited a Euclidean distance-based approach through the resolution of neighbor-joining (NJ) clustering, which projects the relationships among samples in phylogenetic trees

(Figure 3c). The NJ dendrogram was able to disclose finer details than the previous approaches, and it revealed inherent substructures and their connections in each cluster. By visual inspection, most Cl1 samples were segregated into clearly different branches from Cl2 and Cl3 branches, which, in contrast, appeared tightly correlated.

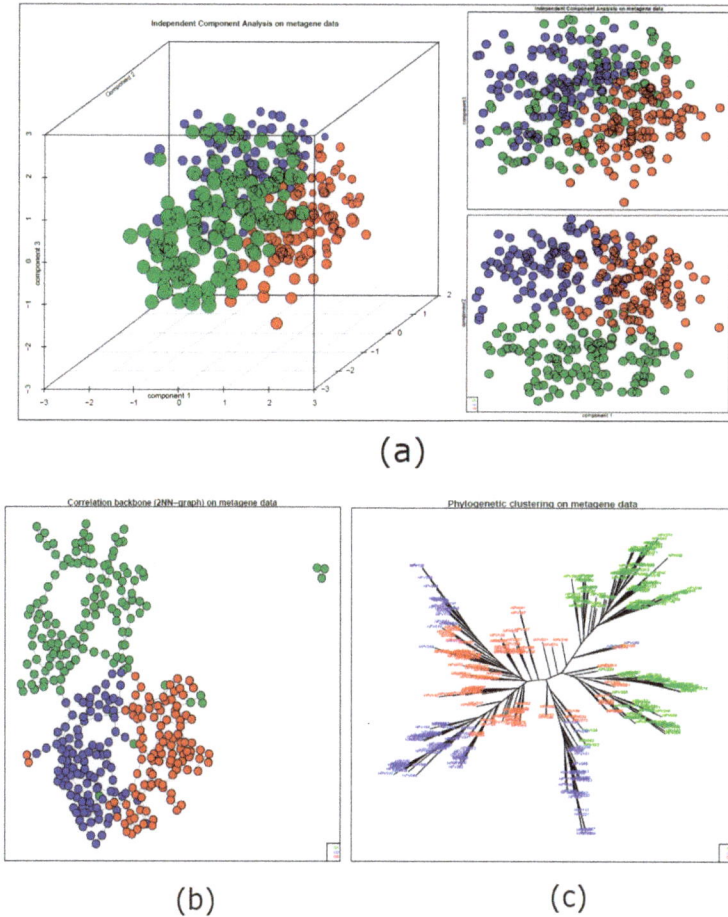

(a)

(b)   (c)

Figure 3. HPV-positive HNSCC cluster similarity relationships: second-level SOM. (**a**) Independent component analysis of meta-gene data. Samples were distributed along the three leading independent components; the plots show the three-dimensional distribution and the projections into the component 1/component 2 (lower panel) and component 1/component 3 (upper panel) dimensions. (**b**) Sample correlation network. The samples are visualized by nodes connected by edges with a backbone structure linking samples with the highest correlation. The similarity between samples is represented by their reciprocal distance; closer nodes have higher similarity and distant nodes have lower similarity. (**c**) Neighbor-joining analysis. The sample similarities are summarized in a phylogenetic tree structure computed using Euclidean distance. The neighbor-joining (NJ) analysis visualizes "bush-like" groups of similar samples by assessing their mutual dissimilarity.

Finally, we investigated the relationship among meta-genes characterizing the three identified subtypes. The process of detection of coherent expression of meta-genes in SOM portraits highlighted specific molecular features for each subtype. Indeed, the resulting map defined three over-expression regions, each of them located in distinct corners of the map. These regions corresponded to SOM clusters of co-regulated meta-genes (Figure 4a). The association of meta-genes to each cluster in precise map locations (left panels) and to a bar plot of expression intensity (right panels) better confirmed and defined the differences between subtypes: 54, 93, and 57 meta-genes had positive correlations with Clusters 1, 2, and 3, respectively ($r = 0.77$, $r = 0.53$, $r = 0.67$) (Figure 4b).

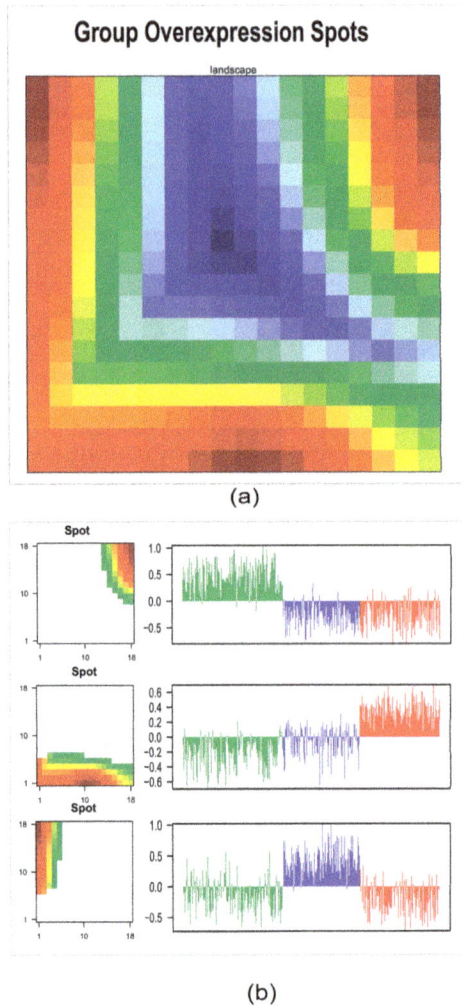

(a)

(b)

Figure 4. Subtype characterization by group overexpression maps. (**a**) The 18×18 map of meta-genes summarizes the expression landscapes over the three subtypes; according to this analysis, co-regulated meta-genes are located in the opposite corners of the map. (**b**) Detailed analysis of metagenes overexpressed in each subtype: map location (left panels) and bar plot of expression intensity (right panels). The bar plot represents the average meta-gene expression of each sample for the selected tiles.

2.4. Tumor Microenvironment Landscape

The xCell tool was applied for the detection and evaluation, if present, of any differences in the three clusters, regarding microenvironment components. According to a dimensionality reduction technique (t-distributed stochastic neighbor embedding, t-SNE), we obtained two-dimensional coordinates that clearly segregated the three molecular clusters. It provided evidence about the existence of unique and defined biological subtypes (Figure 5a). To better disclose the properties of each subtype, the composite scores of immune cells (ImmuneScore), stromal cells (StromaScore), and the score of keratinocytes were calculated. Cl1, compared to Cl2 and Cl3, was characterized by enrichment of immune components (*p*-value = 9.9×10^{-29}) (Figure 5b) and under-expression of keratinocytes (*p*-value = 2.03×10^{-32}) (Figure 5c). On the contrary, Cl2 and Cl3 showed similar enrichment in keratinocytes, but a lower immunoscore. Cl2 and Cl3 were clearly separated when compared in terms of stromal components, with Cl3 significantly decreased (*p*-value = 6.3×10^{-18}) compared with the two other two subtypes (Figure 5d).

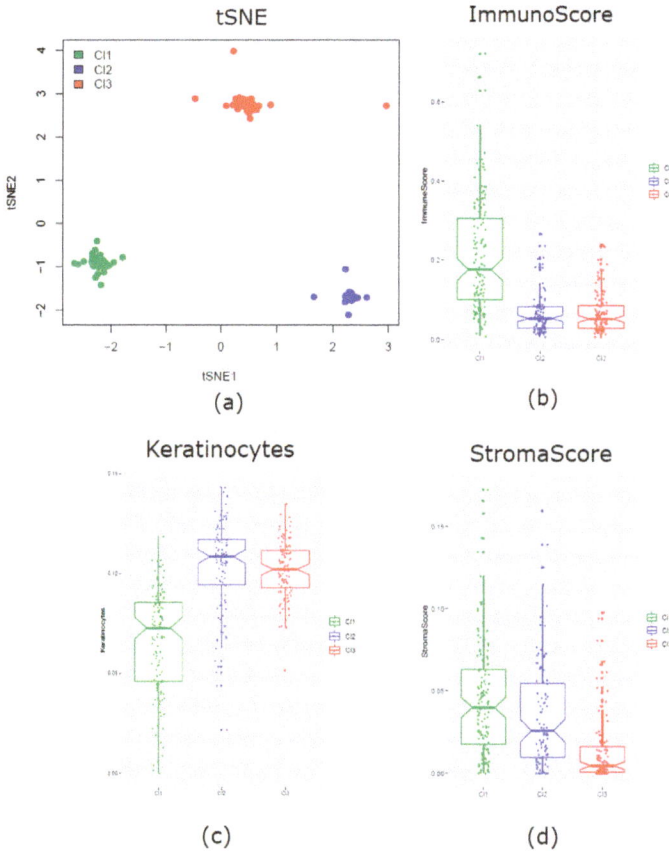

Figure 5. Tumor microenvironment landscape. (**a**) Visualization of the immune and "other cell" infiltrates assessed by xCell. Individual patients are summarized based on two-dimensional coordinates from the t-distributed stochastic neighbor embedding (t-SNE) method. The notched boxplots show the ImmuneScores (*p*-value = 9.9×10^{-29}) (**b**), keratinocytes scores (*p*-value = 2.03×10^{-32}) (**c**), and stromal cell infiltrates (*p*-value = 6.3×10^{-18}) (**d**) split into the three different subtypes.

2.5. Functional Analyses of Subtypes

To disclose the biological properties associated with each of the three resulting clusters, further functional characterization was performed using Gene Set Enrichment Analysis (GSEA). GSEA is a method used to test the overrepresentation of genes in gene sets, which are characterized by independent studies. We investigated the "Hallmark" gene set collection representing specific well-defined biological processes. In particular, our analysis provided evidence of a specific enrichment for each cluster. Cl1 showed enrichment in immune-related hallmarks, such as "allograft rejection", "IFN, interferon gamma", and "IL6 JAK STAT3 signaling"; Cl2 overexpressed genes related to the hallmarks "epithelial–mesenchymal transition" (EMT), "myogenesis", and "hypoxia"; Cl3 displayed enrichment in proliferation-related hallmarks, e.g., "E2F targets" and "G2M checkpoint" (Table 2 and Figure 6).

Table 2. Gene-sets significantly up-regulated in each cluster.

Gene-set ID	HALLMARK Gene-Set Name	Genes [a]	NES [b]	Nom *p*-Value	FDR q-val
		Cl1 vs. Cl2 and Cl3			
GS-1	ALLOGRAFT REJECTION *(immune resp)*	130	2.89	<0.00001	<0.00001
GS-2	INTERFERON GAMMA RESPONSE	151	2.18	<0.00001	<0.00001
GS-3	IL6 JAK STAT3 SIGNALING	60	1.94	<0.00001	<0.00001
GS-4	INFLAMMATORY RESPONSE	132	1.76	<0.00001	0.0018
GS-5	KRAS SIGNALING UP	114	1.75	<0.00001	0.0019
		Cl2 vs. Cl1 and Cl3			
GS-1	EPITHELIAL MESENCHYMAL TRANSITION	140	3.01	<0.00001	<0.00001
GS-2	MYOGENESIS	119	2.42	<0.00001	<0.00001
GS-3	COAGULATION	77	2.23	<0.00001	<0.00001
GS-4	ANGIOGENESIS	19	2.02	<0.00001	<0.00001
GS-5	HYPOXIA	133	1.90	<0.00001	<0.00001
GS-6	HEDGEHOG SIGNALING	17	1.89	0.0020	<0.00001
GS-7	UV RESPONSE DN	97	1.78	<0.00001	0.0020
GS-8	APICAL JUNCTION	137	1.78	<0.00001	0.0020
		Cl3 vs. Cl1 and Cl2			
GS-1	E2F TARGETS	143	2.56	<0.00001	<0.00001
GS-2	G2M CHECKPOINT	150	2.24	<0.00001	0.0020

GS: geneset; thresholds: FDR ≤ 0.005; NES≥1.75, [a] Number of total genes present in the geneset, [b] NES = normalized enrichment score.

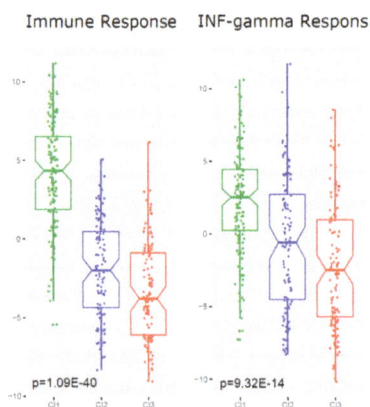

Figure 6. *Cont.*

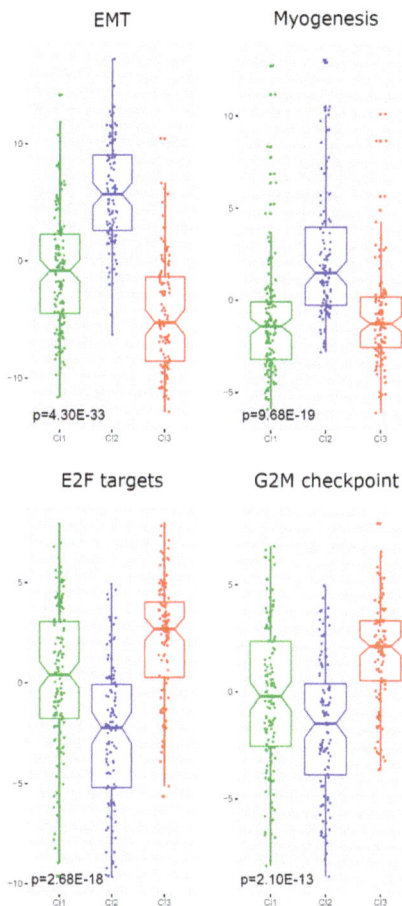

Figure 6. Visualization of the Gene Set Enrichment Analysis (GSEA) functional analysis for each of the three clusters. The boxplots show how the gene set Z score (GSZ) values (depicted in *y*-axis) are distributed within each of the three clusters (Cl1, green; Cl2, blue; Cl3 red). In each row, comparisons of the GSZ score values for the two most enriched hallmark gene sets are shown: for Cl1, over-expression is shown for the "immune response" hallmark (*p*-value 1.09×10^{-40}) and "interferon (IFN)-gamma response" hallmark (*p*-value = 9.32×10^{-14}); for Cl2, enrichment is shown in the "epithelial–mesenchymal transition (EMT)" hallmark (*p*-value = 4.30×10^{-33}) and "myogenesis" hallmark (*p*-value = 9.68×10^{-19}); for Cl3, over-expression is shown in the "E2F targets" hallmark (*p*-value = 2.68×10^{-18}) and "G2M checkpoint" (*p*-value 2.10×10^{-13}). The *p*-values were obtained by means of Kruskal–Wallis tests.

2.6. HPV Presence/Integration and Its Association with Clusters

We investigated the association between HPV viral integration and our three clusters, using the data provided by Koneva et al. [20]. Table S2 (Supplementary Materials) shows the contingency table for the TCGA cases analyzed in Koneva et al., reaching a significant association of χ^2 =12.32 and a *p*-value = 0.00212; the relative presence of HPV integrated cases in each subtype increased in the order Cl1 < Cl3 < Cl2, with relative frequencies of 0.45, 0.77, and 1, respectively. Moreover, we explored the expression of viral genes (E2, E4, and E5). The expression patterns in Cluster 2 are consistent with viral integration. When integrated, the expression of the E2 gene is reduced, since it is truncated along with downstream genes such as E4 and E5 (Figure S3).

2.7. Prognostic Values of the Three-Subtype Classification

Due to the robust analysis revealing three distinct HPV-positive HNSCC subtypes, we aimed to investigate their associations with overall survival as the clinical endpoint. Outcome data (i.e., overall survival; OS) were available for 75/134 Cl1 patients, 56/108 Cl2 patients, and 66/104 Cl3 patients, for a total of 197 patients. As depicted in Figure 7a, the results showed a significantly better outcome for Cl1 subtype patients, with a survival probability at 60 months of 0.809, and a worst outcome for Cl3 and Cl2 subtypes, with a survival probability at 60 months of 0.47 and 0.197, respectively (log-rank *p*-value = 4.76×10^{-9}).

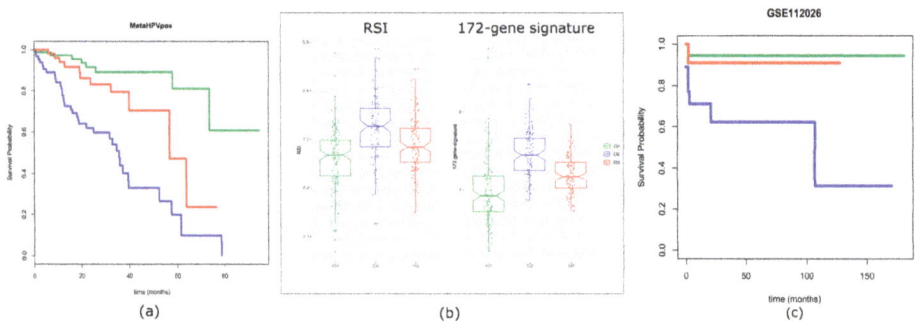

Figure 7. Prognostic evaluation of the three-subtype stratification. (**a**) Survival analysis on the meta-analysis dataset (MetaHPVpos). The 197 cases, entered into the three subtypes (75/134 Cl1 patients; 56/108 Cl2 patients; 66/104 Cl3 patients), were used for the Kaplan–Meier analysis, yielding a log-rank score of *p*-value = 4.76×10^{-9}. The endpoint was overall survival. (**b**) Gene-signature. Two models were evaluated: (i) radiosensitivity index (RSI), (ii) the 172-gene prognostic model. RSI is directly proportional to radioresistance (high index = radioresistance), while the 172-gene model is directly proportional to the risk of recurrence. Stratification by both signatures reached *p*-value = 8.76×10^{-13} and *p*-value = 7.98×10^{-22} for the RSI and 172-gene model, respectively. (**c**) Validation on GSE112026. The 47 cases belonging to GSE112026 were stratified based on our three subtypes: 18, 18, and 11 cases were predicted as belonging to Cl1, Cl2, and Cl3, respectively. The cases, entered into the three identified subtypes, were used for the Kaplan–Meier analysis, yielding a *p*-value = 0.0152 (log-rank test).

Furthermore, we applied two different gene expression published signatures to the 197 HPV-positive HNSCC patients with available follow-up information: (i) the 172-gene model, a prognostic model for HNSCC [21]; (ii) the radiosensitivity index (RSI) [22], a gene signature developed as a pan-marker of cellular radiosensitivity. In order to assess whether and to what extent the signatures were associated with HPV-related subtypes, we applied the algorithms developed [21,22] to our cohort. The resulting scores were compared to the three-subtype stratification. A significant relationship was found between our stratification and these molecular signatures (Figure 7b). In detail, the Cl1 subtype showed the lowest 172-gene signature related score, meaning that Cl1 has the minimum predicted risk, as confirmed by OS. Furthermore, Cl1 displayed the lowest RSI value, which predicted its radiosensitivity. On the contrary, Cl2 subtype exhibited the highest score in the 172-gene signature, and the maximum RSI score, compared with the other two subtypes, predicting its high risk and intrinsic radioresistance, respectively. The Cl3 subtype showed an "intermediate" behavior, with all three analyses (OS, 172-gene signature score, and RSI).

The clinical relevance of our classification was additionally investigated and associated with the outcome in an external validation dataset. For our analysis, we retrieved the RNA-sequencing (RNA-seq) data of Ando et al. [23], which included 47 HPV-positive oropharyngeal squamous cell carcinomas. With this external validation, we confirmed that the three-subtype stratification provides useful prognostic information. As a matter of fact, better outcomes were associated with patients belonging to Cl1/Cl3 subtypes, and worse outcomes were associated with patients belonging to Cl2 subtype (Figure 7c) (log-rank *p*-value = 0.0152). Finally, we investigated the association between clinal features and our molecular stratification. Table S3 (Supplementary Materials) reports the data related to gender, age, smoking habit, site, and TNM v7 stage. We found a significant association with site having Cl2 a higher percentage of cases other than oropharynx. In addition, due to its potential prognostic role, smoking habit was associated with the three subtypes. There was a trend in the different distribution of the smoking habit with higher percentage of smokers in Cl2. Table S4 (Supplementary Materials) reports the association for Ando's dataset including gender, age, smoking, Ang et al. (2010) classification system, smoked packs per year, alcohol use, t-stage, and n-stage. We found a significant association with t-stage, having Cl2 cases a higher percentage of T3–4.

3. Discussion

Among HNSCCs, the HPV-positive tumors are an independent entity with specific clinical and molecular characteristics. Moreover, inside the HPV-positive subgroup, it is additionally possible to observe an intrinsic heterogeneity, in terms of patients' outcomes. This assumption questions whether treatment de-intensification could be applied to all HPV-positive HNSCCs. Clinical factors, such as large tumor burden and smoking history, correlate with a worse prognosis, but the biological mechanisms elucidating the complexity of the HPV-positive subgroup are still not fully understood. In the present meta-analysis of transcriptomic data, we applied a rigorous and up-to-date bioinformatics analysis to 346 HPV-positive HNSCCs with published sample data. To the best of our knowledge, this is the largest cohort of HPV-positive HNSCCs analyzed up until now. Specifically, our study identified three tumor subtypes, and it further dissected a population, which was previously divided into only two subgroups by published studies [12,13,24]. In agreement with these findings, we clearly identified an immune-associated cluster (named Cl1 in our analysis). In addition, we stratified the remaining patients (previously described as one "keratinocyte subtype" cluster [13,24]) into two well distinct subtypes with clearly defined biological and prognostic characteristics. The stratification refinement could be attributed not only to the dimension of the analyzed cohort (from two to three times larger than in previous studies), but also to the application of the NJ analysis, which revealed a degree of heterogeneity moving from Cl2 to Cl3 samples with disjointed branches.

In general, HPV-related HNSCCs are known to have better outcomes when compared with HPV-negative HNSCCs [25]. The observed overall survival of our cohort of patients is aligned with the reported prognostic data. However, our analysis displayed a specific prognosis for each cluster, identifying those HPV-positive cases with the best, intermediate, and poorest prognoses. Interestingly, the subtype stratification did not provide evidence of a significant association with smoking habit, but highlighted some specific biological traits for each cluster that could help in interpreting their different outcomes.

Cluster 1 patients exhibited the best outcome at five years and it showed similar behavior to those patients identified as having low-risk HPV-related HNSCC [25]. Additionally, Cl1 was clearly separated from the other two clusters by its high immune score in the xCell analysis, and by upregulation of the hallmarks "IFN, interferon gamma signaling" and "IL6 JAK STAT3 signaling". The high immune score, associated with a good outcome, could be in agreement with the hypothesis that, in these patients, the immune system plays an important role in the clearance of viral proteins expressed in HPV-positive cancers [26]. Indeed, tumors enriched by the IFN-gamma signature may benefit from immunotherapy [27]. On the contrary, the IL6/JAK/STAT3 pathway hyper-activation is more difficult to interpret in the context of a better prognosis. In fact, IL6/JAK/STAT3 signaling is expected to drive proliferation, survival, and invasiveness of tumor cells, and to suppress the anti-tumor immune response. Overall, we could assume that, in Cl1, the immune infiltrate, as determined by the ImmuneScore, and the high "IFN, interferon gamma signaling" could counterbalance the pro-tumoral action of IL6 JAK STAT3 signaling; however, specific functional assays are necessary to confirm this assumption. Considering the better prognosis and the biological profile, we could hypothesize that Cl1 patients would be the best candidate for de-escalating treatment strategies, even including checkpoint inhibitors.

Cluster 2 exhibited the worst outcomes, and it strongly differed from the other two subtypes by its high stromal score. Essentially, this score reflects fibroblast infiltration, and it frequently leads to deregulation of EMT-inducing factors, EMT upregulation, and hallmark "hypoxia" overexpression. The EMT changes in tumor cells were reported to be linked to the acquisition of aggressive behaviors including (i) increased invasive properties, (ii) resistance to DNA damage, (iii) chemotherapy-induced apoptosis, (iv) immunosuppression, and (v) acquisition of stem-like features [28]. In addition, the increase in the hallmark "hypoxia" is in agreement with the radioresistance detected by RSI [29]. We hypothesize that treatment intensification could be beneficial for these patients. As an example, an accelerated fractionation schedule of radiotherapy should be considered as a strategy to overcome radioresistance.

Cluster 3, characterized by an intermediate outcome compared with the other two clusters, was clearly defined by upregulation of the hallmarks "E2F targets" and "G2M checkpoint", both associated with increased proliferation. A possible explanation for these data may be the interpretation of boosted proliferation as a result of the integration of the viral genome in the host cell. Moreover, upregulation of the hallmarks "E2F targets" and "G2M checkpoints" is in agreement with the observation that the HPV genome does not encode enzymes necessary for viral replication [26]. Instead, the virus utilizes host cell proteins to replicate its DNA. Therefore, basal cells containing HPV genomes remain active in the pathway related to the cell cycle, also due to Rb degradation. The E2F transcription factor, without Rb function, is free to drive the expression of S-phase genes [26,30]. A first explorative investigation, between the viral integration and our three clusters using data provided by Koneva et al. [20], revealed a significant association between the integration of HPV in the host genome and each of our subtypes in the following order: Cl1 < Cl3 < Cl2 (Figure S2, Supplementary Materials). Despite the analysis being performed on a limited number of samples, Cl2 seemed to be in accordance with cases already described in literature, in which HPV was integrated and viral integration was associated with a poor prognosis [31]. Nevertheless, in this regard, Cl3 shows an intermediate behavior, which may possibly be explained through Nulton discovery [32]. Indeed, HPV infection is described not only as its usual integrated and episomal state but, additionally, as a third state where the viral genome exists as both episomal and integrated states. Anyway, the proposed associations require further evaluation, for not only exploring the HPV state, in terms of integration, episomal, and intermediate states, but also to examine possible target amplification.

Some limitations of this study and some differences with more recent data should be mentioned. Based on the clinical characteristics of the analyzed patients, we observed a relatively high number of missing clinical data (near to 30% in age and stage). The possible explanation for the unavailability of these data could reside in the nature of the studies included in our meta-analysis, which had the biological description of the HPV tumors as a primary endpoint and, accordingly, an inconsistent collection of clinical data was performed.

It is noteworthy that HPV-related tumors in subsites, other than the oropharynx, reached a higher percentage than expected (10%). We hypothesize that this difference could be attributed to the sample collection in the years before the clear prognostic role of HPV infection in oropharynx cancers. In fact, the new TNM staging system (American Joint Committee on Cancer, 8th edition) distinguishes, for the first time, HPV-related from HPV-unrelated oropharynx cancers by stratifying according to p16 expression. The prognostic value for other subsites (i.e., oral cavity, hypopharynx, larynx) other than the oropharynx is still debatable, although a recent review demonstrated a prognostic role for HPV infection in all HNSCC subsites [33].

Considering the prognostic role of our stratification, three subtypes, with different outcomes, were described for the first time. An identified limitation could be the fact that treatment was not systematically recorded, and the overall survival of our case series was poorer than the expected outcome [25]. Moreover, another limitation was identified: the association of subtypes and prognoses should be underscored, although we should highlight that the follow-up was only available for 197 out of 346 (57%) cases. A further bias is related to the differences in treatment techniques used in the last 15 years (e.g., three-dimensional (3D) vs. intensity-modulated radiotherapy; trans-oral robotic surgery, TORS, robotics vs. traditional open surgery).

In conclusion, ongoing trials on de-escalation treatment approaches in HPV-positive HNSCC are based only on HPV status and do not take the contributions of genomics and molecular profiles into consideration [34]. It is conceivable that, upon rigorous validation, our stratification could help develop a "precision treatment approach" based on the genomic profile of HPV-related HNSCC to select patients.

4. Materials and Methods

4.1. Case Material: Gene Expression and Clinical Data

A survey of gene-expression data on HNSCC (available at 31 August 2018) was accomplished. The cases entered into our study were selected based on the following eligibility criteria: (i) primary lesions of squamous cell carcinoma; (ii) reported HPV status, according to the clinical practice in the reference center; (iii) MIAME (Minimum Information about a Microarray Experiment) [35] complaint data with the availability of raw data deposited on publicly accessible repositories and full gene annotation (Gene Bank accession or EntrezID). After literature revision, there were 11 datasets [12,36–45]. See Table S1 (Supplementary Materials) for details regarding the datasets including the accession numbers and methods of HPV detection. Raw microarray data were retrieved from the NCBI (National Center for Biotechnology Information) Gene Expression Omnibus (GEO) database [46], ArrayExpress (the EMBL European Bioinformatics Institute, UK) [47], MIAME-Vice [48], and TCGA repositories [49] and were integrated into a unique dataset through a meta-analysis approach, as previously described [50].

In addition, we collected available clinical data related to this case material, comprising age at diagnosis, gender, smoking habits, tumor subsite, stage, and overall survival.

For validation purposes, we retrieved the data from Ando et al. [23], which are publicly available on the GEO repository (identifier (ID): GSE112026). A cohort of 47 primary tumor tissues with HPV-related oropharyngeal squamous cell carcinoma was collected for RNA-seq analysis and microdissected to yield at least 80% tumor purity. HPV tumor status was confirmed by in situ hybridization for high-risk HPV subtypes or p16 immunohistochemistry. According to the TCGA RSEM (RNA-Seq by Expectation Maximization) pipeline, RNA-seq data were processed using RSEM version 1.2.9 and upper quartile normalization. For class prediction purposes, analyses were performed through R-based BRB-ArrayTools software (version 3.5.0) developed by Richard Simon and the BRB-ArrayTools development team [51]. A class prediction method based on a supervised learning method was applied for classifying GSE112026 cases. Prediction was based on the support vector machine (SVM) method by incorporating genes at the univariate significance level ($\alpha = 0.001$) in a binary tree classification framework, which was chosen due to its ability to classify more than two classes. SVM is specifically designed to address binary classification; however, it can be adapted to handle multi-class classification by building a sequence of binary classifiers. The prediction error of the binary tree classifier was estimated by the leave-one-out cross-validation method.

4.2. Data Preprocessing for Meta-Analysis Dataset Generation

The selected studies were analyzed with four platforms, including three microarray platforms (Affymetrix, Agilent, and Nimblegene) and one RNA-seq (Illumina). For Affymetrix data, signal intensities were normalized within each individual dataset using a robust multi-array average (RMA) tool. For Agilent data, the normexp background correction and loess normalization were used for two-channel arrays, while quantile normalization procedures were applied to the probe-level data. For Illumina microarray data, quantile normalization was applied. For RNA-seq data, TCGA level 3 files were downloaded along with the clinical annotations and used for the analysis. The redundancy of probes mapping the same EntrezID was removed by selecting the probe with the highest variance among multiple probe-sets by identifying the same gene; collapse was performed using WGCNA package 1.63 (function: *collapseRows*) and the "*maxRowVariance*" method [52]. To reduce the likelihood of systemic non-biological technical experimental biases among data from different platforms, after log2 transformation, the ComBat algorithm was applied [53]. Then, the expression value of each gene was averaged over all samples of our data matrix, converting the expression data into the change in log-expression ($\Delta e_{i,m}$) of gene i in sample m; $\Delta e_{i,m} = 0$ implies an expression level according to its mean value, while a relative positive or negative value refers to over- or under-expression, respectively, according to the mean gene expression.

4.3. Tumor Clusters: First-Level SOM

The $\Delta e_{i,m}$ data matrix was used to train a SOM, an unsupervised machine learning method based on the artificial neural network, enabling the dimensionality reduction of complex data structures of size N × M (N: number of genes; M: number of samples) to K × M (K: number of meta-genes), where K << N, promoting the discovery of qualitative relationships among samples [54]. Each meta-gene represents a cluster of genes sharing similar expression profiles and was selected by an interactive machine learning process by SOM; the process was trained until the meta-genes captured the entire range of expression patterns present in the data matrix. SOM algorithm data analysis and landscape visualization were performed using the "*oposSOM*" R package (version 1.18.0) [55], which uses the "som" R package [56]. A statistical significance criterion based on expression variance was applied to discard the non-informative features in our data matrix through the BRB-ArrayTools developed by Dr. Richard Simon and the BRB-ArrayTools Development Team [57]. The procedure assigns each input gene measured in M samples into a meta-gene of the same length, and each gene is included in a meta-gene, $\Delta e_{i,m}{}^{meta}$, of closest similarity established by the Euclidian distance. The meta-genes are organized in a two-dimensional grid of K = x × y tiles with the most similar expression profiles of meta-genes adjacent each to another, while the dissimilar ones are more distant. In the present study, we adopted a tile size with an average of $n_k \approx 10$ genes per meta-gene, corresponding to a two-dimensional grid of size K = 18 × 18 meta-genes with square topology and the Gaussian neighborhood function [14]. The meta-genes were normalized to fit into the range $-1 \leq e_{i,m}{}^{meta} \leq 1$ and coded by a color scale from blue (low expression) to red (high expression).

4.4. Tumor Clusters: Unsupervised Clustering Analysis

The R-package "*ConsensusClusterPlus*" [58] was applied to portion the samples into molecular coherent subtypes. The meta-data $\Delta e_{i,m}{}^{meta}$ were used as input for unsupervised class identification using partition around medoids (PAM) clustering with 1-Pearson correlation as the distance matrix. The PAM algorithm [59] is similar to the K-means algorithm, with both being partitional algorithms that split the dataset into clusters and try to minimize the error. However, while K-means works with centroids, which are artificially created entities that are representative of each cluster, PAM chooses real data-points as cluster centers. An unsupervised clustering procedure was applied to the data through 1000 re-sampling interactions by randomly selecting a fraction of the samples. Cluster numbers ranging from 2 to 10 were tested, and the empirical cumulative distribution function (CDF) and delta area plots displaying consensus distributions were assessed to identify the number of clusters giving maximum stability with a negligible increase in the CDF area [60]. To estimate the accuracy of the classification, the silhouette correlation width values were calculated for all samples (R-package: "*oposSOM*"), providing a graphical representation of how well the samples lay within their assigned cluster. The silhouette values ranged from +1 to −1, indicating the degree of similarity of a sample to the assigned cluster (cohesion) or to other clusters (separation). The evaluation of sample size adequacy of the identified clusters was assessed according to Warnes and Liu (R-package: "*ssize*") [61] and computed by imposing the type I error rate (false discovery rate, FDR), $\alpha = 0.05$, and a minimum effect size (log fold-change) of $\Delta = 1$. Cluster-specific portraits represent the mean value of each meta-gene of the samples belonging to the cluster in detail. The portraits are depicted in a log (fold-change) scale where the fold-change is the expression difference compared with the mean expression in all samples. To ascertain to what degree technical variability (i.e., study of origin and platform) affects our subtype clustering analysis, we used the "alluvial diagram", a variant of the parallel coordinates plot that is helpful for exploring categorical data by grouping them into flows that can easily be traced in the diagram [62]. The plots were generated using the R-package "*alluvial*". In addition, we used a linear mixed model to quantify the extent of technical variability in each sample through the "*variancePartition*" R package [63]. To visualize the contribution of each variable, violin plots were depicted to show the trend and rank the distribution of variance explained by each variable across all genes. The plots summarize the results in terms of the percentage of variance explained.

4.5. Cluster Similarity Relationships: Second-Level SOM Cartography

Second-level SOM analysis aims to address the issue of similarity relationships among groups of samples. It estimates the hierarchy of similarities and mutual distances based on the expression of meta-genes, and it provides improved visualization and representativeness of the results. To infer the main structures present in our data, we applied three approaches for computing the distance metrics.

Independent component analysis (ICA) [64] was applied to the SOM meta-genes using the "*fastICA*" R package [65], a method based on the covariance matrix assessed by Pearson's correlation to decompose the input meta-genes into independent and non-Gaussian components in order to ensure that each one is statistically as independent from the others as possible.

The correlation backbone through a two-nearest-neighbor graph is a correlation network approach where Pearson correlations are computed between all pairwise combinations of samples, and their structures are visualized in a graph.

The NJ algorithm ("*ape*" R package [66]) is a distance-based method offering phylogenetic tree reconstruction where similarity trees are defined between samples into an Euclidian space, allowing "bush-like clusters" displaying mutual dissimilarity to be revealed [67].

To visualize the main meta-genes related to subtype stratification, we assessed the group over-expression spots. We exploited SOM portraits by detection of the coherent expression of meta-genes. Using group overexpression maps, we linked selected meta-genes (correlation with $r > 0.5$) in different regions of the SOM with groups of samples. The group overexpression portrait was calculated as the mean map profile by averaging the meta-gene expression over the three subtypes. To identify the over-expression tiles, a 98th percentile criterion was applied to the meta-gene expression SOM training aggregate meta-genes with similar profiles in the adjacent neighbored tiles of the map. These tiles' profiles grouped over-expressed (or under-expressed) samples that differed from the others. The samples belonging to each subtype were summarized in an average representative portrait. The mining of biological functions from SOM portraits was performed using "*oposSOM*" R package (version 1.18.0).

4.6. Tumor Microenvironment Landscape

To evaluate the heterogeneity in the tumor microenvironment, the immune, stromal, and other cell components were inferred by an in silico approach using the xCell tool [68,69]. This approach enables the assessment of 64 cell types using the bulk gene expression profiles of the tumors as input and comparing them across samples, as described by the authors of Reference [69]. The tool outputs include the transformed xCell scores for the immune, stromal, and other cell types. The adjusted ImmuneScore included 10 populations (B-cells, CD4+ T-cells, CD8+ T-cells, DC, eosinophils, macrophages, monocytes, mast cells, neutrophils, and NK cells) and StromaScore 3 populations (adipocytes, endothelial cells, fibroblasts). In addition, to identify potential keratinocyte differentiation, the xCell score for keratynocytes was computed. To visualize the cellular heterogeneity of the clusters, we applied a dimension reduction method by t-distributed stochastic neighbor embedding (t-SNE) using the "*Rtsne*" package [70], which projected the cell type enrichment scores onto two-dimensional axes [71]. We presented the scores of each subtype in notched boxplots using the "*ggplot2*" R package. Notch boxplots display a confidence interval around the median based on the median ±1.58 × IQR (interquartile range) /sqrt(n). They are useful graphs for comparing groups of samples, because an absence in notch overlapping provides strong visual evidence that the medians differ. The *p*-values were calculated by the Kruskal–Wallis test, a nonparametric test that compares the means among three or more groups, as in our subtype classification.

4.7. Functional Analyses

To disclose the biological functional properties associated with the proposed molecular subtypes, gene set analysis was applied. This approach estimates gene set over-representation (probability of finding genes in a list compared to their random appearance) and over-expression (difference in expression compared to the mean expression over the samples). The gene sets were defined from a priori knowledge from independent studies and they were summarized in a list of genes specifically related to molecular pattern/biological function. A large collection of gene sets was retrieved from the Gene Set Enrichment Analysis (GSEA Broad Institute; software.broadinstitute.org/gsea/) and the Molecular Signatures Database (MSigDB) repository, including 50 hallmark gene sets. We used the gene set Z-score (GSZ) to summarize the profile of a gene set across all samples [72]. GSZ is a Z-score function that merges both over-representation and over-expression features from a gene set to give a defined gene set and provides a representative score of the gene set for each sample. Boxplots were generated using the "*ggplot2*" R package with the notched boxplot function (see Section 4.6).

4.8. Analysis of Viral Presence/Integration and Its Association with Clusters

The association between viral integration and our subtype stratification was investigated using the results provided by Koneva et al. [20]. Based on TCGA RNA-seq data and exploiting VirusSeq software [73], they detected known virus strains and identified the integration sites. Thus, the authors disclosed the HPV integration status of 65 TCGA cases present in our meta-analysis and assessed viral gene expression (E2, E4, and E5). We investigated the relative presence of integrated HPV cases defined as integrated cases/(integrated + non-integrated cases) in each subtype, and significance was calculated by the χ^2 test. Counts per million (CPM) were retrieved from Koneva et al. and transformed into the log scale by $\log_2(\text{CPM} + 1)$ [74]. Associations with viral gene expression were visualized by a heatmap. The samples were ranked by the Gene Set Variation Analysis (GSVA [75]) based on the three viral genes. GSVA was used to estimate the variation of a gene set over the samples in an unsupervised manner. The *p*-values were calculated by the Kruskal–Wallis test.

4.9. Evaluation of Prognostic Signatures

Statistical analysis was performed using R (version 3.5.1) [76] and Bioconductor (release 3.7) [77]. Survival curves were assessed according to the Kaplan–Meier method, and overall survival was used as the endpoint. Differences between the subtypes were assessed using the log-rank test and R package "*survival*". Two signatures were evaluated: (i) the 172-gene prognostic model [21]; (ii) the radiosensitivity index (RSI) [22]. The list of genes and the algorithm used for model assessment were retrieved from the original papers.

Supplementary Materials: Supplementary materials can be found at http://www.mdpi.com/2072-6694/11/8/1057/s1: Figure S1: Estimation of sample size adequacy. The relationship between the genes in our data matrix and power to detect a sample size defined by our three-subtype stratification (Cl1 = 134; Cl2 = 104; Cl3 = 108) is shown in the plots. The percentage of genes achieving a power level of at least 0.9 is displayed by the red bars and was calculated by performing a pairwise comparison between subtypes; Figure S2: Violin and boxplot of the percent variation in gene expression explained by the study of origin, platform, and our three-cluster stratification. Median percentage variation explained: cluster = 50.4%; study <1%; platform <1%; Figure S3: Expression heatmap of viral genes. The expression values for HPV E2, E4, and E5 in the TCGA cases were retrieved from Koneva et al. For visualization purposes, samples were ranked based on Gene Set Variation Analysis (GSVA) from low to high viral gene enrichment. The membership of each TCGA sample is depicted in the bar below the heatmap. Low E2, E4, and E5 expression was found in Cl2 cases compared with Cl1 and Cl3 (*p*-value = 0.00156, *p*-value = 0.00204, and *p*-value = 0.00147 determined by Kruskal–Wallis Tests, respectively); Table S1: List of used datasets. Dataset name, platform used, provider, technology, repository (included websource), number of samples, assignment to the three clusters, and methods of HPV detection are detailed in the table for each of the 11 sources utilized; Table S2: Contingency table for TCGA HPV cases annotated for HPV integration status by Koneva et al; Table S3: Association to clinical parameters in the meta-analysis dataset. The table includes the evaluation of the following clinical parameters: (i) gender; (ii) age; (iii) smoking habit (current or former smokers vs. never smoke); (iv) site (oropharynx vs. other sites); (v) stage. *p*-values by χ^2 test, with the exception for age determined by Kruskal–Wallis Tests; Table S4: Association to clinical parameters in the validation dataset (GSE112026). The table includes the evaluation of the following clinical parameters: (i) gender; (ii) age; (iii) smoking, (iv) Ang et al. (2010) classification system; (v) smoked packs per year; (vi) alcohol use; (vii) t-stage; (viii) n-stage. *p*-values by χ^2 test, with the exception for age determined by Kruskal–Wallis Tests.

Author Contributions: Conceptualization, L.D.L. and L.D.C.; Data curation, L.D.C., E.O., S.C., P.B., S.C. and L.D.C.; Formal analysis, M.S.S., M.F.I. and A.C.; Funding acquisition, L.L. and L.D.C.; Investigation, C.R.; Methodology, M.S.S., A.C. and L.D.C.; Writing—original draft, L.D.C., M.S.S. and S.C.; Writing—review & editing, L.D.L., M.S.S. and L.D.C.

Funding: This work was supported by Associazione Italiana Ricerca Cancro (AIRC IG 18519 to L.D.C.) and by the European Union's Horizon 2020 research and innovation program under grant agreement No. 689715.

Conflicts of Interest: The authors declare no conflicts of interest. The funders had no role in the design of the study; in the collection, analyses, or interpretation of data; in the writing of the manuscript, and in the decision to publish the results.

References

1. Fitzmaurice, C.; Allen, C.; Barber, R.M.; Barregard, L.; Bhutta, Z.A.; Brenner, H.; Dicker, D.J.; Chimed-Orchir, O.; Dandona, R.; Dandona, L.; et al. Global, regional, and national cancer incidence, mortality, years of life lost, years lived with disability, and disability-adjusted life-years for 32 cancer groups, 1990 to 2015: A systematic analysis for the global burden of disease study. *JAMA Oncol.* **2017**, *3*, 524–548. [PubMed]
2. Chaturvedi, A.K.; Engels, E.A.; Anderson, W.F.; Gillison, M.L. Incidence trends for human papillomavirus-related and -unrelated oral squamous cell carcinomas in the United States. *J. Clin. Oncol.* **2008**, *26*, 612–619. [CrossRef] [PubMed]
3. Rettig, E.M.; D'Souza, G. Epidemiology of head and neck cancer. *Surg. Oncol. Clin. N. Am.* **2015**, *24*, 379–396. [CrossRef] [PubMed]
4. Gillison, M.L.; Castellsagué, X.; Chaturvedi, A.; Goodman, M.T.; Snijders, P.; Tommasino, M.; Arbyn, M.; Franceschi, S. Eurogin Roadmap: Comparative epidemiology of HPV infection and associated cancers of the head and neck and cervix. *Int. J. Cancer* **2014**, *134*, 497–507. [CrossRef] [PubMed]
5. Marur, S.; Forastiere, A.A. Head and neck cancer: Changing epidemiology, diagnosis, and treatment. *Mayo Clin. Proc.* **2008**, *83*, 489–501. [CrossRef]
6. Fakhry, C.; Westra, W.H.; Li, S.; Cmelak, A.; Ridge, J.A.; Pinto, H.; Forastiere, A.; Gillison, M.L. Improved survival of patients with human papillomavirus-positive head and neck squamous cell carcinoma in a prospective clinical trial. *J. Natl. Cancer Inst.* **2008**, *100*, 261–269. [CrossRef] [PubMed]
7. Martín-Hernán, F.; Sánchez-Hernández, J.G.; Cano, J.; Campo, J.; del Romero, J. Oral cancer, HPV infection and evidence of sexual transmission. *Med. Oral Patol. Oral Cir. Bucal* **2013**, *18*, e439–e444. [CrossRef]
8. Lechner, M.; Fenton, T.; West, J.; Wilson, G.; Feber, A.; Henderson, S.; Thirlwell, C.; Dibra, H.K.; Jay, A.; Butcher, L.; et al. Identification and functional validation of HPV-mediated hypermethylation in head and neck squamous cell carcinoma. *Genome Med.* **2013**, *5*, 15. [CrossRef]
9. Sepiashvili, L.; Bruce, J.P.; Huang, S.H.; O'Sullivan, B.; Liu, F.F.; Kislinger, T. Novel insights into head and neck cancer using next-generation "omic" technologies. *Cancer Res.* **2015**, *75*, 480–486. [CrossRef]

10. Leemans, C.R.; Snijders, P.J.F.; Brakenhoff, R.H. The molecular landscape of head and neck cancer. *Nat. Rev. Cancer* **2018**, *18*, 269–282. [CrossRef]

11. Mirghani, H.; Blanchard, P. Treatment de-escalation for HPV-driven oropharyngeal cancer: Where do we stand? *Clin. Transl. Radiat. Oncol.* **2017**, *8*, 4–11. [CrossRef] [PubMed]

12. Keck, M.K.; Zuo, Z.; Khattri, A.; Stricker, T.P.; Brown, C.D.; Imanguli, M.; Rieke, D.; Endhardt, K.; Fang, P.; Brägelmann, J.; et al. Integrative analysis of head and neck cancer identifies two biologically distinct HPV and three non-HPV subtypes. *Clin. Cancer Res.* **2015**, *21*, 870–881. [CrossRef] [PubMed]

13. Zhang, Y.; Koneva, L.A.; Virani, S.; Arthur, A.E.; Virani, A.; Hall, P.B.; Warden, C.D.; Carey, T.E.; Chepeha, D.B.; Prince, M.E.; et al. Subtypes of HPV-Positive Head and Neck Cancers Are Associated with HPV Characteristics, Copy Number Alterations, PIK3CA Mutation, and Pathway Signatures. *Clin. Cancer Res.* **2016**, *22*, 4735–4745. [CrossRef] [PubMed]

14. Wirth, H.; Loffler, M.; von Bergen, M.; Binder, H. Expression cartography of human tissues using self organizing maps. *BMC Bioinform.* **2011**, *12*, 306. [CrossRef] [PubMed]

15. Tamayo, P.; Slonim, D.; Mesirov, J.; Zhu, Q.; Kitareewan, S.; Dmitrovsky, E.; Lander, E.S.; Golub, T.R. Interpreting patterns of gene expression with self-organizing maps: Methods and application to hematopoietic differentiation. *Proc. Natl. Acad. Sci. USA* **1999**, *96*, 2907–2912. [CrossRef] [PubMed]

16. Törönen, P.; Kolehmainen, M.; Wong, G.; Castrén, E. Analysis of gene expression data using self-organizing maps. *FEBS Lett.* **1999**, *451*, 142–146. [CrossRef]

17. Loeffler-Wirth, H.; Kreuz, M.; Hopp, L.; Arakelyan, A.; Haake, A.; Cogliatti, S.B.; Feller, A.C.; Hansmann, M.L.; Lenze, D.; Möller, P.; et al. A modular transcriptome map of mature B cell lymphomas. *Genome Med.* **2019**, *11*, 27. [CrossRef]

18. Kunz, M.; Löffler-Wirth, H.; Dannemann, M.; Willscher, E.; Doose, G.; Kelso, J.; Kottek, T.; Nickel, B.; Hopp, L.; Landsberg, J.; et al. RNA-seq analysis identifies different transcriptomic types and developmental trajectories of primary melanomas. *Oncogene* **2018**, *37*, 6136–6151. [CrossRef]

19. Venuti, A.; Paolini, F. HPV detection methods in head and neck cancer. *Head Neck Pathol.* **2012**, *6* (Suppl. 1), S63–S74. [CrossRef]

20. Koneva, L.A.; Zhang, Y.; Virani, S.; Hall, P.B.; McHugh, J.B.; Chepeha, D.B.; Wolf, G.; Carey, T.E.; Rozek, L.S.; Sartor, M.A. HPV Integration in HNSCC Correlates with Survival Outcomes, Immune Response Signatures, and Candidate Drivers. *Mol. Cancer Res.* **2017**. [CrossRef]

21. De Cecco, L.; Bossi, P.; Locati, L.; Canevari, S.; Licitra, L. Comprehensive gene expression meta-analysis of head and neck squamous cell carcinoma microarray data defines a robust survival predictor. *Ann. Oncol.* **2014**, *25*, 1628–1635. [CrossRef] [PubMed]

22. Eschrich, S.A.; Pramana, J.; Zhang, H.; Zhao, H.; Boulware, D.; Lee, J.H.; Bloom, G.; Rocha-Lima, C.; Kelley, S.; Calvin, D.P.; et al. A gene expression model of intrinsic tumor radiosensitivity: Prediction of response and prognosis after chemoradiation. *Int. J. Radiat. Oncol. Biol. Phys.* **2009**, *75*, 489–496. [CrossRef]

23. Ando, M.; Saito, Y.; Xu, G.; Bui, N.Q.; Medetgul-Ernar, K.; Pu, M.; Fisch, K.; Ren, S.; Sakai, A.; Fukusumi, T.; et al. Chromatin dysregulation and DNA methylation at transcription start sites associated with transcriptional repression in cancers. *Nat. Commun.* **2019**, *10*, 2188. [CrossRef]

24. Gleber-Netto, F.O.; Rao, X.; Guo, T.; Xi, Y.; Gao, M.; Shen, L.; Erikson, K.; Kalu, N.N.; Ren, S.; Xu, G.; et al. Variations in HPV function are associated with survival in squamous cell carcinoma. *JCI Insight* **2019**. [CrossRef] [PubMed]

25. Ang, K.K.; Harris, J.; Wheeler, R.; Weber, R.; Rosenthal, D.I.; Nguyen-Tân, P.F.; Westra, W.H.; Chung, C.H.; Jordan, R.C.; Lu, C.; et al. Human papillomavirus and survival of patients with oropharyngeal cancer. *N. Engl. J. Med.* **2010**, *363*, 24–35. [CrossRef] [PubMed]

26. Blitzer, G.C.; Smith, M.A.; Harris, S.L.; Kimple, R.J. Review of the clinical and biologic aspects of human papillomavirus-positive squamous cell carcinomas of the head and neck. *Int. J. Radiat. Oncol. Biol. Phys.* **2014**, *88*, 761–770. [CrossRef]

27. Chen, Y.P.; Wang, Y.Q.; Lv, J.W.; Li, Y.Q.; Chua, M.L.K.; Le, Q.T.; Lee, N.; Colevas, A.D.; Seiwert, T.; Hayes, D.N.; et al. Identification and validation of novel microenvironment-based immune molecular subgroups of head and neck squamous cell carcinoma: Implications for immunotherapy. *Ann. Oncol.* **2019**. [CrossRef]

28. Suarez-Carmona, M.; Lesage, J.; Cataldo, D.; Gilles, C. EMT and inflammation: Inseparable actors of cancer progression. *Mol. Oncol.* **2017**, *11*, 805–823. [CrossRef]

29. Nordsmark, M.; Bentzen, S.M.; Rudat, V.; Brizel, D.; Lartigau, E.; Stadler, P.; Becker, A.; Adam, M.; Molls, M.; Dunst, J.; et al. Prognostic value of tumor oxygenation in 397 head and neck tumors after primary radiation therapy. An international multi-center study. *Radiother. Oncol.* **2005**, *77*, 18–24. [CrossRef]

30. Speel, E.J. HPV Integration in Head and Neck Squamous Cell Carcinomas: Cause and Consequence. *Recent Results Cancer Res.* **2017**, *206*, 57–72.

31. Nulton, T.J.; Nak-Kyeong, K.; DiNardo, L.J.; Morgan, I.M.; Windle, B. Patients with integrated HPV16 in head and neck cancer show poor survival. *Oral Oncol.* **2018**, *80*, 52–55. [CrossRef] [PubMed]

32. Nulton, T.J.; Olex, A.L.; Dozmorov, M.; Morgan, I.M.; Windle, B. Analysis of The Cancer Genome Atlas sequencing data reveals novel properties of the human papillomavirus 16 genome in head and neck squamous cell carcinoma. *Oncotarget* **2017**, 17684–17699. [CrossRef]

33. Li, H.; Torabi, S.J.; Yarbrough, W.G.; Mehra, S.; Osborn, H.A.; Judson, B. Association of Human Papillomavirus Status at Head and Neck Carcinoma Subsites With Overall Survival. *JAMA Otolaryngol. Head Neck Surg.* **2018**, *144*, 519–525. [CrossRef] [PubMed]

34. Orlandi, E.; Alfieri, S.; Simon, C.; Trama, A.; Licitra, L.; RARECAREnet Working Group. Treatment challenges in and outside a network setting: Head and neck cancers. *Eur. J. Surg. Oncol.* **2019**, *45*, 40–45. [CrossRef] [PubMed]

35. Brazma, A.; Hingamp, P.; Quackenbush, J.; Sherlock, G.; Spellman, P.; Stoeckert, C.; Aach, J.; Ansorge, W.; Ball, C.A.; Causton, H.C.; et al. Minimum information about a microarray experiment (MIAME)-toward standards for microarray data. *Nat. Genet.* **2001**, *29*, 365–371. [CrossRef]

36. Slebos, R.J.; Yi, Y.; Ely, K.; Carter, J.; Evjen, A.; Zhang, X.; Shyr, Y.; Murphy, B.M.; Cmelak, A.J.; Burkey, B.B.; et al. Gene expression differences associated with human papillomavirus status in head and neck squamous cell carcinoma. *Clin. Cancer Res.* **2006**, *12 Pt 1*, 701–709. [CrossRef]

37. Pyeon, D.; Newton, M.A.; Lambert, P.F.; den Boon, J.A.; Sengupta, S.; Marsit, C.J.; Woodworth, C.D.; Connor, J.P.; Haugen, T.H.; Smith, E.M.; et al. Fundamental differences in cell cycle deregulation in human papillomavirus-positive and human papillomavirus-negative head/neck and cervical cancers. *Cancer Res.* **2007**, *67*, 4605–4619. [CrossRef]

38. Walter, V.; Yin, X.; Wilkerson, M.D.; Cabanski, C.R.; Zhao, N.; Du, Y.; Ang, M.K.; Hayward, M.C.; Salazar, A.H.; Hoadley, K.A.; et al. Molecular subtypes in head and neck cancer exhibit distinct patterns of chromosomal gain and loss of canonical cancer genes. *PLoS ONE* **2013**, *8*, e56823. [CrossRef]

39. Sun, W.; Gaykalova, D.A.; Ochs, M.F.; Mambo, E.; Arnaoutakis, D.; Liu, Y.; Loyo, M.; Agrawal, N.; Howard, J.; Li, R.; et al. Activation of the NOTCH pathway in head and neck cancer. *Cancer Res.* **2014**, *74*, 1091–1104. [CrossRef]

40. Thibodeau, B.J.; Geddes, T.J.; Fortier, L.E.; Ahmed, S.; Pruetz, B.L.; Wobb, J.; Chen, P.; Wilson, G.D.; Akervall, J.A. Gene Expression Characterization of HPV Positive Head and Neck Cancer to Predict Response to Chemoradiation. *Head Neck Pathol.* **2015**, *9*, 345–353. [CrossRef]

41. Tomar, S.; Graves, C.A.; Altomare, D.; Kowli, S.; Kassler, S.; Sutkowski, N.; Gillespie, M.B.; Creek, K.E.; Pirisi, L. Human papillomavirus status and gene expression profiles of oropharyngeal and oral cancers from European American and African American patients. *Head Neck* **2016**, *38* (Suppl. 1), E694–E704. [CrossRef]

42. Wichmann, G.; Rosolowski, M.; Krohn, K.; Kreuz, M.; Boehm, A.; Reiche, A.; Scharrer, U.; Halama, D.; Bertolini, J.; Bauer, U.; et al. The role of HPV RNA transcription, immune response-related gene expression and disruptive TP53 mutations in diagnostic and prognostic profiling of head and neck cancer. *Int. J. Cancer* **2015**, *137*, 2846–2857. [CrossRef]

43. Mirghani, H.; Ugolin, N.; Ory, C.; Lefèvre, M.; Baulande, S.; Hofman, P.; St Guily, J.L.; Chevillard, S.; Lacave, R. A predictive transcriptomic signature of oropharyngeal cancer according to HPV16 status exclusively. *Oral Oncol.* **2014**, *50*, 1025–1034. [CrossRef]

44. Thurlow, J.K.; Peña Murillo, C.L.; Hunter, K.D.; Buffa, F.M.; Patiar, S.; Betts, G.; West, C.M.; Harris, A.L.; Parkinson, E.K.; Harrison, P.R.; et al. Spectral clustering of microarray data elucidates the roles of microenvironment remodeling and immune responses in survival of head and neck squamous cell carcinoma. *J. Clin. Oncol.* **2010**, *28*, 2881–2888. [CrossRef]

45. Cancer Genome Atlas Network. Comprehensive genomic characterization of head and neck squamous cell carcinomas. *Nature* **2015**, *517*, 576–582. [CrossRef]

46. Edgar, R.; Domrachev, M.; Lash, A.E. Gene Expression Omnibus: NCBI gene expression and hybridization array data repository. *Nucleic Acids Res.* **2002**, *30*, 207–210. [CrossRef]

47. Kolesnikov, N.; Hastings, E.; Keays, M.; Melnichuk, O.; Tang, Y.A.; Williams, E.; Dylag, M.; Kurbatova, N.; Brandizi, M.; Burdett, T.; et al. ArrayExpress update—Simplifying data submissions. *Nucleic Acids Res.* **2015**, *43*, D1113–D1116. [CrossRef]

48. BIOINFORMATICS @ MANCHESTER. Available online: http://bioinformatics.picr.man.ac.uk/vice/Welcome.vice (accessed on 31 March 2016).

49. National Cancer Institute GDC Data Portal. Available online: https://portal.gdc.cancer.gov/repository (accessed on 30 April 2018).

50. De Cecco, L.; Nicolau, M.; Giannoccaro, M.; Daidone, M.G.; Bossi, P.; Locati, L.; Licitra, L.; Canevari, S. Head and neck cancer subtypes with biological and clinical relevance: Meta-analysis of gene-expression data. *Oncotarget* **2015**, *6*, 9627–9642. [CrossRef]

51. Simon, R.; Lam, A.; Li, M.C.; Ngan, M.; Menenzes, S.; Zhao, Y. Analysis of gene expression data using BRB-ArrayTools. *Cancer Inform.* **2007**, *3*, 11–17. [CrossRef]

52. Langfelder, P.; Horvath, S. WGCNA: An R package for weighted correlation network analysis. *BMC Bioinform.* **2008**, *9*, 559. [CrossRef]

53. Johnson, W.E.; Li, C.; Rabinovic, A. Adjusting batch effects in microarray expression data using empirical Bayes methods. *Biostatistics* **2007**, *8*, 118–127. [CrossRef]

54. Kohonen, T. Self-organized formation of topologically correct feature maps. *Biol. Cybern.* **1982**, *43*, 59–69. [CrossRef]

55. Löffler-Wirth, H.; Kalcher, M.; Binder, H. oposSOM: R-package for high-dimensional portraying of genome-wide expression landscapes on bioconductor. *Bioinformatics* **2015**, *31*, 3225–3227. [CrossRef]

56. Yan, J. Som: Self-Organizing Map. 2010 R Package. Available online: Cran.r-project.org/web/packages/som (accessed on 30 November 2018).

57. National Cancer Institute. Available online: https://brb.nci.nih.gov/BRB-ArrayTools/index.html (accessed on 30 November 2018).

58. Wilkerson, M.D.; Hayes, D.N. ConsensusClusterPlus: A class discovery tool with confidence assessments and item tracking. *Bioinformatics* **2010**, *26*, 1572–1573. [CrossRef]

59. Kaufman, L.; Rousseeuw, P. Clustering by Means of Medoids. In Proceedings of the Statistical Data Analysis Based on the L1 Norm and Related Methods, Neuchâtel, Switzerland, 31 August–4 September 1987; Dodge, Y., Ed.; Elsevier Science Pub. Co.: Amsterdam, The Netherlands, 1987; pp. 405–416.

60. Monti, S.; Tamayo, P.; Mesirov, J.; Todd, G. Consensus Clustering: A Resampling-Based Method for Class Discovery and Visualization of Gene Expression Microarray Data. *Mach. Learn.* **2003**, *52*, 91–118. [CrossRef]

61. Warnes, G.; Liu, P.; Li, F. Ssize: Estimate Microarray Sample Size. R Package Version 1.54.0. Available online: http://bioconductor.org/packages/release/bioc/html/ssize.html (accessed on 31 May 2017).

62. Rosvall, M.; Bergstrom, C.T. Mapping Change in Large Networks. *PLoS ONE* **2010**, *5*, e8694. [CrossRef]

63. Hoffman, G.E.; Schadt, E.E. variancePartition: Interpreting drivers of variation in complex gene expression studies. *BMC Bioinform.* **2016**, *17*. [CrossRef]

64. Hyvärinen, A.; Oja, E. Independent component analysis: Algorithms and applications. *Neural Netw.* **2000**, *13*, 411–430. [CrossRef]

65. FastICA. Available online: https://CRAN.R-project.org/package=fastICA (accessed on 30 November 2018).

66. Paradis, E.; Claude, J.; Strimmer, K. APE: Analyses of Phylogenetics and Evolution in R language. *Bioinformatics* **2004**, *20*, 289–290. [CrossRef]

67. Saitou, N.; Nei, M. The neighbor-joining method: A new method for reconstructing phylogenetic trees. *Mol. Biol. Evol.* **1987**, *4*, 406–425.

68. xCell. Available online: http://xcell.ucsf.edu/ (accessed on 28 February 2019).

69. Aran, D.; Hu, Z.; Butte, A.J. xCell: Digitally portraying the tissue cellular heterogeneity landscape. *Genome Biol.* **2017**, *18*, 220. [CrossRef]

70. Krijthe, J.H. Rtsne: T-Distributed Stochastic Neighbor Embedding Using a Barnes-Hut Implementation. Available online: https://github.com/jkrijthe/Rtsne (accessed on 28 February 2019).

71. van der Maaten, L.; Hinton, G. Visualizing data using t-SNE. *J. Mach. Learn. Res.* **2008**, *9*, 2579–2605.

72. Törönen, P.; Ojala, P.J.; Marttinen, P.; Holm, L. Robust extraction of functional signals from gene set analysis using a generalized threshold free scoring function. *BMC Bioinform.* **2009**, *10*, 307. [CrossRef]

73. Chen, Y.; Yao, H.; Thompson, E.J.; Tannir, N.M.; Weinstein, J.N.; Su, X. VirusSeq: Software to identify viruses and their integration sites using next-generation sequencing of human cancer tissue. *Bioinformatics* **2013**, *29*, 266–267. [CrossRef]
74. Law, C.W.; Chen, Y.; Shi, W.; Smyth, G.K. voom: Precision weights unlock linear model analysis tools for RNA-seq read counts. *Genome Biol.* **2014**, *15*, R29. [CrossRef]
75. Hänzelmann, S.; Castelo, R.; Guinney, J. GSVA: Gene set variation analysis for microarray and RNA-Seq data. *BMC Bioinform.* **2013**, *14*, 7. [CrossRef]
76. R Development Core Team. R: A Language and Environment for Statistical Computing. Vienna, Austria: R Foundation for Statistical Computing 2007. Available online: http://www.R-project.org (accessed on 30 September 2018).
77. Gentleman, R.C.; Carey, V.J.; Bates, D.M.; Bolstad, B.; Dettling, M.; Dudoit, S.; Ellis, B.; Gautier, L.; Ge, Y.; Gentry, J.; et al. Bioconductor: Open software development for computational biology and bioinformatics. *Genome Biol.* **2004**, *5*, R80. [CrossRef]

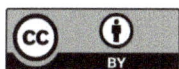

cancers

MDPI

Article

Pathological and Molecular Characteristics of Colorectal Cancer with Brain Metastases

Pauline Roussille [1,2,3], **Gaelle Tachon** [2,3,4], **Claire Villalva** [4], **Serge Milin** [5], **Eric Frouin** [3,5], **Julie Godet** [5], **Antoine Berger** [1], **Sheik Emambux** [2,3,4,6], **Christos Petropoulos** [2,3,4], **Michel Wager** [2,3,7], **Lucie Karayan-Tapon** [2,3,4,†] and **David Tougeron** [3,6,8,*,†]

[1] Department of Radiation Oncology, University Hospital of Poitiers, 86021 Poitiers, France; pauline.roussille@chu-poitiers.fr (P.R.); antoine.berger@chu-poitiers.fr (A.B.)
[2] INSERM 1084, Experimental and Clinical Neurosciences Laboratory, University of Poitiers, 86073 Poitiers, France; gaelle.tachon@chu-poitiers.fr (G.T.); sheik.emambux@chu-poitiers.fr (S.E.); christospetropoulos81@hotmail.com (C.P.); michel.wager@chu-poitiers.fr (M.W.); lucie.karayan-tapon@chu-poitiers.fr (L.K.-T.)
[3] Faculty of Medicine, University of Poitiers, 86021 Poitiers, France; eric.frouin@chu-poitiers.fr
[4] Cancer Biology Department, University Hospital of Poitiers, 86021 Poitiers, France; claire.villalva-gregoire@chu-poitiers.fr
[5] Pathology Department, University Hospital of Poitiers, 86021 Poitiers, France; serge.milin@chu-poitiers.fr (S.M.); julie.godet@chu-poitiers.fr (J.G.)
[6] Medical Oncology Department, University Hospital of Poitiers, 86021 Poitiers, France
[7] Department of Neurosurgery, University Hospital of Poitiers, 86021 Poitiers, France
[8] Department of Gastroenterology, University Hospital of Poitiers, 86021 Poitiers, France
*   Correspondence: david.tougeron@chu-poitiers.fr; Tel.: +33-5-49-44-37-51
†   These authors have contributed equally to this article.

Received: 17 November 2018; Accepted: 5 December 2018; Published: 10 December 2018

Abstract: *Background:* Colorectal cancers (CRC) with brain metastases (BM) are scarcely described. The main objective of this study was to determine the molecular profile of CRC with BM. *Methods:* We included 82 CRC patients with BM. *KRAS*, *NRAS*, *BRAF* and mismatch repair (MMR) status were investigated on primary tumors ($n = 82$) and BM ($n = 38$). ALK, ROS1, cMET, HER-2, PD-1, PD-L1, CD3 and CD8 status were evaluated by immunohistochemistry, and when recommended, by fluorescence in situ hybridization. *Results:* In primary tumors, *KRAS*, *NRAS* and *BRAF* mutations were observed in 56%, 6%, and 6% of cases, respectively. No *ROS1*, *ALK* and *cMET* rearrangement was detected. Only one tumor presented *HER-2* amplification. Molecular profiles were mostly concordant between BM and paired primary tumors, except for 9% of discordances for *RAS* mutation. CD3, CD8, PD-1 and PD-L1 expressions presented some discordance between primary tumors and BM. In multivariate analysis, multiple BM, lung metastases and PD-L1+ tumor were predictive of poor overall survival. *Conclusions:* CRCs with BM are associated with high frequency of *RAS* mutations and significant discordance for *RAS* mutational status between BM and paired primary tumors. Multiple BM, lung metastases and PD-L1+ have been identified as prognostic factors and can guide therapeutic decisions for CRC patients with BM.

Keywords: brain metastases; colorectal cancer; *KRAS* mutation; PD-L1; tumor infiltrating lymphocytes

1. Introduction

Brain metastases (BM) from colorectal cancer (CRC) are rare with an incidence ranging from 0.6 to 3.2% and are associated with a poor prognosis with an overall survival (OS) of about 5.0 months [1,2]. Patients with BM from CRC present a specific clinical profile with predominant rectosigmoid primary tumor location and lung metastases [3–6]. Nevertheless, the molecular profile of BMs from CRC has only been partially explored [7,8]. Some small series have suggested a high rate of *KRAS* mutation in CRC with BM, but no study has evaluated complete *RAS* (*KRAS* and *NRAS*), *BRAF* and mismatch repair (MMR) status [1].

In metastatic CRC (mCRC), molecular profiles of liver and lung metastases have already been tested and revealed a high concordance between the metastases and paired primary tumor (PPT) (95–100%) [9]. Brastianos et al., by performing a whole-exome sequencing of 86 BM and PPT from various sites, reported 53% of discordances in genetic profile, and found actionable mutations (EGFR, HER-2 and PI3K/AKT/mTOR pathways) in BM that were not detected in PPT [10]. However, only four CRCs were analyzed. Therefore, it is of major interest to evaluate molecular abnormalities of CRC with BM in a larger cohort.

The main objective of this study was to evaluate the molecular profile of CRC with BM. The secondary objectives were to evaluate the concordance of molecular profiles between BM and their PPT and to determine the prognostic factors of CRC patients with BM.

2. Results

2.1. Patient and Tumor Characteristics

Eighty-two CRC patients with BM were included, mostly radiologically confirmed (*n* = 44/82), with a median follow-up of 45.1 months (95% Confidence Interval (CI) 26.6–45.5 months). Median age at CRC diagnosis was 64.0 years and most of the patients were male (63%) (Table 1).

Table 1. Clinical characteristics of patients, primary tumors and brain metastases (BM).

Characteristics	Patients (*n* = 82)
Age at primary tumor diagnostic, years	
Median (range)	64 (35–85)
Gender, *n* (%)	
Male	52 (63)
Female	30 (37)
Site of primary tumor, *n* (%)	
Ascending colon	19 (23)
Descending colon	24 (29)
Rectum	35 (42)
Bifocal tumor	5 (6)
Tumor grade, *n* (%)	
Well or moderately differentiated	61 (87)
Poorly differentiated	9 (13)
Missing	12
Stage at initial CRC diagnostic, *n* (%)	
I	4 (5)
II	13 (16)
III	26 (32)
IV	39 (47)
Primary tumor resection, *n* (%)	
No	11 (13)
Yes	71 (87)
ECOG performance status at BM diagnosis, *n* (%)	
< 2	43 (54)
≥ 2	36 (46)
Missing	3
Number of BM, *n* (%)	
Single	43 (52)
Multiple	39 (48)
Site of BM, *n* (%)	
Supratentorial	46 (56)
Subtentorial	18 (22)
Both	18 (22)

Table 1. *Cont.*

Characteristics	Patients (*n* = 82)
Delay between BM and CRC diagnosis, *n* (%)	
Synchronous	8 (10)
Metachronous	74 (90)
ECM at BM diagnosis, *n* (%)	
No	11 (14)
Yes	70 (86)
Missing	1
Lung metastases at BM diagnosis, *n* (%)	
No	23 (28)
Yes	58 (72)
Missing	1
Liver metastases at BM diagnosis, *n* (%)	
No	45 (56)
Yes	36 (44)

Abbreviations: BM, brain metastasis(es); CRC, colorectal cancer; ECM, extracranial metastasis(es); ECOG, Eastern Cooperative Oncology Group score.

2.2. Molecular and Pathological Profiles of Colorectal Cancer with Brain Metastases

In primary tumors (*n* = 82), RAS mutations were observed in 62% of cases with 56% of *KRAS* mutations and 6% of *NRAS* mutations (Table 2). *KRAS* mutations in codon 12 of exon 2 were observed in 48% and the most frequent were G12D and G12V. *BRAF* mutation was observed in 6%. Concerning BM (*n* = 38), RAS was mutated in 85% of cases (74% of *KRAS* mutations and 11% of *NRAS* mutations) and BRAF in 5%. Both primary tumors and BM were mostly MMR-proficient (pMMR) (95%). Four patients had dMMR tumors, one patient had a Lynch syndrome (*MSH2* germline mutation) and the three others patients had sporadic dMMR tumors.

Table 2. Molecular profile of primary tumors and brain metastases.

Molecular Status	Primary Tumors (*n* = 82)	BM (*n* = 38)
***KRAS* status**		
Wild-type, *n* (%)	35 (44)	10 (26)
Mutant, *n* (%)	44 (56)	28 (74)
KRAS exon 2 at codon 12		
G12D	14 (18)	9 (23)
G12V	14 (18)	8 (21)
G12A	5 (6)	3 (8)
G12S	3 (4)	0
G12C	1 (1)	1 (3)
G12R	1 (1)	1 (3)
KRAS exon 2 at codon 13		
G13D	2 (3)	3 (8)
G13R	1 (1)	1 (3)
KRAS exon 3 at codon 61	3 (4)	2 (5)
KRAS exon 4 at codon 146	0	0
Missing, *n*	3	0
***NRAS* status**		
Wild-type, *n* (%)	74 (94)	34 (89)
Mutant, *n* (%)	5 (6)	4 (11)
NRAS exon 2 at codon 12 or 13	1 (1)	1 (3)
NRAS exon 3 at codon 61	4 (5)	3 (8)
Missing, *n*	3	0
***BRAF* exon 15 at codon 600**		
Wild-type, *n* (%)	74 (94)	36 (95)
Mutant, *n* (%)	5 (6)	2 (5)
Missing, *n* (%)	3	0

Table 2. *Cont.*

Molecular Status	Primary Tumors (*n* = 82)	BM (*n* = 38)
MMR status		
pMMR, *n* (%)	70 (95)	36 (95)
dMMR, *n* (%)	4 (5)	2 (5)
Missing, *n*	8	0
cMET expression		
Negative (0, 1+, 2+/3+ with FISH negative), *n* (%)	76 (100)	37 (100)
Positive (2+, 3+ with FISH positive), *n* (%)	0	0
Missing, *n*	6	1
HER-2 expression		
Negative (0, 1+, 2+ with FISH negative), *n* (%)	74 (99)	37 (100)
Positive (2+ with FISH positive, 3+), *n* (%)	1 (1)	0
Missing, *n*	7	1
ALK expression		
Negative (0, 1+/2+/3+ with FISH negative), *n* (%)	76 (100)	37 (100)
Positive (1+/2+/3+ with FISH positive), *n* (%)	0	0
Missing, *n* (%)	6	1
ROS1 expression		
Negative (0, 1+/2+/3+ with FISH negative), *n* (%)	74 (100)	37 (100)
Positive (1+/2+/3+ with FISH positive), *n* (%)	0	0
Missing, *n*	8	1
PD-1 expression		
Negative, *n* (%)	64 (86)	37 (100)
Positive, *n* (%)	10 (14)	0
Missing, *n*	8	1
PD-L1 expression		
Negative, *n* (%)	68 (93)	35 (95)
Positive, *n* (%)	5 (7)	2 (5)
Missing, *n*	9	1
CD3 expression		
Median rate, % (range)	30 (0–80)	11 (0–60)
Missing, *n*	11	1
CD8 expression		
Median rate, % (range)	11 (0–70)	3 (0–50)
Missing, *n*	7	2

Abbreviations: IHC, Immunohistochemistry; FISH, Fluorescence in situ hybridization; MMR, Mismatch repair; pMMR, Proficient Mismatch Repair; dMMR, Deficient Mismatch Repair.

No primary tumor overexpressed ROS1 protein according to immunohistochemistry (IHC) analysis. ALK IHC 1+ was detected in six primary tumors, but was negative by Fluorescence in situ hybridization (FISH) analysis. Concerning HER-2 IHC, three primary tumors were positive, but HER-2 amplification was confirmed by FISH only for one sample. cMET positive staining was detected by IHC in 61% of primary CRC, but none was confirmed by FISH. Concerning BM, ROS1, ALK and HER-2 staining were all negative (score 0). cMET positive staining was detected in 84% of BM, but none was confirmed by FISH.

Ten primary tumors (14%) were programmed death-1 positive (PD-1+), but no BM. Five primary tumors (7%) and two BMs (5%) were programmed death-ligand 1 positive (PD-L1+). Among the five PD-L1+ primary tumors, three were MMR-deficient (dMMR) and two were pMMR. The median percentage of CD3 and CD8 lymphocyte infiltrates were 30% and 11% in primary tumors, 11% and 3% in BM respectively. The mean percentages of CD3 and CD8 lymphocyte infiltrates in primary tumors were 46% and 38% in dMMR tumors and 33% and 11% in pMMR tumors ($p = 0.23$ for CD3 and $p < 0.01$ for CD8) respectively. The mean percentages of CD3 and CD8 lymphocyte infiltrates in primary tumors were 49% and 41% in PD-L1+ tumors and 33% and 12% in PD-L1- tumors ($p = 0.09$ for CD3 and $p < 0.01$ for CD8), respectively.

2.3. Concordance of Molecular and Pathological Profiles between Brain Metastases and Their Paired Primary Tumors

The molecular profiles of BM were compared with their PPT (Table 3), when available (*n* = 35). Discordances in *RAS* and *BRAF* status were observed in four patients (11%), three for *RAS* and one for *BRAF*. In each case, PPT was wild-type and BM was mutated. According to IHC evaluation, PPT and BM were discordant for cMET in nine cases (28%). However, all cases were negative according to FISH analyses.

Table 3. Molecular and pathological profiles of brain metastases and paired primary tumors.

Brain Metastases			
RAS status			
Primary tumors	Wild-type	Mutant	Total
Wild-type, *n* (%)	6 (17)	3 (9)	9 (26)
Mutant, *n* (%)	0	26 (74)	26 (74)
Total, *n* (%)	6 (17)	29 (83)	35
BRAF status			
Primary tumors	Wild-type	Mutant	Total
Wild-type, *n* (%)	33 (94)	1 (3)	34 (97)
Mutant, *n* (%)	0	1 (3)	1 (3)
Total, *n* (%)	33 (94)	2 (6)	35
MMR status			
Primary tumors	pMMR	dMMR	Total
pMMR, *n* (%)	30 (94)	0	30 (94)
dMMR, *n* (%)	0	2 (6)	2 (6)
Total, *n* (%)	30 (94)	2 (6)	32
HER-2 expression			
Primary tumors	Negative	Positive	Total
Negative, *n* (%)	35 (100)	0	35 (100)
Positive, *n* (%)	0	0	0 (0)
Total, *n* (%)	35 (100)	0 (0)	35
cMET expression (IHC)			
Primary tumors	Negative	Positive	Total
Negative, *n* (%)	4 (13)	7 (22)	11 (34)
Positive, *n* (%)	2 (6)	19 (59)	21 (66)
Total, *n* (%)	6 (19)	26 (81)	32
PD-1 expression			
Primary tumors	Negative	Positive	Total
Negative, *n* (%)	30 (94)	0	30 (94)
Positive, *n* (%)	2 (6)	0	2 (6)
Total, *n* (%)	32 (100)	0	32
PD-L1 expression			
Primary tumors	Negative	Positive	Total
Negative, *n* (%)	29 (91)	2 (6)	31 (97)
Positive, *n* (%)	1 (3)	0	1 (3)
Total, *n* (%)	30 (94)	2 (6)	32
CD3 expression	**Primary tumor**	**Brain metastases**	
Median rate, % (range)	34 (0–80)	15 (0–60)	
CD8 expression	**Primary tumor**	**Brain metastases**	
Median rate, % (range)	10 (0–70)	3 (0–50)	

Abbreviations: IHC, immunohistochemistry; MMR, Mismatch repair; pMMR, Proficient Mismatch Repair; dMMR, Deficient Mismatch Repair.

Concerning PD-1+ tumor, discordance was observed in two paired samples (6%). We found three discordances for PD-L1 status (9%). Median percentages of CD3+ and CD8+ lymphocytes were significantly more important in PPT (34% and 10%) compared to BM (15% and 3%) (both $p < 0.01$). In addition, there was a positive correlation between levels of CD8+ infiltrates in BM and PTT ($p = 0.01$), but not for CD3+ infiltrates ($p = 0.40$).

2.4. Overall Survival

79 patients died at the time of data analysis. Median Overall Survival (OS) from BM diagnosis was 4.1 months (95%CI 3.6–5.4 months) (Figure 1). Median OS from diagnosis of metastatic disease was 28.6 months (95%CI 18.0–35.5 months). Age, BRAF mutation, PD-L1+ tumors, Eastern cooperative oncology group (ECOG) performance status $\geq$ 2, multiple BM and lung metastases were significantly associated with poor OS in univariate analysis (Table 4). In multivariate analysis, PD-L1+ primary tumors, multiple BM and lung metastases were significantly associated with poor OS.

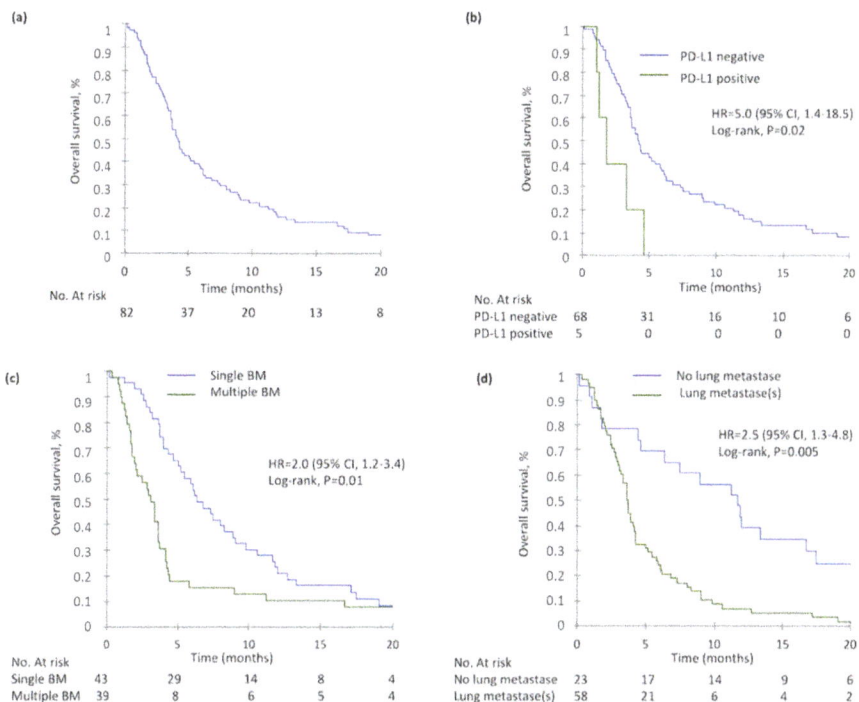

Figure 1. Overall Survival at brain metastasis(es) diagnosis in the whole population and according to PD-L1 expression, number of brain metastasis(es) and the presence of lung metastasis(es): (**a**) Overall survival of 82 patients at BM diagnosis, (**b**) Overall survival according to PD-L1 expression in primary tumor, (**c**) Overall survival according to the BM number, (**d**) Overall survival according to the presence of lung metastasis(es) at BM diagnosis.

Table 4. Univariate and multivariate analysis of overall survival in patients with brain metastases from colorectal cancer.

Variables	n	Univariate Analysis		Multivariate Analysis		
		Median (Months)	p Value	HR	95% CI	p Value
Gender (n = 82)			0.79 *			0.38
Male	52	3.9		1		
Female	30	4.3		0.8	0.5–1.4	
Age at BM diagnosis (n = 82)	82		0.02 *	1.0	1.0–1.0	0.62
Site of primary tumor (n = 82)			0.23			
Ascending colon	20	4.5				
Descending colon	24	5.9				
Rectum	35	2.9				
Tumor grade (n = 70)			0.05			
Well or moderately differentiated	61	3.9				
Poorly differentiated	9	4.6				
RAS status (n = 79)			0.65			
Wild-type	30	3.6				
Mutant	49	4.3				
BRAF status (n = 79)			0.03 *			0.76
Wild-type	74	4.2		1		
Mutant	5	3.3		1.2	0.3–4.2	
MMR status (n = 74)			0.68			
pMMR	70	4.1				
dMMR	4	4.0				
PD-1 expression (n = 74)			0.79			
Negative	64	4.2				
Positive	10	3.6				
PD-L1 expression (n = 73)			0.009 *			0.02
Negative	68	4.2		1		
Positive	5	1.8		5.0	1.4–18.5	
CD3 expression (n = 71)	71		0.08			
CD8 expression (n = 75)	75		0.45			
ECOG performance status (n = 79)			0.0003 *			0.07
<2	43	7.3		1		
≥2	36	3.2		1.8	1.0–3.4	
Number of BM (n = 82)			0.003 *			0.01
Single	43	6.3		1		
Multiple	39	3.1		2.0	1.2–3.4	
Lung metastases at BM diagnosis (n = 81)			0.0003 *			0.005
No	23	11.7		1		
Yes	58	3.6		2.5	1.3–4.8	
Liver metastases at BM diagnosis (n = 81)						
No	45	4.3	0.31			
Yes	36	3.7				

Abbreviations: HR, hazard ratio; BM, brain metastasis(es); 95% CI, 95% confidence interval; ECOG, Eastern Cooperative Oncology Group score. * variables included in multivariate analysis

3. Discussion

In our study, molecular features of CRC with BM were in accordance with rates observed in all-comers mCRC except for *RAS* mutations that appear to be higher than rates commonly observed in mCRC [11]. Surprisingly, we observed some differences of molecular profiles between BM and PPT, especially for *RAS* and PD-L1 status. Finally, we identified multiple BM, lung metastases and PD-L1 positivity as prognostic factors in patients with BM from CRC.

As compared to all-comers mCRC patients, in our study, patients with BM from CRC seemed to be younger, with more frequent rectal tumor and lung metastases. Other studies had previously identified frequent lung metastases and young age as particular characteristics of CRC patients with BM [1]. In accordance with the literature, the interval between primary tumor diagnosis and BM diagnosis reached more than 30 months, probably because the brain is a late sanctuary site for chemo-resistant tumor cells [12]. Moreover, the rate of *RAS* mutation was high (62%) in comparison to what is usually observed in mCRC ($\approx$50%) [11]. This observation is in agreement with other studies, which also showed that *KRAS* mutations could be a predictive factor of BM [13]. The rates of CD3 and CD8 tumor-infiltrating lymphocytes (TILs) observed in our study were in accordance with the rates observed in other mCRC cohorts [14,15]. Also, our study showed comparable proportions of PD-L1+ and PD-1+ tumors, mostly in dMMR tumors, when compared with other studies in the literature [16,17].

There is a high discrepancy observed between IHC and FISH results for cMET status in our study, as described in the literature. In a recent study using IHC, 57.5% of CRC were found to be positive for MET protein IHC, but only 4.4% were FISH positive [18]. Overexpression of MET has been established in CRC [19], with MET protein levels ranging from 12% to 81% (median, 61%) [20]. Zeng et al. established that *MET* gene amplification was present in 2% of localized CRC tumors, 9% of tumors with distant metastases, and 18% of liver metastases using the quantitative PCR/ligase detection reaction technique [21]. In our study cMET positive staining was detected by IHC in 61% of primary CRC, but none was confirmed by FISH.

Comparison of BM and PPT has been scarcely explored in mCRC, but discordances have been observed between BM and PPT in lung and breast cancers [10]. In our study, we found a higher rate of *RAS* mutation in BM (85%) compared to PPT (62%) and three discordant cases (9%). El-Deiry et al. determined *KRAS* status from 2510 primary CRC and 30 BM from CRC and found significantly higher rates of *KRAS* mutation in BM (65%) compared to the primary tumor (45%), but the samples were not paired [13]. In another cohort of 41 BM with PPT, two cases presented discordant *KRAS* status [22]. Discordances between PPT and BM could be explained by intra and/or inter-tumoral heterogeneity, as we recently demonstrated in CRC [23]. Indeed, if CRC patients have had BM surgery, *RAS* should be evaluated in this sample in order to define treatment (anti-EGFR). BM are more frequently observed in breast and gastric cancers with HER-2 overexpression compared to HER-2 negative tumors [24,25], which does not seem to be the case in mCRC.

To our knowledge, no previous study has compared the expression of PD-1, PD-L1, CD3 and CD8 in paired primary CRC and BM. In BM, we identified low rates of immune infiltrates compared to PPT. These results were concordant with the study by Harter et al., which showed low rates of PD-L1+ and PD-1+ tumors (1%) and low rates of CD3+ (3%) and CD8+ T-cells (2%) in BM samples from CRC [26]. In the literature, whatever the tumor type, less immune infiltrate is observed in BM compared to PPT [27]. Moreover, in our study, there was some discordance between PD-1 and PD-L1 status in BM compared to PPT. Recent studies have identified BM as a sanctuary site for tumor cells to escape immunosurveillance [28]. Up until now, there has been only limited data concerning immune checkpoint inhibitor efficacy in BM, but no clinical evidence of lesser efficacy compared to other metastatic sites [29]. Nevertheless, it is important to consider the spatial heterogeneity of the tumor immune microenvironment in BM compared to PPT, especially PD-L1 expression, when cancer patients are treated with PD-1 or PD-L1 inhibitors.

Overall survival of patients with BM from CRC is poor. It is important to identify prognostic factors to help therapeutic decision-making. Some prognostic classifications exist, but most are not designed specifically for patients with mCRC. A recent Italian retrospective study identified age, performance status, BM site and BM number as prognostic factors associated with OS of CRC patients with BM [30]. In our study, we found no association between *RAS* or *BRAF* status and OS. However, OS of patients with PD-L1 negative primary tumors was significantly higher than patients with PD-L1+ tumors. This result should be interpreted with caution considering the small number of patients with PDL1+ tumors, the potential tumor heterogeneity and the absence of standard cut-off for this marker. High PD-L1 expression has been associated with longer OS in pMMR mCRC in some studies, but not all [31]. In addition, in lung cancer with BM, PD-L1 expression has been associated with worse OS [32]. Our study highlighted two other prognostic markers, single BM and the absence of lung metastases that had already been reported for patients with BM whatever the primary tumor.

The main limitation of the study is its retrospective nature, but there are few missing data (≈10%). Results concerning the comparison of BM and PPT should be confirmed given the small size of our study, since most patients did not have surgery of BM. Nevertheless, it is the largest study up until now concerning the molecular profile of CRC with BM.

4. Materials and Methods

4.1. Patients

All patients with BM from CRC, diagnosed from 2001 to 2016, were identified in our institution using our clinical report database. All patients with a histologically confirmed CRC and histologically or radiologically confirmed BM by computed tomography scan (CT-scan) and/or magnetic resonance imaging (MRI) were included. BM was defined as synchronous if they occur within three months of mCRC diagnosis. Our institution's Ethics Committee approved the study (DC-2008-565).

4.2. Molecular Analyses

Genomic DNA from tumor samples was extracted using Maxwell 16 FFPE Plus LEV DNA purification kit© (Promega, Charbonnières-les-Bains, France). *KRAS/NRAS* codons 12, 13, 61, 146 and *BRAF* (V600E) were analyzed by pyrosequencing (TheraScreenPyroKit©, Qiagen, Hilden, Germany) using homemade specific primers as previously described [33]. MMR status was determined by microsatellite analysis using MD1641 Promega kit© (Promega).

4.3. Tissue Microarray Construction and Immunohistochemistry

Formalin-fixed paraffin-embedded blocks were used for tissue microarray (TMA) construction using four biopsy cores of 1 mm diameter per tumor in the tumor center (MTA Booster© version 1.01, Alphelys, Paris, France).

IHCwas carried out on paraffin-embedded 3-μm thick TMA sections with antibodies directed against ALK, ROS1, cMet, HER-2, PD-1, PD-L1, CD3 and CD8 according to the manufacturer's instructions.

IHC is a prescreening test commonly used for the detection of ALK rearrangement in lung carcinoma [34] and the same scoring was used here. Immunostaining scores were assigned from 0 to 3. For ALK cytoplasmic staining, a score of 1+ (weak), 2+ (moderate) or 3+ (strong) in more than 10% of tumor cells and for ROS1 staining, any percentage of tumor cells with cytoplasmic staining intensity of 1+, 2+ or 3+ were considered as IHC-positive and then evaluated by FISH [35]. Indeed, FISH is considered the "gold standard" to confirm IHC results, due to possible false-positive signals with IHC testing [36]. For MET only 2+ or 3+ in more than 10% of tumor cells were defined as positive and subsequently evaluated by FISH [37]. HER-2 IHC positive status was defined as tumors with a 2+ or 3+ staining in more than 10% of the cells and then evaluated by FISH [38].

PD-1 IHC was considered positive when ≥1% of intra-epithelial TILs were stained. PD-L1 immunostaining was considered positive when ≥1% of tumor cells had membranous staining [39]. CD3 and CD8 staining were also analyzed as the percentage of both intra-tumoral and stromal CD3 and CD8 positive lymphocytes over the total immune cells [14,15].

4.4. Fluorescent In Situ Hybridization (FISH)

Vysis ALK Break Apart FISH probes© (Abbott Molecular, Abbott Park, IL, USA), HER-2/CEP17 DNA Probe Kit II probes© (Abbott Molecular) and ZytoLight SPEC MET/CEN 7 Dual Color Probes© (ZytoVision, Bremerhaven, Germany) were used respectively for the detection of *ALK* rearrangement, *HER-2* and *cMET* amplification.

ALK locus rearrangement was considered translocated if ≥15% of tumor cells showed isolated red signal(s) and/or split red and green signals. *ALK* appeared amplified and required further verification if an average copy number ≥6 copies per nucleus was detected [40]. HER-2 was considered amplified

Cancers **2018**, *10*, 504

if average *HER-2/CEP17* ratio was higher than 2.0 [38]. Tumors with *MET*/CEP7 ratio $\geq$2 or with an average number of *MET* signals per nucleus >6 were scored as positive for *MET* amplification [41].

4.5. Statistical Analysis

Survival curves and 95% confidence intervals were determined using the Kaplan-Meier method. Predictive factors of OS were evaluated using the log-rank test for univariate analysis and statistically significant variables were included in multivariate analysis using a Cox regression model. The level of significance was set at a p value of 0.05. Statistical analyses were performed using XLSTAT 2017 software (Addinsoft, New York, NY, USA).

5. Conclusions

Our study provided relevant and specific features of CRC patients with BM, such as frequent lung metastasis, frequent rectal tumor site and high rate of *RAS* mutation. These results suggest a need for BM screening in this mCRC patients subgroup, but will require further prospective investigations to determine if early identification of BM improves survival and/or quality of life. We have highlighted the usefulness of BM number, the presence of lung metastases and the expression of PD-L1 as prognostic markers. For the first time, we found that PD-L1 expression was associated with poor prognostic in CRC patients with BM. All of these new data can guide therapeutic decision-making in patients with BM from CRC.

Author Contributions: Conceptualization, P.R., L.K.-T. and D.T.; methodology, P.R., G.T., C.V., S.M., E.F., L.K.-T. and D.T.; validation, P.R., L.K.-T. and D.T.; formal analysis, P.R., G.T., C.V., S.M., E.F., J.G., A.B., S.E., C.P., M.W., L.K.-T. and D.T.; investigation, P.R., G.T., L.K.-T. and D.T.; data curation, P.R., L.K.-T. and D.T.; writing—original draft preparation, P.R., G.T., L.K.-T. and D.T.; writing—review and editing, P.R., G.T., C.V., S.M., E.F., J.G., A.B., S.E., C.P., M.W., L.K.-T. and D.T.; supervision, L.K.-T. and D.T.; project administration, L.K.-T. and D.T.

Funding: This work was supported by a grant from the associations "Sport et Collection" and "Ligue Contre le Cancer, Comités départementaux de la Vienne, Charente et Charente-Maritime".

Acknowledgments: The authors thank all of the clinical research technicians who participated in DNA extraction. Our original English-language manuscript was reread and revised by Jeffrey Arsham, an American medical translator. Finally, the authors would like to thank Vanessa Le Berre and Laetitia Rouleau for their assistance in preparing the submission of the article.

Conflicts of Interest: The authors declare no conflict of interest.

Abbreviations

BM	Brain Metastases
CI	Confidence Interval
CT-scan	Computed Tomography scan
CRC	Colorectal Cancer
ECM	Extracranial Metastasis(es)
ECOG	Eastern Cooperative Oncology Group score
FISH	Fluorescence In Situ Hybridization
HR	Hazard Ratio
IHC	Immunohistochemistry
OS	Overall Survival
mCRC	Metastatic Colorectal Cancer
MMR	Mismatch Repair
MRI	Magnetic Resonance Imaging
pMMR	Proficient Mismatch Repair
dMMR	Deficient Mismatch Repair
PPT	Paired Primary Tumor
TMA	Tissue Microarray
TILs	Tumor-Infiltrating Lymphocytes

References

1. Christensen, T.D.; Spindler, K.-L.G.; Palshof, J.A.; Nielsen, D.L. Systematic review: Brain metastases from colorectal cancer—Incidence and patient characteristics. *BMC Cancer* **2016**, *16*, 260. [CrossRef]
2. Jung, M.; Ahn, J.B.; Chang, J.H.; Suh, C.O.; Hong, S.; Roh, J.K.; Shin, S.J.; Rha, S.Y. Brain metastases from colorectal carcinoma: Prognostic factors and outcome. *J. Neurooncol.* **2011**, *101*, 49–55. [CrossRef] [PubMed]
3. Tanriverdi, O.; Kaytan-Saglam, E.; Ulger, S.; Bayoglu, I.V.; Turker, I.; Ozturk-Topcu, T.; Cokmert, S.; Turhal, S.; Oktay, E.; Karabulut, B.; et al. The clinical and pathological features of 133 colorectal cancer patients with brain metastasis: A multicenter retrospective analysis of the Gastrointestinal Tumors Working Committee of the Turkish Oncology Group (TOG). *Med. Oncol.* **2014**, *31*, 152. [CrossRef] [PubMed]
4. Yaeger, R.; Cowell, E.; Chou, J.F.; Gewirtz, A.N.; Borsu, L.; Vakiani, E.; Solit, D.B.; Rosen, N.; Capanu, M.; Ladanyi, M.; et al. RAS mutations affect pattern of metastatic spread and increase propensity for brain metastasis in colorectal cancer. *Cancer* **2015**, *121*, 1195–1203. [CrossRef] [PubMed]
5. Christensen, T.D.; Palshof, J.A.; Larsen, F.O.; Høgdall, E.; Poulsen, T.S.; Pfeiffer, P.; Jensen, B.V.; Yilmaz, M.K.; Christensen, I.J.; Nielsen, D. Risk factors for brain metastases in patients with metastatic colorectal cancer. *Acta Oncol.* **2017**, *56*, 639–645. [CrossRef] [PubMed]
6. Michl, M.; Thurmaier, J.; Schubert-Fritschle, G.; Wiedemann, M.; Laubender, R.P.; Nüssler, N.C.; Ruppert, R.; Kleeff, J.; Schepp, W.; Reuter, C.; et al. Brain Metastasis in Colorectal Cancer Patients: Survival and Analysis of Prognostic Factors. *Clin. Colorectal. Cancer* **2015**, *14*, 281–290. [CrossRef] [PubMed]
7. Liu, J.; Zeng, W.; Huang, C.; Wang, J.; Yang, D.; Ma, D. Predictive and Prognostic Implications of Mutation Profiling and Microsatellite Instability Status in Patients with Metastatic Colorectal Carcinoma. Available online: https://www.hindawi.com/journals/grp/2018/4585802/abs/ (accessed on 27 November 2018).
8. Prasanna, T.; Karapetis, C.S.; Roder, D.; Tie, J.; Padbury, R.; Price, T.; Wong, R.; Shapiro, J.; Nott, L.; Lee, M.; et al. The survival outcome of patients with metastatic colorectal cancer based on the site of metastases and the impact of molecular markers and site of primary cancer on metastatic pattern. *Acta Oncol.* **2018**, *57*, 1438–1444. [CrossRef] [PubMed]
9. Vakiani, E.; Janakiraman, M.; Shen, R.; Sinha, R.; Zeng, Z.; Shia, J.; Cercek, A.; Kemeny, N.; D'Angelica, M.; Viale, A.; et al. Comparative genomic analysis of primary versus metastatic colorectal carcinomas. *J. Clin. Oncol.* **2012**, *30*, 2956–2962. [CrossRef]
10. Brastianos, P.K.; Carter, S.L.; Santagata, S.; Cahill, D.P.; Taylor-Weiner, A.; Jones, R.T.; Van Allen, E.M.; Lawrence, M.S.; Horowitz, P.M.; Cibulskis, K.; et al. Genomic Characterization of Brain Metastases Reveals Branched Evolution and Potential Therapeutic Targets. *Cancer Discov.* **2015**, *5*, 1164–1177. [CrossRef]
11. Douillard, J.-Y.; Oliner, K.S.; Siena, S.; Tabernero, J.; Burkes, R.; Barugel, M.; Humblet, Y.; Bodoky, G.; Cunningham, D.; Jassem, J.; et al. Panitumumab-FOLFOX4 treatment and RAS mutations in colorectal cancer. *N. Engl. J. Med.* **2013**, *369*, 1023–1034. [CrossRef]
12. Berghoff, A.S.; Schur, S.; Füreder, L.M.; Gatterbauer, B.; Dieckmann, K.; Widhalm, G.; Hainfellner, J.; Zielinski, C.C.; Birner, P.; Bartsch, R.; et al. Descriptive statistical analysis of a real life cohort of 2419 patients with brain metastases of solid cancers. *ESMO Open* **2016**, *1*, e000024. [CrossRef] [PubMed]
13. El-Deiry, W.S.; Vijayvergia, N.; Xiu, J.; Scicchitano, A.; Lim, B.; Yee, N.S.; Harvey, H.A.; Gatalica, Z.; Reddy, S. Molecular profiling of 6,892 colorectal cancer samples suggests different possible treatment options specific to metastatic sites. *Cancer Biol. Ther.* **2015**, *16*, 1726–1737. [CrossRef] [PubMed]
14. Tougeron, D.; Fauquembergue, E.; Rouquette, A.; Le Pessot, F.; Sesboüé, R.; Laurent, M.; Berthet, P.; Mauillon, J.; Di Fiore, F.; Sabourin, J.-C.; et al. Tumor-infiltrating lymphocytes in colorectal cancers with microsatellite instability are correlated with the number and spectrum of frameshift mutations. *Mod. Pathol.* **2009**, *22*, 1186–1195. [CrossRef] [PubMed]
15. Maby, P.; Tougeron, D.; Hamieh, M.; Mlecnik, B.; Kora, H.; Bindea, G.; Angell, H.K.; Fredriksen, T.; Elie, N.; Fauquembergue, E.; et al. Correlation between Density of CD8+ T-cell Infiltrate in Microsatellite Unstable Colorectal Cancers and Frameshift Mutations: A Rationale for Personalized Immunotherapy. *Cancer Res.* **2015**, *75*, 3446–3455. [CrossRef] [PubMed]
16. Gatalica, Z.; Snyder, C.; Maney, T.; Ghazalpour, A.; Holterman, D.A.; Xiao, N.; Overberg, P.; Rose, I.; Basu, G.D.; Vranic, S.; et al. Programmed cell death 1 (PD-1) and its ligand (PD-L1) in common cancers and their correlation with molecular cancer type. *Cancer Epidemiol. Biomark. Prev.* **2014**, *23*, 2965–2970. [CrossRef] [PubMed]

17. Lee, L.H.; Cavalcanti, M.S.; Segal, N.H.; Hechtman, J.F.; Weiser, M.R.; Smith, J.J.; Garcia-Aguilar, J.; Sadot, E.; Ntiamoah, P.; Markowitz, A.J.; et al. Patterns and prognostic relevance of PD-1 and PD-L1 expression in colorectal carcinoma. *Mod. Pathol.* **2016**, *29*, 1433–1442. [CrossRef]

18. Zhang, M.; Li, G.; Sun, X.; Ni, S.; Tan, C.; Xu, M.; Huang, D.; Ren, F.; Li, D.; Wei, P.; et al. MET amplification, expression, and exon 14 mutations in colorectal adenocarcinoma. *Hum. Pathol.* **2018**, *77*, 108–115. [CrossRef]

19. Abou-Bakr, A.A.; Elbasmi, A. c-MET overexpression as a prognostic biomarker in colorectal adenocarcinoma. *Gulf. J. Oncol.* **2013**, *1*, 28–34.

20. Liu, Y.; Yu, X.-F.; Zou, J.; Luo, Z.-H. Prognostic value of c-Met in colorectal cancer: A meta-analysis. *World J. Gastroenterol.* **2015**, *21*, 3706–3710. [CrossRef]

21. Zeng, Z.-S.; Weiser, M.R.; Kuntz, E.; Chen, C.-T.; Khan, S.A.; Forslund, A.; Nash, G.M.; Gimbel, M.; Yamaguchi, Y.; Culliford, A.T.; et al. c-Met gene amplification is associated with advanced stage colorectal cancer and liver metastases. *Cancer Lett.* **2008**, *265*, 258–269. [CrossRef]

22. Aprile, G.; Casagrande, M.; De Maglio, G.; Fontanella, C.; Rihawi, K.; Bonotto, M.; Pisa, F.E.; Tuniz, F.; Pizzolitto, S.; Fasola, G. Comparison of the molecular profile of brain metastases from colorectal cancer and corresponding primary tumors. *Future Oncol.* **2017**, *13*, 135–144. [CrossRef] [PubMed]

23. Jeantet, M.; Tougeron, D.; Tachon, G.; Cortes, U.; Archambaut, C.; Fromont, G.; Karayan-Tapon, L. High Intra- and Inter-Tumoral Heterogeneity of RAS Mutations in Colorectal Cancer. *Int. J. Mol. Sci.* **2016**, *17*, 2015. [CrossRef] [PubMed]

24. Feilchenfeldt, J.; Varga, Z.; Siano, M.; Grabsch, H.I.; Held, U.; Schuknecht, B.; Trip, A.; Hamaguchi, T.; Gut, P.; Balague, O.; et al. Brain metastases in gastro-oesophageal adenocarcinoma: Insights into the role of the human epidermal growth factor receptor 2 (HER2). *Br. J. Cancer* **2015**, *113*, 716–721. [CrossRef] [PubMed]

25. Gabos, Z.; Sinha, R.; Hanson, J.; Chauhan, N.; Hugh, J.; Mackey, J.R.; Abdulkarim, B. Prognostic significance of human epidermal growth factor receptor positivity for the development of brain metastasis after newly diagnosed breast cancer. *J. Clin. Oncol.* **2006**, *24*, 5658–5663. [CrossRef]

26. Harter, P.N.; Bernatz, S.; Scholz, A.; Zeiner, P.S.; Zinke, J.; Kiyose, M.; Blasel, S.; Beschorner, R.; Senft, C.; Bender, B.; et al. Distribution and prognostic relevance of tumor-infiltrating lymphocytes (TILs) and PD-1/PD-L1 immune checkpoints in human brain metastases. *Oncotarget* **2015**, *6*, 40836–40849. [CrossRef] [PubMed]

27. Mansfield, A.S.; Aubry, M.C.; Moser, J.C.; Harrington, S.M.; Dronca, R.S.; Park, S.S.; Dong, H. Temporal and spatial discordance of programmed cell death-ligand 1 expression and lymphocyte tumor infiltration between paired primary lesions and brain metastases in lung cancer. *Ann. Oncol.* **2016**, *27*, 1953–1958. [CrossRef] [PubMed]

28. Puhalla, S.; Elmquist, W.; Freyer, D.; Kleinberg, L.; Adkins, C.; Lockman, P.; McGregor, J.; Muldoon, L.; Nesbit, G.; Peereboom, D.; et al. Unsanctifying the sanctuary: Challenges and opportunities with brain metastases. *Neuro-Oncology* **2015**, *17*, 639–651. [CrossRef] [PubMed]

29. Goldberg, S.B.; Gettinger, S.N.; Mahajan, A.; Chiang, A.C.; Herbst, R.S.; Sznol, M.; Tsiouris, A.J.; Cohen, J.; Vortmeyer, A.; Jilaveanu, L.; et al. Pembrolizumab for patients with melanoma or non-small-cell lung cancer and untreated brain metastases: Early analysis of a non-randomised, open-label, phase 2 trial. *Lancet Oncol.* **2016**, *17*, 976–983. [CrossRef]

30. Pietrantonio, F.; Aprile, G.; Rimassa, L.; Franco, P.; Lonardi, S.; Cremolini, C.; Biondani, P.; Sbicego, E.L.; Pasqualetti, F.; Tomasello, G.; et al. A new nomogram for estimating survival in patients with brain metastases secondary to colorectal cancer. *Radiother. Oncol.* **2015**, *117*, 315–321. [CrossRef]

31. Droeser, R.A.; Hirt, C.; Viehl, C.T.; Frey, D.M.; Nebiker, C.; Huber, X.; Zlobec, I.; Eppenberger-Castori, S.; Tzankov, A.; Rosso, R.; et al. Clinical impact of programmed cell death ligand 1 expression in colorectal cancer. *Eur. J. Cancer* **2013**, *49*, 2233–2242. [CrossRef]

32. Téglási, V.; Reiniger, L.; Fábián, K.; Pipek, O.; Csala, I.; Bagó, A.G.; Várallyai, P.; Vízkeleti, L.; Rojkó, L.; Tímár, J.; et al. Evaluating the significance of density, localization, and PD-1/PD-L1 immunopositivity of mononuclear cells in the clinical course of lung adenocarcinoma patients with brain metastasis. *Neuro-Oncology* **2017**, *19*, 1058–1067. [CrossRef] [PubMed]

33. Cortes, U.; Guilloteau, K.; Rouvreau, M.; Archaimbault, C.; Villalva, C.; Karayan-Tapon, L. Development of pyrosequencing methods for the rapid detection of RAS mutations in clinical samples. *Exp. Mol. Pathol.* **2015**, *99*, 207–211. [CrossRef] [PubMed]

34. Lindeman, N.I.; Cagle, P.T.; Beasley, M.B.; Chitale, D.A.; Dacic, S.; Giaccone, G.; Jenkins, R.B.; Kwiatkowski, D.J.; Saldivar, J.-S.; Squire, J.; et al. Molecular testing guideline for selection of lung cancer patients for EGFR and ALK tyrosine kinase inhibitors: Guideline from the College of American Pathologists, International Association for the Study of Lung Cancer, and Association for Molecular Pathology. *J. Mol. Diagn.* **2013**, *15*, 415–453. [CrossRef] [PubMed]

35. Houang, M.; Toon, C.W.; Clarkson, A.; Sioson, L.; de Silva, K.; Watson, N.; Singh, N.R.; Chou, A.; Gill, A.J. ALK and ROS1 overexpression is very rare in colorectal adenocarcinoma. *Appl. Immunohistochem. Mol. Morphol.* **2015**, *23*, 134–138. [CrossRef] [PubMed]

36. Yatabe, Y. ALK FISH and IHC: You cannot have one without the other. *J. Thorac. Oncol.* **2015**, *10*, 548–550. [CrossRef]

37. Bardelli, A.; Corso, S.; Bertotti, A.; Hobor, S.; Valtorta, E.; Siravegna, G.; Sartore-Bianchi, A.; Scala, E.; Cassingena, A.; Zecchin, D.; et al. Amplification of the MET receptor drives resistance to anti-EGFR therapies in colorectal cancer. *Cancer Discov.* **2013**, *3*, 658–673. [CrossRef]

38. Valtorta, E.; Martino, C.; Sartore-Bianchi, A.; Penaullt-Llorca, F.; Viale, G.; Risio, M.; Rugge, M.; Grigioni, W.; Bencardino, K.; Lonardi, S.; et al. Assessment of a HER2 scoring system for colorectal cancer: Results from a validation study. *Mod. Pathol.* **2015**, *28*, 1481–1491. [CrossRef]

39. Overman, M.J.; McDermott, R.; Leach, J.L.; Lonardi, S.; Lenz, H.-J.; Morse, M.A.; Desai, J.; Hill, A.; Axelson, M.; Moss, R.A.; et al. Nivolumab in patients with metastatic DNA mismatch repair-deficient or microsatellite instability-high colorectal cancer (CheckMate 142): An open-label, multicentre, phase 2 study. *Lancet Oncol.* **2017**, *18*, 1182–1191. [CrossRef]

40. Zito Marino, F.; Rocco, G.; Morabito, A.; Mignogna, C.; Intartaglia, M.; Liguori, G.; Botti, G.; Franco, R. A new look at the ALK gene in cancer: Copy number gain and amplification. *Expert Rev. Anticancer Ther.* **2016**, *16*, 493–502. [CrossRef]

41. Pietrantonio, F.; Oddo, D.; Gloghini, A.; Valtorta, E.; Berenato, R.; Barault, L.; Caporale, M.; Busico, A.; Morano, F.; Gualeni, A.V.; et al. MET-Driven Resistance to Dual EGFR and BRAF Blockade May Be Overcome by Switching from EGFR to MET Inhibition in BRAF-Mutated Colorectal Cancer. *Cancer Discov.* **2016**, *6*, 963–971. [CrossRef]

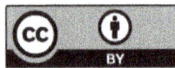

cancers

MDPI

Article

Genomic Profiling of the Steroidogenic Acute Regulatory Protein in Breast Cancer: In Silico Assessments and a Mechanistic Perspective

Pulak R. Manna [1],*, Ahsen U. Ahmed [1], Shengping Yang [2], Madhusudhanan Narasimhan [3], Joëlle Cohen-Tannoudji [4], Andrzej T. Slominski [5,6] and Kevin Pruitt [1]

[1] Departments of Immunology and Molecular Microbiology, School of Medicine, Texas Tech University Health Sciences Center, Lubbock, TX 79430, USA; ahsen.ahmed@ttuhsc.edu (A.U.A.); kevin.pruitt@ttuhsc.edu (K.P.)

[2] Internal Medicine, School of Medicine, Texas Tech University Health Sciences Center, Lubbock, TX 79430, USA; shengping.yang@ttuhsc.edu

[3] Pharmacology and Neuroscience, School of Medicine, Texas Tech University Health Sciences Center, Lubbock, TX 79430, USA; madhu.narasimhan@ttuhsc.edu

[4] Physiologie de l'axe gonadotrope U1133, Institut National de la Santé et de la Recherche Médicale, CNRS, Biologie Fonctionnelle et Adaptative UMR 8251, Université Paris Diderot, 75205 Paris, France; tannoudji@univ-paris-diderot.fr

[5] Department of Dermatology and Laboratory Medicine, Comprehensive Cancer Center, Cancer Chemoprevention Program, University of Alabama at Birmingham, Birmingham, AL 35294, USA; aslominski@uabmc.edu

[6] Veterans Administration Medical Center, Birmingham, AL 35294, USA

* Correspondence: pulak.manna@ttuhsc.edu; Tel.: +1-806-743-3542; Fax: +1-806-743-2334

Received: 18 April 2019; Accepted: 30 April 2019; Published: 4 May 2019

Abstract: Cancer is a multifactorial condition with aberrant growth of cells. A substantial number of cancers, breast in particular, are hormone sensitive and evolve due to malfunction in the steroidogenic machinery. Breast cancer, one of the most prevalent form of cancers in women, is primarily stimulated by estrogens. Steroid hormones are made from cholesterol, and regulation of steroid/estrogen biosynthesis is essentially influenced by the steroidogenic acute regulatory (StAR) protein. Although the impact of StAR in breast cancer remains a mystery, we recently reported that StAR protein is abundantly expressed in hormone sensitive breast cancer, but not in its non-cancerous counterpart. Herein, we analyzed genomic profiles, hormone receptor expression, mutation, and survival for StAR and steroidogenic enzyme genes in a variety of hormone sensitive cancers. These profiles were specifically assessed in breast cancer, exploiting The Cancer Genome Atlas (TCGA) datasets. Whereas StAR and key steroidogenic enzyme genes evaluated (*CYP11A1*, *HSD3B*, *CYP17A1*, *CYP19A1*, and *HSD17B*) were altered to varying levels in these hormone responsive cancers, amplification of the *StAR* gene was correlated with poor overall survival of patients afflicted with breast cancer. Amplification of the *StAR* gene and its correlation to survival was also verified in a number of breast cancer studies. Additionally, TCGA breast cancer tumors associated with aberrant high expression of *StAR* mRNA were found to be an unfavorable risk factor for survival of patients with breast cancer. Further analyses of tumors, nodal status, and metastases of breast cancer tumors expressing *StAR* mRNA displayed cancer deaths in stage specific manners. The majority of these tumors were found to express estrogen and progesterone receptors, signifying a link between StAR and luminal subtype breast cancer. Collectively, analyses of genomic and molecular profiles of key steroidogenic factors provide novel insights that StAR plays an important role in the biologic behavior and/or pathogenesis of hormone sensitive breast cancer.

Keywords: hormone sensitive cancers; breast cancer; StAR; estrogen; steroidogenic enzymes

1. Introduction

The rate-limiting step in the regulation of steroid hormone biosynthesis is the transport of the substrate of all steroid hormones, cholesterol, from the outer to the inner mitochondrial membrane, a process that is predominantly mediated by the steroidogenic acute regulatory (StAR; also called STARD1) protein [1–4]. There is wealth of information that regulation of steroid biosynthesis is mediated by mechanisms that enhance the transcription, translation, or activity of StAR [2,4–6]. Noteworthy, whereas phosphorylation of StAR is associated with the optimal cholesterol transferring ability of the StAR protein in steroid biosynthesis, mutations in the *StAR* gene results in a protein that is nonfunctional and inactive in transporting cholesterol. In almost every system studied, agents/factors that influence StAR expression also influence steroid biosynthesis through endocrine, autocrine, and paracrine regulation in a variety of classical and non-classical steroidogenic tissues [2,4,7–11]. Following the transport of cholesterol, by StAR, to the inner mitochondrial membrane, the P450 side chain cleavage (P450scc) enzyme, encoded by the *CYP11A1* gene, catalyzes the first enzymatic step in steroidogenesis i.e., the conversion of cholesterol to pregnenolone [4,6]. In addition, CYP11A1 converts 7-dehydrocholesterol to 7-dehydropregneolone and activates vitamin D, emphasizing the importance of StAR to transport other substrates for non-canonical activity of CYP11A1 [12,13]. The first steroid, pregnenolone, is then metabolized to various sex steroids by a series of enzymes in target tissues. These enzymes include 3β-hydroxysteroid dehydrogenase (3β-HSD), 17α-monooxygenase, 17α-hydroxylase, 17,20-lyase (P45017α), aromatase, and 17β-HSD, which are encoded by the *HSD3B*, *CYP17A1*, *CYP19A1*, and *HSD17B* genes, respectively [4,8].

Steroid hormones are synthesized not only in endocrine tissues, but also in a variety of extra-gonadal/adrenal tissues, and they play crucial roles in diverse processes, ranging from development to homeostasis to carcinogenesis [4,10,11,14–16]. Of note, StAR mediates steroid biosynthesis by controlling the transport of cholesterol and, thus, its entry to the mitochondrial inner membrane is a key event in influencing various cholesterol/steroid led functions. Conversely, inappropriate regulation of StAR, involving cholesterol transport, might influence hormone dependent disorders. Accordingly, cholesterol and its metabolites have been shown to be involved in the etiology of a number of cancers [17,18]. Moreover, dysregulation of androgen and estrogen biosynthesis has long been implicated in the pathogenesis a variety of hormone sensitive cancers [16,19].

One of the most common malignancies in women is breast cancer, which is activated by estrogens, especially 17β-estradiol (E2), and it accounts for over one-fourth of all cancer cases [16,20–22]. The American Cancer Society estimated that 266,120 women were expected to be diagnosed with invasive breast cancer, with 40,920 deaths in 2018. Breast cancers are classified into four subtypes, i.e., luminal A, luminal B, HER2/ErbB2+ (human epidermal growth factor receptor 2/the erythroblastosis oncogene-B2 positive), and TNBC (triple negative breast cancer), based on estrogen receptor (ER), progesterone receptor (PR), and HER2 expression [23]. Hormone sensitive breast cancers predominantly express ER, especially ERα, and/or PR, and account for ~80% of all breast cancer cases. The remaining 15–20% cancers include HER2+ that expresses HER2, and TNBC that does not express ER, PR, and HER2 [24,25]. In this connection, it is worth noting that expression of the StAR protein has been shown to be markedly high in ER+/PR+ breast cancer, modest in TNBC, but little to none in normal mammary epithelial cells [5]. Additionally, accumulation of E2 mirrored StAR protein expression in both noncancerous and cancerous breast cell lines, suggesting that StAR plays a key role in the development of ER+/PR+ breast cancer. To obtain more insight into the association of StAR in breast cancer, genomic profiling of StAR and key steroidogenic enzyme genes were analyzed by exploiting two publicly available research databases: The Cancer Genome Atlas (TCGA, provisional for different cancer types) and cBioPortal (for independent breast cancer studies).

2. Materials and Methods

2.1. TCGA Hormone Responsive Cancer Tumors and Their Correlation to Copy Number Alterations of StAR and Steroidogenic Enzyme Genes

TCGA genomic research databases were assessed for the following hormone sensitive cancers: breast (1080 tumors), colorectal (616 tumors), melanoma (367 tumors), ovarian (579 tumors), pancreatic (184 tumors), prostate (492 tumors), and uterine endometrial (539 tumors) [26–29]. These tumors were analyzed for DNA copy number alterations (CNAs) for StAR and key steroidogenic enzyme genes using the GISTIC 2.0. algorithm. CNA data were categorized as high-level amplification (+2 copies), gain (+1 copy), diploid (normal/no change), homozygous deletion (−2 copies), and hemizygous deletion (−1 copy). These analyses were performed using UCSC Xena [30] and/or cBioPortal Cancer Genomics [31,32] platforms. StAR CNA data were further evaluated for their correlation to StAR mRNA expression with RNA-Seq data, using the RSEM algorithm [33]. The correlation between StAR CNA and StAR mRNA levels was verified by Spearman's rank coefficient analysis.

2.2. Expression of ER, PR, and HER2 in Breast Cancer Tumors

The predictive immunohistochemical (IHC) markers, employed in clinical settings to classify breast cancer tumors into biologically distinct subtypes with unique pathogenesis, were examined. The use of IHC to assess ER, PR, and HER2 expression status in breast cancer has been routinely performed in clinics. IHC based tumor classification was analyzed for ER, PR, and HER2 expression using TCGA breast cancer datasets. These receptors were also evaluated in a number of breast cancer publications and/or projects that are available in cBioPortal website [31,32].

2.3. Amplification of the StAR Gene in Breast Cancer Studies

Amplification of the *StAR* gene was assessed in a variety of breast cancer publications/projects with cBioPortal browser. In particular, *StAR* gene amplification was analyzed in the following breast cancer studies: METABRIC (Molecular Taxonomy of Breast Cancer International Consortium), *Nature Communication* [34], (2173 tumors); breast cancer patient xenografts [35], (29 tumors); breast invasive carcinoma [36], (TCGA Cell 2015, 816 tumors); breast invasive carcinoma, [27], (TCGA Provisional; *Nature* 2012, 1080 tumors); metastatic breast cancer, *PLoS Medicine* [37], (216 tumors); and metastatic breast cancer (MBC) project (TCGA 2017, 103 tumors). These studies include mixed tumor types with variable numbers, in which amplification of the *StAR* gene and its correlation to overall survival, were evaluated, using available datasets.

2.4. Mutational Portraits of the StAR Gene in TCGA Hormone Responsive Cancers

Mutation in the *StAR* gene was examined in different hormone responsive cancers by analyzing exome sequencing, utilizing TCGA datasets. Mutational analyses were limited for functional forms. Intronic, silent, or other forms of mutations were not considered. These analyses were performed using UCSC Xena platform [30]. Gene mutation frequency is described as a percentage of total number of tumors.

2.5. Expression of StAR mRNA in TCGA Breast Cancer Tumors and Their Correlation to TNM Stages

Expression of StAR mRNA, evaluated from RNA-Seq data, available for breast cancer tumors, was downloaded from TCGA and UCSC Xena websites. StAR mRNA expressed as upper quartile-normalized fragments per kilobase of transcript per million mapped reads (fpkm+uq+1), generated by TCGA, was plotted using the Box and Whisker plot [38]. The Box and Whisker plot depicts normal distribution of StAR mRNA and determines the median and quartiles in a statistical population.

The T (tumor), N (node), and M (metastasis) staging, is a globally recognized system for defining the extent of stage and/or spread of solid tumors for prognosis and treatment [39,40]. The TNM staging of TCGA breast cancer tumors, expressing StAR mRNA, was performed using the American Joint

Committee on cancer classifications [39,40]. StAR mRNA/RNA-Seq data analyzed for various purposes are provided as an Excel file under Supplemental Materials.

2.6. Generation of Kaplan-Meier Curves and Overall Survival Analyses

Kaplan-Meier curve is frequently used to determine survival analysis for clinical outcomes such as recovery rates, probability of death, and disappearance of a tumor [41]. Utilizing TCGA and/or cBioportal breast cancer tumor CNA data, Kaplan-Meier survival curves were generated using with (high level amplification) and without (diploid) amplification [42–44] for *StAR, CYP11A1, HSD3B1, CYP17A1, CYP19A1, HSD17B1,* and *HSD17B2* genes. For StAR, survival curve was also generated with and without (all tumors excluding homozygous deletion) amplification. Both *HSD17B1* and *HSD17B2* gene isoforms evaluated were based on their association with breast cancer [45]. Additionally, Kaplan-Meier survival curves were generated by dividing tumors into non-overlapping upper and lower groups based on two reports, with StAR mRNA values up to 50th percentile as low and above 50th as high [46]; and up to 25th percentile as low and above 25th percentile as high [47,48].

2.7. Statistical Analysis

Statistical analyses were performed using GraphPad Prism software (GraphPad, San Diego, CA, USA). Data represented are the mean ± SEM and analyzed using one-way analysis of variance (ANOVA) followed by post-hoc test. Spearman's rank coefficient analysis was performed to determine the correlation between StAR CNA and StAR mRNA levels. The analysis of overall survival between groups was performed by log-rank Mantel-Cox method. A *p*-value less than 0.05 was considered statistically significant.

3. Results

3.1. Assessment of StAR CNAs in Various Hormone Sensitive Cancers

Gene amplification, comprising oncogene activation, is a fundamental event in tumor progression [42]. The hypothesis that estrogen and/or androgen sensitive cancers involve gain of function of StAR in the transport of cholesterol, and thereby influence hormone sensitive cancers, was examined. Utilizing TCGA datasets, StAR CNA data were analyzed in a variety of hormone dependent cancers (Table 1). Breast cancer CNA data for StAR demonstrated ~13% high level amplification (138 tumors), ~25% gain (268 tumors), ~38% diploid (406 tumors), ~23% hemizygous deletion (252 tumors), and ~1.5% homozygous deletion (16 tumors). Tumor numbers altered in each category are shown in parentheses. Analysis of colorectal cancer CNA data for StAR resulted in ~2.5%, ~30%, ~44%, ~23%, and ~8% high level amplification, gain, diploid, hemizygous deletion, and homozygous deletion, respectively. Whereas StAR CNA data were found to be altered at varying levels, high level amplification was observed at 4.4% in pancreatic cancer. Likewise, melanoma, ovarian, prostate, and uterine endometrial cancer CNA data for StAR displayed ~0.3%, ~3.5%, ~2.9%, and ~1.9% high level amplification in these malignant tumors, respectively (Table 1). These data are consistent with previous detection of StAR in peripheral tissues and malignant tumors [4,49]. Higher amplification of the *StAR* gene (~13%) was next evaluated for its impact on breast cancer.

Table 1. DNA copy number alterations of the steroidogenic acute regulatory (*StAR*) gene in different hormone responsive cancers.

CNAs	Breast N (%)	Colorectal N (%)	Melanoma N (%)	Ovarian N (%)	Pancreatic N (%)	Prostate N (%)	Uterine Endometrial N (%)
Homozygous Deletion	16 (1.48)	8 (1.30)	3 (0.82)	7 (1.21)	0 (0.00)	32 (6.50)	7 (1.30)
Hemizygous Deletion	252 (23.33)	140 (22.73)	69 (18.80)	215 (37.13)	42 (22.83)	133 (27.03)	66 (12.24)
Diploid	406 (37.59)	271 (43.99)	184 (50.14)	220 (38.00)	109 (59.24)	258 (52.44)	345 (64.01)
Gain	268 (24.81)	182 (29.55)	110 (29.97)	117 (20.21)	25 (13.59)	55 (11.18)	111 (20.59)
High Level Amplification	138 (12.78)	15 (2.44)	1 (0.27)	20 (3.45)	8 (4.35)	14 (2.85)	10 (1.86)
Total Number of Tumors	1080	616	367	579	184	492	539

StAR CNA data were assessed for the following cancer tumors: breast (1080 cases), colorectal (616 cases), melanoma (367 cases), ovarian (579 cases), pancreatic (184 cases), prostate (492 cases), and uterine endometrial (539 cases). The CNA level was categorized as homozygous deletion, hemizygous deletion, diploid, gain, and high level amplification, as described under Section 2. N (%) = number of tumors with percentages in parentheses.

3.2. Expression of ER, PR and HER2 in TCGA Breast Cancer Tumors

To assess breast cancer subtype(s) in TCGA tumor datasets, expression of ER, PR and HER2 was examined. IHC data revealed differential expression of ER (74% positive, 21% negative, 5% unknown), PR (64% positive, 31% negative, 5% unknown), and HER2 (15% positive, 51% negative, 34% unknown) (Figure 1). These results indicate that TCGA breast cancer tumors are mostly ER+/PR+, representing they are largely luminal subtypes.

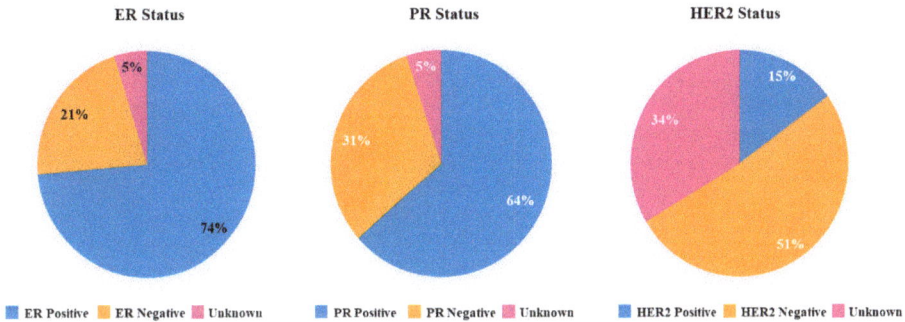

Figure 1. Expression of ER, PR and HER2 in The Cancer Genome Atlas (TCGA) breast cancer tumors. These tumors were previously stained with specific IHC markers in a clinical setting to classify into biologically distinct subtypes. Pie charts illustrate ER, PR, and HER2 expression in breast cancer tumors, which are presented as percentage of total numbers. Expression of these receptors was categorized as positive, negative, and unknown. The unknown category includes tumors in which IHC analysis was either not done or indeterminate or equivocal or data was not available.

3.3. Amplification of the StAR Gene in Breast Cancer and Its Correlation to Overall Survival

Utilizing TCGA breast cancer data cohort, amplification of the *StAR* gene was examined for cancer survival. As illustrated in Figure 2A, StAR CNA data in different categories were positively correlated with StAR mRNA expression (RNA-Seq data). The correlation between StAR CNA and StAR mRNA levels was verified with Spearman's correlation coefficient, i.e., 0.463. The analysis of Kaplan-Meier curve demonstrated that amplification of the *StAR* gene (~13%) was correlated with poor survival of breast cancer patients (*p*-value = 0.020). The median survival rate was noticeably reduced with amplification of the *StAR* gene when compared without amplification (Figure 2B). Similarly, the survival of breast cancer was affected (*p*-value = 0.045) when Kaplan-Meier curve was generated with and without (in which all tumors, excluding homozygous deletion, was included) *StAR* gene amplification (Figure 2C).

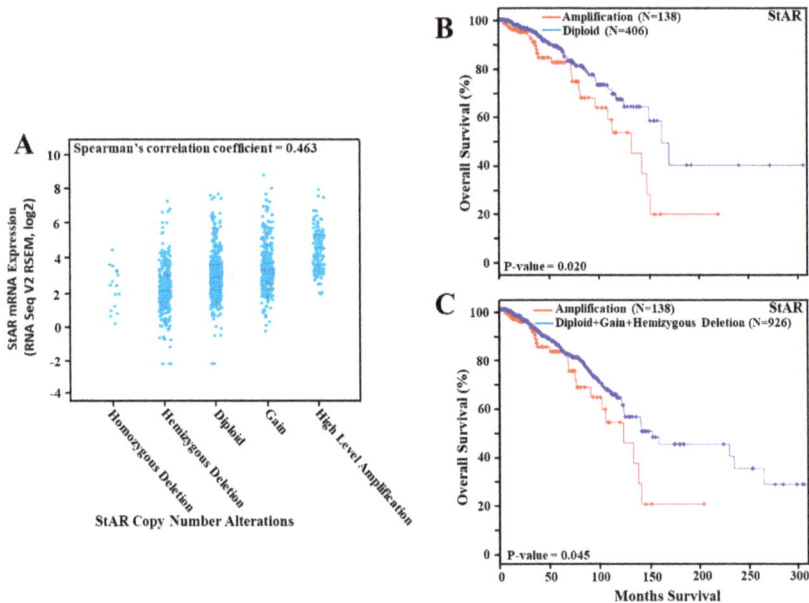

Figure 2. Frequency of StAR CNA data in breast cancer tumors and its correlation to overall survival. StAR CNA data were obtained from TCGA breast cancer tumor datasets with 1080 tumors. The CNA level was categorized as homozygous deletion, hemizygous deletion, diploid, gain, and high level amplification (**A**), utilizing cBioPortal browser, as described under Section 2. Breast cancer RNA-Seq data were assessed for StAR mRNA expression that positively correlated with StAR CNA data in different categories (**A**), which were presented in Y-axis and X-axis, respectively. Amplification of the *StAR* gene was evaluated for overall breast cancer survival (**B**,**C**). Kaplan-Meier curve was generated with TCGA breast cancer tumor CNA data, using with amplification (138 tumors) vs. without amplification (diploid, 406 tumors; **B**), or with a category (926 tumors; **C**) excluding homozygous deletion (16 tumors) of the *StAR* gene. Red and blue lines in panels B and C represent with and without amplification of the *StAR* gene, respectively.

3.4. StAR Gene Amplification, Hormone Receptor Expression, and Their Correlation to Cancer Survival in a Number of Breast Cancer Studies

To better understand involvement of *StAR* gene amplification in breast cancer deaths, genomic data from a number of publications/projects, as available in cBioPortal, were analyzed. As depicted in Figure 3A, amplification of the *StAR* gene was observed between 12% and 26% in all breast cancer studies examined. Specifically, amplification of the *StAR* gene was 26% in a breast cancer patient xenografts study, 12% in breast cancer METABRIC, and 13% and 14% in two independent publications associated with breast invasive carcinomas, and 15% each in two independent metastatic breast cancer studies (specified in Section 2).

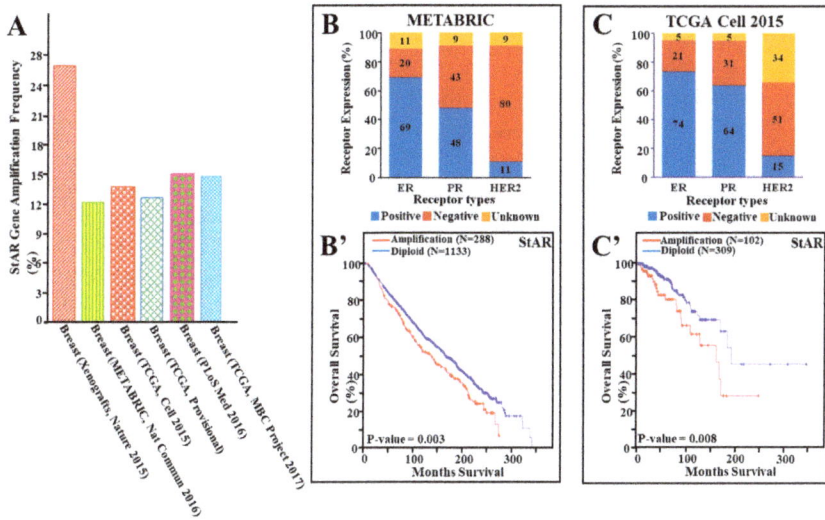

Figure 3. Amplification of the *StAR* gene, expression of hormone receptors, and their correlation to breast cancer survival in a number of publications/projects. Amplification of the *StAR* gene in different breast cancer studies, as available in cBioPortal, was analyzed. (**A**), amplification of the *StAR* gene was evaluated in the following breast cancer studies: breast cancer patient xenografts, Nature 2015 (29 tumors), [35]; breast METABRIC, *Nature Communication* 2016 (2173 tumors) [34]; breast TCGA Cell 2015, (816 tumors), [36]: TCGA Provisional (1080 tumors), [27]; breast *PLoS Medicine* 2016 (216 tumors), [37]; and TCGA Metastatic Breast Cancer (MBC) Project 2017 (103 tumors). Receptor expression was categorized as positive, negative, and unknown, and presented as percentages of total number of tumors (**B,C**), as described in the legend of Figure 1. Levels of ER, PR, and HER2 expression and their correlation to overall survival were analyzed for METABRIC (**B,B'**) and TCGA Cell 2015 (**C,C'**) studies. Kaplan-Meier survival curves were generated with METABRIC (red line, 288 tumors; blue line, 1133 tumors) and *Cell* 2015 (red line, 102 tumors; blue line, 309 tumors) CNA data, using tumors with amplification and without amplification (diploid) of the *StAR* gene.

In additional analyses, ER, PR, and HER2 expression, amplification of the *StAR* gene and its correlation to overall survival, were evaluated. In METABRIC study, breast cancer tumors (2173 tumors) were 69% ER+, 48% PR+, and 80% HER−, representing a mixed subtype, in which amplification of the *StAR* gene (~12%) affected the survival (*p*-value = 0.003) of breast cancer (Figure 3B,B'). In a breast invasive carcinoma study (Cell 2015, 816 tumors), amplification of the *StAR* gene (~14%), associated with 74% ER+, 64% PR+, and 51% HER2− (15% HER2+), was found to correlate (*p*-value = 0.008) with poor breast cancer survival (Figure 3C,C'). These data corroborate the findings presented in Figure 2B,C, and demonstrate that amplification of the *StAR* gene is correlated with poor survival of patients with luminal subtype breast cancer. Survival data were not available for other studies included in Figure 3A.

3.5. Amplification of Steroidogenic Enzyme Genes and Their Correlation to Overall Breast Cancer Survival

Estrogen plays an important role in stimulating breast cancer. The involvement of key steroidogenic enzyme genes (Supplementary Figure S1) to estrogen synthesis was next evaluated for their association to breast cancer survival utilizing TCGA data cohort. The data presented in Figure 4A–F illustrate bar graphs of different CNA frequencies (high level amplification (red), gain (blue), hemizygous deletion (green), and homozygous deletion (pink) for *CYP11A1*, *CYP17A1*, *HSD3B1*, *CYP19A1*, *HSD17B1*, and *HSD17B2* enzyme genes in different hormone sensitive cancers. Diploid category is not shown in these bar diagrams for easier visualization. CNA data demonstrate that the *CYP11A1* gene was amplified at ~1.5%, ~1.4%, ~3%, ~1.6%, and ~1.1% in breast, melanoma, ovarian, pancreatic, and uterine endometrial cancers, respectively (Figure 4A). No amplification of the *CYP11A1* gene was observed in prostate and colorectal cancers. The *CYP17A1* gene was amplified less than 1% in all cancer types analyzed (Figure 4B). Amplification of the *HSD3B1* gene was highest (~5%) in melanoma and none in colorectal cancer (Figure 4C). In breast cancer, this gene was amplified at ~2.3%. Amplification of the *CYP19A1* gene (aromatase) was ~1%, ~0.5%, ~0.3%, ~0.2%, ~1.6%, 0%, and ~0.2% in breast, colorectal, melanoma, ovarian, pancreatic, prostate, and uterine endometrial cancers, respectively (Figure 4D). Additionally, both *HSD17B1* and *HSD17B2* gene isoforms were found to be amplified minimally (0–1.4%) in different hormone sensitive cancers studied (Figure 4E,F). These *HSD17B1* and *HSD17B2* isoforms were amplified at ~1.4% and ~0.6% in breast cancer, respectively. These results are in support of previous studies that demonstrated upregulation of aberrant steroidogenesis during tumor progression [49,50].

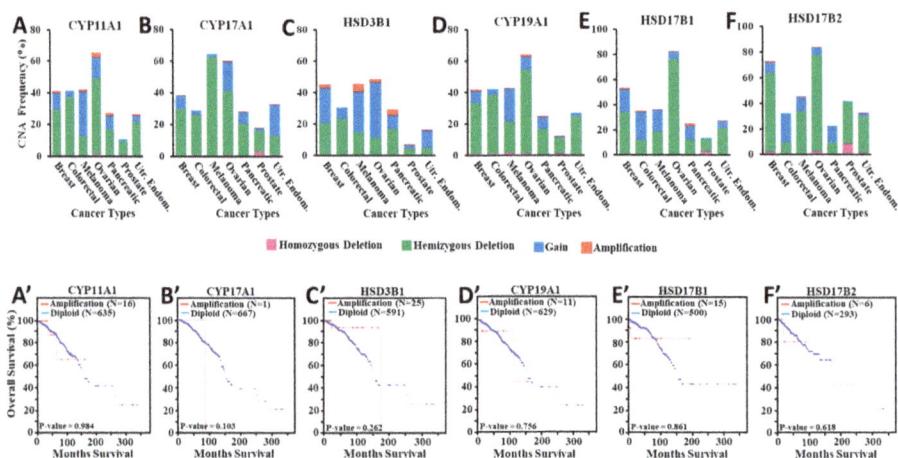

Figure 4. Analyses of CNA data for various steroidogenic enzyme genes in different hormone sensitive cancers and their correlation to breast cancer survival. TCGA CNA data analyzed for different cancers were the following: breast cancer tumors (1080 cases), colorectal (616 cases), melanoma (367 cases), ovarian (579 cases), pancreatic (184 cases), prostate (492 cases), and uterine endometrial (539 cases). Bar graphs illustrate CNA data for steroidogenic enzyme genes: *CYP11A1* (**A**), *CYP17A1* (**B**), *HSD3B1* (**C**), *CYP19A1* (**D**), *HSD17B1* (**E**), and *HSD17B2* (**F**). Amplification of these genes was analyzed for overall breast cancer survival (**A'**–**F'**). Kaplan-Meier survival curves were generated with and without (diploid) amplification of the following steroidogenic enzyme genes: *CYP11A1* (**A'**; red line, 16 tumors; blue line, 635 tumors), *CYP17A1* (**B'**; red line, 1 tumor; blue line, 667 tumors), *HSD3B1* (**C'**; red line, 25 tumors; blue line, 591 tumors), *CYP19A1* (**D'**; red line, 11 tumors; blue line, 629 tumors), *HSD17B1* (**E'**; red line, 15 tumors; blue line, 500 tumors), and *HSD17B2* (**F'**; red line, 6 tumors; blue line, 293 tumors). Red and blue lines represent with and without amplification of target genes, respectively. Utr. Endom., Uterine Endometrial.

The amplification of these steroidogenic enzyme genes in breast cancer survival was next evaluated. As determined by Kaplan-Meier survival analyses, amplification of the *CYP11A1* gene was not associated (p-value = 0.984) with breast cancer survival (Figure 4A'). Similarly, both *CYP17A1* and *HSD3B1* gene amplifications were not found to affect the survival of breast cancer, in which p-values were 0.103 and 0.262, respectively (Figure 4B',C'). Kaplan-Meier survival analysis revealed that amplification of the *CYP19A1* gene was not correlated (p-value = 0.756) with breast cancer survival (Figure 4D'). Additionally, amplification of both *HSD17B1* and *HSD17B2* gene isoforms did not affect the survival of breast cancer, where p-values were 0.861 and 0.618, respectively (Figure 4E',F'). These data indicate that none of these steroidogenic enzyme genes were either substantially amplified or affected the survival of ER+/PR+ breast cancer.

3.6. Assessment of StAR Gene Mutation in Hormone Sensitive Cancers

TCGA hormone responsive cancer datasets were analyzed for identifying mutation(s) in the *StAR* gene, which has been shown to affect the biological activity of the StAR protein in steroid biosynthesis [4,51]. As determined by exome sequencing, no mutations in the *StAR* gene were observed in breast (982 tumors) and prostate (499 tumors) cancers, suggesting StAR is functionally active in mobilizing cholesterol to the mitochondria. However, one mutation in the *StAR* gene was identified in each of the following cancers: colorectal (one out of 223 tumors; 0.45%), pancreatic (one out of 150 tumors; 0.67%), and ovarian (one out of 316 tumors; 0.32%). In melanoma and uterine endometrial carcinomas, five (368 tumors; 1.36%) and four (248 tumors; 1.61%) mutations were observed in the *StAR* gene, respectively (Supplementary Figure S2). The absence of mutation in the *StAR* gene, especially in breast cancer, suggests that amplification of the *StAR* gene is culpable in the transport of excess cholesterol to the inner mitochondrial membrane, resulting in increased estrogen synthesis which would promote tumorigenesis.

3.7. Expression of StAR mRNA in TCGA Breast Cancer Tumors and Its Association to Overall Survival

TCGA breast cancer tumor datasets were assessed for StAR mRNA expression. As illustrated by the Box and Whisker plot, StAR mRNA expression was represented as fkpm+uq+1 (obtained from RNA-Seq data), in which normal distribution across the population was visualized as 25th (9.114) and 75th (11.32) percentiles with a median of 10.2 (Figure 5A).

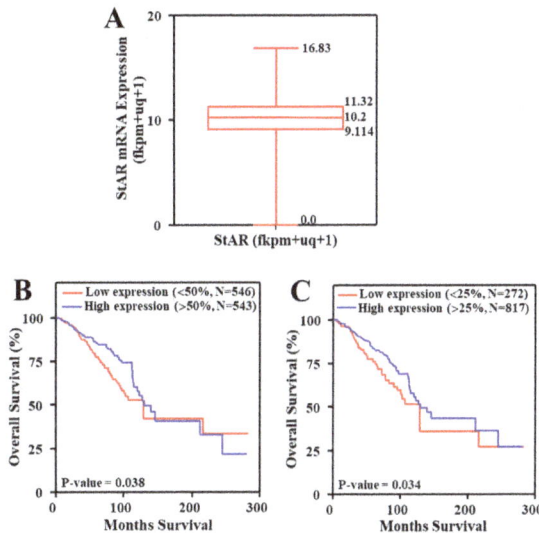

Figure 5. Expression of StAR mRNA in TCGA breast cancer tumors using the Box and Whisker Plot, and generation of Kaplan-Meier curves with low vs. high StAR levels. StAR mRNA expression was illustrated as fkpm+uq+1, generated by TCGA (1089 tumors), and visualized with the Box and Whisker Plot (**A**), as described in Section 2. Shown are 25th (9.114) and 75th (11.32) percentiles with a median of 10.2 (indicated by a horizontal line). Kaplan-Meier survival curves were generated with StAR mRNA values up to 50th percentile (<10.2; 546 tumors) as low and above 50th percentile (>10.2; 543 tumors) as high (**B**), and up to 25th percentile as low (<9.114; 272 tumors) and above 25th percentile (>9.114; 817 tumors) as high (**C**). Red and blue lines represent low and high StAR mRNA expression, respectively.

To better understand the involvement of StAR in breast cancer, TCGA breast cancer tumors expressing StAR mRNA were verified for survival analyses with two different quartile combinations. As depicted in Figure 5B, Kaplan-Meier curve generated with StAR mRNA values up to 50th percentile (<10.2) as low and above 50th percentile (>10.2) as high [46], was found to correlate with poor survival (*p*-value = 0.038) of patients with breast cancer. In a different category, StAR mRNA values up to 25th percentile (<9.114) as low and above 25th percentile (>9.114) as high [48], showed qualitatively similar effect (*p* = 0.034) on the survival of breast cancer (Figure 5C). These data suggest that higher expression of StAR mRNA can be a risk factor for poor survival of patients with breast cancer.

3.8. TNM Staging and Its Correlation to Breast Cancer Deaths

To obtain more insight in to the impact of StAR in breast cancer deaths, TCGA breast cancer tumors expressing StAR mRNA were analyzed in conjunction with the TNM staging. Specifically, different TNM stages were evaluated with low and high StAR mRNA levels with two quantile combinations as those utilized in Figure 5B,C. The results presented in Table 2 demonstrate TNM stage specific effects of tumors and their correlation to breast cancer deaths. These results show that breast cancer deaths were found to be coordinately associated with not only to increased tumor sizes, but also to lymph nodes in stage dependent manners. Additionally, tumor metastasis (M1) markedly affected the survival of breast cancer when compared with no metastasis (M0) in both low and high categories (Table 2). Specifically, the results obtained with TNM stages confirm the Kaplan-Meier survival data presented in Figure 5B,C. Altogether, genomic analyses of key steroidogenic factors, within the context of TCGA breast cancer datasets, indicated that aberrant amplification/ expression of the *StAR* gene is involved, at least in part, in poor survival of ER+/PR+ breast cancer patients. These results are in support of our recent finding that demonstrated that StAR protein is abundantly expressed in hormone sensitive breast cancer [5].

Table 2. T, N, M staging of TCGA breast cancer tumors segregated for low and high StAR mRNA expression based on two different quartile combinations, and their correlation to patient deaths.

TNM Staging	Low Expression (<50%)			High Expression (>50%)			Low Expression (<25%)			High Expression (>25%)		
	Tumor Nos.	Death Nos.	% Deaths	Tumor Nos.	Death Nos.	% Deaths	Tumor Nos.	Death Nos.	% Deaths	Tumor Nos.	Death Nos.	% Deaths
T1	120	17	14.2	158	16	10.1	54	8	14.8	224	25	11.2
T2	336	44	13.1	294	33	11.2	169	25	14.8	461	52	11.3
T3	63	11	17.5	75	14	18.7	32	9	28.1	106	16	15.1
T4	26	8	30.8	14	7	50	16	5	31.3	24	10	41.7
N0	257	22	8.6	257	22	8.6	120	15	12.5	394	29	7.4
N1	169	31	18.3	190	28	14.7	91	19	20.1	268	40	14.9
N2	75	16	21.3	45	6	13.3	38	6	15.8	82	16	19.5
N3	33	5	15.2	45	12	26.7	16	4	25.0	60	11	18.3
M0	459	62	13.5	621	32	5.2	224	26	11.6	672	83	12.4
M1	13	10	76.9	8	5	62.5	4	2	50	12	9	75.0

TCGA breast cancer tumors expressing low and high StAR mRNA levels (as specified) were categorized based on tumor sizes (T1–T4), nodal variations (N0–N3), and metastasis and non-metastasis (M0–M1), as described in Section 2.

4. Discussion

Abnormality in gene expression is responsible for anomalous growth of cells connecting tumor progression. The majority of the human genome is transcribed, but not translated, and gene amplification, involving oncogene activation, is a fundamental event in cancers. Hormone responsive cancers, especially breast cancer, are most common globally. Since StAR plays an indispensable role in the regulation of steroidogenesis, its expression must be finely regulated to appropriate functioning of steroid led activities. Conversely, dysregulation of steroid biosynthesis has been implicated in the pathophysiology of a number of relevant cancers. While StAR's involvement in breast malignancy remains obscure, we recently reported that both StAR protein expression and E2 synthesis are profoundly higher in ER+/PR+ breast cancer cell lines, when compared their levels with either non-cancerous mammary epithelial cells or TNBC [5]. By analyzing genomic profiles of StAR and steroidogenic enzyme genes for several hormone sensitive cancers, our data extend previous observations and provide novel insight that aberrant high amplification/expression of the *StAR* gene is correlated with poor survival of patients with breast cancer.

The comprehensive analyses of TCGA and cBioPortal research datasets for various hormone responsive cancers demonstrate that *StAR* gene is amplified (associated with a positive correlation between StAR CNA and StAR mRNA levels), but not mutated, in luminal subtype breast cancer. Specifically, the association of StAR with ER+/PR+ breast cancer indicates that StAR acts as a tumor promoter in the most prevalent hormone sensitive breast cancer. Several lines of evidence demonstrate a close correlation between StAR mRNA and StAR protein synthesis which parallels the synthesis of steroids in a variety of target tissues [4,7,10,52]. The involvement of StAR in breast cancer appeared specific, as translocator protein (TSPO), a mitochondrial factor involved in steroidogenesis [53,54], was not connected (*TSPO* gene was amplified at 0.7% with a *p*-value = 0.540) with cancer deaths (data not illustrated). The mechanism accounting for estrogen sensitive ovarian and endometrial cancers, connecting mutations in the *StAR* gene, remains unclear, and may involve one or more compensatory event(s), including involvement of StAR related lipid transfer proteins 3-6 (STARD3-6) and/or other factors involved in cholesterol trafficking [55,56]. Of note, the late endosomal membrane protein STARD3 (also known as metastatic lymph node 64), with ~37% C-terminal homology to StAR, was initially cloned as a gene amplified in the breast, gastric, and esophageal cancers [57,58]. It has previously been shown that overexpression of STARD3 is associated with increased cholesterol biosynthesis in HER2+ breast cancer subtype [59,60]. Regardless of the influence of these transporters, cholesterol and its oxygenated derivatives were demonstrated to be involved in the pathophysiology of a number of hormone sensitive malignancies, including breast cancer [17,18]. Studies have also reported that both cholesterol and its metabolites, including 27-hydroxycholesterol (27-HC) and 6-oxocholestan-diol, are capable to accelerate and/or enhance breast tumorigenesis [17,61,62]. Noteworthy, 27-HC is a ligand for ER and liver X receptor (LXR), in which the effects of 27-HC on tumor formation and growth are dependent on ER, while the action of this oxysterol involves LXR in tumor metastasis in mouse breast cancer models [17]. Whereas an overwhelming amount of evidence indicates the involvement of cholesterol in hormone sensitive breast cancer, epidemiologic findings are contradictory, requiring future studies to assess whether total cholesterol and its metabolites, high-density lipoprotein, or low-density lipoprotein influence cancer development and progression.

Almost all proteins in eukaryotic cells are modified by various post-translational modifications (PTMs) that influence protein function. We recently identified that StAR is a novel acetylated protein in ER+ breast cancer cells, in which three acetyl lysine residues were recognized endogenously, surmising they contribute to higher accumulation E2 in these cells [5]. It is plausible that both higher expression and activity of StAR facilitate abnormal cholesterol delivery to the mitochondrial inner membrane and, as a consequence, precursor availability for estrogen in promoting breast tumorigenesis. This reinforces the notion that estrogen levels in the majority of hormone sensitive malignant breast tumors can be 10–30 times higher than those found in either circulation or non-cancerous counterparts [16,21,63,64]. Previously, we [14,65,66] and others [67,68] have reported that cAMP mediated mechanisms phosphorylate StAR and this PTM enhances the optimal cholesterol transferring ability of the StAR protein in steroid biosynthesis. Despite the regulatory events involved, the impact of StAR to serve as a risk factor in affecting the survival of ER+/PR+ breast cancer opens up a new avenue in breast cancer research.

A notable aspect of the present findings is that amplification of the *CYP19A1* gene (aromatase), within the context of TCGA data cohort, was not correlated with breast cancer death [16], even though aromatase is the rate-limiting enzyme in estrogen biosynthesis. Expression of aromatase has been shown to be high in both non-cancerous and cancerous breast cell lines, suggesting its relevance in a number of physiological and pathophysiological events [5,69]. There is increasing evidence that enhanced expression/activity of aromatase is one of the key events for elevated intra-tumoral production of estrogen in malignant breast tissues [16,21,70,71]. Estrogen is also produced by the action of the 17β-HSD enzyme, and CNA data revealed that the *HSD17B* gene was neither significantly amplified nor connected with the survival of hormone sensitive breast cancer. These data imply that StAR mediated delivery of excess cholesterol, resulting in a substantial increase in estrogen accumulation, appears to be a fundamental event in the development of hormone sensitive breast cancer. In accordance with this, preliminary data obtained reveal that the expression of both StAR mRNA and StAR protein was markedly high in transgenic (Tg) mouse models of breast cancer, activated by MMTV promoter driven cNeu and H-Ras oncogenes, and polyomavirus, in comparison to nearly undetectable level of StAR in normal Tg mammary tissue.

Estrogen is primarily produced in the ovaries via the classical steroidogenic pathway through the synthesis of androstenedione and testosterone from cholesterol (in which StAR plays a permissive role) in the theca cells. These androgens are then converted to estrogens in granulosa cells. In peri- and post-menopausal women, extra ovarian tissues become a major source for estrogen synthesis [72]. This transition is critical since most hormone sensitive cancers, including breast, occur over the age of 50, in which estrogens synthesized in peripheral tissues are believed to play pivotal roles [63,64]. The plasma androgen level in post-menopausal women, with the loss of ovarian estrogen production, remains stable for years. Utilizing the non-classical pathway, these androgens are converted to estrogens in peripheral tissues. In addition to peripheral estrogen that reaches the tumor site through systemic circulation, estrogen is also synthesized locally in malignant breast tumors [16,21,63,64]. Breast cancer tumors in TCGA datasets were predominantly ER+/PR+, in which aberrant high expression of *StAR* mRNA, was found to affect poor survival of breast cancer. Further analyses of these tumors, expressing StAR mRNA, demonstrated increasing patterns of breast cancer deaths with advanced TNM stages. It should be noted, however, while breast cancer deaths were steadily increased with various TNM stages, they were not coordinately associated with StAR mRNA expression, which could be due to tumor numbers, tumor stages, or involvement of additional factors.

5. Conclusions

Analyses of molecular genomic profiling of steroidogenic factors associated with TCGA and cBioPortal research datasets revealed that abundant amplification and/or expression of the StAR gene is connected with poor survival of patients with luminal subtype breast cancer. This is in support of our recent report that demonstrated that StAR protein, concomitant with E2 synthesis, is markedly expressed in ER+/PR+ breast cancer, in comparison to nearly undetectable to modest StAR and E2 levels in non-cancerous mammary epithelial cells [5]. Based on these data (albeit limited), it is highly likely that StAR facilitates abnormal delivery of cholesterol to the inner mitochondria, resulting in adequate availability of precursors for E2 overproduction, which could be a plausible mechanism in the development and growth of hormone sensitive breast cancer. Furthermore, the results of in silico analyses, together with our in vitro data reported recently, attest that StAR can serve as a novel prognostic marker in ER+/PR+ breast cancer, whereas its inhibition, involving E2 synthesis, by a number of histone deacetylase inhibitors, might have therapeutic implications in the prevention/treatment of this devastating disease. The present data indicating the involvement of the classical pathway in intra-tumoral androgen/estrogen synthesis points to an additional new mechanism in growth and development of ER+/PR+ breast and/or other pertinent cancers, even though overexpression of aromatase, resulting in an increase in estrogen synthesis through the non-classical pathway is well established. Whereas *StAR* gene is highly amplified/expressed in hormone sensitive breast cancer, its association with HER2 and TNBC subtypes remains to be elucidated.

Supplementary Materials: The following are available online at http://www.mdpi.com/2072-6694/11/5/623/s1, Figure S1: Steroid biosynthetic pathway. Figure S2: Assessment of mutation in the StAR gene in a variety of hormone sensitive cancers. Supplementary Excel file: StAR mRNA (RNA-Seq) data for overall survival analysis.

Author Contributions: Conceptualization, P.R.M.; Methodology, P.R.M., A.U.A., S.Y. and M.N.; Project Administration and Supervision, P.R.M.; Validation, P.R.M., A.U.A., S.Y. and M.N.; Formal Analysis, P.R.M., A.U.A., S.Y., M.N., J.C.-T., A.T.S. and K.P.; Investigation, P.R.M., A.U.A., S.Y., A.T.S. and M.N.; Writing—Original Draft Preparation, P.R.M.; Visualization, P.R.M., A.U.A., M.N., J.C.-T., A.T.S. and K.P.; Funding acquisition, A.T.S. and K.P.; Writing—Review & Editing, P.R.M., A.U.A., S.Y., M.N., J.C.-T., A.T.S. and K.P.

Funding: This work was supported in part by a Cancer Prevention Research Institute of Texas (CPRIT) Award RR140008 to K.P., and National Institutes of Health grants (1R01AR073004-01A1 and 1RO1AR071189-01A1) and a V.A. grant (1I01BX004293-01A1) to A.T.S.

Acknowledgments: The authors would like to acknowledge the utilization of TCGA (https://tcga-data.nci.nih.gov), cBioPortal (http://www.cbioportal.org), and UCSC Xena (http://www.xenabrowser.net) research network datasets in this study.

Conflicts of Interest: The authors declare that there is no conflict of interest that could be perceived as prejudicing the impartiality of this work.

References

1. Manna, P.R.; Stocco, D.M. Regulation of the steroidogenic acute regulatory protein expression: Functional and physiological consequences. *Curr. Drug Targets Immune Endocr. Metabol. Disord.* **2005**, *5*, 93–108. [CrossRef] [PubMed]

2. Manna, P.R.; Dyson, M.T.; Stocco, D.M. Regulation of the steroidogenic acute regulatory protein gene expression: Present and future perspectives. *Mol. Hum. Reprod.* **2009**, *15*, 321–333. [CrossRef]

3. Papadopoulos, V.; Miller, W.L. Role of mitochondria in steroidogenesis. *Best Pract. Res. Clin. Endocrinol. Metab.* **2012**, *26*, 771–790. [PubMed]

4. Manna, P.R.; Stetson, C.L.; Slominski, A.T.; Pruitt, K. Role of the steroidogenic acute regulatory protein in health and disease. *Endocrine* **2016**, *51*, 7–21. [CrossRef] [PubMed]

5. Manna, P.R.; Ahmed, A.U.; Vartak, D.; Molehin, D.; Pruitt, K. Overexpression of the steroidogenic acute regulatory protein in breast cancer: Regulation by histone deacetylase inhibition. *Biochem. Biophys. Res. Commun.* **2019**, *509*, 476–482. [CrossRef] [PubMed]

6. Miller, W.L.; Bose, H.S. Early steps in steroidogenesis: Intracellular cholesterol trafficking. *J. Lipid Res.* **2011**, *52*, 2111–2135. [CrossRef]

7. Manna, P.R.; Dyson, M.T.; Eubank, D.W.; Clark, B.J.; Lalli, E.; Sassone-Corsi, P.; Zeleznik, A.J.; Stocco, D.M. Regulation of steroidogenesis and the steroidogenic acute regulatory protein by a member of the cAMP response-element binding protein family. *Mol. Endocrinol.* **2002**, *16*, 184–199. [CrossRef] [PubMed]

8. Miller, W.L.; Auchus, R.J. The molecular biology, biochemistry, and physiology of human steroidogenesis and its disorders. *Endocr. Rev.* **2011**, *32*, 81–151. [CrossRef]

9. Manna, P.R.; Cohen-Tannoudji, J.; Counis, R.; Garner, C.W.; Huhtaniemi, I.; Kraemer, F.B.; Stocco, D.M. Mechanisms of action of hormone sensitive lipase in mouse Leydig cells: Its role in the regulation of the steroidogenic acute regulatory protein. *J. Biol. Chem.* **2013**, *288*, 8505–8518. [CrossRef] [PubMed]

10. Manna, P.R.; Stetson, C.L.; Daugherty, C.; Shimizu, I.; Syapin, P.J.; Garrel, G.; Cohen-Tannoudji, J.; Huhtaniemi, I.; Slominski, A.T.; Pruitt, K.; et al. Up-regulation of steroid biosynthesis by retinoid signaling: Implications for aging. *Mech. Ageing. Dev.* **2015**, *150*, 74–82. [CrossRef] [PubMed]

11. Slominski, A.T.; Manna, P.R.; Tuckey, R.C. On the role of skin in the regulation of local and systemic steroidogenic activities. *Steroids* **2015**, *103*, 72–88. [CrossRef] [PubMed]

12. Slominski, A.; Semak, I.; Zjawiony, J.; Wortsman, J.; Li, W.; Szczesniewski, A.; Tuckey, R.C. The cytochrome P450scc system opens an alternate pathway of vitamin D3 metabolism. *FEBS J.* **2005**, *272*, 4080–4090. [CrossRef]

13. Slominski, A.T.; Li, W.; Kim, T.K.; Semak, I.; Wang, J.; Zjawiony, J.K.; Tuckey, R.C. Novel activities of CYP11A1 and their potential physiological significance. *J. Steroid Biochem. Mol. Biol.* **2015**, *151*, 25–37. [CrossRef] [PubMed]

14. Manna, P.R.; Slominski, A.T.; King, S.R.; Stetson, C.L.; Stocco, D.M. Synergistic Activation of Steroidogenic Acute Regulatory Protein Expression and Steroid Biosynthesis by Retinoids: Involvement of cAMP/PKA Signaling. *Endocrinology* **2014**, *155*, 576–591. [CrossRef]

15. Slominski, A.T.; Manna, P.R.; Tuckey, R.C. Cutaneous glucocorticosteroidogenesis: Securing local homeostasis and the skin integrity. *Exp. Dermatol.* **2014**, *23*, 369–374. [CrossRef]

16. Manna, P.R.; Molehin, D.; Ahmed, A.U. Dysregulation of Aromatase in Breast, Endometrial, and Ovarian Cancers: An Overview of Therapeutic Strategies. *Prog. Mol. Biol. Transl. Sci.* **2016**, *144*, 487–537. [PubMed]

17. Nelson, E.R.; Wardell, S.E.; Jasper, J.S.; Park, S.; Suchindran, S.; Howe, M.K.; Carver, N.J.; Pillai, R.V.; Sullivan, P.M.; Sondhi, V.; et al. 27-Hydroxycholesterol links hypercholesterolemia and breast cancer pathophysiology. *Science* **2013**, *342*, 1094–1098. [CrossRef] [PubMed]

18. Silvente-Poirot, S.; Dalenc, F.; Poirot, M. The Effects of Cholesterol-Derived Oncometabolites on Nuclear Receptor Function in Cancer. *Cancer Res.* **2018**, *78*, 4803–4808. [CrossRef]

19. Brodie, A.; Njar, V.; Macedo, L.F.; Vasaitis, T.S.; Sabnis, G. The Coffey Lecture: Steroidogenic enzyme inhibitors and hormone dependent cancer. *Urol. Oncol.* **2009**, *27*, 53–63. [CrossRef]

20. Richie, R.C.; Swanson, J.O. Breast cancer: A review of the literature. *J. Insur. Med.* **2003**, *35*, 85–101.

21. Bulun, S.E.; Lin, Z.; Zhao, H.; Lu, M.; Amin, S.; Reierstad, S.; Chen, D. Regulation of aromatase expression in breast cancer tissue. *Ann. N. Y. Acad. Sci.* **2009**, *1155*, 121–131. [CrossRef]

22. Folkerd, E.; Dowsett, M. Sex hormones and breast cancer risk and prognosis. *Breast* **2013**, *22* (Suppl. 2), S38–S43. [CrossRef]

23. Cheang, M.C.; Martin, M.; Nielsen, T.O.; Prat, A.; Voduc, D.; Rodriguez-Lescure, A.; Ruiz, A.; Chia, S.; Shepherd, L.; Ruiz-Borrego, M.; et al. Defining breast cancer intrinsic subtypes by quantitative receptor expression. *Oncologist* **2015**, *20*, 474–482. [CrossRef] [PubMed]

24. Prat, A.; Pineda, E.; Adamo, B.; Galvan, P.; Fernandez, A.; Gaba, L.; Diez, M.; Viladot, M.; Arance, A.; Munoz, M. Clinical implications of the intrinsic molecular subtypes of breast cancer. *Breast* **2015**, *24* (Suppl. 2), S26–S35. [CrossRef]

25. Dai, X.; Li, T.; Bai, Z.; Yang, Y.; Liu, X.; Zhan, J.; Shi, B. Breast cancer intrinsic subtype classification, clinical use and future trends. *Am. J. Cancer Res.* **2015**, *5*, 2929–2943.

26. Cancer Genome Atlas Research Network. Integrated genomic analyses of ovarian carcinoma. *Nature* **2011**, *474*, 609–615. [CrossRef]

27. Cancer Genome Atlas Network. Comprehensive molecular portraits of human breast tumours. *Nature* **2012**, *490*, 61–70. [CrossRef] [PubMed]

28. Cancer Genome Atlas, N. Comprehensive molecular characterization of human colon and rectal cancer. *Nature* **2012**, *487*, 330–337. [CrossRef] [PubMed]

29. Kandoth, C.; Schultz, N.; Cherniack, A.D.; Akbani, R.; Liu, Y.; Shen, H.; Robertson, A.G.; Pashtan, I.; Shen, R.; Benz, C.C.; et al. Integrated genomic characterization of endometrial carcinoma. *Nature* **2013**, *497*, 67–73.

30. Casper, J.; Zweig, A.S.; Villarreal, C.; Tyner, C.; Speir, M.L.; Rosenbloom, K.R.; Raney, B.J.; Lee, C.M.; Lee, B.T.; Karolchik, D.; et al. The UCSC Genome Browser database: 2018 update. *Nucleic Acids Res.* **2018**, *46*, D762–D769. [PubMed]

31. Cerami, E.; Gao, J.; Dogrusoz, U.; Gross, B.E.; Sumer, S.O.; Aksoy, B.A.; Jacobsen, A.; Byrne, C.J.; Heuer, M.L.; Larsson, E.; et al. The cBio cancer genomics portal: An open platform for exploring multidimensional cancer genomics data. *Cancer Discov.* **2012**, *2*, 401–404. [CrossRef] [PubMed]

32. Gao, J.; Aksoy, B.A.; Dogrusoz, U.; Dresdner, G.; Gross, B.; Sumer, S.O.; Sun, Y.; Jacobsen, A.; Sinha, R.; Larsson, E.; et al. Integrative analysis of complex cancer genomics and clinical profiles using the cBioPortal. *Sci. Signal.* **2013**, *6*, pl1. [CrossRef]

33. Li, B.; Dewey, C.N. RSEM: Accurate transcript quantification from RNA-Seq data with or without a reference genome. *BMC Bioinform.* **2011**, *12*, 323. [CrossRef] [PubMed]

34. Pereira, B.; Chin, S.F.; Rueda, O.M.; Vollan, H.K.; Provenzano, E.; Bardwell, H.A.; Pugh, M.; Jones, L.; Russell, R.; Sammut, S.J. The somatic mutation profiles of 2,433 breast cancers refines their genomic and transcriptomic landscapes. *Nat. Commun.* **2016**, *7*, 11479. [CrossRef]

35. Eirew, P.; Steif, A.; Khattra, J.; Ha, G.; Yap, D.; Farahani, H.; Gelmon, K.; Chia, S.; Mar, C.; Wan, A.; et al. Dynamics of genomic clones in breast cancer patient xenografts at single-cell resolution. *Nature* **2015**, *518*, 422–426. [CrossRef] [PubMed]

36. Ciriello, G.; Gatza, M.L.; Beck, A.H.; Wilkerson, M.D.; Rhie, S.K.; Pastore, A.; Zhang, H.; McLellan, M.; Yau, C.; Kandoth, C.; et al. Comprehensive Molecular Portraits of Invasive Lobular Breast Cancer. *Cell* **2015**, *163*, 506–519. [CrossRef] [PubMed]

37. Lefebvre, C.; Bachelot, T.; Filleron, T.; Pedrero, M.; Campone, M.; Soria, J.C.; Massard, C.; Levy, C.; Arnedos, M.; Lacroix-Triki, M.; et al. Mutational Profile of Metastatic Breast Cancers: A Retrospective Analysis. *PLoS Med.* **2016**, *13*, e1002201. [CrossRef]

38. Bullard, J.H.; Purdom, E.; Hansen, K.D.; Dudoit, S. Evaluation of statistical methods for normalization and differential expression in mRNA-Seq experiments. *BMC Bioinform.* **2010**, *11*, 94. [CrossRef]

39. O'Sullivan, B.; Brierley, J.; Byrd, D.; Bosman, F.; Kehoe, S.; Kossary, C.; Pineros, M.; Van Eycken, E.; Weir, H.K.; Gospodarowicz, M. The TNM classification of malignant tumours-towards common understanding and reasonable expectations. *Lancet Oncol.* **2017**, *18*, 849–851. [CrossRef]

40. Lydiatt, W.M.; Patel, S.G.; O'Sullivan, B.; Brandwein, M.S.; Ridge, J.A.; Migliacci, J.C.; Loomis, A.M.; Shah, J.P. Head and Neck cancers-major changes in the American Joint Committee on cancer eighth edition cancer staging manual. *CA Cancer J. Clin.* **2017**, *67*, 122–137. [CrossRef]

41. Sedgwick, P. How to read a Kaplan-Meier survival plot. *BMJ* **2014**, *349*, g5608. [CrossRef] [PubMed]

42. Slamon, D.J.; Clark, G.M.; Wong, S.G.; Levin, W.J.; Ullrich, A.; McGuire, W.L. Human breast cancer: Correlation of relapse and survival with amplification of the HER-2/neu oncogene. *Science* **1987**, *235*, 177–182. [CrossRef]

43. Schneiderman, J.; London, W.B.; Brodeur, G.M.; Castleberry, R.P.; Look, A.T.; Cohn, S.L. Clinical significance of MYCN amplification and ploidy in favorable-stage neuroblastoma: A report from the Children's Oncology Group. *J. Clin. Oncol.* **2008**, *26*, 913–918. [CrossRef] [PubMed]

44. Liu, L.; Kimball, S.; Liu, H.; Holowatyj, A.; Yang, Z.Q. Genetic alterations of histone lysine methyltransferases and their significance in breast cancer. *Oncotarget* **2015**, *6*, 2466–2482. [CrossRef] [PubMed]

45. Hilborn, E.; Stal, O.; Jansson, A. Estrogen and androgen-converting enzymes 17beta-hydroxysteroid dehydrogenase and their involvement in cancer: With a special focus on 17beta-hydroxysteroid dehydrogenase type 1, 2, and breast cancer. *Oncotarget* **2017**, *8*, 30552–30562. [CrossRef] [PubMed]

46. Giovannetti, E.; Wang, Q.; Avan, A.; Funel, N.; Lagerweij, T.; Lee, J.H.; Caretti, V.; van der Velde, A.; Boggi, U.; Wang, Y.; et al. Role of CYB5A in pancreatic cancer prognosis and autophagy modulation. *J. Natl. Cancer Inst.* **2014**, *106*, djt346. [CrossRef] [PubMed]

47. Yoshihara, K.; Shahmoradgoli, M.; Martinez, E.; Vegesna, R.; Kim, H.; Torres-Garcia, W.; Trevino, V.; Shen, H.; Laird, P.W.; Levine, D.A.; et al. Inferring tumour purity and stromal and immune cell admixture from expression data. *Nat. Commun.* **2013**, *4*, 2612. [CrossRef]

48. Geng, X.; Liu, Y.; Diersch, S.; Kotzsch, M.; Grill, S.; Weichert, W.; Kiechle, M.; Magdolen, V.; Dorn, J. Clinical relevance of kallikrein-related peptidase 9, 10, 11, and 15 mRNA expression in advanced high-grade serous ovarian cancer. *PLoS ONE* **2017**, *12*, e0186847. [CrossRef]

49. Slominski, A.T.; Zmijewski, M.A.; Semak, I.; Zbytek, B.; Pisarchik, A.; Li, W.; Zjawiony, J.; Tuckey, R.C. Cytochromes p450 and skin cancer: Role of local endocrine pathways. *Anticancer Agents Med. Chem.* **2014**, *14*, 77–96. [CrossRef]

50. Slominski, A.; Gomez-Sanchez, C.E.; Foecking, M.F.; Wortsman, J. Metabolism of progesterone to DOC, corticosterone and 18OHDOC in cultured human melanoma cells. *FEBS Lett.* **1999**, *455*, 364–366. [CrossRef]

51. Camats, N.; Pandey, A.V.; Fernandez-Cancio, M.; Fernandez, J.M.; Ortega, A.M.; Udhane, S.; Andaluz, P.; Audi, L.; Fluck, C.E. STAR splicing mutations cause the severe phenotype of lipoid congenital adrenal hyperplasia: Insights from a novel splice mutation and review of reported cases. *Clin. Endocrinol.* **2014**, *80*, 191–199. [CrossRef]

52. Miller, W.L. Steroidogenic acute regulatory protein (StAR), a novel mitochondrial cholesterol transporter. *Biochim. Biophys. Acta* **2007**, *1771*, 663–676. [CrossRef]

53. Papadopoulos, V.; Aghazadeh, Y.; Fan, J.; Campioli, E.; Zirkin, B.; Midzak, A. Translocator protein-mediated pharmacology of cholesterol transport and steroidogenesis. *Mol. Cell. Endocrinol.* **2015**, *408*, 90–98. [CrossRef]

54. Fan, J.; Wang, K.; Zirkin, B.; Papadopoulos, V. CRISPR/Cas9Mediated Tspo Gene Mutations Lead to Reduced Mitochondrial Membrane Potential and Steroid Formation in MA-10 Mouse Tumor Leydig Cells. *Endocrinology* **2018**, *159*, 1130–1146. [CrossRef]

55. Strauss, J.F., 3rd; Kishida, T.; Christenson, L.K.; Fujimoto, T.; Hiroi, H. START domain proteins and the intracellular trafficking of cholesterol in steroidogenic cells. *Mol. Cell. Endocrinol.* **2003**, *202*, 59–65. [CrossRef]

56. Alpy, F.; Legueux, F.; Bianchetti, L.; Tomasetto, C. START domain-containing proteins: A review of their role in lipid transport and exchange. *Med. Sci. Paris* **2009**, *25*, 181–191.

57. Tomasetto, C.; Regnier, C.; Moog-Lutz, C.; Mattei, M.G.; Chenard, M.P.; Lidereau, R.; Basset, P.; Rio, M.C. Identification of four novel human genes amplified and overexpressed in breast carcinoma and localized to the q11-q21.3 region of chromosome 17. *Genomics* **1995**, *28*, 367–376. [CrossRef]

58. Akiyama, N.; Sasaki, H.; Ishizuka, T.; Kishi, T.; Sakamoto, H.; Onda, M.; Hirai, H.; Yazaki, Y.; Sugimura, T.; Terada, M. Isolation of a candidate gene, CAB1, for cholesterol transport to mitochondria from the c-ERBB-2 amplicon by a modified cDNA selection method. *Cancer Res.* **1997**, *57*, 3548–3553.

59. Alpy, F.; Boulay, A.; Moog-Lutz, C.; Andarawewa, K.L.; Degot, S.; Stoll, I.; Rio, M.C.; Tomasetto, C. Metastatic lymph node 64 (MLN64), a gene overexpressed in breast cancers, is regulated by Sp/KLF transcription factors. *Oncogene* **2003**, *22*, 3770–3780. [CrossRef]

60. Vassilev, B.; Sihto, H.; Li, S.; Holtta-Vuori, M.; Ilola, J.; Lundin, J.; Isola, J.; Kellokumpu-Lehtinen, P.L.; Joensuu, H.; Ikonen, E. Elevated levels of StAR-related lipid transfer protein 3 alter cholesterol balance and adhesiveness of breast cancer cells: Potential mechanisms contributing to progression of HER2-positive breast cancers. *Am. J. Pathol.* **2015**, *185*, 987–1000. [CrossRef]

61. Llaverias, G.; Danilo, C.; Mercier, I.; Daumer, K.; Capozza, F.; Williams, T.M.; Sotgia, F.; Lisanti, M.P.; Frank, P.G. Role of cholesterol in the development and progression of breast cancer. *Am. J. Pathol.* **2011**, *178*, 402–412. [CrossRef]

62. Voisin, M.; de Medina, P.; Mallinger, A.; Dalenc, F.; Huc-Claustre, E.; Leignadier, J.; Serhan, N.; Soules, R.; Segala, G.; Mougel, A.; et al. Identification of a tumor-promoter cholesterol metabolite in human breast cancers acting through the glucocorticoid receptor. *Proc. Natl. Acad. Sci. USA* **2017**, *114*, E9346–E9355. [CrossRef] [PubMed]

63. Simpson, E.; Santen, R.J. Celebrating 75 years of oestradiol. *J. Mol. Endocrinol.* **2015**, *55*, T1–T20. [CrossRef]

64. Zhao, H.; Zhou, L.; Shangguan, A.J.; Bulun, S.E. Aromatase expression and regulation in breast and endometrial cancer. *J. Mol. Endocrinol.* **2016**, *57*, 19–33. [CrossRef]

65. Manna, P.R.; Chandrala, S.P.; King, S.R.; Jo, Y.; Counis, R.; Huhtaniemi, I.T.; Stocco, D.M. Molecular mechanisms of insulin-like growth factor-I mediated regulation of the steroidogenic acute regulatory protein in mouse leydig cells. *Mol. Endocrinol.* **2006**, *20*, 362–378. [CrossRef]

66. Manna, P.R.; Soh, J.W.; Stocco, D.M. The involvement of specific PKC isoenzymes in phorbol ester-mediated regulation of steroidogenic acute regulatory protein expression and steroid synthesis in mouse Leydig cells. *Endocrinology* **2011**, *152*, 313–325. [CrossRef]

67. Arakane, F.; King, S.R.; Du, Y.; Kallen, C.B.; Walsh, L.P.; Watari, H.; Stocco, D.M.; Strauss, J.F., 3rd. Phosphorylation of steroidogenic acute regulatory protein (StAR) modulates its steroidogenic activity. *J. Biol. Chem.* **1997**, *272*, 32656–32662. [CrossRef]

68. Clark, B.J.; Ranganathan, V.; Combs, R. Steroidogenic acute regulatory protein expression is dependent upon post-translational effects of cAMP-dependent protein kinase A. *Mol. Cell. Endocrinol.* **2001**, *173*, 183–192. [CrossRef]

69. Castro-Piedras, I.; Sharma, M.; den Bakker, M.; Molehin, D.; Martinez, E.G.; Vartak, D.; Pruitt, W.M.; Deitrick, J.; Almodovar, S.; Pruitt, K. DVL1 and DVL3 differentially localize to CYP19A1 promoters and regulate aromatase mRNA in breast cancer cells. *Oncotarget* **2018**, *9*, 35639–35654. [CrossRef]

70. Simpson, E.R.; Misso, M.; Hewitt, K.N.; Hill, R.A.; Boon, W.C.; Jones, M.E.; Kovacic, A.; Zhou, J.; Clyne, C.D. Estrogen–the good, the bad, and the unexpected. *Endocr. Rev.* **2005**, *26*, 322–330. [CrossRef] [PubMed]

71. Molehin, D.; Castro-Piedras, I.; Sharma, M.; Sennoune, S.R.; Arena, D.; Manna, P.R.; Pruitt, K. Aromatase Acetylation Patterns and Altered Activity in Response to Sirtuin Inhibition. *Mol. Cancer Res.* **2018**, *16*, 1530–1542. [CrossRef] [PubMed]

72. Bulun, S.E.; Lin, Z.; Imir, G.; Amin, S.; Demura, M.; Yilmaz, B.; Martin, R.; Utsunomiya, H.; Thung, S.; Gurates, B.; et al. Regulation of aromatase expression in estrogen-responsive breast and uterine disease: From bench to treatment. *Pharmacol. Rev.* **2005**, *57*, 359–383. [CrossRef] [PubMed]

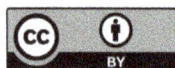

cancers

MDPI

Article

Identification of Novel MicroRNAs and Their Diagnostic and Prognostic Significance in Oral Cancer

Luca Falzone [1,†], Gabriella Lupo [1,2,†], Giusy Rita Maria La Rosa [3], Salvatore Crimi [4], Carmelina Daniela Anfuso [1,2], Rossella Salemi [1], Ernesto Rapisarda [3], Massimo Libra [1,2,*] and Saverio Candido [1,2]

1   Department of Biomedical and Biotechnological Sciences, Oncologic, Clinic and General Pathology Section, University of Catania, 95123 Catania, Italy; luca.falzone@unict.it (L.F.); lupogab@unict.it (G.L.); anfudan@unict.it (C.D.A.); rossellasalemi@alice.it (R.S.); scandido@unict.it (S.C.)
2   Research Center for Prevention, Diagnosis and Treatment of Cancer, University of Catania, 95123 Catania, Italy
3   Department of General Surgery and Surgical-Medical Specialties, University of Catania, 95125 Catania, Italy; g_larosa92@live.it (G.R.M.L.R.); errapis@tin.it (E.R.)
4   Department of Surgical and Biomedical Sciences, University of Catania, 95123 Catania, Italy; torecrimi@gmail.com
*   Correspondence: mlibra@unict.it; Tel.: +39-095-478-1271
†   The authors contribute equally to this work.

Received: 1 April 2019; Accepted: 30 April 2019; Published: 30 April 2019

Abstract: *Background*: Oral cancer is one of the most prevalent cancers worldwide. Despite that the oral cavity is easily accessible for clinical examinations, oral cancers are often not promptly diagnosed. Furthermore, to date no effective biomarkers are available for oral cancer. Therefore, there is an urgent need to identify novel biomarkers able to improve both diagnostic and prognostic strategies. In this context, the development of innovative high-throughput technologies for molecular and epigenetics analyses has generated a huge amount of data that may be used for the identification of new cancer biomarkers. *Methods*: In the present study, GEO DataSets and TCGA miRNA profiling datasets were analyzed in order to identify miRNAs with diagnostic and prognostic significance. Furthermore, several computational approaches were adopted to establish the functional roles of these miRNAs. *Results*: The analysis of datasets allowed for the identification of 11 miRNAs with a potential diagnostic role for oral cancer. Additionally, eight miRNAs associated with patients' prognosis were also identified; six miRNAs predictive of patients' overall survival (OS) and one, hsa-miR-let.7i-3p, associated with tumor recurrence. *Conclusions*: The integrated analysis of different miRNA expression datasets allows for the identification of a set of miRNAs that, after validation, may be used for the early detection of oral cancers.

Keywords: oral cancer; miRNA; bioinformatics; datasets; biomarkers; TCGA; GEO DataSets

---

1. Introduction

Oral cancer is one of the most prevalent cancers worldwide, accounting for about 354,864 new diagnoses and approximately 177,384 new deaths annually [1]. Generally, the term oral cancer identifies a subset of head and neck cancers arising in the lips, hard palate, upper and lower alveolar ridges, anterior two-thirds of the tongue, sublingual region, buccal mucosa, retro-molar trigone and floor of the mouth [2]. Among these cancers, the most frequent histotype is oral squamous cell carcinoma (OSCC) representing about 95% of all oral cancers [3]. Recent epidemiological data demonstrated that despite the development of novel screening strategies together with the advancement of pharmacological treatments, the incidence and mortality rates of head and neck cancer, and in particular that of oral cancer, are almost stable or increased during the last years [4,5].

Behind the increase of both oral cancer incidence and mortality rates, there are several modifiable factors, including dietary and lifestyles habits, together contributing to cancer development. Among these factors, alcohol consumption and smoking represent the most recognized factors predisposing to OSCC [6,7]. Additionally, viruses and other microbes have been intensively associated with a higher increase of OSCC development, such as infections sustained by human papilloma viruses (HPVs), Epstein-Barr virus (EBV) or Candida albicans [8–10]. Although the majority of the studies are focused on the investigation of microbial factors as cancer risk factors, recently several studies were pursued with the aim of establishing a potential role of the human microbiota in protecting the host from several tumors, including those of the oral cavity [11–13].

Along with these well-recognized risk factors, oral cancer development is also associated with several molecular alterations affecting key genes involved in the regulation of pivotal cellular processes, such as cell cycle, cell proliferation and apoptosis. The most frequent gene alterations found linked with OSCC affect *TP53*, *NOTCH1*, *CDKN2A*, *SYNE1*, *PIK3CA*, as well as the EGFR pathway-related genes (including *TGF-β*, fibroblastic growth factor-BP (*FGF-BP*) and *MMK6*) [14,15]. Recently, epigenetic modifications, including promoter/intragenic methylation and microRNAs (miRNAs) de-regulation, have been linked to the development of oral cancers by mediating the alteration of cellular homeostasis and physiological processes [16–18].

Despite that the oral cavity is readily explorable, most oral tumors are diagnosed at an advanced stage reducing the survival rate of patients [19,20]. Currently, there are no effective biomarkers for the early diagnosis of oral cancer. Several studies have proposed the evaluation of the salivary and serum levels of IL-6 and/or IL-8 as promising biomarkers for oral cancer lesions, however, the sensitivity and specificity of these markers were low because they increase also in presence of various oral cavity inflammatory conditions [21,22]. Other studies focused the attention on tumor markers already used for the diagnosis of other solid tumors, such as the salivary levels of the carcino-embryonic antigen (CEA; 68.9% sensitivity, 73.3% specificity) [23], carcinoantigen 19-9 (CA19-9; no diagnostic value) [24] and CA125 (80.0% sensitivity, 66.0% specificity) [25]. However, the sensitivity and specificity of these markers were not high enough to diagnose effectively all oral tumors.

Therefore, there is an urgent need to identify novel biomarkers for the early diagnosis of oral cancer. In this context, the role of non-coding RNAs, of which miRNAs are the most studied, has been recently acquiring remarkable importance in the development of several pathologies, including cancer [26–28]. In particular, several studies demonstrated that miRNAs, a class of small non-coding RNAs with a length of 20–22 nucleotides, are involved in cancer, including that of oral cavity cancer, inducing epigenetic modifications altering key cellular processes, such as cell differentiation, growth, apoptosis and drug resistance [29,30]. Notably, miRNAs are able to regulate gene expression by controlling mRNA translation, either by translational repression of the targeted mRNA or by enhancing its degradation through an RNA interference mechanism [31]. Furthermore, a growing body of evidence demonstrated that dysregulated miRNAs may be used for diagnostic and prognostic purposes. In fact, it is well established that certain miRNAs are specifically associated with the presence of tumors, even in the early stages, or associated with a worse prognosis [32,33].

Therefore, miRNAs may represent good candidate biomarkers also for oral cancer. On this matter, during the last decade, a huge amount of molecular and bioinformatics data has been generated, with the final goal of characterizing miRNAs' expression profile in several cancers. These databases were therefore used to identify new effective biomarkers identified through computational approaches [34]. Several studies analyzed the data deriving from miRNAs microarray or sequencing profiling in oral cancer samples. However, the lack of integration between the different data matrix generated has generated confusing data on this matter. For instance, Manikandan M and colleagues (2016) have performed a miRNA microarray analysis in a discovery cohort (*n* = 29) and validation cohort (*n* = 61) of primary OSCC tissue specimens identifying a set of miRNAs (let-7a, let-7d, let-7f, miR-16, miR-29b, miR-142-3p, miR-144, miR-203, miR-223 and miR-1275) potentially involved in oral cancer development and progression [35]. Other microarray studies have identified miRNAs different from those identified by Manikandan et al. In particular, Chamorro Petronacci and colleagues (2019) have recently identified two potential miRNAs, miR-497-5p and miR-4417 associated with the presence of OSCC [36]. Yan ZY and co-workers (2017) have identified seven key miRNAs (miR-21, miR-31, miR-338, miR-125b, hsa-miR-133a, miR-133b and miR-139) associated with the tumor [37]. Therefore, it is evident that there are no concordant data generated by the single and independent analysis of different miRNA microarray datasets for oral cancer.

To our best knowledge, no previous studies have analyzed simultaneously different oral cancer tissue miRNAs profiling datasets. In the present study, miRNA expression datasets, contained in both the Gene Expression Omnibus DataSets (GEO DataSets) and The Cancer Genome Atlas (TCGA) Head and Neck Cancer (HNSC), were analyzed to identify a panel of miRNAs used as potential diagnostic and/or prognostic biomarkers for oral cancer.

2. Results

2.1. Identification of Oral Cancer-Associated miRNAs

The differential analysis performed by GEO2R on the two datasets of the GEO DataSets database allowed the identification of two lists of de-regulated miRNAs in oral tumors compared to non-tumor controls. By comparing these two lists of miRNAs, it was possible to identify 28 miRNAs differentially expressed in the tumor tissue, 12 of which were up-regulated and 16 were down-regulated (Table 1).

Table 1. Up-regulated and down-regulated miRNAs in tumor samples compared to the healthy controls.

miRNA ID	GSE45238		GSE31277	
	Fold Change	*p*-Value *	Fold Change	*p*-Value *
Up-regulated miRNAs				
hsa-miR-196a-5p	8.096	9.45×10^{-12}	8.132	1.42×10^{-6}
hsa-miR-503-5p	5.010	4.83×10^{-21}	2.622	4.69×10^{-4}
hsa-miR-7-5p	3.505	9.41×10^{-20}	2.297	5.00×10^{-4}
hsa-miR-542-5p	3.348	9.21×10^{-12}	2.700	1.10×10^{-4}
hsa-miR-142-5p	3.323	3.98×10^{-8}	2.633	2.12×10^{-3}
hsa-miR-19a-3p	3.068	3.81×10^{-7}	2.910	4.75×10^{-4}
hsa-miR-18a-5p	2.646	2.34×10^{-10}	1.554	2.66×10^{-3}
hsa-miR-19b-3p	2.179	1.28×10^{-5}	2.415	7.73×10^{-4}
hsa-miR-32-5p	1.997	1.76×10^{-5}	3.874	3.28×10^{-5}
hsa-miR-196b-5p	1.791	2.05×10^{-8}	1.874	2.00×10^{-4}
hsa-miR-33b-5p	1.581	9.26×10^{-4}	2.541	2.00×10^{-3}
hsa-miR-34b-3p	1.558	1.95×10^{-4}	2.079	1.13×10^{-3}
Down-Regulated miRNAs				
hsa-miR-195-5p	−1.778	1.25×10^{-12}	−1.620	1.71×10^{-6}
hsa-miR-378a-5p	−1.799	9.47×10^{-12}	−2.194	4.45×10^{-3}
hsa-miR-363-3p	−1.869	1.56×10^{-5}	−1.951	4.16×10^{-5}
hsa-miR-100-5p	−1.883	8.04×10^{-14}	−2.199	1.19×10^{-4}
hsa-miR-328-5p	−2.471	1.18×10^{-8}	−1.599	2.32×10^{-4}
hsa-miR-99a-5p	−2.732	4.83×10^{-16}	−2.441	7.82×10^{-5}
hsa-miR-218-5p	−3.021	1.08×10^{-10}	−1.853	1.72×10^{-4}
hsa-miR-432-5p	−3.155	1.55×10^{-13}	−1.718	3.14×10^{-3}
hsa-miR-379-5p	−3.513	1.83×10^{-11}	−2.345	9.63×10^{-4}
hsa-miR-154-5p	−4.021	4.01×10^{-13}	−1.826	2.00×10^{-3}
hsa-miR-133a-3p	−4.202	6.37×10^{-9}	−3.446	8.47×10^{-3}
hsa-miR-487b-5p	−4.366	6.96×10^{-15}	−1.899	9.71×10^{-3}
hsa-miR-135a-5p	−4.910	1.11×10^{-14}	−3.324	1.90×10^{-3}
hsa-miR-411-5p	−5.574	3.25×10^{-16}	−2.542	6.18×10^{-3}
hsa-miR-1-3p	−9.783	3.47×10^{-9}	−5.786	2.16×10^{-3}
hsa-miR-375	−16.589	1.95×10^{-17}	−3.198	5.12×10^{-4}

* *p*-values were automatically obtained by using the GEO2R software by performing Student's *t*-test.

The analysis of the expression data of miRNAs contained in the TCGA HNSC dataset allowed us to obtain a list of 514 de-regulated miRNAs associated with the presence of a tumor ($p < 0.01$;

Table S1). Furthermore, 21 of the 28 miRNAs identified with the GEO DataSets analysis were contained in this list of 514 miRNAs (Table S1), thus confirming that the results obtained from the two analyses were overlapping.

To further narrow the search towards miRNAs showing a strong diagnostic significance, the 25 most up-regulated and the 25 most down-regulated miRNAs were selected from the list of 514 miRNAs. The analysis of the TCGA HNSC dataset showed a list of 50 miRNAs that were strongly associated with the presence of the tumor (Table 2).

Table 2. TCGA analysis of up-regulated and down-regulated miRNAs in the tumor compared to the normal samples.

miRNA ID	miRNA Name	FC Cancer vs Normal	*p*-Value *
Up-regulated			
MIMAT0000226	**hsa-miR-196a-5p**	**12.145**	3.12×10^{-19}
MIMAT0001080	**hsa-miR-196b-5p**	**11.639**	5.43×10^{-20}
MIMAT0000267	hsa-miR-210-3p	9.733	1.18×10^{-9}
MIMAT0000089	hsa-miR-31-5p	7.684	8.42×10^{-12}
MIMAT0004784	hsa-miR-455-3p	7.165	9.21×10^{-18}
MIMAT0005923	hsa-miR-1269a	5.899	1.99×10^{-11}
MIMAT0000102	hsa-miR-105-5p	5.510	9.64×10^{-13}
MIMAT0004504	hsa-miR-31-3p	5.298	1.59×10^{-9}
MIMAT0003882	hsa-miR-767-5p	5.294	5.40×10^{-13}
MIMAT0000281	hsa-miR-224-5p	4.789	5.39×10^{-11}
MIMAT0002874	**hsa-miR-503-5p**	**4.044**	$\mathbf{3.86 \times 10^{-19}}$
MIMAT0002819	hsa-miR-193b-3p	3.407	8.17×10^{-15}
MIMAT0005951	hsa-miR-1307-3p	3.395	1.14×10^{-11}
MIMAT0000076	hsa-miR-21-5p	3.209	3.05×10^{-10}
MIMAT0000266	hsa-miR-205-5p	3.040	1.64×10^{-5}
MIMAT0016895	hsa-miR-2355-5p	3.023	6.22×10^{-14}
MIMAT0004987	hsa-miR-944	3.020	7.56×10^{-7}
MIMAT0005797	hsa-miR-1301-3p	2.902	6.39×10^{-17}
MIMAT0000761	hsa-miR-324-5p	2.878	7.41×10^{-12}
MIMAT0000758	hsa-miR-135b-5p	2.859	4.08×10^{-8}
MIMAT0001341	hsa-miR-424-5p	2.856	4.57×10^{-13}
MIMAT0000072	**hsa-miR-18a-5p**	**2.829**	$\mathbf{8.10 \times 10^{-10}}$
MIMAT0001545	hsa-miR-450a-5p	2.828	1.20×10^{-15}
MIMAT0000688	hsa-miR-301a-3p	2.807	5.32×10^{-13}
MIMAT0003150	hsa-miR-455-5p	2.799	3.50×10^{-12}
Down-regulated			
MIMAT0002870	hsa-miR-499a-5p	−3.296	3.76×10^{-5}
MIMAT0000733	**hsa-miR-379-5p**	**−3.298**	$\mathbf{1.29 \times 10^{-10}}$
MIMAT0002890	hsa-miR-299-5p	−3.504	8.97×10^{-7}
MIMAT0000461	**hsa-miR-195-5p**	**−3.510**	$\mathbf{7.79 \times 10^{-14}}$
MIMAT0022721	hsa-miR-1247-3p	−3.553	3.40×10^{-7}
MIMAT0016847	hsa-miR-378c	−3.670	4.61×10^{-8}
MIMAT0002171	hsa-miR-410-3p	−3.684	9.33×10^{-12}
MIMAT0004603	hsa-miR-125b-2-3p	−3.694	1.52×10^{-18}
MIMAT0004606	hsa-miR-136-3p	−3.797	1.08×10^{-12}
MIMAT0004550	hsa-miR-30c-2-3p	−3.881	1.03×10^{-12}
MIMAT0004552	hsa-miR-139-3p	−3.937	3.02×10^{-14}
MIMAT0000099	hsa-miR-101-3p	−4.017	3.64×10^{-23}
MIMAT0000087	hsa-miR-30a-5p	−4.132	6.93×10^{-14}
MIMAT0003329	**hsa-miR-411-5p**	**−4.160**	$\mathbf{2.03 \times 10^{-10}}$
MIMAT0000265	hsa-miR-204-5p	−4.519	1.28×10^{-17}
MIMAT0000681	hsa-miR-29c-3p	−4.539	5.24×10^{-17}
MIMAT0000064	hsa-let-7c-5p	−4.674	3.68×10^{-22}
MIMAT0000462	hsa-miR-206	−5.228	4.62×10^{-3}
MIMAT0000736	hsa-miR-381-3p	−5.293	5.06×10^{-8}
MIMAT0000770	hsa-miR-133b	−5.580	3.66×10^{-4}
MIMAT0000088	hsa-miR-30a-3p	−5.696	2.66×10^{-13}
MIMAT0000097	**hsa-miR-99a-5p**	**−5.746**	$\mathbf{1.85 \times 10^{-27}}$
MIMAT0000427	**hsa-miR-133a-3p**	**−7.055**	2.93×10^{-4}
MIMAT0000416	**hsa-miR-1-3p**	**−10.663**	8.80×10^{-6}
MIMAT0000728	**hsa-miR-375-3p**	**−18.183**	1.33×10^{-11}

In bold the miRNAs in common with the results of the GEO DataSets analysis; * *p*-values were calculated by Student's *t*-test.

In Table 2, in bold, are reported the miRNAs matching between the analyses of GEO DataSets and TCGA datasets. These common-shared miRNAs are presumably more involved in neoplastic transformation mechanisms underlying the development of oral cancers. As shown in Table 2, most of these miRNAs presented the highest levels of up-regulation (miR-196a-5p and miR-196b-5p) and down-regulation (miR-99a-5p, miR-133a-3p, miR-1-3p and miR-375-3p).

In summary, the two differential analyses between tumor samples and normal samples performed on GEO DataSets and TCGA datasets, showed that 11 miRNAs, of which four up-regulated and seven down-regulated, were strictly related to the presence of a tumor (Table 3).

Table 3. Summary table of GEO DataSets and TCGA HNSC datasets "Cancer vs Normal" differential analyses.

| miRNA Name | GEO DataSets | | | | TCGA HNSC Datasets | |
| | GSE45238 | | GSE31277 | | | |
	FC Cancer vs Normal	*p*-Value *	FC Cancer vs Normal	*p*-Value *	FC Cancer vs Normal	*p*-Value **
Up-regulated						
hsa-miR-196a-5p	8.096	9.45×10^{-12}	8.132	1.42×10^{-6}	12.145	3.12×10^{-19}
hsa-miR-196b-5p	1.791	2.05×10^{-8}	1.874	2.00×10^{-4}	11.639	5.43×10^{-20}
hsa-miR-503-5p	5.010	4.83×10^{-21}	2.622	4.69×10^{-4}	4.044	3.86×10^{-19}
hsa-miR-18a-5p	2.646	2.34×10^{-10}	1.554	2.66×10^{-3}	2.829	8.10×10^{-10}
Down-regulated						
hsa-miR-379-5p	−3.513	1.83×10^{-11}	−2.345	9.63×10^{-4}	−3.298	1.29×10^{-10}
hsa-miR-195-5p	−1.778	1.25×10^{-12}	−1.620	1.71×10^{-6}	−3.510	7.79×10^{-14}
hsa-miR-411-5p	−5.574	3.25×10^{-16}	−2.542	6.18×10^{-3}	−4.160	2.03×10^{-10}
hsa-miR-99a-5p	−2.732	4.83×10^{-16}	−2.441	7.82×10^{-5}	−5.746	1.85×10^{-27}
hsa-miR-133a-3p	−4.202	6.37×10^{-9}	−3.446	8.47×10^{-3}	−7.055	2.93×10^{-4}
hsa-miR-1-3p	−9.783	3.47×10^{-9}	−5.786	2.16×10^{-3}	−10.663	8.80×10^{-6}
hsa-miR-375-3p	−16.589	1.95×10^{-17}	−3.198	5.12×10^{-4}	−18.183	1.33×10^{-11}

* *p*-values were already calculated by GEO2R software; ** *p*-values were calculated by applying Student's *t*-test.

As shown in Table 3, the miRNA miR-196a-5p and the two miRNAs miR-1-3p and miR-375-3p, respectively up-regulated and down-regulated, presented the higher levels of over-expression or down-regulation in all three datasets (two GEO DataSets and one TCGA).

For the further prediction analyses of target genes and altered molecular pathways, the 11 miRNAs reported in Table 3 were considered: hsa-miR-196a-5p, hsa-miR-196b-5p, hsa-miR-503-5p, hsa-miR-18a-5p, hsa-miR-379-5p, hsa-miR-195-5p, hsa-miR-411-5p, hsa-miR-99a-5p, hsa-miR-133a-3p, hsa-miR- 1-3p and hsa-miR-375-3p.

2.2. Levels of Interaction Between the 11 Selected miRNAs and Oral Cancer Altered Genes

Through the use of COSMIC and mirDIP, the majority of mutated and altered genes in oral cavity tumors were identified and miRNA-gene interaction specificity was determined, respectively. First, by using COSMIC the 10 most frequent mutations and gene alteration found in oral cancers were identified. These altered genes were the *TP53* genes (43%), *FAT1* (28%), *CASP8* (23%), *TERT* (22%), *NOTCH1* (20%), *CDKN2A* (16%), *HRAS* (10%), *KMT2D* (10%), *FGFR3* (8%) and *PIK3CA* (8%).

Then, through mirDIP it was possible to establish the interaction levels with the selected 11 oral cancer-associated miRNAs and the genes identified by using COSMIC (Table S2). For the 10 interacting genes, also gene expression levels were analyzed using the TCGA HNSC IlluminaHiSeq pancan normalized dataset (Table S3). This analysis revealed that all the identified miRNAs were able to target the commonly mutated genes in oral cancers. In fact, the majority of the interactions occurred with medium-high specificity underlining the strong correlation between deregulated miRNAs in cancer patients and the aforementioned genes involved in fundamental cellular and cancer pathways (Figure 1). However, the analysis of the TCGA HNSC IlluminaHiSeq pancan normalized dataset showed that only six out of the 10 (*TP53, FAT1, CASP8, TERT, CDKN2A* and *PIK3CA*) genes were significantly de-regulated in oral cancers (Table S3).

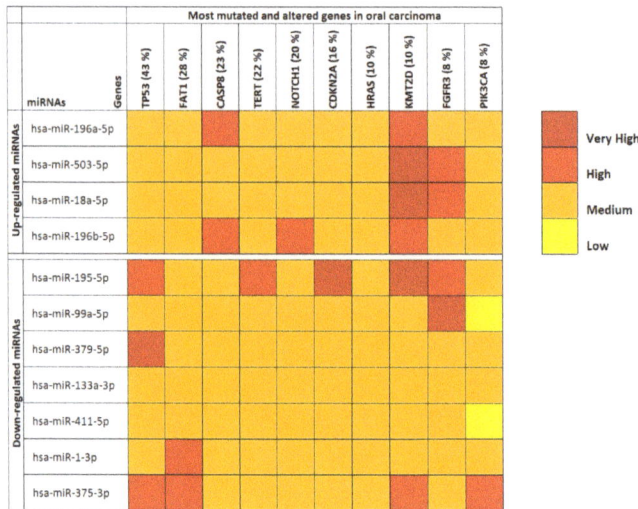

Figure 1. mirDIP analysis of interaction levels between selected miRNAs and the main mutated and altered genes in oral cavity tumors.

The most interesting data showed in Figure 1 were relative to the *KMT2D* gene where it is possible to note how all up-regulated miRNAs were able to target this gene by reducing its expression levels. This is important if we consider that KMT2D is a tumor suppressor gene, therefore its down-regulation due to the suppressive action of up-regulated miRNAs triggers cellular neoplastic transformation. Taking into account the miRNAs, it can instead be noted that, generally, the 11 selected miRNAs have medium levels of interaction with the target genes (medium interaction orange). However, the down-regulated hsa-miR-195-5p and hsa-miR-375-3p miRNAs showed the highest interaction levels with the analyzed genes (Figure 1). The expression levels of the 10 targeted genes showed that the *FAT1, CASP8, TERT, CDKN2A* and *PIK3CA* genes were significantly up-regulated in tumor samples, while *TP53* was significantly down-regulated.

2.3. Correlation Analysis Between the 11 Selected Tumor-Associated miRNAs and Ene Expression

The correlation value of each miRNA with different genes was obtained by using the bioinformatics tool miRCancerdb. This tool is a free easy-to-use database of microRNA-gene/protein expression and correlation in cancer where the correlation levels are calculated using the Pearson correlation coefficient (ρ). Therefore, the correlation levels are denoted by "*r*" [38].

In particular, for each miRNA a list of miRNAs-correlated genes, ranging from 4493 to 9042, was obtained through miRCancerdb analysis. Subsequently, these lists of genes were compared showing a total of 121 genes in common and altered by the 11 selected miRNAs. However, only the genes shared by the 11 miRNAs and belonging to the first quartile of the genes most positively and negatively correlated to each miRNA were considered (Figure 2). This selection unveiled the correlation levels of 105 different genes (Figure 2A).

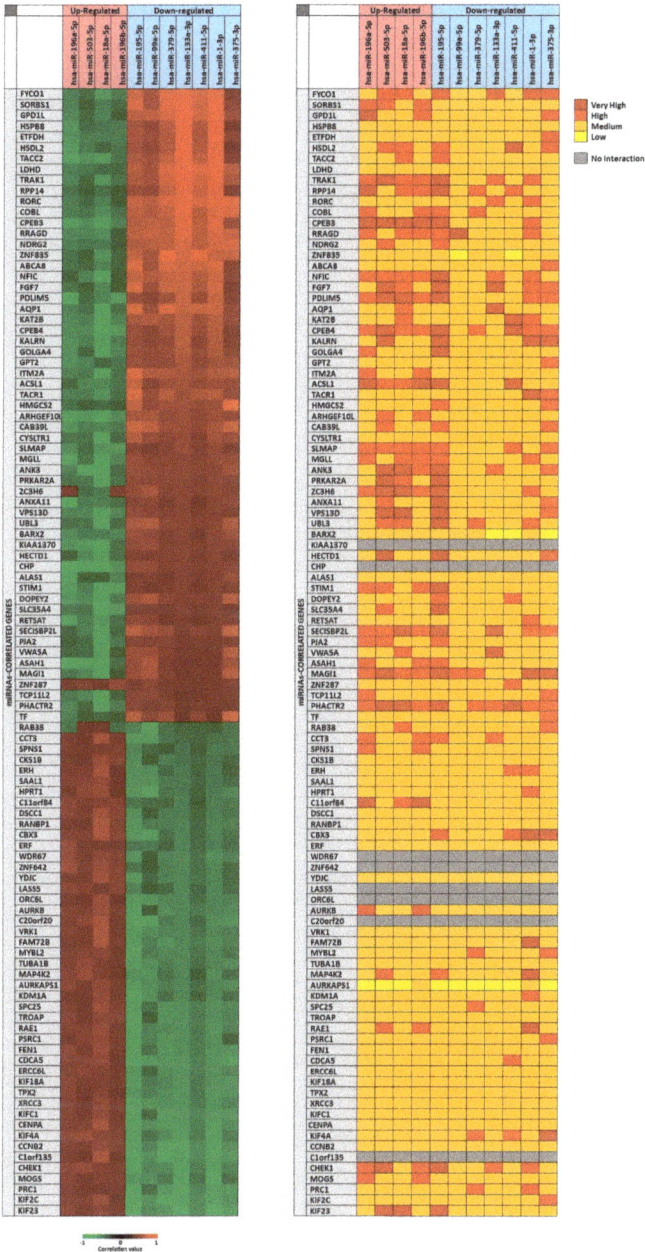

Figure 2. Panel (**A**) miRCancerdb analysis of genes whose expression is positively and negatively related to the 11 selected miRNAs; panel (**B**) mirDIP analysis of interaction levels between miRNAs and related genes.

In Figure 2A, the heat map showed that the down-regulated miRNAs miR-133a-3p and miR-1-3p were those with the highest positive correlation levels; instead, the miRNA with lower negative correlation levels was the up-regulated miRNA miR-18a-5p. Moreover, it can be observed that *FYCO1*,

SORBS1 and *GPD1L* genes were strongly positively correlated with the selected miRNAs; on the other hand, *ASA1*, *NFIC* and *SECISBP2L* genes were the least correlated with the analyzed miRNAs.

To further confirm the correlation levels existing among miRNAs and genes, the mirDIP tool was used. In Figure 2B, the interaction levels between the 11 selected miRNAs and the positively and negatively correlated genes are showed (Figure 2B). The figure shows that for eight genes there were no interactions with the selected miRNAs (*KIAA1370*, *CHP*, *WDR67*, *ZNF642*, *LASS5*, *ORC6L*, *C20orf20*, *C1orf135*). Overall, such analysis revealed that miR-195-5p, miR-503-5p, miR-18a-5p (up-regulated) and miR-375-3p (down-regulated) showed highest interaction levels with the 105 genes. On the other hand, the genes *CPEB3*, *CPEB4*, *MAGI1*, *PHACTR2*, *PDLIM5*, *NFIC*, *SLMAP* and *SECISBP2L* were strongly targeted by the 11 selected miRNAs (Figure 2B).

2.4. Determination of the Functional Roles of Tumor-Associated MiRNAs Through Pathway and GO Enrichment Analyses

For the pathway prediction analysis, all the 11 tumor-associated miRNAs were inputted into the bioinformatics prediction tool DIANA-mirPath. The analysis revealed that for the miRNAs miR-503-5p, miR-133a-3p and miR-1-3p there were not modulated pathways and targeted genes according to the TarBase Version 7.0 database of DIANA-mirPath. For the remaining miRNAs the cumulative pathway analysis showed that, overall, the miRNAs were able to alter 48 different pathways and over 2100 genes. However, the pathways involved in the tumor processes were 22 and the modulated genes amounted to 345 univocal genes (Table 4).

Table 4. Pathways involved in neoplastic transformation and modulated by the 11 computationally selected miRNAs.

No.	KEGG Pathway	Up-Regulated miRNAs			Down-Regulated miRNAs		
		p-Value *	#Genes	#miRNAs	*p*-Value *	#Genes	#miRNAs
1	Bladder cancer (hsa05219)	2.25×10^{-3}	14	3	2.78×10^{-3}	19	5
2	Cell cycle (hsa04110)	1.11×10^{-2}	27	3	5.48×10^{-3}	43	6
3	Central carbon metabolism in cancer (hsa05230)	/	/	/	4.59×10^{-2}	20	5
4	Chronic myeloid leukemia (hsa05220)	3.61×10^{-4}	22	3	1.99×10^{-2}	25	5
5	Colorectal cancer (hsa05210)	7.53×10^{-5}	18	3	/	/	/
6	FoxO signaling pathway (hsa04068)	7.64×10^{-3}	28	3	4.50×10^{-3}	44	6
7	Glioma (hsa05214)	2.56×10^{-3}	16	3	3.70×10^{-3}	23	5
8	Hippo signaling pathway (hsa04390)	1.74×10^{-11}	41	3	4.22×10^{-8}	51	6
9	Melanoma (hsa05218)	1.48×10^{-2}	15	3	/	/	/
10	mTOR signaling pathway (hsa04150)	/	/	/	1.82×10^{-2}	22	5
11	Non-small cell lung cancer (hsa05223)	2.54×10^{-2}	14	3	/	/	/
12	p53 signaling pathway (hsa04115)	1.84×10^{-3}	19	3	6.53×10^{-4}	28	6
13	Pancreatic cancer (hsa05212)	2.90×10^{-2}	17	3	4.79×10^{-2}	23	5
14	Pathways in cancer (hsa05200)	1.33×10^{-3}	62	3	1.68×10^{-4}	111	6
15	Prostate cancer (hsa05215)	3.73×10^{-3}	19	3	3.83×10^{-3}	33	6
16	Proteoglycans in cancer (hsa05205)	2.13×10^{-4}	35	3	1.11×10^{-12}	73	6
17	Renal cell carcinoma (hsa05211)	/	/	/	1.65×10^{-2}	23	6
18	Small cell lung cancer (hsa05222)	2.34×10^{-2}	19	3	1.65×10^{-2}	29	5
19	TGF-beta signaling pathway (hsa04350)	8.01×10^{-6}	19	3	6.45×10^{-3}	26	6
20	Thyroid cancer (hsa05216)	3.68×10^{-2}	7	3	/	/	/
21	TNF signaling pathway (hsa04668)	/	/	/	1.88×10^{-2}	36	6
22	Viral carcinogenesis (hsa05203)	1.53×10^{-2}	35	3	3.77×10^{-6}	65	6

* *p*-values were already calculated by the DIANA-mirPath by automatically applying the Fisher's Exact Test.

As shown in Table 4, the identified miRNAs play a key role in the modulation of different pathways involved in neoplastic development and in different types of tumors, highlighting their potential pro-oncogenic role when de-regulated (Table 4). The pathways found highly modulated were: "Pathways in cancer (hsa05200)", "Cell cycle (hsa04110)", various signal transduction pathways, including "FoxO signaling pathway (hsa04068)", "p53 signaling pathway (hsa04115)" and "Hippo signaling pathways (hsa04390)".

Within these pathways, *MAPK1* (18 counts), *CCND1* (17 counts), *AKT3* and *PIK3CA* (15 counts), *PIK3CB* (14 counts), *NRAS* (13 counts), *BRAF* (12 counts), *CDK4* and *CDKN1A* (11 counts) and *E2F2* (10 counts) genes were found commonly altered by the selected miRNAs. All these genes, when de-regulated, were notoriously involved in cancer development and progression.

To further confirm the functional roles of miRNAs and their modulated genes, gene enrichment analyses were performed on both miRCancerdb and DIANA-mirPath lists of genes by using both GO PANTHER and STRING software.

Both enrichment analyses were performed on the list of the 105 miRCancerdb genes correlated to the 11 cancer-associated miRNAs giving back similar results regarding the three ontological categories "biological process", "molecular function" and "cellular component". Figure 3 shows the results of the GO PANTHER and STRING analyses (Figure 3).

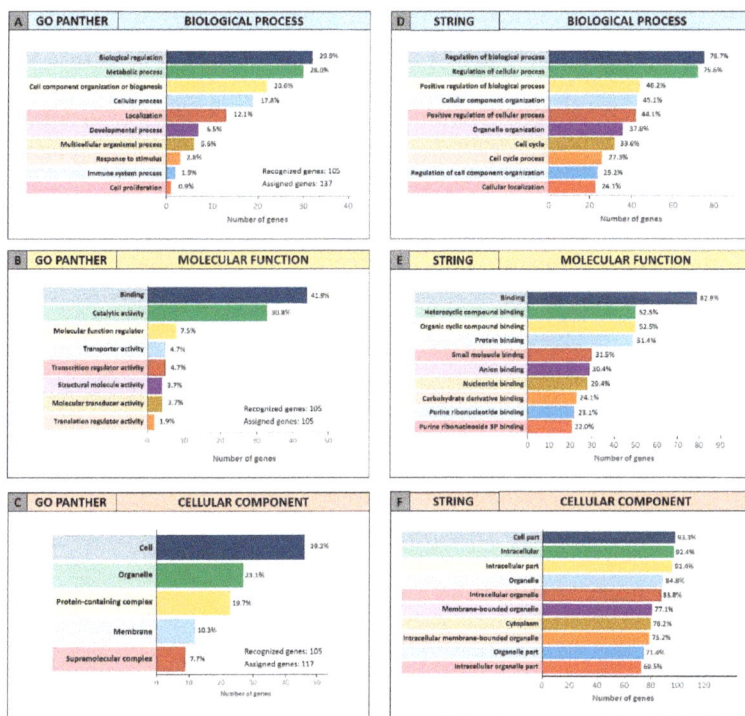

Figure 3. Gene Ontology enrichment of the 105 genes identified through miRCancerdb. Panel (**A,D**) GO PANTHER and STRING analyses of the "biological process" category; panel (**B,E**) GO PANTHER and STRING analyses of the "molecular function" category; panel (**C,F**) GO PANTHER and STRING analyses of the "cellular component" category.

Regarding the "biological process" category, it was demonstrated that most of the miRNAs-modulated genes are involved in the regulation of biological (29.9% and 78.7%, GO PANTHER and STRING, respectively) and cellular (17.8% and 75.6%, GO PANTHER and STRING, respectively) processes (Figure 3A,D). In Figure 3B,E, the genes were clustered according to their "molecular function" and the results showed that the genes were all involved in protein binding, cyclic compounds and nucleotides binding (STRING analysis Figure 3E). While the GO PANTHER analysis for the same category (molecular function) showed that the genes were mainly involved in the binding and, to a lesser extent, in the catalytic, molecular and transport activities (Figure 3B). Finally, with regard to the "cellular component" category, the majority of the genes were components of the cell (39.3% and

93.3, GO PANTHER and STRING, respectively) and organelles (23.1% and 84.8%, GO PANTHER and STRING, respectively; Figure 3C,F).

The same GO enrichment analyses were performed on the 345 genes identified by DIANA-mirPath showing similar results to those described above (Figure 4).

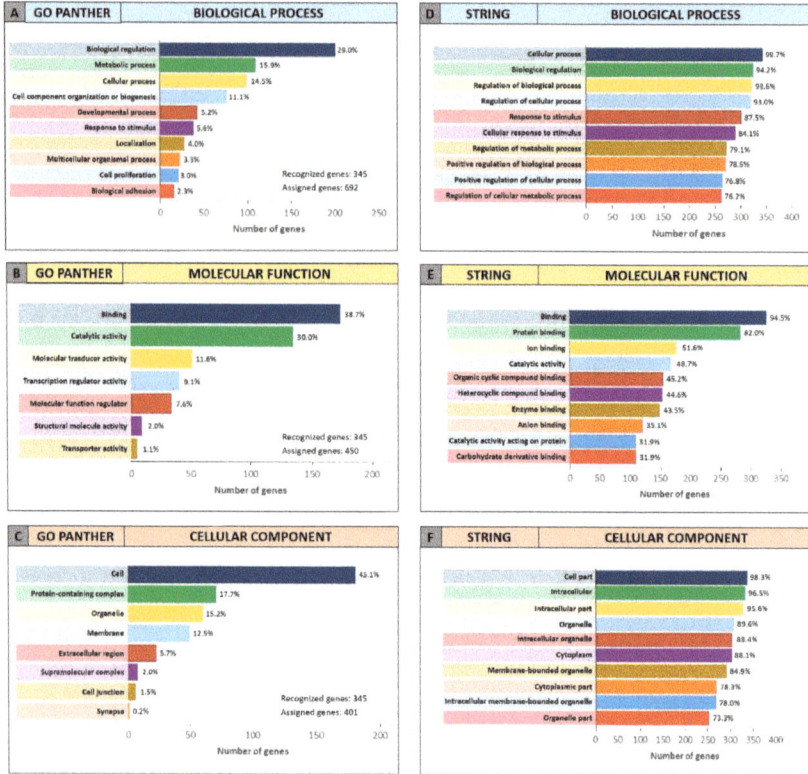

Figure 4. Gene Ontology enrichment of the 345 genes identified through DIANA-mirPath. Panel (**A,D**) GO PANTHER and STRING analyses of the "biological process" category; panel (**B,E**) GO PANTHER and STRING analyses of the "molecular function" category; panel (**C,F**) GO PANTHER and STRING analyses of the "cellular component" category.

Figure 4 (Panel A and D) shows that, in the "biological process" category, the genes identified by DIANA-mirPath were involved in the regulation of the biological and cellular processes as observed in Figure 3. Similarly, in the "molecular function" and "cellular component" categories, the 345 genes were involved, respectively, in molecular binding and catalytic activities (Figure 4B,E), and were components of the cell and intracellular organelles (Figure 4C,F).

2.5. Identification of Oral Cancer Stage-Related miRNAs

The same differential analysis performed to find the oral cancer-associated miRNAs was also performed between high-grade tumor samples (254 stage III and IV samples—high-grade) and low-grade tumor samples (94 Stage I and II samples—low-grade) in order to find oral cancer stage-related miRNAs with a prognostic significance. This second differential analysis showed that 36 miRNAs were de-regulated in high-grade samples compared to low-grade ($p < 0.01$; Table 5).

Table 5. TCGA analysis of up-regulated and down-regulated miRNAs in high-grade compared with low-grade tumors.

miRNA ID	miRNA Name	FC High-Grade vs Low-Grade	*p*-Value **
Up-regulated			
MIMAT0001536	hsa-miR-429	1.279	3.20×10^{-3}
MIMAT0003233	hsa-miR-551b-3p	1.205	1.31×10^{-3}
MIMAT0004697	hsa-miR-151a-5p	1.172	3.78×10^{-3}
MIMAT0003246	hsa-miR-581	1.078	3.88×10^{-3}
MIMAT0019931	hsa-miR-4775	1.064	1.31×10^{-3}
Down-regulated			
MIMAT0004594	hsa-miR-132-5p	−1.141	4.88×10^{-3}
MIMAT0000727	hsa-miR-374a-5p	−1.148	7.65×10^{-3}
MIMAT0022272	hsa-miR-664b-3p	−1.159	9.42×10^{-4}
MIMAT0000415	hsa-let-7i-5p	−1.180	2.57×10^{-3}
MIMAT0003338	hsa-miR-660-5p	−1.202	5.19×10^{-3}
MIMAT0004775	hsa-miR-502-3p	−1.206	4.61×10^{-3}
MIMAT0000082	hsa-miR-26a-5p	−1.209	4.96×10^{-3}
MIMAT0004694	hsa-miR-342-5p	−1.213	4.45×10^{-3}
MIMAT0004766	hsa-miR-146b-3p	−1.222	7.84×10^{-3}
MIMAT0025849	hsa-miR-6718-5p	−1.223	3.61×10^{-4}
MIMAT0004682	hsa-miR-361-3p	−1.224	8.00×10^{-4}
MIMAT0004597	hsa-miR-140-3p	−1.232	5.38×10^{-5}
MIMAT0004673	hsa-miR-29c-5p	−1.234	1.88×10^{-3}
MIMAT0002808	hsa-miR-511-5p	−1.246	9.53×10^{-3}
MIMAT0000250	hsa-miR-139-5p	−1.248	2.75×10^{-3}
MIMAT0004585	hsa-let-7i-3p	−1.251	7.09×10^{-3}
MIMAT0019071	hsa-miR-4532	−1.256	3.56×10^{-3}
MIMAT0019927	hsa-miR-4772-3p	−1.258	6.01×10^{-3}
MIMAT0000258	hsa-miR-181c-5p	−1.267	1.17×10^{-3}
MIMAT0004570	hsa-miR-223-5p	−1.285	7.97×10^{-3}
MIMAT0000086	hsa-miR-29a-3p	−1.290	1.94×10^{-3}
MIMAT0004552	**hsa-miR-139-3p**	**−1.314**	$\mathbf{2.04 \times 10^{-3}}$
MIMAT0000433	**hsa-miR-142-5p**	**−1.329**	$\mathbf{3.76 \times 10^{-3}}$
MIMAT0000646	hsa-miR-155-5p	−1.349	5.08×10^{-3}
MIMAT0000274	hsa-miR-217-5p	−1.354	6.83×10^{-3}
MIMAT0000449	hsa-miR-146a-5p	−1.375	1.56×10^{-3}
MIMAT0000280	hsa-miR-223-3p	−1.397	1.40×10^{-3}
MIMAT0000681	**hsa-miR-29c-3p**	**−1.430**	$\mathbf{1.90 \times 10^{-3}}$
MIMAT0000451	hsa-miR-150-5p	−1.644	3.98×10^{-4}
* **MIMAT0000427**	**hsa-miR-133a-3p**	**−2.168**	$\mathbf{6.39 \times 10^{-3}}$
MIMAT0000462	hsa-miR-206	−3.070	1.29×10^{-3}

In bold, miRNAs detected in the differential analysis "Cancer vs Normal" performed in both the TCGA and GEO Datasets; * miRNA included in the list of 11 selected miRNAs; ** *p*-values were calculated by Student's *t*-test.

As shown in Table 5, among the 36 identified miRNAs, 31 were down-regulated and five were up-regulated. Furthermore, among the 31 down-regulated miRNAs, three were in common with those obtained by the lists of differentially expressed miRNAs in tumor samples compared to the normal one, i.e. miRNAs miR-139-3p, miR-142-5p and miR-29c-3p, which therefore may have both diagnostic and prognostic significance in oral cancers. Furthermore, the down-regulated miRNA miR-133a-3p was in common with the list of 11 miRNAs obtained from the comparison between GEO DataSets and TCGA analyses (Table 3) suggesting that these miRNAs may have both a diagnostic and prognostic role for oral cancer.

2.6. Prognostic Value of Oral Cancer Stage-Related miRNAs

The OncoLnc analysis performed on the 36 differently expressed miRNAs in high-grade oral cancers revealed the real prognostic significance of each miRNA in terms of patients' overall survival (OS). As shown in Figure 5, of 36 miRNAs analyzed only nine were statistically associated with patients' OS (log-rank test, $p < 0.05$). These prognostic miRNAs were all down-regulated miRNAs, i.e., miR-181c-5p, miR-342-5p, miR-361-3p, miR-29c-5p, miR-142-5p, miR-146a-5p, miR-150-5p, miR-146b-3p and miR-206 (Figure 5).

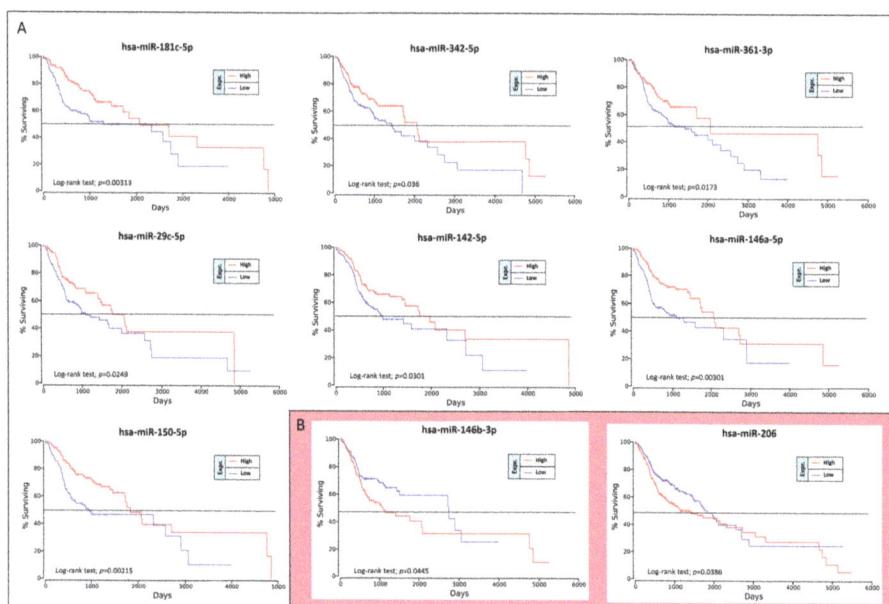

Figure 5. Survival analysis performed by OncoLnc. Panel (**A**) down-regulated miRNAs statistically associated with patients' overall survival (OS) whose expression is concordant with survival curves; panel (**B**) miRNAs statistically associated with patients' OS whose expression levels are not concordant with the survival curves.

However, two of these miRNAs, miR-146b-3p and miR-206, have shown results of dubious interpretation. In fact, despite these miRNAs are down-regulated in high-grade tumors, their down-regulation is not associated with a worse OS, but with a better prognosis (Figure 5B).

To confirm the Kaplan-Meier results obtained by using OncoLnc, the OS curves were also calculated by using GraphPad v.6 and analyzing the TGCA HNSC survival data previously downloaded from the UCSC Xena Browser. Overall, this analysis revealed the same results previously obtained.

The TCGA HNSC data were also used for the identification of miRNAs able to predict the risk of oral cancer recurrence. For this purpose, GraphPad Kaplan-Meier curves showed that two out of 36 tumor stage-related miRNAs were statistically linked to the patients' recurrence-free survival (RFS). Of these miRNAs, miR-581 was up-regulated and miR-let-7i-3p was down-regulated. Unexpectedly the over-expression of the up-regulated miR-581 was not associated with a worse prognosis, but with a minor RFS (Figure 6).

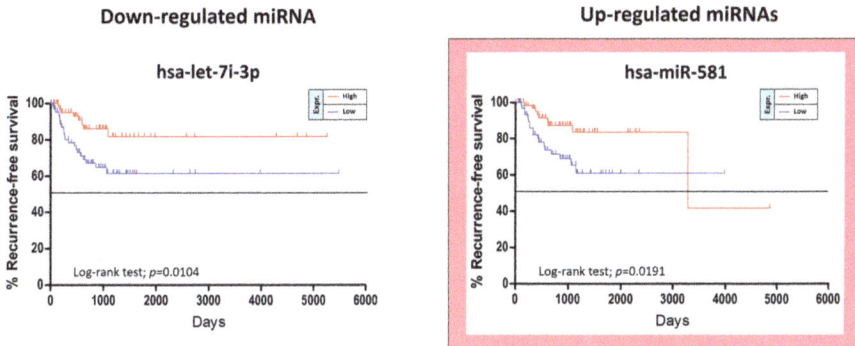

Figure 6. Recurrence-free survival analysis performed on the TCGA HNSC data.

Other five miRNAs, miR-151a-5p, miR-6718-5p, miR-660-5p, miR-4772-3p and miR-217-5p, showed a weak correlation with RFS when de-regulated, however no statistical significance was reached.

These analyses allowed us to identify 11 miRNAs significantly associated to both tumor grade and patients' OS and RFS, of these only eight were related to patients' OS (seven miRNAs) and RFS (one miRNA), respectively.

2.7. Determination of the Functional Roles of the 11 Tumor-Grade Associated miRNAs Through Pathway and GO Enrichment Analyses

As previously described for the analysis of the 11 selected miRNAs associate to the presence of tumor, the miRCancerdb and mirDIP analyses were performed for the 11 miRNAs associated to patients' prognosis in order to identify the miRNAs-correlated and -targeted genes. The miRCancerdb analysis showed that 19 different genes were positively and negatively correlated to the 11 selected miRNAs (Figure 7A).

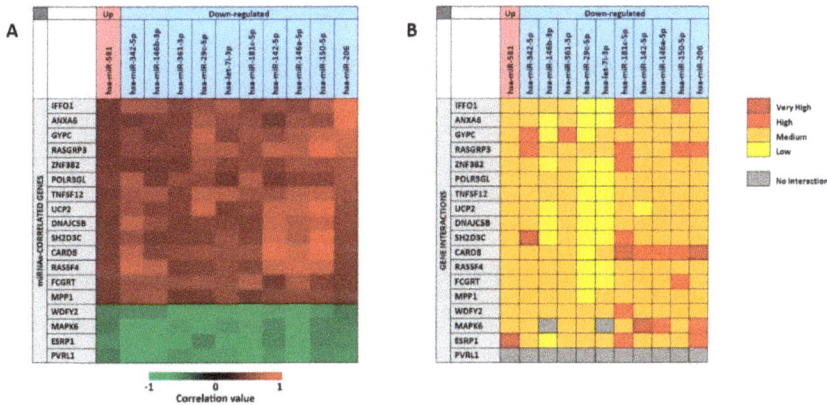

Figure 7. Panel (**A**) miRCancerdb analysis of genes whose expression is positively and negatively related to the 11 selected miRNAs; panel (**B**) mirDIP analysis of interaction levels between miRNAs and related genes.

The heat map showed that the down-regulated miRNAs miR-150-5p and miR-206 are those with the highest positive correlation levels. Of note, these two miRNAs were also those with the higher levels of down-regulation among the 36 differentially expressed miRNAs showed in Table 5. Figure 7 also shows that the miRNAs miR-181c-5p and miR-146a-5p were those more negatively correlated with the identified genes. By considering the genes, it was observed that *CARD8* and *RASGAP3* genes were those that were more positively correlated with the selected miRNAs, while the four genes *WDFY2, MAPK6, ESRP1* and *PVRL1* were all negatively correlated with the 11 miRNAs with similar correlation levels.

The mirDIP analysis performed on the 19 genes and the 11 miRNAs showed that for the *PVRL1* gene no interaction levels were available. Overall, the analysis revealed the existence of medium interaction levels between miRNAs and genes. However, the down-regulated miR-29c-5p and let-7i-3p showed lower interaction levels with most of the 19 genes, while the miR-181c-5p was the miRNA with the higher interaction levels. On the other hand, the *CARD8* gene was the most targeted by the 11 selected miRNAs, while the *UCP2* was the less targeted (Figure 7B).

After the gene targets analysis, the DIANA-mirPath analysis of the 11 prognostic miRNAs revealed that for the miRNA miR-581 there were not modulated pathways and targeted genes according to the TarBase Version 7.0 database of the mirPath tool. For the other 10 miRNAs the cumulative pathway analysis showed that, the miRNAs were able to modulate 44 different pathways and over than 1300 genes. The selection of the 21 pathways involved in the tumor processes showed that the selected miRNAs were able to modulate 292 univocal genes (Table 6).

Table 6. Tumor pathways modulated by the 11 computationally selected miRNAs associated to patients' prognosis.

N.	KEGG Pathway	*p*-Value *	#Genes	#miRNAs
1	PI3K-Akt signaling pathway (hsa04151)	8.22×10^{-3}	82	10
2	Cell cycle (hsa04110)	1.91×10^{-5}	45	10
3	Proteoglycans in cancer (hsa05205)	6.81×10^{-5}	48	9
4	Transcriptional misregulation in cancer (hsa05202)	2.00×10^{-2}	46	9
5	FoxO signaling pathway (hsa04068)	2.66×10^{-3}	43	9
6	Hippo signaling pathway (hsa04390)	9.14×10^{-4}	39	9
7	Melanoma (hsa05218)	7.56×10^{-3}	22	9
8	Viral carcinogenesis (hsa05203)	1.08×10^{-6}	62	8
9	Prostate cancer (hsa05215)	6.33×10^{-3}	29	8
10	Small cell lung cancer (hsa05222)	2.63×10^{-3}	29	8
11	Renal cell carcinoma (hsa05211)	6.92×10^{-6}	27	8
12	Chronic myeloid leukemia (hsa05220)	7.67×10^{-4}	26	8
13	Glioma (hsa05214)	1.74×10^{-4}	23	8
14	TGF-beta signaling pathway (hsa04350)	7.03×10^{-4}	23	8
15	Pancreatic cancer (hsa05212)	3.18×10^{-2}	21	8
16	Non-small cell lung cancer (hsa05223)	8.22×10^{-3}	18	8
17	p53 signaling pathway (hsa04115)	2.00×10^{-3}	26	7
18	Central carbon metabolism in cancer (hsa05230)	1.96×10^{-5}	24	7
19	Colorectal cancer (hsa05210)	4.50×10^{-2}	19	6
20	Acute myeloid leukemia (hsa05221)	3.52×10^{-2}	17	6
21	Endometrial cancer (hsa05213)	4.46×10^{-2}	16	6

* *p*-values were already calculated by the DIANA-mirPath by automatically applying the Fisher's Exact Test.

The DIANA-mirPath analysis showed that all the selected miRNAs were involved in the modulation of the "PI3K-Akt signaling pathway (hsa04151)" and the "Cell cycle (hsa04110)", both involved in various neoplastic processes when altered (Table 6). Of note, "Cell cycle (hsa04110)" pathways were also strongly altered by the 11 cancer-associated miRNAs previously analyzed (Table 4). The genes altered by these miRNAs were all involved in neoplastic processes, such as *CCND1* (18 counts), *MAPK1* (16 counts), *MAP2K1* (14 counts), *PIK3CB* and *PIK3R3* (16 counts), *AKT2* and *AKT3* (15 counts), *CDK4* and *CDK6* (11 counts), etc.

The genes identified through miRCancerdb and DIANA-mirPath analyses were finally analyzed with GO PANTHER and STRING to establish for which molecular processes and functions these miRNAs were enriched.

For the 19 genes identified by miRCancerdb analysis only the GO PANTHER evaluation was performed because the gene ontology enrichment performed by STRING requires a wide number of analyzed genes. The GO PANTHER analysis showed that most of selected genes were involved in the cellular processes (23.3% of genes) and in biological regulation (20.0% of genes) for the "biological process" category (Figure 8A). Regarding the "molecular function" category, the analysis demonstrated that the 43.5% and 17.4% of genes were involved in binding and molecular regulatory functions, respectively (Figure 8B); while for the "cellular component" category, the results showed that the 19 genes constitute mainly part of the cell, of the organelles and of the cell junctions (37.5%, 25.0% and 18.8% respectively; Figure 8C).

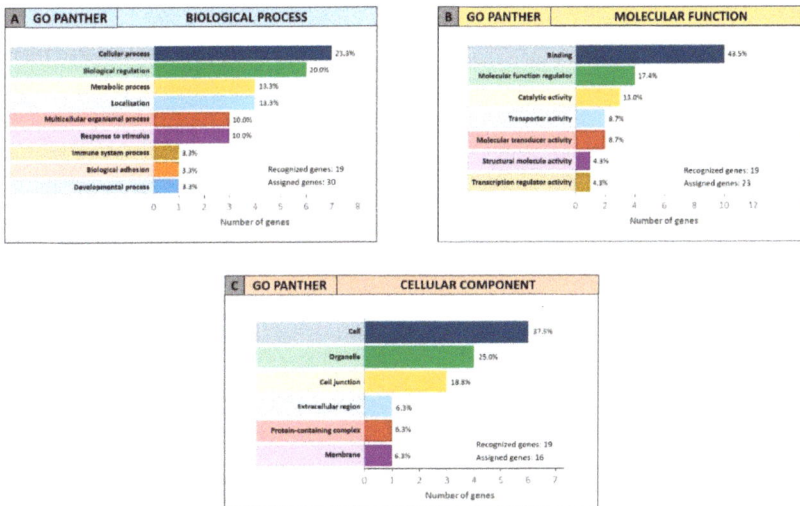

Figure 8. Gene Ontology enrichment of the 19 genes identified through miRCancerdb. Panel (**A**) GO PANTHER analysis of the "biological process" category; panel (**B**) GO PANTHER analysis of the "molecular function" category; panel (**C**) GO PANTHER analysis of the "cellular component" category.

The same enrichment analysis was performed on the 292 genes identified by DIANA-mirPath carrying out both GO PANTHER and STRING analyses.

The results obtained for the "biological process" category showed that the identified genes were mainly involved in the cellular processes (23.3% of genes) and in biological regulation (20.0% of genes) as observed for the 19 genes identified by miRCancerdb (Figure 9A,D). Furthermore, both the analyses (GO PANTHER and STRING) showed that the 292 genes were involved in molecular binding and catalytic activities (Figure 9B,E), as observed in the previous evaluations. Regarding the "cellular component" category, it was finally demonstrated that the genes were part of the cell and of the intracellular organelles (Figure 9C,F).

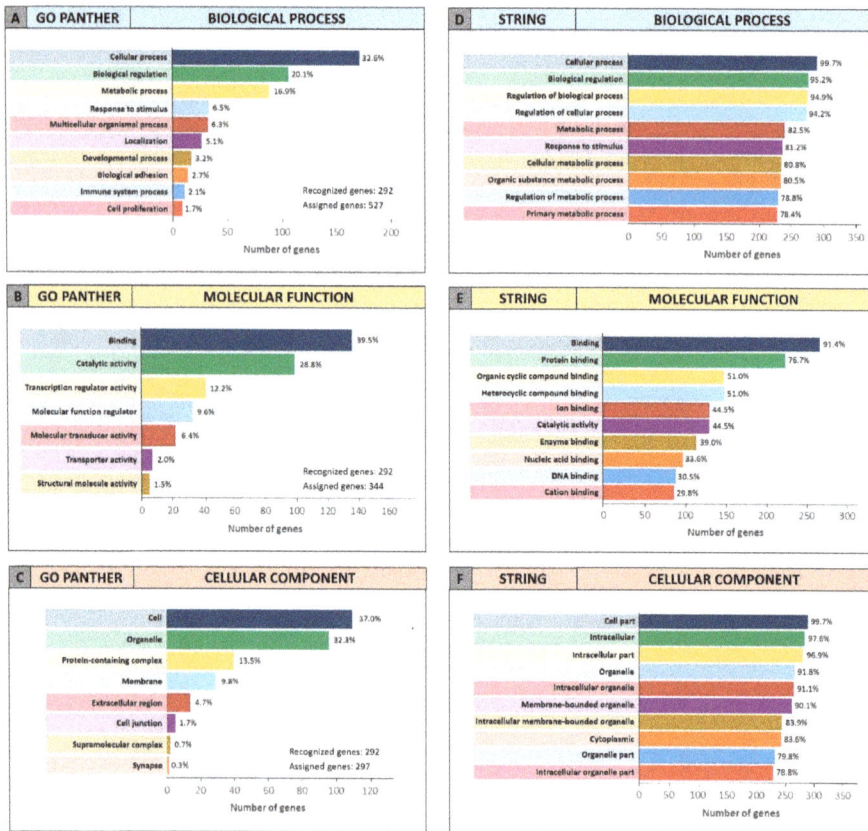

Figure 9. Gene Ontology enrichment of the 345 genes identified through DIANA-mirPath. Panel (**A,D**) GO PANTHER and STRING analyses of the "biological process" category; panel (**B,E**) GO PANTHER and STRING analyses of the "molecular function" category; panel (**C,F**) GO PANTHER and STRING analyses of the "cellular component" category.

3. Discussion

During the last decade, the advancement of bioinformatics and high-throughput technologies led to the development of omics sciences, as well as to the collection of thousands of petabytes of molecular data related to various human diseases, including tumors [39].

The increase in the number of available bioinformatics data allowing the understanding of various physio-pathological aspects of tumors. However, the huge amount of data, either deriving from individual basic science experiments, or collected by large international consortia, such as TCGA and ENCODE, are often incorrectly analyzed, thus generating conflicting results [40–42].

In order to best analyze the so-called "Big Data", in recent years different researchers have created several bioinformatics software useful for a fast and efficient analysis of a large number of data thus interpretation through a process named "data mining" [43,44].

Thanks to the availability of new software for the computational analysis of Big Data, numerous studies tried to establish the molecular mechanisms responsible for neoplastic transformation, as well as to identify novel molecular targets or biomarkers useful for the management of tumors [45].

In recent years, several genetic, epigenetic and proteomic data were also generated for oral cancer. These data allowed the researchers to obtain important information regarding the main molecular and clinical-pathological characteristics of this kind of tumor. However, the analysis of the data contained in the various oral cancer datasets generated conflicting data difficult to interpret due to the lack of data integration among the different data matrices [46]. Furthermore, despite the increasing number of bioinformatics studies, no effective diagnostic and prognostic biomarkers have been yet identified for oral cancers, making this pathology one of the most aggressive, since in most cases it is not promptly diagnosed [47].

Therefore, the aim of the present study was to identify new specific diagnostic and prognostic biomarkers for oral cancer through the analysis and integration of different miRNAs profiling datasets, using several computational approaches.

For this purpose, two of the biggest worldwide genomics databases, TCGA and GEO DataSets were analyzed in order to select miRNA expression profiling datasets. In particular, the analysis of the TCGA HNSC "miRNA mature strand expression RNAseq by Illumina Hiseq" dataset and of two GEO DataSets miRNA microarray matrices allowed the identification of a panel of miRNAs with diagnostic and prognostic value for oral cancer patients. From these datasets, a group of 11 de-regulated miRNAs was identified by comparing cancer patients with healthy controls. Among these miRNAs, the up-regulated miR-196a-5p and miR-196b-5p and the down-regulated miR-99a-5p, miR-133a-3p, miR-1-3p and miR-375-3p were the most de-regulated and therefore these miRNAs may be used to improve the actual diagnostic strategies for oral cancers. Indeed, different research groups are currently investigating all these miRNAs because their deregulation is associated with the development of different cancers. In particular, Sutliff and colleagues (2019) demonstrated that the de-regulation miR-196 family (miR-196a-5p and miR-196b-5p) is associated with the development of lung cancer [48].

Furthermore, other studies have demonstrated that the miR-196 family and other miRNAs, including miR-375 and miR-133a-3p, may play a key role as diagnostic biomarkers for head and neck cancers, especially for the tumors of the oral cavity [49–51]. In addition to these five miRNAs, the miRNAs miR-139-3p, miR-142-5p and miR-29c-3p are also noteworthy because beyond their diagnostic role, they have also an important prognostic role. On this regard, the analysis of miRNA expression levels in high-grade tumors compared to the low-grade tumors contained in the TCGA HNSC dataset revealed that the down-regulation of these three miRNAs, together with the aforementioned miRNA miR-133a-3p, was associated with a more aggressive and infiltrating phenotype. Accordingly, these results are supported by several studies performed on different tumors where it has been shown that the de-regulation of these miRNAs is associated with a more aggressive tumor phenotype [32,52–54].

Furthermore, the OncoLnc analysis revealed that among the 36 tumor-stage associated miRNAs only eight were related to patients' OS and RFS (seven and one, respectively). Of note, all these miRNAs were found all down-regulated in high-grade tumors compared to low-grade. In particular, the most statistically significant miRNAs associated with OS, and therefore to a worse prognosis, were the miRNAs miR-150-5p, miR-181c-5p and miR-146a-5p. Regarding the RFS, only the miRNA miR-let-7i-3p was a good indicator of disease recurrence. These data are also supported by several studies since the miR-7i (both 3p and 5p strands) is associated with a poorer prognosis when down-regulated [55]. Furthermore, other studies showed that the down-regulation of other miRNAs, such as miR-375 and miR-181c, is associated with a cancer aggressive phenotype [56,57].

Therefore, these first computational data demonstrated that by using an integrated computational approach for the analysis of miRNAs datasets it is possible to identify a set of miRNAs potentially used as specific biomarkers for oral cancers. As described above, the validity of the obtained results is further strengthened by the results obtained by other research groups in independent experimental studies.

Once identified which miRNAs bear a diagnostic and/or prognostic significance, it was also established which genes and pathways they were able to modulate to uncover their functional roles. As described in previous studies, the DIANA-mirPath analysis showed that the computationally selected miRNAs were strictly related to cancer development since they were able to alter key oncogenic pathways [32–34,58]. On this regard, the oral cancer-associated miRNAs identified in the present study were able to alter several intracellular signal transduction pathways, including mTOR, p53 and TGF-β pathways, whose implication in the development of oral carcinoma has been widely demonstrated [59–61]. Similarly, the selected miRNAs were also able to target genes frequently down-regulated or over-expressed in oral cancers. Some of these genes, including *AKT*, *BRAF*, *PIK3CA*, *NRAS*, *GSK3*, *CNND1*, etc., are involved not only in oral cancers but, generally, in several solid tumors [62–65]. The subsequent gene ontology enrichment analyses further demonstrated that the miRNAs' targeted genes were involved in the biological process linked to the cell proliferation, biological regulation, protein binding, catalytic activities and metabolic processes.

Similarly, the prediction and GO enrichment analyses performed on the 11 miRNAs associated to the patients' OS and RFS revealed that all the miRNAs with a significant diagnostic and/or prognostic role were able to modulate several cancer pathways by modulating numerous genes known to be involved in neoplastic transformation.

Overall, the computational approaches adopted in the present studies allowed us to identify a set of specific miRNAs for the diagnosis of oral cancer and the definition of patients' prognosis through the integrated analysis of different bioinformatics datasets that allowed us to understand the functional role of each miRNA. However, the results obtained from this study represent only the starting point for identifying effective markers for oral carcinoma. Therefore, further experimental and functional studies will have to be performed on a large number of samples in order to evaluate the expression levels of these putative miRNAs biomarkers and to validate their predictive role for oral cancer. With the advancement of both bioinformatics and high-throughput and high-sensitive molecular technologies this future goal can be easily achieved thanks to the detection of even small variations in the expression levels of selected miRNAs indicative of the presence of a possible pathological state [66–68].

4. Materials and Methods

4.1. Oral Cancer MicroRNA Datasets Selection

In order to identify miRNAs potentially involved in the development and progression of oral cancer, several oral cancer miRNAs datasets were taken into account. Firstly, the oral cancer datasets of microRNA profiling by array were selected by checking within the datasets registered in the GEO DataSets portal publicly available on NCBI (www.ncbi.nlm.nih.gov/geo/) [69]. In particular, for the selection of the suitable datasets an advanced search was carried out by inserting the search terms "(("non coding RNA profiling by array"[DataSet Type]) and oral carcinoma) and "Homo sapiens"[porgn:__txid9606]". With this first approach, a list of all oral cancer datasets containing miRNA expression levels was obtained. Of these datasets, only those that respect the following inclusion and exclusion criteria were selected for the subsequent evaluations:

Inclusion criteria, i) datasets containing miRNA expression levels of oral cancer tissues, excluding tumor arising in the hypopharynx, larynx, esophagus and tonsil; ii) datasets reporting miRNAs expression levels of both tumor and normal tissue samples; iii) datasets containing the miRNA expression data of at least 30 samples (tumor + normal).

Exclusion criteria, i) datasets constructed only with tumor samples; ii) datasets containing information about miRNAs of oral cancer or normal cell lines; iii) datasets containing information on miRNAs expression levels of serum samples.

The search criteria for the selection of the datasets contained in the GEO DataSets database allowed us to preliminarily identify 37 different datasets of oral carcinoma microRNA profiling by array (published up to December 2018). However, most of these datasets did not respect the exclusion and inclusion criteria because they were datasets reporting the miRNA expression data relative to tumor cell lines and not from oral cancer patients. Hence, after the application of the abovementioned criteria only two datasets were selected for performing the differential analyses (Table 7).

Table 7. Features of the two selected datasets from GEO DataSets.

Series Accession	n. Normal	n. Cancer	Samples	Platform	Author Ref	Total Number
GSE45238	40	40	Fresh Frozen Tissues	GPL8179 Illumina Human v2 MicroRNA expression beadchip	Shiah SG et al, Cancer Res 2014	80
GSE31277	15	15	Fresh Frozen Tissues	GPL9770 Illumina miR arrays version 1.0	Severino P et al, BMC Cancer 2013	30

In addition to the datasets contained in the GEO DataSets database, also the TCGA Head and Neck Cancer (HNSC) database was selected. Among the 25 datasets available in the TCGA HNSC database, the "Phenotype" and "miRNA mature strand expression RNAseq by Illumina Hiseq" HNSC datasets were downloaded for the analyses by using the UCSC Xena Browser (https://xenabrowser.net/) portal where all the HNSC molecular profiling data, generated by the TCGA consortium, were deposited, including those of oral cancer. In particular, the first dataset contained the clinical-pathological data of 604 samples (530 cancer patients and 74 normal individuals) while the second one contained the miRNAs expression profile of 529 samples. Since the TCGA HNSC database also contains tumor samples obtained not only from the oral cavity but also from other sites (oropharynx, hypopharynx, larynx and tonsil), for the purposes of this study only the data of samples derived from alveolar ridge, base of tongue, buccal mucosa, floor of mouth, hard palate, lip, oral cavity and oral tongue were analyzed. In this way, the number of analyzed samples was reduced to 399. By selecting only samples of the oral cavity also the number of samples with available miRNAs expression profile it was reduced passing from 529 to 351 samples.

4.2. Differential Analysis of miRNAs Expression Between Groups

Two distinct differential analyses were performed by using the datasets selected from the GEO DataSets and TCGA databases. A first differential analysis was performed to both GEO DataSets and TCGA data matrices by integrating the different GEO DataSets platform and by comparing the miRNAs expression levels of tumor samples with a normal one in order to identify new diagnostic biomarkers.

The second differential analysis was conducted only for the TCGA dataset comparing the expression levels of miRNAs of advanced tumors with that of low-grade tumors to identify miRNAs able to define the prognosis of patients.

In particular, the data matrices of each dataset selected from GEO DataSets were downloaded to identify the down-regulated or up-regulated miRNAs in oral cancer. The differential analysis between cancer and normal samples was performed by using the GEO2R tool [69]. The fold change value (FC) obtained for each miRNA was indicated as base-2 logarithm of FC (logFC) in order to normalize the data derived from different microarray platforms. Then, for each dataset only the differentially expressed miRNAs with a statistical significance $p < 0.01$ were taken into account. The lists of the de-regulated miRNAs of the two selected GEO DataSets platforms were subsequently compared in order to select only the miRNAs shared by the two datasets and with a logFC value greater than ±1.5.

In parallel, other differential analyses of miRNAs expression levels between tumor vs normal samples and between high-grade vs low-grade tumors of TCGA HNSC dataset were performed.

For the differential analyses, the samples were clustered according to the presence or absence of tumor (Tumor (348 samples) vs Normal (51 samples)) and according to the tumor stage (T3–T4 (319 samples) vs. T1–T2 (32 samples)). After patients' stratification, the down-regulated and up-regulated miRNAs were identified by calculating the fold change value obtained through the differential analysis between the different clusters of samples. Of note, for some of the oral cancer patients the miRNA expression levels were missing (NA value). Therefore, in order to avoid the identification of non-representative miRNAs, for further analysis only the differentially expressed miRNAs with reported expression data for at least 50% of the patients and with *p*-value of $p < 0.01$ were selected.

Moreover, with reference to the differential analysis between tumor and normal samples, only the 25 most up-regulated and down-regulated miRNAs were considered to obtain more significant data; while for the differential analysis between high-grade and low-grade tumors all the differentially expressed miRNAs were considered.

Finally, the annotation of the TCGA HNSC miRNAs was performed using miRBase V.22 (http://www.mirbase.org/) by converting the miRNA IDs 'MIMAT00' in 'hsa-miR-'.

4.3. Analysis of the Interaction Levels Between the Selected miRNAs and Oral Cancer-Altered Genes

After the identification of the most de-regulated miRNAs in tumor samples compared to normal samples, their functional roles were studied using different bioinformatics approaches. At first, using the data reported in the Catalogue of Somatic Mutations in Cancer (COSMIC) (http://cancer.sanger.ac.uk/cosmic), the most mutated and altered genes of oral cavity tumors were identified. Subsequently, for each of the COSMIC genes, the specificity of miRNA-gene interaction was highlighted by using the bioinformatics prediction software miRNA Data Integration Portal (mirDIP; (http://ophid.utoronto.ca/mirDIP). In particular, this software is able to integrate the data related to 26 different databases for miRNAs (including miRBase, microrna.org and DIANA microT-CDS v5) allowing the users to centralize the data related to the miRNAs-target genes interactions obtaining more robust data. The levels of interaction between the miRNAs and the targeted gene are expressed as very high, high, medium and low according to the integrated score calculated by the mirDIP algorithm that combines the confidence scores from all available predictions data of the 26 different databases [70,71]. Furthermore, the expression levels of the 10 interacting genes identified with COSMIC were analyzed by performing the differential analysis of the gene expression data contained in the TCGA HNSC IlluminaHiSeq pancan normalized dataset.

4.4. Analysis of TCGA HNSC Genes Positively and Negatively Correlated with the Selected Tumor-Associated/Grade-Associated miRNAs

In addition to the COSMIC analysis, a global correlation analysis was also performed on the genes contained in the TCGA HNSC dataset whose expression is modulated, positively or negatively, by the selected tumor-associated miRNAs. In particular, for this analysis the bioinformatics tool miRCancerdb (https://mahshaaban.shinyapps.io/miRCancerdb/) was used. miRCancerdb is a free R software for the correlation analysis between gene expression and miRNAs levels with a web interface based on data contained in the TCGA and TargetScan databases [38]. In particular, through miRCancerdb, for each selected miRNA was obtained the correlation value (ρ) with different genes. The lists of genes generated for each miRNA were subsequently combined using the tool Draw Venn Diagrams of the Bioinformatics & Evolutionary Genomics (BEG) (http://bioinformatics.psb.ugent.be/webtools/Venn/) to identify the genes correlated and shared among all miRNAs.

However, since miRCancerdb uses interaction data between miRNAs and genes derived exclusively from the TargetScan database, the previously described mirDIP tool, that uses 26 different miRNA databases, was also used to establish the levels of miRNAs-genes interaction. These analyses were performed for the 11 miRNAs associated to the presence of oral cancer and for the 11 miRNAs that after OncoLnc analysis were associated to both tumor grade and patients' OS and RFS.

4.5. Prediction Pathway Analysis, Gene Ontology (GO) and Functional Roles of Tumor-Associated Selected miRNAs

To better understand the functional role of the tumor-associated selected miRNAs, a pathway prediction analysis was performed. For this purpose, the bioinformatics tool DIANA-mirPath v.3 was used [72]. With this computational approach it was possible to identify the main molecular pathways altered by selected miRNAs, especially those related to tumor development and hence to oral carcinoma.

Finally, the functional role of the selected miRNAs was determined by performing the pathways enrichment analysis of the lists of genes obtained from the miRCancerdb and DIANA-mirPath v.3 analyses. For this purpose, both GO PANTHER version 14.0 (http://pantherdb.org/) and STRING version 11.0 (https://string-db.org/) software were used [73,74]. The two software were used to perform a more robust analysis. In fact, STRING database uses a number of functional classification systems including GO, Pfam and KEGG and therefore provide more comprehensive results than those obtained with the GO PANTHER analysis. Furthermore, the data derived from the biological functional prediction analyses performed with DIANA-mirPath, GO PANTHER and STRING tools are already normalized with data used as reference or negative control, therefore, no additional datasets were used for the normalization of the data.

The DIANA-mirPath, GO PANTHER and STRING analyses were performed for the 11 selected miRNAs associated to the presence of oral cancer and for the 11 miRNAs that after OncoLnc analysis were associated to both tumor grade and patients' OS and RFS.

4.6. Kaplan-Meier Estimate of Overall Survival (OS) and Recurrence-Free Survival (RFS) in Patients with Down-regulated and Up-regulated Tumor Stage-Related miRNAs

In order to establish the prognostic significance of the tumor stage-related miRNAs identified, the bioinformatics tool OncoLnc (http://www.oncolnc.org/) was used [75]. OncoLnc is a tool able to derive the mortality data from the TCGA datasets, including that of HNSC, allowing the user to obtain the Kaplan-Meier survival curves for each miRNA. The software identifies which of the selected tumor stage-related miRNAs were correlated to a patients' overall survival (OS). The OncoLnc analysis was performed according to the instruction given by the software developers that suggest to perform the analysis between the expression levels of bottom quartile samples and top quartile samples.

To further confirm the OS Kaplan-Meier results obtained by OncoLnc, the survival curves were also calculated by using the TGCA survival data downloaded only for the oral cancer (excluding tumor arising in hypopharynx, oropharynx, larynx and tonsil) analyzed with GraphPad v.6.

Furthermore, to our best knowledge no bioinformatics tools are available for the analysis of TCGA recurrence-free survival data; therefore, the RFS curves were calculated by using the TGCA HNSC progression data analyzed with a GraphPad survival curve sheet. In particular, RFS was calculated from the date of diagnosis to patient progression, or to the end of follow-up, whichever occurred first. The times of follow-up were different from patient to patient up to a maximum follow-up time of 5480 days, however, for some patients RFS data were not available.

4.7. Statistical Analyses

The miRNAs expression data derived from the GEO DataSets were already normalized by the GEO2R software, while the fold change values of TCGA HNSC miRNA expression levels were calculated through differential analysis. Student's t-test was performed to select the differentially expressed miRNAs of the TCGA dataset with a statistical significance. The GEO2R software already calculated the p-values of the GEO DataSets data. For the Kaplan-Meier analyses, GraphPad survival sheet and log-rank non-parametric test were used. Data with a *p*-value of ≤0.05 and ≤0.01 were considered statistically significant.

5. Conclusions

In conclusion, in the present study the integrated analysis of different miRNA expression datasets and the use of several tools for the interpretation of bioinformatics data allowed us to identify a set of miRNAs that, after in vitro and in vivo validations, may be used in clinical practice for the early detection of pre-cancerous and cancerous oral lesions.

Supplementary Materials: The following are available online at http://www.mdpi.com/2072-6694/11/5/610/s1, Table S1: List of 514 de-regulated TCGA HNSC miRNAs associated with the presence of tumor; Table S2: mirDIP number of prediction source and interaction levels between the 11 oral cancer-associated miRNAs and the genes identified by using COSMIC; Table S3: TCGA HNSC gene expression values of the 10 miRNA interacting genes.

Author Contributions: Conceptualization, L.F., M.L. and S.C.; Formal analysis, G.R.M.L.R.; Investigation, L.F. and G.R.M.L.R.; Supervision, E.R. and M.L.; Writing – original draft, L.F.; Writing—review & editing, G.L., S.C., C.D.A., R.S., E.R. and M.L. All authors have approved the final version of the manuscript.

Funding: The authors would like to thank the 'Lega Italiana per la Lotta contro i Tumori (LILT)' for providing funding.

Acknowledgments: The authors would like to thank the support kindly provided by the researcher of the Research Center for Prevention, Diagnosis and Treatment of Cancer, University of Catania, Catania.

Conflicts of Interest: The authors declare no conflict of interest.

References

1. Bray, F.; Ferlay, J.; Soerjomataram, I.; Siegel, R.L.; Torre, L.A.; Jemal, A. Global cancer statistics 2018: GLOBOCAN estimates of incidence and mortality worldwide for 36 cancers in 185 countries. *CA Cancer J. Clin.* **2018**, *68*, 394–424. [CrossRef]

2. Dhanuthai, K.; Rojanawatsirivej, S.; Thosaporn, W.; Kintarak, S.; Subarnbhesaj, A.; Darling, M.; Kryshtalskyj, E.; Chiang, C.P.; Shin, H.I.; Choi, S.Y.; et al. Oral cancer: A multicenter study. *Med. Oral Patol. Oral Cir. Bucal* **2018**, *23*, e23–e29. [CrossRef]

3. Rivera, C.; Venegas, B. Histological and molecular aspects of oral squamous cell carcinoma (Review). *Oncol. Lett.* **2014**, *8*, 7–11. [CrossRef] [PubMed]

4. Falzone, L.; Salomone, S.; Libra, M. Evolution of Cancer Pharmacological Treatments at the Turn of the Third Millennium. *Front. Pharmacol.* **2018**, *9*, 1300. [CrossRef] [PubMed]

5. Gupta, N.; Gupta, R.; Acharya, A.K.; Patthi, B.; Goud, V.; Reddy, S.; Garg, A.; Singla, A. Changing Trends in oral cancer—A global scenario. *Nepal. J. Epidemiol.* **2016**, *6*, 613–619.

6. Santos, H.B.; dos Santos, T.K.; Paz, A.R.; Cavalcanti, Y.W.; Nonaka, C.F.; Godoy, G.P.; Alves, P.M. Clinical findings and risk factors to oral squamous cell carcinoma in young patients: A 12-year retrospective analysis. *Med. Oral Patol. Oral Cir. Bucal* **2016**, *21*, e151–e156. [CrossRef] [PubMed]

7. Polesel, J.; Franceschi, S.; Talamini, R.; Negri, E.; Barzan, L.; Montella, M.; Libra, M.; Vaccher, E.; Franchin, G.; La Vecchia, C.; et al. Tobacco smoking, alcohol drinking, and the risk of different histological types of nasopharyngeal cancer in a low-risk population. *Oral. Oncol.* **2011**, *47*, 541–545. [CrossRef] [PubMed]

8. Yete, S.; D'Souza, W.; Saranath, D. High-Risk Human Papillomavirus in Oral Cancer: Clinical Implications. *Oncology.* **2018**, *94*, 133–141. [CrossRef] [PubMed]

9. She, Y.; Nong, X.; Zhang, M.; Wang, M. Epstein-Barr virus infection and oral squamous cell carcinoma risk: A meta-analysis. *PLoS ONE* **2017**, e0186860. [CrossRef]

10. Mohd Bakri, M.; Mohd Hussaini, H.; Rachel Holmes, A.; David Cannon, R.; Mary Rich, A. Revisiting the association between candidal infection and carcinoma, particularly oral squamous cell carcinoma. *J. Oral Microbiol.* **2010**, *2*. [CrossRef] [PubMed]

11. Vivarelli, S.; Salemi, R.; Candido, S.; Falzone, L.; Santagati, M.; Stefani, S.; Torino, F.; Banna, G.L.; Tonini, G.; Libra, M. Gut Microbiota and Cancer: From Pathogenesis to Therapy. *Cancers (Basel)* **2019**, *11*, 38. [CrossRef]

12. Karpiński, T.M. Role of Oral Microbiota in Cancer Development. *Microorganisms.* **2019**, *7*, 20. [CrossRef] [PubMed]

13. Banna, G.L.; Torino, F.; Marletta, F.; Santagati, M.; Salemi, R.; Cannarozzo, E.; Falzone, L.; Ferraù, F.; Libra, M. Lactobacillus rhamnosus GG: An Overview to Explore the Rationale of Its Use in Cancer. *Front. Pharmacol.* **2017**, *8*, 603. [CrossRef]

14. Nakagaki, T.; Tamura, M.; Kobashi, K.; Koyama, R.; Fukushima, H.; Ohashi, T.; Idogawa, M.; Ogi, K.; Hiratsuka, H.; Tokino, T.; et al. Profiling cancer-related gene mutations in oral squamous cell carcinoma from Japanese patients by targeted amplicon sequencing. *Oncotarget* **2017**, *8*, 59113–59122. [CrossRef] [PubMed]

15. Bavle, R.M.; Venugopal, R.; Konda, P.; Muniswamappa, S.; Makarla, S. Molecular Classification of Oral Squamous Cell Carcinoma. *J. Clin. Diagn. Res.* **2016**, *10*, ZE18–ZE21. [CrossRef]

16. Irimie, A.I.; Ciocan, C.; Gulei, D.; Mehterov, N.; Atanasov, A.G.; Dudea, D.; Berindan-Neagoe, I. Current Insights into Oral Cancer Epigenetics. *Int. J. Mol. Sci.* **2018**, *19*, 670. [CrossRef] [PubMed]

17. Hema, K.N.; Smitha, T.; Sheethal, H.S.; Mirnalini, S.A. Epigenetics in oral squamous cell carcinoma. *J. Oral Maxillofac. Pathol.* **2017**, *21*, 252–259. [CrossRef] [PubMed]

18. Falzone, L.; Salemi, R.; Travali, S.; Scalisi, A.; McCubrey, J.A.; Candido, S.; Libra, M. MMP-9 overexpression is associated with intragenic hypermethylation of MMP9 gene in melanoma. *Aging (Albany NY)* **2016**, *8*, 933–944. [CrossRef] [PubMed]

19. Grafton-Clarke, C.; Chen, K.W.; Wilcock, J. Diagnosis and referral delays in primary care for oral squamous cell cancer: a systematic review. *Br. J. Gen. Pract.* **2019**, *69*, e112–e126. [CrossRef] [PubMed]

20. Akbulut, N.; Oztas, B.; Kursun, S.; Evirgen, S. Delayed diagnosis of oral squamous cell carcinoma: A case series. *J. Med. Case. Rep.* **2011**, *5*, 291. [CrossRef]

21. Sahibzada, H.A.; Khurshid, Z.; Khan, R.S.; Naseem, M.; Siddique, K.M.; Mali, M.; Zafar, M.S. Salivary IL-8, IL-6 and TNF-α as Potential Diagnostic Biomarkers for Oral Cancer. *Diagnostics (Basel)* **2017**, *7*, 21. [CrossRef] [PubMed]

22. St John, M.A.; Li, Y.; Zhou, X.; Denny, P.; Ho, C.M.; Montemagno, C.; Shi, W.; Qi, F.; Wu, B.; Sinha, U.; et al. Interleukin 6 and interleukin 8 as potential biomarkers for oral cavity and oropharyngeal squamous cell carcinoma. *Arch. Otolaryngol. Head Neck Surg.* **2004**, *130*, 929–935. [CrossRef] [PubMed]

23. Zheng, J.; Sun, L.; Yuan, W.; Xu, J.; Yu, X.; Wang, F.; Sun, L.; Zeng, Y. Clinical value of Naa10p and CEA levels in saliva and serum for diagnosis of oral squamous cell carcinoma. *J. Oral Pathol. Med.* **2018**, *47*, 830–835. [CrossRef]

24. Yuan, C.; Yang, K.; Tang, H.; Chen, D. Diagnostic values of serum tumor markers Cyfra21-1, SCCAg, ferritin, CEA, CA19-9, and AFP in oral/oropharyngeal squamous cell carcinoma. *Onco. Targets Ther.* **2016**, *9*, 3381–3386.

25. Geng, X.F.; Du, M.; Han, J.X.; Zhang, M.; Tang, X.F.; Xing, R.D. Saliva CA125 and TPS levels in patients with oral squamous cell carcinoma. *Int. J. Biol. Markers.* **2013**, *28*, 216–220. [CrossRef] [PubMed]

26. Yang, C.X.; Sedhom, W.; Song, J.; Lu, S.L. The Role of MicroRNAs in Recurrence and Metastasis of Head and Neck Squamous Cell Carcinoma. *Cancers (Basel)* **2019**, *11*, 395. [CrossRef]

27. Dias, F.; Morais, M.; Teixeira, A.L.; Medeiros, R. Involving the microRNA Targetome in Esophageal-Cancer Development and Behavior. *Cancers (Basel)* **2018**, *10*, 381. [CrossRef]

28. Wang, M.; Yu, F.; Li, P. Circular RNAs: Characteristics; Function and Clinical Significance in Hepatocellular Carcinoma. *Cancers (Basel)* **2018**, *10*, 258. [CrossRef]

29. Russo, D.; Merolla, F.; Varricchio, S.; Salzano, G.; Zarrilli, G.; Mascolo, M.; Strazzullo, V.; Di Crescenzo, R.M.; Celetti, A.; Ilardi, G. Epigenetics of oral and oropharyngeal cancers. *Biomed. Rep.* **2018**, *9*, 275–283.

30. Castilho, R.M.; Squarize, C.H.; Almeida, L.O. Epigenetic Modifications and Head and Neck Cancer: Implications for Tumor Progression and Resistance to Therapy. *Int. J. Mol. Sci.* **2017**, *18*, 1506. [CrossRef] [PubMed]

31. Duchaine, T.F.; Fabian, M.R. Mechanistic Insights into MicroRNA-Mediated Gene Silencing. *Cold Spring Harb. Perspect. Biol.* **2019**, *11*. [CrossRef]

32. Falzone, L.; Romano, G.L.; Salemi, R.; Bucolo, C.; Tomasello, B.; Lupo, G.; Anfuso, C.D.; Spandidos, D.A.; Libra, M.; Candido, S. Prognostic significance of deregulated microRNAs in uveal melanomas. *Mol. Med. Rep.* **2019**, *19*, 2599–2610. [CrossRef]

33. Hafsi, S.; Candido, S.; Maestro, R.; Falzone, L.; Soua, Z.; Bonavida, B.; Spandidos, D.A.; Libra, M. Correlation between the overexpression of Yin Yang 1 and the expression levels of miRNAs in Burkitt's lymphoma: A computational study. *Oncol. Lett.* **2016**, *11*, 1021–1025. [CrossRef]

34. Falzone, L.; Scola, L.; Zanghì, A.; Biondi, A.; Di Cataldo, A.; Libra, M.; Candido, S. Integrated analysis of colorectal cancer microRNA datasets: identification of microRNAs associated with tumor development. *Aging (Albany NY)* **2018**, *10*, 1000–1014. [CrossRef]

35. Manikandan, M.; Deva Magendhra Rao, A.K.; Arunkumar, G.; Manickavasagam, M.; Rajkumar, K.S.; Rajaraman, R.; Munirajan, A.K. Oral squamous cell carcinoma: microRNA expression profiling and integrative analyses for elucidation of tumourigenesis mechanism. *Mol. Cancer* **2016**, *15*, 28. [CrossRef]

36. Chamorro Petronacci, C.M.; Pérez-Sayáns, M.; Padín Iruegas, M.E.; Suárez Peñaranda, J.M.; Lorenzo Pouso, A.I.; Blanco Carrión, A.; García García, A. miRNAs expression of oral squamous cell carcinoma patients: Validation of two putative biomarkers. *Medicine (Baltimore)* **2019**, *98*, e14922. [CrossRef]

37. Yan, Z.Y.; Luo, Z.Q.; Zhang, L.J.; Li, J.; Liu, J.Q. Integrated Analysis and MicroRNA Expression Profiling Identified Seven miRNAs Associated With Progression of Oral Squamous Cell Carcinoma. *J. Cell Physiol.* **2017**, *232*, 2178–2185. [CrossRef]

38. Ahmed, M.; Nguyen, H.; Lai, T.; Kim, D.R. miRCancerdb: A database for correlation analysis between microRNA and gene expression in cancer. *BMC Res. Notes* **2018**, *11*, 103. [CrossRef]

39. Greene, C.S.; Tan, J.; Ung, M.; Moore, J.H.; Cheng, C. Big data bioinformatics. *J. Cell Physiol.* **2014**, *22*, 1896–1900. [CrossRef]

40. Cheng, P.F.; Dummer, R.; Levesque, M.P. Data mining The Cancer Genome Atlas in the era of precision cancer medicine. *Swiss Med. Wkly.* **2015**, *145*, w14183. [CrossRef]

41. Cancer Genome Atlas Research Network; Weinstein, J.N.; Collisson, E.A.; Mills, G.B.; Shaw, K.R.; Ozenberger, B.A.; Ellrott, K.; Shmulevich, I.; Sander, C.; Stuart, J.M. The Cancer Genome Atlas Pan-Cancer analysis project. *Nat. Genet.* **2013**, *45*, 1113–1120. [CrossRef]

42. ENCODE Project Consortium. An integrated encyclopedia of DNA elements in the human genome. *Nature* **2012**, *489*, 57–74. [CrossRef]

43. Gauthier, J.; Vincent, A.T.; Charette, S.J.; Derome, N. A brief history of bioinformatics. *Brief. Bioinform.* **2018**, *3*. [CrossRef]

44. Gill, S.K.; Christopher, A.F.; Gupta, V.; Bansal, P. Emerging role of bioinformatics tools and software in evolution of clinical research. *Perspect. Clin. Res.* **2016**, *7*, 115–122.

45. Shukla, H.D. Comprehensive Analysis of Cancer-Proteogenome to Identify Biomarkers for the Early Diagnosis and Prognosis of Cancer. *Proteomes.* **2017**, *5*, 28. [CrossRef]

46. Giacomelli, L.; Covani, U. Bioinformatics and data mining studies in oral genomics and proteomics: new trends and challenges. *Open. Dent. J.* **2010**, *4*, 67–71. [CrossRef] [PubMed]

47. Santosh, A.B.; Jones, T.; Harvey, J. A review on oral cancer biomarkers: Understanding the past and learning from the present. *J. Cancer Res. Ther.* **2016**, *12*, 486–492. [CrossRef] [PubMed]

48. Sutliff, A.K.; Watson, C.J.W.; Chen, G.; Lazarus, P. Regulation of UGT2A1 by miR-196a-5p and miR-196b-5p and its implications for lung cancer risk. *J. Pharmacol. Exp. Ther.* **2019**. [CrossRef] [PubMed]

49. Mazumder, S.; Datta, S.; Ray, J.G.; Chaudhuri, K.; Chatterjee, R. Liquid biopsy: miRNA as a potential biomarker in oral cancer. *Cancer Epidemiol.* **2019**, *58*, 137–145. [CrossRef]

50. Gissi, D.B.; Morandi, L.; Gabusi, A.; Tarsitano, A.; Marchetti, C.; Cura, F.; Palmieri, A.; Montebugnoli, L.; Asioli, S.; Foschini, M.P.; et al. A Noninvasive Test for MicroRNA Expression in Oral Squamous Cell Carcinoma. *Int. J. Mol. Sci.* **2018**, *19*, 1789. [CrossRef]

51. He, B.; Lin, X.; Tian, F.; Yu, W.; Qiao, B. MiR-133a-3p Inhibits Oral Squamous Cell Carcinoma (OSCC) Proliferation and Invasion by Suppressing COL1A1. *J. Cell. Biochem.* **2018**, *119*, 338–346. [CrossRef]

52. Mizuno, K.; Mataki, H.; Seki, N.; Kumamoto, T.; Kamikawaji, K.; Inoue, H. MicroRNAs in non-small cell lung cancer and idiopathic pulmonary fibrosis. *J. Hum. Genet.* **2017**, *62*, 57–65. [CrossRef]

53. Li, Z.; Yu, X.; Shen, J.; Law, P.T.; Chan, M.T.; Wu, W.K. MicroRNA expression and its implications for diagnosis and therapy of gallbladder cancer. *Oncotarget* **2015**, *6*, 13914–13921.

54. Srivastava, S.K.; Arora, S.; Singh, S.; Bhardwaj, A.; Averett, C.; Singh, A.P. MicroRNAs in pancreatic malignancy: Progress and promises. *Cancer Lett.* **2014**, *347*, 167–174. [CrossRef]

55. Du, M.; Giridhar, K.V.; Tian, Y.; Tschannen, M.R.; Zhu, J.; Huang, C.C.; Kilari, D.; Kohli, M.; Wang, L. Plasma exosomal miRNAs-based prognosis in metastatic kidney cancer. *Oncotarget* **2017**, *8*, 63703–63714. [CrossRef]

56. Yamazaki, N.; Koga, Y.; Taniguchi, H.; Kojima, M.; Kanemitsu, Y.; Saito, N.; Matsumura, Y. High expression of miR-181c as a predictive marker of recurrence in stage II colorectal cancer. *Oncotarget.* **2017**, *8*, 6970–6983. [CrossRef]

57. Feng, X.; Matsuo, K.; Zhang, T.; Hu, Y.; Mays, A.C.; Browne, J.D.; Zhou, X.; Sullivan, C.A. MicroRNA Profiling and Target Genes Related to Metastasis of Salivary Adenoid Cystic Carcinoma. *Anticancer Res.* **2017**, *37*, 3473–3481.

58. Falzone, L.; Candido, S.; Salemi, R.; Basile, M.S.; Scalisi, A.; McCubrey, J.A.; Torino, F.; Signorelli, S.S.; Montella, M.; Libra, M. Computational identification of microRNAs associated to both epithelial to mesenchymal transition and NGAL/MMP-9 pathways in bladder cancer. *Oncotarget* **2016**, *7*, 72758–72766. [CrossRef]

59. Lakshminarayana, S.; Augustine, D.; Rao, R.S.; Patil, S.; Awan, K.H.; Venkatesiah, S.S.; Haragannavar, V.C.; Nambiar, S.; Prasad, K. Molecular pathways of oral cancer that predict prognosis and survival: A systematic review. *J. Carcinog.* **2018**, *17*, 7. [CrossRef]

60. Ji, L.; Xu, J.; Liu, J.; Amjad, A.; Zhang, K.; Liu, Q.; Zhou, L.; Xiao, J.; Li, X. Mutant p53 promotes tumor cell malignancy by both positive and negative regulation of the transforming growth factor β (TGF-β) pathway. *J. Biol. Chem.* **2015**, *290*, 11729–11740. [CrossRef]

61. Vander Broek, R.; Mohan, S.; Eytan, D.F.; Chen, Z.; Van Waes, C. The PI3K/Akt/mTOR axis in head and neck cancer: functions; aberrations; cross-talk; and therapies. *Oral Dis.* **2015**, *21*, 815–825. [CrossRef]

62. Salemi, R.; Falzone, L.; Madonna, G.; Polesel, J.; Cinà, D.; Mallardo, D.; Ascierto, P.A.; Libra, M.; Candido, S. MMP-9 as a Candidate Marker of Response to BRAF Inhibitors in Melanoma Patients with BRAFV600E Mutation Detected in Circulating-Free DNA. *Front. Pharmacol.* **2018**, *9*, 856. [CrossRef]

63. Leonardi, G.C.; Falzone, L.; Salemi, R.; Zanghì, A.; Spandidos, D.A.; Mccubrey, J.A.; Candido, S.; Libra, M. Cutaneous melanoma: From pathogenesis to therapy (Review). *Int. J. Oncol.* **2018**, *52*, 1071–1080. [CrossRef]

64. McCubrey, J.A.; Fitzgerald, T.L.; Yang, L.V.; Lertpiriyapong, K.; Steelman, L.S.; Abrams, S.L.; Montalto, G.; Cervello, M.; Neri, L.M.; Cocco, L.; et al. Roles of GSK-3 and microRNAs on epithelial mesenchymal transition and cancer stem cells. *Oncotarget* **2017**, *8*, 14221–14250. [CrossRef] [PubMed]

65. Vogelstein, B.; Papadopoulos, N.; Velculescu, V.E.; Zhou, S.; Diaz, L.A. Jr.; Kinzler, K.W. Cancer genome landscapes. *Science* **2013**, *339*, 1546–1558. [CrossRef]

66. Battaglia, R.; Palini, S.; Vento, M.E.; La Ferlita, A.; Lo Faro, M.J.; Caroppo, E.; Borzì, P.; Falzone, L.; Barbagallo, D.; Ragusa, M.; et al. Identification of extracellular vesicles and characterization of miRNA expression profiles in human blastocoel fluid. *Sci. Rep.* **2019**, *9*, 84. [CrossRef] [PubMed]

67. Hasin, Y.; Seldin, M.; Lusis, A. Multi-omics approaches to disease. *Genome Biol.* **2017**, *18*, 83. [CrossRef]

68. Casamassimi, A.; Federico, A.; Rienzo, M.; Esposito, S.; Ciccodicola, A. Transcriptome Profiling in Human Diseases: New Advances and Perspectives. *Int. J. Mol. Sci.* **2017**, *18*, 1652. [CrossRef] [PubMed]

69. Barrett, T.; Wilhite, S.E.; Ledoux, P.; Evangelista, C.; Kim, I.F.; Tomashevsky, M.; Marshall, K.A.; Phillippy, K.H.; Sherman, P.M.; Holko, M.; et al. NCBI GEO: Archive for functional genomics data sets—Update. *Nucleic Acids Res.* **2013**, *41*, D991–D995. [CrossRef]

70. Tokar, T.; Pastrello, C.; Rossos, A.E.M.; Abovsky, M.; Hauschild, A.C.; Tsay, M.; Lu, R.; Jurisica, I. mirDIP 4.1-integrative database of human microRNA target predictions. *Nucleic Acids Res.* **2018**, *46*, D360–D370. [CrossRef] [PubMed]

71. Shirdel, E.A.; Xie, W.; Mak, T.W.; Jurisica, I. NAViGaTing the Micronome. Using Multiple MicroRNA Prediction Databases to Identify Signalling Pathway-Associated MicroRNAs. *PLoS ONE* **2011**, *6*, e17429. [CrossRef]

72. Vlachos, I.S.; Zagganas, K.; Paraskevopoulou, M.D.; Georgakilas, G.; Karagkouni, D.; Vergoulis, T.; Dalamagas, T.; Hatzigeorgiou, A.G. DIANA-miRPath v3.0: Deciphering microRNA function with experimental support. *Nucleic Acids Res.* **2015**, *43*, W460–W466. [CrossRef]

73. Mi, H.; Muruganujan, A.; Ebert, D.; Huang, X.; Thomas, P.D. PANTHER version 14: More genomes, a new PANTHER GO-slim and improvements in enrichment analysis tools. *Nucleic Acids Res.* **2019**, *47*, D419–D426. [CrossRef]

74. Szklarczyk, D.; Gable, A.L.; Lyon, D.; Junge, A.; Wyder, S.; Huerta-Cepas, J.; Simonovic, M.; Doncheva, N.T.; Morris, J.H.; Bork, P.; et al. STRING v11: Protein-protein association networks with increased coverage, supporting functional discovery in genome-wide experimental datasets. *Nucleic Acids Res.* **2019**, *47*, D607–D613. [CrossRef] [PubMed]

75. Anaya, J. OncoLnc: Linking TCGA survival data to mRNAs, miRNAs, and lncRNAs. *PeerJ. Comput. Sci.* **2016**, *2*, e67. [CrossRef]

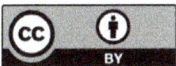

cancers

MDPI

Article

Validation of miRNAs as Breast Cancer Biomarkers with a Machine Learning Approach

Oneeb Rehman [1], Hanqi Zhuang [1,*], Ali Muhamed Ali [1], Ali Ibrahim [1] and Zhongwei Li [2]

[1] College of Engineering and Computer Science, Florida Atlantic University, Boca Raton, FL 33431, USA; orehman@fau.edu (O.R.); amuhamedali2014@fau.edu (A.M.A.); aibrahim2014@fau.edu (A.I.)
[2] Charles E. Schmidt College of Medicine, Florida Atlantic University, Boca Raton, FL 33431, USA; zli@health.fau.edu
* Correspondence: zhuang@fau.edu; Tel.: +1-561-756-5372

Received: 28 February 2019; Accepted: 20 March 2019; Published: 26 March 2019

Abstract: Certain small noncoding microRNAs (miRNAs) are differentially expressed in normal tissues and cancers, which makes them great candidates for biomarkers for cancer. Previously, a selected subset of miRNAs has been experimentally verified to be linked to breast cancer. In this paper, we validated the importance of these miRNAs using a machine learning approach on miRNA expression data. We performed feature selection, using Information Gain (IG), Chi-Squared (CHI2) and Least Absolute Shrinkage and Selection Operation (LASSO), on the set of these relevant miRNAs to rank them by importance. We then performed cancer classification using these miRNAs as features using Random Forest (RF) and Support Vector Machine (SVM) classifiers. Our results demonstrated that the miRNAs ranked higher by our analysis had higher classifier performance. Performance becomes lower as the rank of the miRNA decreases, confirming that these miRNAs had different degrees of importance as biomarkers. Furthermore, we discovered that using a minimum of three miRNAs as biomarkers for breast cancers can be as effective as using the entire set of 1800 miRNAs. This work suggests that machine learning is a useful tool for functional studies of miRNAs for cancer detection and diagnosis.

Keywords: miRNAs; cancer biomarkers; breast cancer detection; machine learning; feature selection; classification

1. Introduction

MicroRNAs (miRNAs) are small non-coding RNA molecules involved in the regulation of gene expression by partially base-pairing to complementary sequences of target messenger RNAs (mRNA), which leads to cleavage and eventual degradation of the target mRNA or translational repression [1]. The objective of this research is to investigate the potential of using a machine learning approach to validate clinically chosen relevant miRNAs as reliable biomarkers for cancer detection and diagnosis.

Calin et al. [2] were among the first who established the relationship between miRNAs and cancers after discovering that mir15 and mir16 are deleted or down-regulated in a majority of chronic lymphocytic leukemia cases. McManus [3] reviewed examples that link miRNA expression to the development of cancer, and proposed a general role of miRNAs in oncogenesis. Further studies conducted on a variety of cancer types reinforced the causal relationship between miRNA and cancer by demonstrating significantly altered expression profiles of miRNAs in cancer as compared to normal tissue [4–6]. It was shown that alteration of only a single miRNA can influence cell identity [7]. These observations led to the increasing interests to test the effectiveness of using miRNAs as biomarkers for diagnosing cancer. However, it has been difficult to identify miRNAs that are clearly important for cancer detection as some miRNAs are up-regulated in certain cancers and function as oncogenes while they are down-regulated in others, acting as tumor suppressors. Furthermore, some miRNAs play pivotal roles in cancer development whereas others are less important. This means that identifying relevant miRNAs will be context-sensitive and dependent on the location and type of cancer that is being considered [7,8]. Therefore, computational analysis of large datasets of miRNA and cancer may greatly improve identification of miRNA biomarkers.

Computational methods, especially machine learning, have been applied for cancer detection and diagnosis using miRNAs as biomarkers. Lu et al. [5] used hierarchical clustering on 73 bone marrow samples and determined that miRNA expression distinguishes tumors of different subtypes within acute lymphoblastic leukemia. They constructed a k-NN classifier using lung cancer samples as well as adjacent healthy samples from mice, which achieved a classification accuracy of 100%. Rosenfeld et al. [9] constructed a miRNA-based tissue classifier to identify the source location of metastatic tumors. By using k-NN and decision trees to classify tumors into 22 different tumor origins (classes), they obtained an accuracy of 89% on the validation set. Prior work was also done by Kotlarchyk et al. [10] on the subject of using feature selection on liver, breast and brain cancer datasets. However, the previous studies were limited by the amount of miRNA data that was readily available and the number of miRNAs that were known at the time. With the emergence of the Genomic Data Commons (GDC) Data Portal provided by the National Cancer Institute, the amount of miRNA expression data increased dramatically. With 34 different types of cancers available, more precise experiments could be performed. Waspada et al. [11] used 22 different miRNA expression datasets from the GDC Data Portal and achieved multiple objectives: (i) a multiclass classification combination of all 22 cancer types, (ii) binary classification using only breast cancer data, (iii) binary classification using breast cancer data with the addition of a feature selection step, and (iv) binary classification with miRNAs selected according to clinical research. Cheerla et al. [12] constructed a SVM-RBF classifier trained with various miRNA expression data across 21 different cancer types, achieving an accuracy of 97.2%. They also used feature selection methods to reduce the number of miRNAs to 60 and still achieved a 95.5% overall classification accuracy. Ali et al. [13] used Neighbourhood Component Analysis to extract relevant miRNA features in order to perform subtype classification, achieving around 95% accuracy. These studies demonstrated the potential of improved cancer detection and diagnosis using miRNAs as biomarkers.

This research aims at using a variety of feature selection techniques to select a subset of miRNAs to identify important miRNA features that are crucial in the diagnosis of breast cancer, a cancer that has accumulated ample amount of miRNA data [14]. The miRBase release 22 (version 22) recorded 1917 confirmed mature human miRNAs [15]. For all practical purposes, it is important to narrow down this large number of miRNAs to find the most discriminative subset of miRNA features for the specific tasks we are working on. Since these miRNAs correspond directly as features, we can employ feature selection methods to remove irrelevant and redundant ones. In machine learning, feature selection is a method of selecting a subset from a given feature set based on a certain set of criteria without transformation of the original features, which preserves the interpretation of the results. This prevents overfitting and improves classification performance especially with gene expression data, which usually has a large number of features. In order to determine the best subset of features, we focus only those miRNAs which have been verified clinically. This allows us to focus on miRNAs that have been deemed relevant in the laboratory. We then apply feature selection methods on this reduced subset of miRNAs to determine which are more important for cancer detection. Even though quite a few miRNAs have been clinically shown to be linked to breast cancer, we aim to show with a machine learning approach that not all miRNAs are equally important as a cancer biomarker, even among those clinically selected ones.

2. Methodology

Our approach for validating clinically selected miRNAs for cancer detection and diagnosis is summarized in Figure 1.

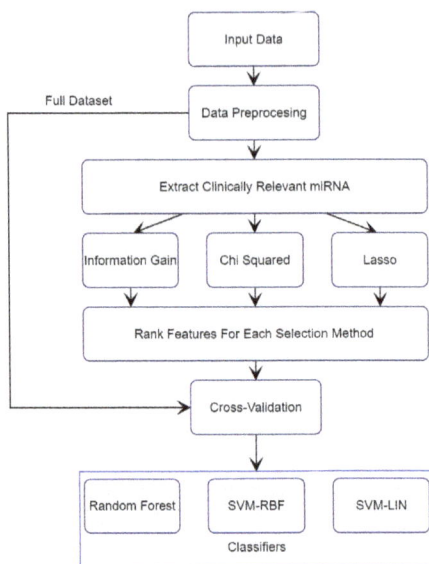

Figure 1. Schematics for Cancer Detection with Machine Learning.

The algorithm is divided into two stages: training and verification. In the training stage, the first step is to clean up the miRNA row data by removing rows with all zero values. We then keep only those miRNAs that have been identified via wet lab as possible biomarkers for breast cancer detection. These biomarkers are classified as clinically verified miRNAs. The list of clinically verified miRNAs identified in the literature is shown in Table 1. Three feature selection methods, Information Gain, Chi Squared, and LASSO, are applied to independently rank the importance of miRNAs. The resulting feature vectors are then fed to classification algorithms. For this purpose, two classifiers, Random Forest and Support Vector Machines (SVMs), are applied to train the model. Feature selection is performed on the selected subset of the breast-cancer dataset and these miRNA features are ranked by each feature selection method individually. From these ranked features, different subsets were selected and were then fed into the classification algorithms. The performance of the miRNAs is then evaluated based on certain performance metrics which will be introduced later.

In the next subsections, we discuss the techniques used for both feature selection and classification.

Table 1. Clinically Verified miRNA.

miRNA [14]			
hsa-mir-10b	hsa-let-7d	hsa-mir-206	hsa-mir-34a
hsa-mir-125b-1	hsa-let-7f-1	hsa-mir-17	hsa-mir-27b
hsa-mir-145	hsa-let-7f-2	hsa-mir-335	hsa-mir-126
hsa-mir-21	hsa-mir-206	hsa-mir-373	hsa-mir-101-1
hsa-mir-125a	hsa-mir-30a	hsa-mir-520c	hsa-mir-101-2
hsa-mir-17	hsa-mir-30b	hsa-mir-27a	hsa-mir-146a
hsa-mir-125b-2	hsa-mir-203a	hsa-mir-221	hsa-mir-146b
hsa-let-7a-2	hsa-mir-203b	hsa-mir-222	hsa-mir-205
hsa-let-7a-3	has-mir-213	hsa-mir-200c	
hsa-let-7c	hsa-mir-155	hsa-mir-31	

2.1. Feature Selection

As has been mentioned before, the objective of feature selection is to identify the specific miRNAs that are most effective in discriminating normal and cancerous tissues. Since the dimensionality of expression data is large in relation to the number of samples, it is easy for classifiers to over-fit, therefore a reduction in feature size will alleviate that problem. Another important aspect of feature selection versus using certain dimensionality reduction techniques, such as Principal Component Analysis, Discrete Cosine Transform and Wavelet Transform, is that we can preserve the original features as opposed to mapping them to a different representation.

In this section, three popular feature selection techniques, Information Gain, Chi-Squared Feature Selection, and Least Absolute Shrinkage and Selection Operator, are reviewed. For a detailed discussion of these methods, readers are referred to [16–18].

2.1.1. Information Gain

Information Gain (IG) is a feature selection method based on Information Theory, which measures the reduction of entropy that occurs by having knowledge of a feature, A. For a dataset X with n class labels, the Shannon entropy, which is a measure of unpredictability, is given by the following equation,

$$H(X) = -\sum_{i=1}^{n} p_i \log_2 p_i. \tag{1}$$

where p_i is the probability of class i in the data set X. IG is the reduction of entropy that is achieved by knowing the feature A, shown by the following equation,

$$IG(X, A) = H(x) - H(X|A). \tag{2}$$

where,

$$H(X|A) = \sum_{i=i}^{v} \frac{X_i}{X} H(X_i). \tag{3}$$

where X_i is a subset of X containing a distinct value of A, v is the number of distinct values present in A and $H(X_i)$ is the entropy of the i-th subset created by splitting X on feature A. Therefore, IG can be seen as the difference between the prior entropy and the entropy after splitting the original dataset based on the feature A.

2.1.2. Chi-Squared Feature Selection

Chi-squared (CHI2) is another feature selection method which evaluates features with respect to the classes. It is a statistical test to determine the dependency of a feature on the class label. We can discard features that do not show dependency and extract the relevant features that are useful for classification. The range of continuous valued features needs to be discretized into intervals.

$$\chi^2 = \sum_{i=1}^{C} \sum_{j=1}^{I} \frac{(A_{ij} - E_{ij})^2}{E_{ij}} \tag{4}$$

where C is the number of classes, I is the number of intervals, E_{ij} is the expected number of samples, A_{ij} is the number of samples of the C_i class within the j-th interval. The larger the value of χ^2, the more information the corresponding feature provides.

2.1.3. Least Absolute Shrinkage and Selection Operator

Least Absolute Shrinkage and Selection Operator (LASSO) is a regularization and variable selection method for statistical models. LASSO minimizes the sum of squared errors while also being subject to a constraint on the sum of the absolute values of the regression coefficients, which is described by,

$$\min_{\beta_0,\beta} \sum_{i=1}^{N} (y_i - \beta_0 - x_i^T \beta)^2 s.t. \sum_{j=1}^{p} |\beta_j| \leq t. \tag{5}$$

Where N is the number of cases, p is the number of features, $(\beta, \beta_0, \beta_j)$ are regression coefficients, y_i is the i-th predicted output and x_i is the i-th set of features. By tuning the parameter t, we can choose the best performing features, as the less predictive coefficients will go to zero.

2.2. Classification

After feature selection, one can apply classification algorithms to determine if the target is cancerous or not. In this section, two classifiers, Random Forest and Support Vector Machine (SVM), are overviewed [11,18].

2.2.1. Random Forest

The Random Forest (RF) algorithm is an ensemble classifier that generates multiple decision trees, including weak classifiers learned on a random sample from the data. The classification of a new sample is done by majority voting of the decision trees. Random Forest is constructed in the following manner. Assume that the given training set has N cases, each with M features. Each decision tree is grown as follows: First, n samples are selected at random with replacement from the training set. At each node of the tree, $m << M$ of the features are selected at random. The best split on these m features, based on some objective function (for instance, Information Gain), is used to perform a binary split on that node. This process is repeated until a predefined minimum node size is reached. Classification of new data is done through majority votes by aggregating the predictions of all the decision trees.

2.2.2. Support Vector Machine

Support Vector Machine (SVM), a supervised machine learning method, aims to design an optimum hyperplane that separates the input features into two difference classes for binary classification. The best solution maximizes the margin, defined by so-called support vectors, between both classes. Given the miRNA data consists of n feature vectors, (x_i, y_i), where $y_i \in \{+1, -1\}$, one can construct an optimization problem in which the distance between the margins is maximized by minimizing the following equation,

$$\frac{1}{2}||w||^2 \tag{6}$$

under the following constraint,

$$y_i(wx_i + b) - 1 \geq 0. \tag{7}$$

where w is the weights vector which dictates the margin size and b is the bias, which shifts the hyperplane boundary. In the case of non-linearly separable data, kernel functions can be used to map the input space to a higher dimensional feature space to allow for a linear separation. A popular kernel function, the Radial Basis Function (RBF), is given as follows:

$$k(x_i, y_i) = \exp\left(-\gamma||x_i - x_j||^2\right) \tag{8}$$

where γ is a hyperparameter that controls the error due to bias and variance. We will use both linear SVM as well as SVM with a radial basis function kernel (RBF) in our experimentation.

3. Results

The microRNA expression dataset for breast cancer was obtained from the National Cancer Institute's Genomic Data Commons Data Portal [19]. This dataset consists of 1207 patient samples with

1881 miRNA features, containing 1103 primary solid tumor samples, 7 metastatic samples and 104 healthy samples. The dataset is imbalanced as there are many more number of cancerous samples compared to healthy samples.

The dataset included raw read counts as well as counts normalized to reads per million mapped reads (RPM). The metastatic samples were combined with the solid tumor samples as one class, since metastatic cancer tissue retained most of the genomic features of the source tumor [20]. The log2 of the RPM values was taken plus a pseudo count of 1 and then the values were standardized to zero mean and unit variance. Zero values were also removed which further reduced the number of miRNA features to 1626. Then miRNAs that were not identified by Table 1 were removed.

The dataset was run through the classifiers first without feature selection and then with feature selection using different feature selection methods (IG, LASSO and CHI2, see Section 2.1). In the experiment, we grouped miRNAs into subsets of 3, 5, and 10 members and test their effectiveness in identifying cancer using different feature selection procedures with different classifiers. Also, 10-fold validation was performed throughout. The 10-fold validation is a technique in which in each trial, 90% of the data samples are used for training and the remaining 10% for testing; the process is repeated 10 times, ensuring that all samples are tested once. We chose to only utilize cross-validation and neglect the other steps outlined by the Data Analysis Protocol (DAP), which is outlined by the US-FDA MAQC-II initiative [21]. This is because the focus of this paper is to demonstrate that a small subset of miRNAs can be used to detect cancer with 10-fold validation [22].

Due to the nature of the unbalanced dataset, using only accuracy as a performance metric may misrepresent the performance of our classifiers. In the experiment, we establish the outcomes using the following measures: True positive (TP), False Positive (FP), True negative (TN) and False negative (FN). Here the positive class means a tumorous sample and the negative class is non-cancerous (healthy). Specificity is defined as,

$$\frac{TN}{TN + FP} \tag{9}$$

which is the proportion of non-cancerous samples correctly identified. Sensitivity is,

$$\frac{TP}{TP + FN} \tag{10}$$

which tests the ability for the cancerous samples to be correctly identified. In addition, Accuracy is simply,

$$\frac{TP + TN}{TP + TN + FP + FN} \tag{11}$$

which tests the overall ability to different between healthy and cancerous samples. We also calculate Area Under Curve (AUC).

Table 2 shows the performance of different feature selection techniques vs different classifiers. In the table, the first column indicates which classifier was used in the experiment. The second one lists the feature selection method along with the number of miRNAs in each group. For instance, IG-10 means that Information Gain is used for feature selection, and miRNAs are grouped into 10 each. Other columns show the performance of the feature selection algorithm teamed up with the classifier.

Examining Table 2, we can see that the performance metric that fluctuates the most is the specificity. Since it is possible to achieve a high accuracy even while misclassifying all of the minority class, we need to look at a performance metric that can give us a more meaningful result. Note that the classification accuracy across all selections is practically the same, which confirms its ineffectiveness as a performance metric. The difficulty of this dataset lies in correctly classifying its minority class. We can see a trend of improved sensitivity values when feature selection is used for the RF and SVM-RBF classifiers. This reinforces the notion that there are redundant and irrelevant features present in the dataset and that we may be able to achieve better results with a handful of features rather than the original 1881. We also observed a marked improvement in terms of Specificity by applying any type of feature selection (across all subsets).

Table 2. Performance Metrics across different thresholds of miRNA Features (3, 5, 10).

Classifier	Method	Accuracy	Sensitivity	Specificity	AUC
RF		0.996	1.000	0.952	0.999
	IG-10	0.995	0.998	0.962	0.996
	IG-5	0.996	0.997	0.977	0.998
	IG-3	0.997	0.997	0.990	0.999
	CHI2-10	0.995	0.999	0.952	0.995
	CHI2-5	0.996	0.999	0.979	0.996
	CHI2-3	0.996	0.997	0.981	0.999
	LASS-10	0.996	0.998	0.971	0.997
	LASS-5	0.995	0.997	0.965	0.998
	LASS-3	0.994	0.997	0.962	0.999
SVM-RBF		0.989	1.000	0.875	0.938
	IG-10	0.994	0.998	0.952	0.995
	IG-5	0.996	1.000	0.990	0.985
	IG-3	0.998	0.998	0.990	0.980
	CHI2-10	0.994	0.999	0.951	0.995
	CHI2-5	0.996	0.998	0.983	0.993
	CHI2-3	0.998	0.999	0.990	0.980
	LASS-10	0.995	0.998	0.962	0.996
	LASS-5	0.995	0.999	0.974	0.985
	LASS-3	0.996	0.999	0.962	0.980
SVM		0.997	0.999	0.971	0.985
	IG-10	0.997	0.999	0.971	0.997
	IG-5	0.997	0.999	0.985	0.989
	IG-3	0.998	0.999	0.990	0.981
	CHI2-10	0.997	0.999	0.971	0.997
	CHI2-5	0.996	1.000	0.988	0.987
	CHI2-3	0.998	0.999	0.990	0.991
	LASS-10	0.994	0.997	0.962	0.996
	LASS-5	0.995	0.999	0.956	0.993
	LASS-3	0.997	1.000	0.962	0.981

Examining the results from Table 2, one can also see that even using a small fraction of the entire feature set, one may obtain very good classification results. This means that clinically one may only need to focus on just a few miRNAs to diagnose a patient. In the next section, we ranked the importance of individual miRNAs under different feature selection techniques. Table 3 show the test results. In this table, miRNAs are ranked in a top-down order under different feature selection algorithms. This means that the miRNAs listed in the top of the table provide better detection performance.

Table 3. Top Ranked Features Under Different Feature Selection Techniques.

Info Gain	CHI2	Lasso
hsa-mir-10b	hsa-mir-10b	hsa-let-7a-3
hsa-let-7c	hsa-let-7c	hsa-let-7c
hsa-mir-145	hsa-mir-145	hsa-let-7d
hsa-mir-125b-1	hsa-mir-125b-2	hsa-mir-101-1
hsa-mir-125b-2	hsa-mir-125b-1	hsa-mir-10b
hsa-mir-335	hsa-mir-335	hsa-mir-125b-2
hsa-mir-126	hsa-mir-126	hsa-mir-145
hsa-mir-125a	hsa-mir-125a	hsa-mir-206
hsa-let-7a-2	hsa-let-7a-2	hsa-mir-27b
hsa-let-7a-3	hsa-let-7a-3	hsa-mir-335

We can see that the subsets of Info Gain and CHI2 are remarkably identical, while overlap six features Lasso, as shown in Table 3.

We can also use feature selection to rank those clinically-selected miRNAs. After ranking, we can verify our results by taking different subsets and testing their performance for cancer detection. We begin by choosing the top four miRNA features in subsets of IG and CHI2, ranked 1–3 as Subset #1. We then slide down by choosing ranked 2–4 miRNAs as Subset #2, and so on. In this way, we obtain eight different subsets, shown in Table 4. We choose four miRNAs as our threshold to mirror our previous experiment as that served as a good limit before performance degradation.

Table 4. Subset Selection of Ranked miRNA.

Subset 1	Subset 2	Subset 3	Subset 4	Subset 5	Subset 6	Subset 7	Subset 8
hsa-mir-10b	hsa-let-7c	hsa-mir-145	hsa-mir-125b-1	hsa-mir-125b-2	hsa-mir-335	hsa-mir-126	hsa-mir-125a
hsa-let-7c	hsa-mir-145	hsa-mir-125b-1	hsa-mir-125b-2	hsa-mir-335	hsa-mir-126	hsa-mir-125a	hsa-let-7a-2
hsa-mir-145	hsa-mir-125b-1	hsa-mir-125b-2	hsa-mir-335	hsa-mir-126	hsa-mir-125a	hsa-let-7a-2	hsa-let-7a-3

We can now evaluate these data sets with both RF and SVM algorithms. The Specificity has been plotted across the eight subsets, shown in Figure 2.

Interestingly, we observe a downward trend as the subset index (the horizontal axis) goes up, which demonstrates a decrease in classifier performance as we go from Subset #1 to #7. The results strongly suggest that miRNAs that are ranked higher are better biomarkers for breast cancer detection than the ones on the bottom in the list.

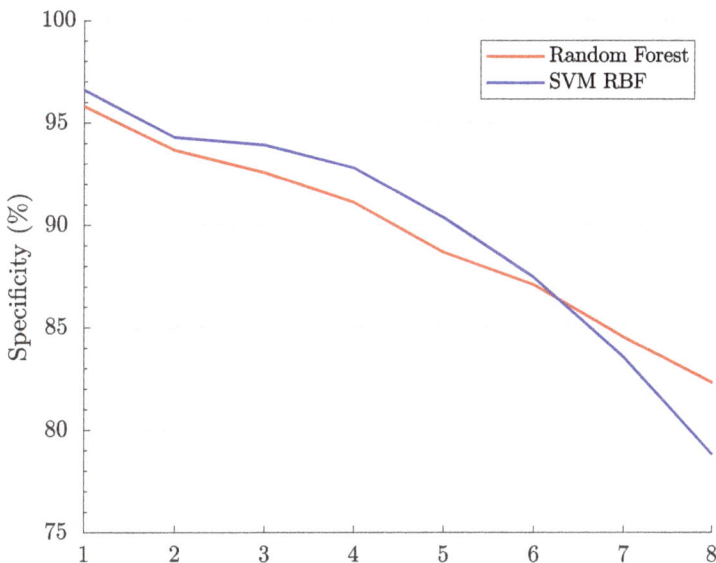

Figure 2. Specificity Across Different Clinical miRNA Subsets.

4. Conclusions

Our results in this work validate clinically-chosen miRNAs as biomarkers for breast cancer detection with a machine learning approach. It demonstrates that by ranking miRNAs using feature selection methods, one is able to determine the best performing miRNAs for breast cancer detection among those clinically verified ones. Our tests have also demonstrated that with merely three selected miRNAs as biomarkers, the classifiers can still produce nearly optimal results in breast cancer detection, in comparison to the use of many more miRNAs.

There are multiple avenues to pursue regarding further work. Specifically, one may extend the framework to identify discriminative miRNAs that indicate different stages of cancer progression if features are available in the datasets. One can also extend these ideas for other cancer types. These other datasets may have common characteristics which can be leveraged using machine learning techniques. With machine learning, one may be able to overcome the problems caused by very small number of samples in cancer datasets. More importantly, the ability of machine learning to classify breast cancer related miRNAs demonstrated here may lead to future development of robotic methods for *de novo* identification of miRNA biomarkers for other diseases with or without laboratory data.

Author Contributions: Conceptualization, O.R., A.M.A., H.Z., and Z.L.; methodology, O.R., A.I., and H.Z.; formal analysis, O.R. and A.I.; writing—original draft preparation, O.R.; writing—review and editing, H.Z., O.R. and Z.L.; supervision, H.Z.; project administration, H.Z.; funding acquisition, H.Z.

Funding: This research was partially funded by US National Science Foundation grant number 1624497. Ali Ibrahim was partially funded by a grant from GtechProcure.

Acknowledgments: We would like to thank National Cancer Institute and National Human Genome Research Institute for providing us with the TCGA data portal and Nvidia for the hardware platform. This work was partially supported by an NSF Phase II I/UCRC grant. Furthermore, we would like to thank GTech Procure and HCED for their sponsorship.

Conflicts of Interest: The authors declare no conflict of interest.

References

1. He, L.; Hannon, G.J. MicroRNAs: Small RNAs with a big role in gene regulation. *Nat. Rev. Genet.* **2004**, *5*, 522–531. [CrossRef] [PubMed]
2. Calin, G.A.; Dumitru, C.D.; Shimizu, M.; Bichi, R.; Zupo, S.; Noch, E.; Aldler, H.; Rattan, S.; Keating, M.; Rai, K.; et al. Frequent deletions and down-regulation of micro- RNA genes miR15 and miR16 at 13q14 in chronic lymphocytic leukemia. *Proc. Natl. Acad. Sci. USA* **2002**, *99*, 15524–15529. [CrossRef] [PubMed]
3. McManus, M.T. MicroRNAs and cancer. *Semin. Cancer Biol.* **2003**, *13*, 253–258. [CrossRef]
4. Croce, C.M. Causes and consequences of microRNA dysregulation in cancer. *Nat. Rev. Genet.* **2009**, *10*, 704–714. [CrossRef] [PubMed]
5. Lu, J.; Getz, G.; Miska, E.A.; Alvarez-Saavedra, E.; Lamb, J.; Peck, D.; Sweet-Cordero, A.; Ebert, B.L.; Mak, R.H.; Ferrando, A.A.; et al. MicroRNA expression profiles classify human cancers. *Nature* **2005**, *435*, 834–838. [CrossRef] [PubMed]
6. Volinia, S.; Calin, G.A.; Liu, C.G.; Ambs, S.; Cimmino, A.; Petrocca, F.; Visone, R.; Iorio, M.; Roldo, C.; Ferracin, M.; et al. A microRNA expression signature of human solid tumors defines cancer gene targets. *Proc. Natl. Acad. Sci. USA* **2006**, *103*, 2257–2261. [CrossRef] [PubMed]
7. Jansson, M.D.; Lund, A.H. MicroRNA and cancer. *Mol. Oncol.* **2012**, *6*, 590–610. [CrossRef] [PubMed]
8. van Schooneveld, E.; Wildiers, H.; Vergote, I.; Vermeulen, P.B.; Dirix, L.Y.; Van Laere, S.J. Dysregulation of microRNAs in breast cancer and their potential role as prognostic and predictive biomarkers in patient management. *Breast Cancer Res.* **2015**, *17*, 21. [CrossRef] [PubMed]
9. Rosenfeld, N.; Aharonov, R.; Meiri, E.; Rosenwald, S.; Spector, Y.; Zepeniuk, M.; Benjamin, H.; Shabes, N.; Tabak, S.; Levy, A.; et al. MicroRNAs accurately identify cancer tissue origin. *Nat. Biotechnol.* **2008**, *26*, 462–469. [CrossRef] [PubMed]
10. Kotlarchyk, A.; Khoshgoftaar, T.; Pavlovic, M.; Zhuang, H.; Pandya, A. Identification of microRna biomarkers for cancer by combining multiple featureselection techniques. *J. Comput. Methods Sci. Eng.* **2011**, *11*, 283–298.
11. Waspada, I.; Wibowo, A.; Meraz, N. Supervised Machine Learing Model for microRNA Expression Data in Cancer. *Jurnal Ilmu Komputer dan Informasi* **2017**, *10*, 108–115. [CrossRef]
12. Cheerla, N.; Gevaert, O. MicroRNA based Pan-Cancer Diagnosis and Treatment Recommendation. *BMC Bioinf.* **2017**, *18*, 32. [CrossRef]
13. Muhamed Ali, A.; Zhuang, H.; Ibrahim, A.; Rehman, O.; Huang, M.; Wu, A. A Machine Learning Approach for the Classification of Kidney Cancer Subtypes Using miRNA Genome Data. *Appl. Sci.* **2018**, *8*, 2422. [CrossRef]
14. Fu, S.W.; Chen, L.; Man, Y.G. miRNA Biomarkers in Breast Cancer Detection and Management. *J. Cancer* **2011**, *2*, 116–122. [CrossRef]

15. miRBase: The microRNA Database. Available online: http://www.mirbase.org/ (accessed on 12 February 2019).
16. Saeys, Y.; Inza, I.; Larranaga, P. A review of feature selection techniques in bioinformatics. *Bioinformatics* **2007**, *23*, 2507–2517. [CrossRef]
17. Ghosh, D.; Chinnaiyan, A.M. Classification and selection of biomarkers in genomic data using LASSO. *J. Biomed. Biotechnol.* **2005**, *2005*, 147–154. [CrossRef] [PubMed]
18. Razak, E.; Yusof, F.; Raus, R.A. Classification of miRNA Expression Data Using Random Forests for Cancer Diagnosis. In Proceedings of the 2016 International Conference on Computer and Communication Engineering (ICCCE), Kuala Lumpur, Malaysia, 26–27 July 2016; pp. 187–190. [CrossRef]
19. The Cancer Genome Atlas. Available online: http://cancergenome.nih.gov/ (accessed on 12 February 2019).
20. Liu, G.; Zhan, X.; Dong, C.; Liu, L. Genomics alterations of metastatic and primary tissues across 15 cancer types. *Sci. Rep.* **2017**, *7*, 13262. [CrossRef] [PubMed]
21. Shi, L.; Campbell, G.; Jones, W.D.; Campagne, F.; Wen, Z.; Walker, S.J.; Su, Z.; Chu, T.M.; Goodsaid, F.M.; Pusztai, L.; et al. The MicroArray Quality Control (MAQC)-II study of common practices for the development and validation of microarray-based predictive models. *Nat. Biotechnol.* **2010**, *28*, 827–838.
22. Cruz, J.A.; Wishart, D.S. Applications of Machine Learning in Cancer Prediction and Prognosis. *Cancer Inf.* **2006**, *2*, 59–77. [CrossRef]

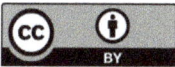

cancers

MDPI

Article

Observed Survival Interval: A Supplement to TCGA Pan-Cancer Clinical Data Resource

Jie Xiong [1], Zhitong Bing [2] and Shengyu Guo [1,3,*]

[1] Department of Epidemiology and Health Statistics, XiangYa School of Public Health, Central South University, Changsha 410078, China; xiongjie86@126.com
[2] Department of Computational Physics, Institute of Modern Physics of Chinese Academy of Sciences, Lanzhou 730000, China; bingzt@impcas.ac.cn
[3] Department of Public Management, College of Economic Management, Changsha University, Changsha 410022, China
* Correspondence: z20100919@ccsu.cn; Tel.: +86-0731-84261438

Received: 24 January 2019; Accepted: 22 February 2019; Published: 26 February 2019

Abstract: To drive high-quality omics translational research using The Cancer Genome Atlas (TCGA) data, a TCGA Pan-Cancer Clinical Data Resource was proposed. However, there is an out-of-step issue between clinical outcomes and the omics data of TCGA for skin cutaneous melanoma (SKCM), due to the majority of metastatic samples. In clinical cases, the survival time started from the initial SKCM diagnosis, while the omics data were characterized at TCGA sampling. This study aimed to address this issue by proposing an observed survival interval (OBS), which was defined as the time interval from TCGA sampling to patient death or last follow-up. We compared the OBS with the usual recommended overall survival (OS) by associating them with both clinical data and microRNA sequencing data of TCGA-SKCM. We found that the OS of primary SKCM was significantly shorter than that of metastatic SKCM, while the opposite happened if OBS was compared. OS was associated with the pathological stage of both primary and metastatic SKCM, while OBS was associated with the pathological stage of primary SKCM but not that of metastatic SKCM. Five previously cross-validated survival-associated microRNAs were found to be associated with the OBS rather than OS in metastatic SKCM. Thus, the OBS was more appropriate for associating microRNA-omics data of TCGA-SKCM than OS, and it is a timely supplement to TCGA Pan-Cancer Clinical Data Resource.

Keywords: overall survival; observed survival interval; skin cutaneous melanoma; The Cancer Genome Atlas; omics

1. Introduction

Skin cutaneous melanoma (SKCM) is the most common malignant skin cancer and its incidence, mortality, and disease burden have been increasing annually [1–3]. Clinically, the American Joint Committee on Cancer (AJCC) staging is now the dominant synthetical index to predict SKCM prognosis [4]. Although useful, on the one hand, significant variability of prognosis in SKCM patients with the same AJCC pathological stage is observed [5]. On the other hand, it is hard to understand the underlying biology of SKCM just based on clinicopathological characteristics, and, further, it is difficult to apply individualized treatment protocols to SKCM patients [6].

By comprehensively characterizing molecular patterns in hundreds of SKCM samples, The Cancer Genome Atlas (TCGA) project has provided a comprehensive way to understand SKCM [7]. Multi-omics data with large sample sizes make the discovery of novel biomarkers that may potentially affect diagnosis, treatment and prognosis of SKCM possible. Several studies have been conducted to identify prognostic biomarkers based on various TCGA-SKCM omics data. Jayawardana et al. and Guo et al. proposed fifteen and five prognostic microRNAs (miRNAs) by mining TCGA-SKCM miRNA sequencing data, respectively [8,9]. Chen et al., Yang et al. and Ma et al. identified, from TCGA-SKCM RNA sequencing data, four, six, and six long non-coding RNAs for SKCM prognosis, respectively [10–12]. Furthermore, Jiang et al. focused on a multi-omics analysis by integration of mutation, copy number variation, methylation, and messenger RNA expression data to achieve this objective [13].

Methodologically, survival analysis (non-parametric methods, such as the Kaplan-Meier method, or the semi-parametric methods, such as Cox regression analysis) is now the dominant method to explore associations between outcome variables and the possible affecting factors. Therefore, the first step of survival analysis was to select an appropriate outcome variable. All previous studies adopted overall survival (OS), defined as the time interval from initial SKCM diagnosis to patient death or last follow-up [14], as the outcome variable. To ensure proper use of the large clinical dataset associated with omics features for TCGA users and to drive high quality survival outcome analytics, Liu et al. proposed an integrated TCGA Pan-Cancer Clinical Data Resource (TCGA-CDR), which includes four clinical outcomes and a list of outcome usage recommendations for each cancer type [14]. For SKCM, TCGA-CDR also recommends the use of OS for large-scale translational research. However, an out-of-step issue (or discordance) between OS and TCGA-SKCM omics data should be noticed. Specifically, TCGA didn't always take the initially diagnosed SKCM samples for sequencing. Instead, SKCM samples from relapses or metastases in the follow-up of SKCM patients were usually adopted (i.e., SKCM samples submitted to TCGA were usually not the samples used for initial SKCM diagnosis). Therefore, omics data measured from TCGA-SKCM samples were out-of-step with the start time point of OS. This discordance will lead to biologically meaningless associations between OS and the omics data of TCGA-SKCM. Furthermore, prognostic biomarkers identified based on these associations will further misguide downstream experimental directions.

In this study, we aimed to address the out-of-step issue by proposing an observed survival interval and comparing it with OS in TCGA-SKCM dataset. Our findings prompted TCGA users to carefully select clinical outcomes when using TCGA-SKCM data for omics translational research.

2. Materials and Methods

2.1. Data Retrieval and Preprocessing

Level 1 clinical data, level 3 miRNA isoform sequencing raw counts, and the corresponding meta-data of SKCM samples were retrieved and downloaded from TCGA repository (https://cancergenome.nih.gov/). The retrieval strategies, exclusion criteria, preprocessing of miRNA sequencing data and clinical data [15] are presented in Section I–IV of the Supplementary Materials, respectively. Hierarchical clustering was performed to detect sample outliers and guided principal component analysis (Supplementary Materials Section V) was used to evaluate the batch effects of the normalized miRNA isoform expression matrix [16].

2.2. Differential Expression Analysis

There were both primary SKCM (PCM) and metastatic SKCM (MCM) samples in TCGA-SKCM cohort. PCM samples with pathological stage I or II were defined as localized PCM (LPCM) samples and those with pathological stage III or IV were considered advanced PCM (APCM) samples [5]. Differential expression analysis was carried out to evaluate differences among LPCM, APCM, and MCM.MicroRNAs with at least a two-fold change of expression were considered to be biologically meaningful. The results of this analysis determined whether we would combine LPCM and APCM samples (i.e., PCM) or further combine PCM and MCM samples (i.e., SKCM) to identify prognostic miRNAs.

2.3. Observed Survival Interval

We defined an observed survival interval (OBS) as the time interval from TCGA sampling to patient death or last follow-up (Figure 1A). Unlike the usually adopted OS, the OBS has the same end time point as OS but different start time points, i.e., TCGA sampling introduced randomization to the start time point of OS. We obtained the DTS (days from initial SKCM diagnosis to TCGA sampling) and INPTS (indicator of new tumor event prior to TCGA sampling) from the parsed clinical files entitled "clinical_data.csv" and "new_tumor.csv", respectively (see Section IV of the Supplementary Materials for parsing clinical files). TCGA may take samples at different time points of SKCM progression. If TCGA took samples at initial SKCM diagnosis (i.e., DTS = 0), the OBS was equal to OS. If TCGA took samples at the first SKCM relapse or metastasis (i.e., DTS > 0 and INPTS = No), the OBS was equal to SAR (survival after the first relapse or metastasis). DTS was equal to PFI (progression-free interval) (Figure 1A) if TCGA took samples at subsequent SKCM relapses or metastases (i.e., the second/third/ ... relapse or metastasis). In practice, we could obtain the OBS by subtracting DTS from OS. For example, patient TCGA-W3-A825 survived for 1917 days from her initial SKCM diagnosis to death (i.e., OS = 1917). Furthermore, a MCM was found in her lung at 1644 days after initial SKCM diagnosis. TCGA didn't obtain her initially diagnosed SKCM sample and therefore the MCM sample was taken for sequencing (i.e., DTS = 998). Thus, her OBS = OS − DTS = 273 days (Figure 1B).

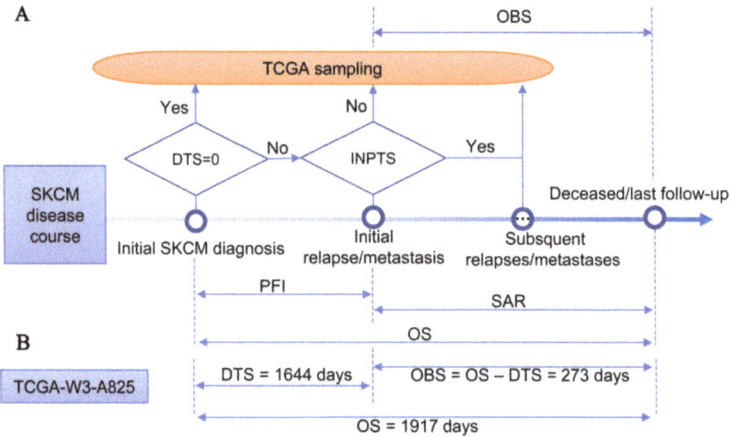

Figure 1. Definition of observed survival interval for TCGA-SKCM cohort. (**A**) Disease course of TCGA-SKCM cohort. DTS—days from initial SKCM diagnosis to TCGA sampling; INPTS—indicator of new tumor event prior to TCGA sampling; SAR—survival after the first relapse/metastasis; OS—overall survival; OBS—observed survival interval; PFI—progression-free interval. The diamond-shaped box denotes the examination of the condition included in the box. (**B**) Disease course of patient TCGA-W3-A825.

2.4. Comparison of OS and OBS in Association with Clinical Data

The Kaplan-Meier survival analysis and log-rank test were applied to evaluate the prognostic effects of demographic and clinicopathological characteristics by considering both OS and OBS as clinical outcomes. The multivariate Cox regression model [17] was used to evaluate the independence of demographic and clinicopathological characteristics.

We also inferred the pathological stage at the time of TCGA sampling for MCM patients based on the 8th edition of the AJCC melanoma staging system [4]. Specifically, if the SKCM patient was initially diagnosed as pathological stage IV, the patient was still stage IV at the time of TCGA sampling; otherwise, if TCGA took a non-distant MCM sample from the patient, the patient was stage III at the time of TCGA sampling; otherwise, TCGA took a distant MCM sample from the patient and the patient should have been stage IV at the time of TCGA sampling. The prognostic effect of the inferred pathological stage was also evaluated by the Kaplan-Meier survival analysis.

2.5. Comparison of OS and OBS in Associating miRNA Sequencing Data

Univariate Cox regression analyses and proportional hazards assumption tests [18] were used to preliminarily explore the associations between OS or OBS and miRNA expression profiles. The Benjamini-Hochberg method was adopted for multiple testing corrections [19]. A stepwise multivariate Cox regression analysis with all preliminarily survival associated miRNAs as covariates was applied to construct an independent miRNA expression signature for SKCM prognosis.

The survival risk score (SRS), defined as the standard form of the prognostic index, was used as the synthetical index to represent the prognostic miRNA expression signature. The prognostic index was defined as a linear combination of the miRNA expression values weighted by the regression coefficients. Specifically,

$$SRS = \frac{PI - mean(PI)}{sd(PI)} \tag{1}$$

where PI is a prognostic index vector and the *j*th element of PI is the prognostic index of the *j*th patient, i.e.,

$$PI_j = \sum_i \beta_i \times E_{ij} \tag{2}$$

where, β_i is the multivariate Cox regression coefficient of the *i*th miRNA and E_{ij} is the expression value of the *i*th miRNA in the *j*th sample. The ability of SRS to predict the SKCM patient survival outcome was assessed by calculating the area under the curve (AUC) of the time dependent receiver operating characteristic (ROC) at 3 years, 5 years, and 10 years, respectively [20].

2.6. Statistical Analysis

All analyses were done using R 3.4.4 [21]. MicroRNA sequencing raw counts normalization and differential expression analyses were conducted by a "DESeq2" package [22]. Guided principal component analysis was implemented by a "gPCA" package [16]. Survival analysis and proportional hazards assumption tests were performed by a "survival" package and a "survminer" package, respectively. Time dependent ROC analyses were done using a "timeROC" package [20]. All *P* values or adjusted *p*-values less than 0.05 were considered to be significant.

3. Results

3.1. TCGA-SKCM Dataset

There were 470 SKCM patients who provided 452 samples to TCGA for miRNA sequencing. Of the 452 SKCM samples, 97 were primary SKCM (PCM) samples, 352 were metastatic SKCM (MCM) samples, one was an additional MCM sample, and two were normal samples. We only analyzed the PCM and MCM samples due to the small number of normal and additional MCM samples. After preprocessing, 357 SKCM samples (82 PCM samples and 275 MCM samples) and 564 miRNAs were retained. To reproduce our analysis, the preprocessed clinical data and normalized miRNA sequencing data are presented in Datasets S1 and S2, respectively. Batch effect analyses of the normalized miRNA expression matrix showed that there was no discernible separation on the first two guided principal components (Figure S1A) with a permutation test *p*-value of 0.472 (Figure S1B). These results revealed that although TCGA-SKCM samples were sequenced in different batches, there was no significant batch effect among them.

3.2. Differences between OBS and OS

Of the 357 patients in TCGA-SKCM cohort, 171 patients were deceased and 186 patients were alive at the time of last follow-up. The median OS time and OBS time of TCGA-SKCM cohort were 2184 days

(95% CI, 1927–3266 days) and 986 days (95% CI, 854–1276 days), respectively. For TCGA-PCM cohort, 18 patients were deceased and 64 patients were alive at the time of the last follow-up. The median OS time and OBS time of TCGA-PCM cohort were 1070 days (95% CI, 857–NA days) and 1276 days (95% CI, 1070–NA days), respectively. For TCGA-MCM cohort, 122 patients were deceased and 153 patients were alive at the time of last follow-up. The median OS time and OBS time of TCGA-MCM cohort were 2402 days (95% CI, 1992–3424 days) and 896 days (95% CI, 732–1175 days), respectively.

There was no obvious difference between OS and the OBS in TCGA-PCM cohort ($p = 0.85$) because the majority of the samples (80.49%) submitted to TCGA in this cohort were samples that were initially SKCM diagnosed. However, the OBS was significantly shorter than OS in TCGA-MCM cohort ($p = 2.51 \times 10^{-11}$) as the majority of the samples (90.55%) submitted to the TCGA in this cohort were not samples that were initially SKCM diagnosed, but samples excised from follow-up metastases (an average of a 1403 day delay after initial SKCM diagnosis). Furthermore, the median OS of TCGA-PCM cohort was significantly shorter than that of TCGA-MCM cohort (Figure 2A) and the opposite was true when the OBS was compared (Figure 2B). Logically, PCM patients were expected to survive longer than MCM patients. According to our analyses, the results were hard to explain if OS was adopted as the survival outcome, while it became explicable by considering the OBS as the survival outcome. These results revealed that OS and the OBS were different and the difference may give rise to distinct associations when used as survival outcomes in omics translational research.

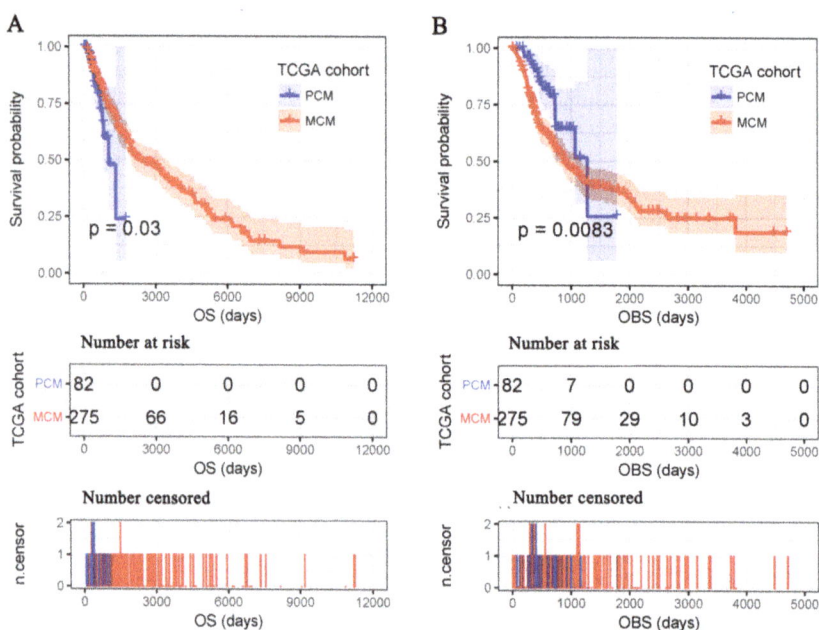

Figure 2. Kaplan-Meier survival analysis between PCM patients and MCM patients. PCM—primary SKCM; MCM—metastatic SKCM. OS (**A**) and the OBS (**B**) were considered clinical outcomes. The upper, middle, and lower parts represent the Kaplan-Meier plot, number of patients at risk for each group, and number of censored patients for each group respectively. OS—overall survival; OBS—observed survival interval.

3.3. OS Deemed More Appropriate to Associate Clinicopathological Characteristics than the OBS

Demographic and clinicopathological characteristics of TCGA-SKCM cohort measured at initial SKCM diagnosis are summarized in Table 1. The age at initial diagnosis, AJCC pathological stage, ulceration, and Breslow depth were significantly associated with OS of SKCM patients (Table 1).

However, none of them were associated with the OBS (Table S1). Furthermore, only the AJCC pathological stage was an independent predictor of OS of SKCM patients (Table 1).

Table 1. Survival analysis of demographic and clinicopathological characteristics based on OS.

Column Header	Deaths/Patients (%)	MS (95% CI)	[U]Log-rank test *p*	[M]HR (95% CI)	[M]Wald test *p*
Age[1]					
≤50 years	58/113 (51.33)	4062 (2022–5370)			
>50 years	115/244 (47.13)	1927 (1524–2927)	0.011	1.27 (0.82–1.96)	0.282
Gender					
Male	60/138 (43.48)	2004 (1640–4507)			
Female	111/219 (50.68)	2402 (1960–3424)	0.736		
Breslow depth[1]					
≤2 mm	55/114 (48.25)	3943 (3139–5318)			
>2 mm	80/169 (47.33)	1424 (1103–2004)	<0.001	1.44 (0.93–2.22)	0.098
Pathological stage[2]					
I–II	81/179 (45.25)	3266 (2402–4601)			
III–IV	75/153 (49.02)	1490 (988–2071)	<0.001	1.82 (1.22–2.72)	0.004
Ulceration[1]					
No	57/111 (51.35)	2402 (1927–4222)			
Yes	58/133 (43.61)	1354 (1059–2028)	<0.001	1.53 (1.00–2.35)	0.052
Primary tumor site					
Extremities	76/158 (48.1)	2071 (1910–4000)			
Head and neck	11/23 (47.83)	2192 (787–NA)			
Trunk	59/128 (46.09)	3139 (1691–5107)	0.787		
Radiation therapy					
No	165/355 (49.25)	2192 (1917–3266)			
Yes	7/14 (50.00)	1341–NA	0.892		
Chemotherapy					
No	121/251 (48.21)	2173 (1832–3564)			
Yes	40/75 (53.33)	2184 (1917–3683)	0.813		

MS—median survival; CI—confidence interval; HR—hazard ratio; [U]—univariate analysis; [M]—multivariate analysis. For the multivariate Cox regression analyses, variable coding are: age (1, ≤50 years; 2, >50 years), pathological stage (1, I–II; 2, III–IV), ulceration (1, No; 2, Yes), and Breslow depth (1, ≤2 mm; 2, >2 mm). [1]Significant in univariate analysis; [2]Significant in multivariate analysis. Patients with missing values were omitted from the table.

Subgroup analysis revealed that SKCM patients with a higher pathological stage had shorter OS in bothTCGA-PCM cohort (HR = 3.63, 95%CI: 1.26–10.42; Figure S2A) and TCGA-MCM cohort (HR = 1.77, 95%CI: 1.25–2.52; Figure S2B). However, for the OBS, it was associated with the pathological stage in TCGA-PCM cohort (HR=3.63, 95%CI: 1.26–10.41; Figure S2C) but not in TCGA-MMC cohort (HR = 0.94, 95%CI: 0.67–1.30; Figure S2D).

As the AJCC pathological stage was the only independent predictor of OS of SKCM patients, we further inferred the pathological stage at the time of TCGA sampling for MCM patients. The inferred pathological stage was significantly associated with the OBS (HR = 2.06, 95%CI: 1.24–3.41; Figure 3B) rather than OS (HR = 1.03, 95%CI: 0.69–1.53; Figure 3A) in TCGA-MCM cohort.

The clinicopathological characteristics provided by TCGA were measured at the time of the initial SKCM diagnosis. Thus, they were in accordance with the start time point of OS, while they were usually out-of-step with respect to the OBS (especially for TCGA-MCM cohort). For TCGA-PCM cohort, OS and the OBS were usually the same, and indiscriminate usage of them will not result in a significant difference. Overall, these results indicated that the clinicopathological characteristics reasonably predicted OS, while they were not appropriate to predict the OBS due to the out-of-step issue.

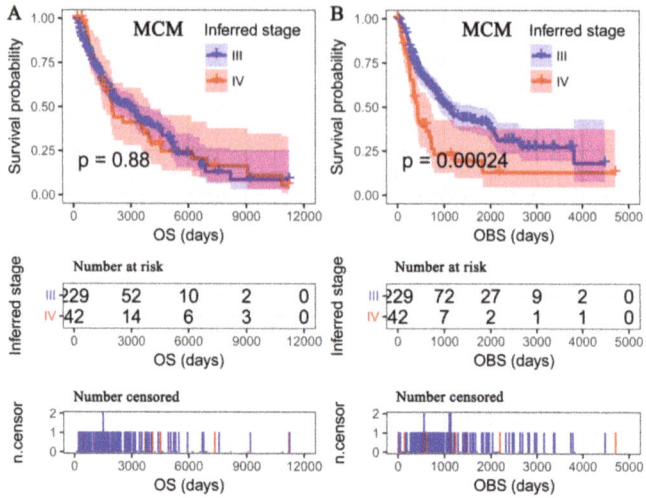

Figure 3. Kaplan-Meier survival analysis of inferred pathological stage. The OBS and inferred pathological stage in TCGA-MCM cohort (**A**), OS and inferred pathological stage in TCGA-MCM cohort (**B**). OS—overall survival; OBS—observed survival interval.

3.4. Differentially Expressed miRNAs

Differentially expressed miRNAs between PCM and MCM were mainly in the hsa-miR-205-5p, hsa-miR-203a-3p, and hsa-miR-200 family (Figure 4). Only hsa-miR-3150b-3p was differentially expressed in APCM (advanced PCM, PCM with pathological stage III and IV) versus LPCM (localized PCM, PCM with pathological stage I and II), while it didn't show any difference in APCM versus MCM or LPCM versus MCM (Figure 4). These results were consistent with the discoveries of Xu et al. on differentially expressed miRNAs in MCM versus PCM [23]. Furthermore, these results revealed that biological differences were mainly between PCM and MCM rather than between LPCM and APCM. Thus, it was appropriate to combine LPCM samples and APCM samples as PCM samples to explore survival associated miRNAs, while it was improper to further combine PCM samples and MCM samples as SKCM samples to identify survival associated miRNAs.

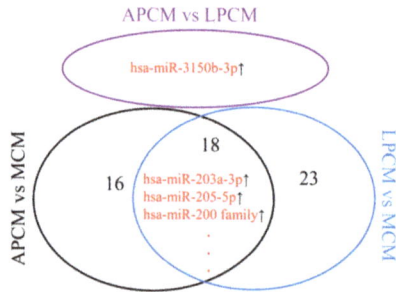

Figure 4. Venn plot of differentially expressed miRNAs of APCM versus LPCM, APCM versus MCM, and LPCM versus MCM. Arrow and number represent regulation direction and number of differentially expressed miRNAs, respectively. LPCM—localized primary SKCM; APCM—advanced primary SKCM; MCM—metastatic SKCM.

3.5. OBS Deemed More Appropriate to Associate miRNA-Omics Data than OS

Segura et al., Caramuta et al. and Tembe et al. proposed several miRNA expression signatures for MCM prognosis based on low sample size microarray data [24–26]. Jayawardana et al. [8] proposed fifteen prognostic miRNAs for stage III MCMs from TCGA miRNA-omics data and, further, systematically cross-validated these fifteen miRNAs with previous studies [24–26]. Five miRNAs (hsa-miR-142-5p, hsa-miR-150-5p, hsa-miR-342-3p, hsa-miR-155-5p, and hsa-miR-146b-5p) were found to be cross-validated (i.e., with greater validation rates across studies). However, none of the fifteen miRNAs identified from TCGA data overlapped with the five cross-validated miRNAs. Thus, Jayawardana et al. claimed that TCGA-MCM data performed the worst. These results were considered priori criteria for comparison of OS and the OBS in miRNA sequencing data.

Univariate Cox regression analysis revealed that there was no miRNA associated with either OS or the OBS in TCGA-PCM cohort. Meanwhile, 27 and nine miRNAs were found to be significantly associated with the OBS and OS of patients in TCGA-MCM cohort, respectively (Table S2). Interestingly, all of the five cross-validated miRNAs were found to be associated with the OBS rather than OS in TCGA-MCM cohort (Table S2) despite all being missed in the analysis of Jayawardana et al. due to the adoption of OS [8].

Unlike the clinicopathological characteristics measured at the time of initial SKCM diagnosis, the molecular patterns were characterized at the time of TCGA sampling. Thus, the miRNA-omics data were in accordance with the start time point of the OBS, while they were out-of-step with respect to OS (especially for TCGA-MCM cohort). Combined with the results from the above clinical analyses, OS and the OBS were usually the same in TCGA-PCM cohort, while they were usually different in TCGA-MCM cohort. Thus, for TCGA-MCM cohort, the OBS should be used for associating miRNA-omics data, and indiscriminate usage of OS and the OBS in TCGA-PCM cohort will not result in a significant difference. Overall, the OBS was more appropriate for identification of prognostic biomarkers than OS. Furthermore, to evaluate the independence and compare the prognostic power of clinicopathological characteristics and biomarkers, the time point of clinical data and omics data must be in accordance. As the time point of the omics data was fixed at TCGA sampling, it is wise to deduce the clinicopathological characteristics at the time point of TCGA sampling.

3.6. A miRNA Expression Signature for MCM Prognosis Based on the OBS

Although Jayawardana et al. have cross-validated five miRNAs for MCM prognosis, the cross-validation was based on differential expression analysis between MCM patients with longer OS and MCM patients with poor OS [8]. Thus, relationships among the five miRNAs were not investigated further. For the identification of prognostic biomarkers, the construction of signatures that included as many independent biomarkers as possible was expected [15]. Correlation analysis showed that the five cross-validated miRNAs were correlated with each other (Figure 5A) and a collinearity existed among them (Kappa value = 70.32). Furthermore, multivariate Cox regression analyses revealed that hsa-miR-155-5p was an appropriate representative for the five cross-validated miRNAs (Table S3).

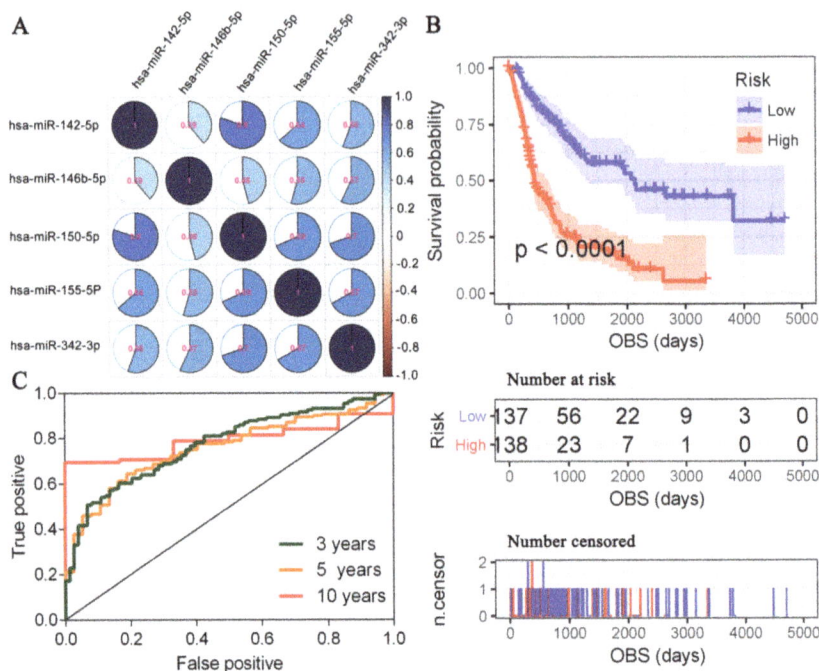

Figure 5. Prognostic miRNAs for MCM based on the OBS. (**A**) Pairwise Spearman correlations of the five cross-validated prognostic miRNAs in MCM. (**B**) Kaplan-Meier survival analysis between high-risk and low-risk MCM patients. (**C**) Time dependent receiver operating characteristic curves of SRS at different times. SRS-survival risk score.

Stepwise multivariate Cox regression analyses, by considering the OBS to be the survival outcome and the 27 OBS associated miRNAs as covariates, revealed that hsa-miR-155-5p, hsa-miR-4461, hsa-miR-504-5p, hsa-miR-625-5p, and hsa-miR-664b-5p were independent prognostic miRNAs for patients with MCM (Table 2, upper part). Model diagnosis revealed that the final regression model (Global Schoenfeld test p = 0.49) and all covariates in the model satisfied the proportional hazards assumption (Figure S3) with negligible collinearity (Kappa value = 2.70).

The survival risk score (SRS) was calculated for each MCM patient and Kaplan-Meier survival analysis showed that high-risk (SRS>0) MCM patients had shorter OBS compared with low-risk (SRS $\leq$ 0) MCM patients (HR = 3.29; 95%CI: 2.37–4.56; Figure 5B). Furthermore, as a continuous variable, the SRS was inversely associated with the OBS (HR = 2.32; 95%CI: 1.93–2.78; Wald test p < 0.001). The area under the curve of the receiver operating characteristic for SRS were 0.77 (95%CI: 0.71–0.84), 0.76 (95%CI: 0.68–0.83), and 0.79 (95%CI: 0.71–0.88) at three years, five years, and 10 years, respectively (Figure 5C). Finally, multivariate Cox regression analysis showed that the SRS was an independent predictor of the OBS of MCM patients while the inferred pathological stage was no longer significant (Table 2, lower part).

Table 2. Independent prognostic miRNAs for MCM patients based on OBS.

Column Header	^{M}HR (95% CI)	^{M}Wald Test P	Type
hsa-miR-155-5p	0.73 (0.63–0.85)	3.15×10^{-5}	Protective[1]
hsa-miR-4461	1.29 (1.13–1.46)	1.07×10^{-4}	Risky[2]
hsa-miR-504-5p	0.80 (0.71–0.92)	1.17×10^{-3}	Protective
hsa-miR-625-5p	0.67 (0.53–0.86)	1.35×10^{-3}	Protective
hsa-miR-664b-5p	0.69 (0.58–0.83)	4.39×10^{-5}	Protective
SRS	2.28 (1.89–2.74)	$<2.00 \times 10^{-16}$	Risky
Inferred stage	1.32 (0.88–1.98)	0.18	Risky

^{M}—multivariate analysis; [1]—HR<1; [2]—HR>1.

4. Discussion

The recently proposed TCGA-CDR includes OS, PFI (progression-free interval), DFI (disease-free survival), DSS (disease-specific survival), and a list of outcome usage recommendations for each cancer type [14]. As indicated by Liu et al., TCGA mainly collected primary tumors for molecular characterization, with the exception of the SKCM study, which included mainly metastatic samples. According to our results, there was no statistically significant difference between OS and the OBS in PCM ($p = 0.85$). Thus, TCGA-CDR prudently recommended using only the limited number of PCM samples for SKCM clinical outcome correlations [14]. However, this recommendation discarded the majority of the MCM samples. Although there was no statistically significant difference between OS and the OBS in TCGA-PCM cohort, OS and the OBS were not always the same for every PCM patient (19.51%). This means that some of the PCM samples submitted to TCGA may not be samples obtained at initial SKCM diagnosis but relapse samples from the follow-up. For example, patient TCGA-ER-A2NB provided a PCM sample to TCGA, but his DTS = 124 days. Although we believe this non-significant difference between OS and the OBS will not lead to significantly different associations when applying to TCGA-PCM omics data, a more precise recommendation is necessary.

Some limitations of the current study should be noticed. (I) We addressed the out-of-step issue of survival outcome but various outcome endpoints based on relapses or metastases were not investigated. With the exception of OS, Liu et al. also recommended PFI and DSS for TCGA-SKCM data. However, there also existed the out-of-step issue for these outcomes in MCM. For example, all outcome endpoints of TCGA-W3-A825 in TCGA-CDR were 1917 days [14]. According to our analyses, the PFI of TCGA-W3-A825 should be 1644 days (i.e., DTS = 1644 days; Figure 1B), but this outcome was not appropriate for the investigation of associations between it and omics data due to no primary sample being available for TCGA-W3-A825. (II) We didn't find any prognostic miRNAs to predict the survival of PCM. Possible explanations are: (a) PCM is a relatively early event in SKCM progression and PCMomics data may be unable to predict the relatively long survival-based outcomes such as OS and the OBS. Thus, relatively shorter outcome endpoints based on relapses or metastases may be appropriate for PCMomics translational research. (b) Single miRNA-omics may not be enough for predicting PCM patient survival, and a multi-omics analysis should be conducted. (III) Despite this study focusing on the outcome endpoints of TCGA-SKCM data, the five identified novel prognostic miRNAs based on the OBS call for additional studies for further validation and mechanism exploration.

5. Conclusions

In conclusion, we defined the OBS, to supplement TCGA-CDR, and recommended it for TCGA-SKCMomics translational research. Our results could remind subsequent TCGA-SKCM data users to pay attention to the out-of-step issue of outcome endpoints. Although our analyses were based on associations between survival-based outcomes and TCGA-SKCM miRNA-omics data, they could be generalized to associate other TCGA-SKCMomics data and relapses, or metastasis-based outcomes. In addition, the five identified prognostic miRNAs may be of value in predicting the OBS of MCM patients and informing future experimental investigations.

Supplementary Materials: The following are available online at http://www.mdpi.com/2072-6694/11/3/280/s1, Figure S1: batch effect evaluation; Figure S2: Kaplan-Meier survival analysis of pathological stage; Figure S3: Schoenfeld residuals; Table S1: survival analysis of the four OS associated clinicopathological characteristics based on the OBS; Table S2: univariate analysis of OS associated and the OBS associated miRNAs in TCGA-MCM cohort; Table S3: univariate and multivariate analysis of the five cross-validated miRNAs based on the OBS; Dataset S1: clinical data; Dataset S2: normalized miRNA expression data.

Author Contributions: Conceptualization, J.X. and S.G.; Data curation, S.G.; Formal analysis, J.X. and Z.B.; Investigation, Z.B.; Methodology, J.X.; Project administration, S.G.and J.X.; Supervision, S.G. and J.X.; Visualization, J.X. and S.G.; Writing—original draft, J.X.; Writing—review and editing, J.X., Z.B. and S.G.

Funding: This research received no external funding.

Acknowledgments: The authors thank TCGA research network for making the omics data of skin cutaneous melanoma available. All data was kept according to the rules for usage and publication of TCGA (https://cancergenome.nih.gov/publications/publicationguidelines). We wish to thank the editors and the anonymous reviewers for their helpful comments.

Conflicts of Interest: The authors declare no conflicts of interest.

References

1. Ali, Z.; Yousaf, N.; Larkin, J. Melanoma epidemiology, biology and prognosis. *Eur. J. Cancer Suppl.* **2013**, *11*, 81–91. [CrossRef] [PubMed]

2. Wang, H.; Naghavi, M.; Allen, C.; Barber, R.M.; Bhutta, Z.A.; Carter, A.; Casey, D.C.; Charlson, F.J.; Chen, A.Z.; Coates, M.M.; et al. Global, regional, and national life expectancy, all-cause mortality, and cause-specific mortality for 249 causes of death, 1980–2015: A systematic analysis for the Global Burden of Disease Study 2015. *Lancet* **2016**, *385*, 117–171. [CrossRef]

3. Siegel, R.L.; Miller, K.D.; Jemal, A. Cancer statistics, 2018. *CA Cancer J. Clin.* **2018**, *68*, 7–30. [CrossRef] [PubMed]

4. Gershenwald, J.E.; Scolyer, R.A.; Hess, K.R.; Sondak, V.K.; Long, G.V.; Ross, M.I.; Lazar, A.J.; Faries, M.B.; Kirkwood, J.M.; McArthur, G.A.; et al. Melanoma staging: Evidence-based changes in the American Joint Committee on Cancer eighth edition cancer staging manual. *CA Cancer J. Clin.* **2017**, *67*, 472–492. [CrossRef] [PubMed]

5. Hanniford, D.; Zhong, J.; Koetz, L.; Gaziel-Sovran, A.; Lackaye, D.J.; Shang, S.; Pavlick, A.; Shapiro, R.; Berman, R.; Darvishian, F.; et al. A miRNA-Based Signature Detected in Primary Melanoma Tissue Predicts Development of Brain Metastasis. *Clin. Cancer Res.* **2015**, *21*, 4903–4912. [CrossRef] [PubMed]

6. Hu, X.; Schwarz, J.K.; Lewis, J.S.J.; Huettner, P.C.; Rader, J.S.; Deasy, J.O.; Grigsby, P.W.; Wang, X. A microRNA expression signature for cervical cancer prognosis. *Cancer Res.* **2010**, *70*, 1441–1448. [CrossRef] [PubMed]

7. Akbani, R.; Akdemir, K.C.; Aksoy, B.A.; Albert, M.; Ally, A.; Amin, S.B.; Arachchi, H.; Arora, A.; Auman, J.T.; Ayala, B.; et al. Genomic Classification of Cutaneous Melanoma. *Cell* **2015**, *161*, 1681–1696. [CrossRef] [PubMed]

8. Jayawardana, K.; Schramm, S.J.; Tembe, V.; Mueller, S.; Thompson, J.F.; Scolyer, R.A.; Mann, G.J.; Yang, J. Identification, Review, and Systematic Cross-Validation of microRNA Prognostic Signatures in Metastatic Melanoma. *J. Investig. Dermatol.* **2016**, *136*, 245–254. [CrossRef] [PubMed]

9. Guo, J.; Yang, M.; Zhang, W.; Lu, H.; Li, J. A panel of miRNAs as prognostic indicators for clinical outcome of skin cutaneous melanoma. *Int. J. Clin. Exp. Med.* **2016**, *9*, 28–39.

10. Chen, X.; Guo, W.; Xu, X.J.; Su, F.; Wang, Y.; Zhang, Y.; Wang, Q.; Zhu, L. Melanoma long non-coding RNA signature predicts prognostic survival and directs clinical risk-specific treatments. *J. Dermatol. Sci.* **2017**, *85*, 226–234. [CrossRef] [PubMed]

11. Yang, S.; Xu, J.; Zeng, X. A six-long non-coding RNA signature predicts prognosis in melanoma patients. *Int. J. Oncol.* **2018**, *52*, 1178–1188. [CrossRef] [PubMed]

12. Ma, X.; He, Z.; Li, L.; Yang, D.; Liu, G. Expression profiles analysis of long non-coding RNAs identified novel lncRNA biomarkers with predictive value in outcome of cutaneous melanoma. *Oncotarget* **2017**, *8*, 77761–77770. [CrossRef] [PubMed]

13. Jiang, Y.; Shi, X.; Zhao, Q.; Krauthammer, M.; Rothberg, B.E.; Ma, S. Integrated analysis of multidimensional omics data on cutaneous melanoma prognosis. *Genomics* **2016**, *107*, 223–230. [CrossRef] [PubMed]

14. Liu, J.; Lichtenberg, T.; Hoadley, K.A.; Poisson, L.M.; Lazar, A.J.; Cherniack, A.J.; Kovatich, A.J.; Benz, C.C.; Levine, D.A.; Lee, A.V.; et al. An Integrated TCGA Pan-Cancer Clinical Data Resource to Drive High-Quality Survival Outcome Analytics. *Cell* **2018**, *173*, 400–416. [CrossRef] [PubMed]

15. Xiong, J.; Guo, S.; Bing, Z.; Su, Y.; Guo, L. A Comprehensive RNA Expression Signature for Cervical Squamous Cell Carcinoma Prognosis. *Front. Genet.* **2018**, *9*, 696. [CrossRef] [PubMed]

16. Reese, S.E.; Archer, K.J.; Therneau, T.M.; Atkinson, E.J.; Vachon, C.M.; de Andrade, M.; Kocher, J.P.; Eckel-Passow, J.E. A new statistic for identifying batch effects in high-throughput genomic data that uses guided principal component analysis. *Bioinformatics* **2013**, *29*, 2877–2883. [CrossRef] [PubMed]

17. Cox, D.R. Regression Models and Life-Tables. *J. Royal Stat. Soc.* **1972**, *34*, 187–220. [CrossRef]

18. Grambsch, P.M.; Therneau, T.M. Proportional hazards tests and diagnostics based on weighted residuals. *Biometrika* **1994**, *81*, 515–526. [CrossRef]

19. Benjamini, Y.; Hochberg, Y. Controlling the false discovery rate: A practical and powerful approach to multiple testing. *J. Royal Stat. Soc. Ser. B* **1995**, *57*, 289–300. [CrossRef]

20. Blanche, P.; Dartigues, J.F.; Jacqmin-Gadda, H. Estimating and comparing time-dependent areas under receiver operating characteristic curves for censored event times with competing risks. *Stat. Med.* **2013**, *32*, 5381–5397. [CrossRef] [PubMed]

21. Ihaka, R.; Gentleman, R.R. A language for data analysis and graphics. *J.Comput. Gr. Stat.* **1996**, *5*, 299–314.

22. Love, M.I.; Huber, W.; Anders, S. Moderated estimation of fold change and dispersion for RNA-seq data with DESeq2. *Genome Biol.* **2014**, *15*, 550. [CrossRef] [PubMed]

23. Xu, Y.; Brenn, T.; Brown, E.R.; Doherty, V.; Melton, D.W. Differential expression of microRNAs during melanoma progression: miR-200c, miR-205 and miR-211 are downregulated in melanoma and act as tumour suppressors. *Br. J. Cancer* **2012**, *106*, 553–561. [CrossRef] [PubMed]

24. Segura, M.F.; Belitskayalévy, I.; Rose, A.E.; Zarkrzewski, J.; Gaziel, A.; Hanniford, D.; Darvishian, F.; Berman, R.S.; Shapiro, R.L.; Pavlick, A.C.; et al. Melanoma microRNA signature predicts post-recurrence survival. *Clin. Cancer Res.* **2010**, *16*, 1577–1586. [CrossRef] [PubMed]

25. Caramuta, S.; Egyha´zi, S.; Rodolfo, M.; Witten, D.; Hansson, J.; Larsson, C.; Lui, W.O. MicroRNA Expression Profiles Associated with Mutational Status and Survival in Malignant Melanoma. *J. Investig. Dermatol.* **2010**, *130*, 2062–2070. [CrossRef] [PubMed]

26. Tembe, V.; Schramm, S.J.; Stark, M.S.; Patrick, E.; Jayaswal, V.; Tang, Y.H.; Barbour, A.; Hayward, N.K.; Thompson, J.F.; Scolyer, R.A.; et al. microRNA and mRNA expression profiling in metastatic melanoma reveal associations with BRAF mutation and patient prognosis. *Pigment. Cell Melanoma Res.* **2014**, *28*, 254–266. [CrossRef] [PubMed]

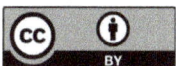

Article

Prognostic Biomarkers in Pancreatic Cancer: Avoiding Errata When Using the TCGA Dataset

Remy Nicolle [1], Jerome Raffenne [2], Valerie Paradis [2,3], Anne Couvelard [2,3], Aurelien de Reynies [1], Yuna Blum [1] and Jerome Cros [2,3,*]

[1] Programme Cartes d'Identité des Tumeurs (CIT), Ligue Nationale Contre le Cancer, 75014 Paris, France; Remy.Nicolle@ligue-cancer.net (R.N.); Aurelien.DeReynies@ligue-cancer.net (A.d.R.); yuna.blum@ligue-cancer.net (Y.B.)

[2] INSERM U1149, Beaujon University Hospital, 92110 Clichy, France; raffenne.jerome@gmail.com (J.R.); valerie.paradis@aphp.fr (V.P.); anne.couvelard@aphp.fr (A.C.)

[3] Department of Pathology, Beaujon-Bichat University Hospital - Paris Diderot University, 100 Bvd Gal Leclerc, 92110 Clichy, France

* Correspondence: jerome.cros@aphp.fr; Tel.: +33-0140875625; Fax: +33-0140875625

Received: 4 December 2018; Accepted: 16 January 2019; Published: 21 January 2019

Abstract: Data from the Cancer Genome Atlas (TCGA) are now easily accessible through web-based platforms with tools to assess the prognostic value of molecular alterations. Pancreatic tumors have heterogeneous biology and aggressiveness ranging from the deadly adenocarcinoma (PDAC) to the better prognosis, neuroendocrine tumors. We assessed the availability of the pancreatic cancer TCGA data (TCGA_PAAD) from several repositories and investigated the nature of each sample and how non-PDAC samples impact prognostic biomarker studies. While the clinical and genomic data ($n = 185$) were fairly consistent across all repositories, RNAseq profiles varied from 176 to 185. As a result, 35 RNAseq profiles (18.9%) corresponded to a normal, inflamed pancreas or non-PDAC neoplasms. This information was difficult to obtain. By considering gene expression data as continuous values, the expression of the 5312 and 4221 genes were significantly associated with the progression-free and overall survival respectively. Considering the cohort was not curated, only 4 and 14, respectively, had prognostic value in the PDAC-only cohort. Similarly, mutations in key genes or well-described miRNA lost their prognostic significance in the PDAC-only cohort. Therefore, we propose a web-based application to assess biomarkers in the curated TCGA_PAAD dataset. In conclusion, TCGA_PAAD curation is critical to avoid important biological and clinical biases from non-PDAC samples.

Keywords: pancreatic cancer; TCGA; curation

1. Introduction

Consortium efforts, such as those of the Cancer Genome Atlas (TCGA) or the International Cancer Genome Consortium (ICGC), to massively sequence thousands of tumors from multiple types have led to a much better understanding of tumor biology. While the data were freely accessible, their use was restricted in practice to teams with great expertise in bioinformatics. Further efforts from centers such as the Broad Institute (https://gdac.broadinstitute.org) or the University of California Santa Cruz (http://xena.ucsc.edu) allowed easy access to TCGA normalized RNAseq, methylation and clinical data, often readily available in excel files. Finally, multiple web-based platforms were launched with "one-click" capabilities to give users direct access to the prognostic role of the gene expression level, the frequency of any mutation, the protein level expression and the networks of genes and proteins, etc. Main platforms include TCGA (https://gdc.cancer.gov), the Broad Institute (https://gdac.broadinstitute.org), the University of California Santa Cruz (http://xena.ucsc.edu), cBioportal (http://www.cbioportal.org) and the Human Protein Atlas (https://www.proteinatlas.org). These platforms have given everyone access to use these data as exploratory or validation sets.

Pancreatic cancer is a generic term often misused as a surrogate for the most common malignant tumor entity in this organ, the ductal adenocarcinoma (PDAC). Other malignant tumor entities such as the neuroendocrine neoplasms or the acinar cell carcinomas can also be found in the pancreas [1]. While these tumors are uncommon, they often fall under the umbrella term of "pancreatic cancer", and are as such defined by completely different biology (mutational and transcriptional profiles) and clinical outcomes from the classical PDAC [2,3]. If such tumors were unnoticeably included within a dataset mainly composed of PDAC, they may introduce a strong bias in data analysis and lead to false conclusions regarding the prognostic value of a DNA mutation or an mRNA expression level. Depending on the source, 176 to 185 samples compose the TCGA study dedicated to the pancreas (TCGA_PAAD) and the multiomic analysis of these samples from the TCGA group was restricted to 150 samples [4]. In a recent study, Peran et al. highlighted that the TCGA_PAAD cohort, which mostly comprised patients who underwent surgery, displayed a much better survival rate than that of the unselected cohort SEER [5]. They further demonstrated that a failure to exclude non-PDAC samples might introduce a bias in the gene expression analyses leading to false conclusions being drawn when assessing the prognostic value of several mRNAs.

In this study, we aim to gather and compare the available data concerning the TCGA_PAAD from all the main repositories and clearly establish a list of suitable TCGA_PAAD samples for the PDAC centered studies. We then compare the TCGA_PAAD cohort to a large multicentric consecutive cohort of surgical PDAC. Using the key DNA mutation and the whole transcriptome, we then assessed the potential for bias based on survival analyses when using an uncurated sample list. Finally, we designed a web-based tool to assess the prognostic value of any gene expression on the curated TCGA_PAAD dataset.

2. Results

2.1. Data Comparison from the Repositories for the TCGA_PAAD

Across most platforms queried, the number of patients within the TCGA_PAAD study was consistent and set at 185 (TCGA data portal $n = 185$, UCSC Xena $n = 185$, Broad Institute Firehose $n = 185$, The Human Protein Atlas $n = 176$ (only patients with available RNAseq data were considered) and cBioportal $n = 185$). In all platforms, clinical data were available for the 185 patients. Depending on the platforms, mutation and copy number data were available for 184 or 185 samples, DNA methylation data were consistent and available for 184 samples, and RNAseq data were the most discordant, ranging from 176 to 185 samples (cBioportal $n = 185$, UCS Xena $n = 183$, Broad Institute Firehose $n = 178$, TCGA data portal $n = 178$ and The Human Protein Atlas $n = 176$). TCGA-derived RNAseq data were the most frequently used. As a result, we carefully investigated the nature of the samples to explain the discrepancy in the available number of samples depending on the platforms. RNAseq data were not available for seven patients and the number of patients with RNAseq data (list in Table S1) was set at 178. For four patients, RNAseq data from the normal adjacent pancreas were available and included in the datasets from the platforms with more than 183 samples. These samples could be identified, as they have the same ID number as the tumor sample but with "-11" at the end of their ID instead of "-01" (TCGA-HV-A5A3-01 and TCGA-HV-A5A3-11, for instance). For one patient, RNAseq data from the primary tumor and the metastasis was available. The metastasis is identifiable by its "-06" at the end of the sample ID TCGA-HZ-A9TJ-01 (primary tumor) and TCGA-HZ-A9TJ-06 (metastasis). This highlighted that data retrieval must be done with care, and confirms that while genomic and clinical data are available for 185 patients, RNAseq data are only available for 178 unique patients.

2.2. Curation of the TCGA_PAAD Dataset

The recent study from the TCGA group focused on pancreatic ductal adenocarcinoma and only included 150 samples. Therefore, we carefully reviewed the clinical and histological data of all the cases gathered through the repositories and by viewing the virtual slides. Ten samples presented the pancreas as normal with atrophy, eight samples were neuroendocrine neoplasms, four samples were tumors derived from other organs (duodenum-ampulla in three cases and undefined location in one case), two samples were intraductal papillary neoplasms, one sample was an acinar cell carcinoma, one was a ductal adenocarcinoma but had received neoadjuvant chemotherapy and one had a normal ampulla. It should be noted that for several patients, while the analyzed specimens were not PDAC (atrophic pancreas, PanIN, etc.), these patients did have a PDAC. These clinical data may therefore be used, but not the omic data. One additional case was excluded, as no single nucleotide variation data was available (TCGA-L1-A7W4-01). This sample was listed as a PDAC and treated with adjuvant gemcitabine, a classical drug for this tumor. The examination of the frozen section showed a poorly differentiated tumor, which was difficult to clearly identify as a PDAC or a neuroendocrine carcinoma. Copy number abnormalities (*SMAD4* deletion, *MYC* amplification, no alteration on *TP53*, *CDKN2A* and *RB1*) did not help in further assuring the diagnosis. The flow chart presenting the TCGA-PAAD sample curation is presented in Figure 1 and the full list of the 150 proper PDAC sample and the 28 non PDAC sample are provided in Table S1.

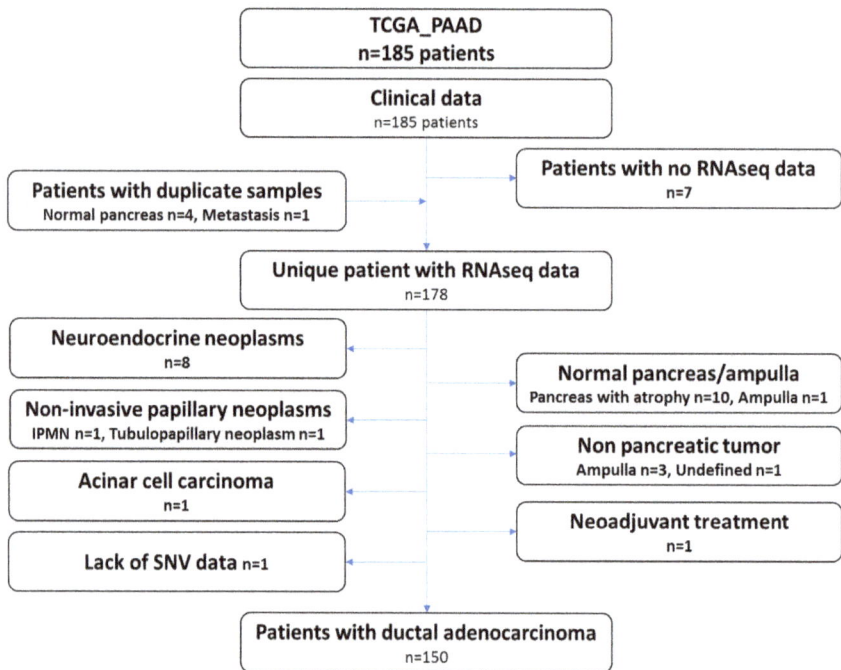

Figure 1. Flow chart depicting the curation of the pancreatic cancer dataset (TCGA_PAAD).

2.3. Clinical Relevance of the TCGA_PAAD Curated Sample List

Samples constituting of the TCGA cohorts were collected from multiple institutions, which may have introduced some heterogeneity in patient management and clinical data collection. In addition, while these cases were all surgical resections, they were not consecutive. To assess how representative the curated TCGA_PAAD cohort was, we compared it to our well characterized cohort of 471 consecutive resected PDAC in five centers collected over a 13 years period [6]. Basic clinical and pathological comparison is presented in Table 1. For this comparison, we used the consensual 150 cases, but the seven PDAC cases with no RNAseq data could have been added (results unchanged, data not shown). Both cohorts were comparable on most criteria. Tumors from the TCGA_PAAD study tended to be slightly more aggressive with larger and more poorly differentiated tumors ($p < 0.05$). Progression-free survival (PFS) was comparable in both cohorts (TCGA_PAAD 16.75 months vs. 14.51 months in our cohort, *ns*) (Figure 2a). In contrast, overall survival (OS) was much shorter in the TCGA_PAAD cohort (19.54 vs. 33.09 months, $p < 0.0001$) (Figure 2b).

Table 1. Clinical comparison of the TCGA_PAAD and the pancreatic adenocarcinoma multicenter cohort.

Clinical/Pathological Features	TCGA_PAAD (*n* = 150)	PDAC Multicenter Cohort (*n* = 471)	*p*-Value
Age at diagnostic (avg. (min, max))	64.89 (35, 88)	63.31 (34, 88)	0.12
Sex (male proportion (female, male))	54% (69, 81)	54% (215, 256)	1
Tumor size (avg. (min, max))	37.97 (18, 120)	32.42 (7, 150)	1.86×10^{-4}
Tumor grade			$< 1 \times 10^{-10}$
G1	5	201	$< 1 \times 10^{-10}$
G2	75	189	0.079
G3	69	67	$< 1 \times 10^{-10}$
G4	1	0	0.5579
Pathology TNM			0.0047
T1	1	17	0.114
T2	20	68	0.861
T3	125	386	0.676
T4	3	0	0.016
N (N1 proportion (N0, N1))	73.8% (39, 110)	74.5% (120, 351)	0.950
M (M0 proportion (M0, M1))	94.4% (68, 0)	100% (471, 0)	1.11×10^{-5}

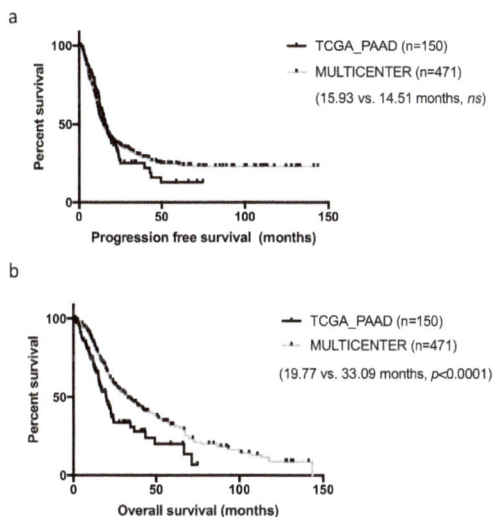

a

b

Figure 2. Progression-free and overall survival of the curated TCGA_PAAD and a PDAC multicenter cohort. Kaplan-Meier curves depicting the progression-free (**a**) and overall survival (**b**) of the curated TCGA-PAAD cohort (*n* = 150) and a multicenter PDAC cohort (*n* = 471).

2.4. Bias in the Prognostic Value when Using the Uncurated Cohort

We assessed whether the clinical or biological data from the non-PDAC patients impacted survival analyses performed on the TCGA_PAAD cohort. While the median PFS and OS of the uncurated cohort was marginally longer than that of the pure PDAC cohort (median PFS: 17.0 versus. 15.9 months and median OS 20.1 vs. 20.2 months respectively), the non-PDAC patients had a much longer PFS and OS compared to the pure PDAC cohort ($n = 150$) (median PFS: 27.3 vs. 15.9 months $p = 0.07$; median OS: unattained vs. 19.6 months $p = 0.03$; five year overall survival: 54.6% vs. 19.7%) (Figure 3a.). When the gene expression data were considered as continuous values; 5312 and 4221 genes were significantly associated (FDR 5%) with the PFS and OS respectively in the uncurated cohort (where a total of 17,302 genes were tested, uncorrected log-rank test: 6618 and 7260 genes at alpha = 5%). In contrast, if the PDAC-only cohort was considered, only 4 and 14 genes were significantly associated with the PFS and OS respectively (at FDR 5%; uncorrected log-rank test: 2632 and 2374 genes at alpha = 5%) (Figure 3b). In the PDAC-only cohort, 2671 genes were significantly over expressed and 1730 genes were significantly under expressed compared to the non-PDAC samples of the cohort (Table S2). Using a median cut off, 594 and 409 genes were associated with progression-free and overall survival, respectively, in the whole cohort (at FDR 5%; uncorrected log-rank test: 3907 and 3776 genes at alpha = 5%), while only 3 and 0 in the PDAC-only subgroup (at FDR 5%; uncorrected log-rank test: 1706 and 2062 genes at alpha = 5%). Within the genes that were differentially expressed in the 2 cohorts, we handpicked genes that were previously described as having a strong impact on prognosis. The progression-free and overall survival of cases with the top and bottom 25% expression were then compared in the uncurated and the curated cohort. While some genes such as *ERBB2, HK2, SLC2A1* were significantly or nearly significantly associated with the prognosis in both cohorts, others such as *MUC1/LOX/TWIST1/PI3K* lost their prognostic significance in the pure PDAC cohort (*TWIST1* as an example in Figure 4a).

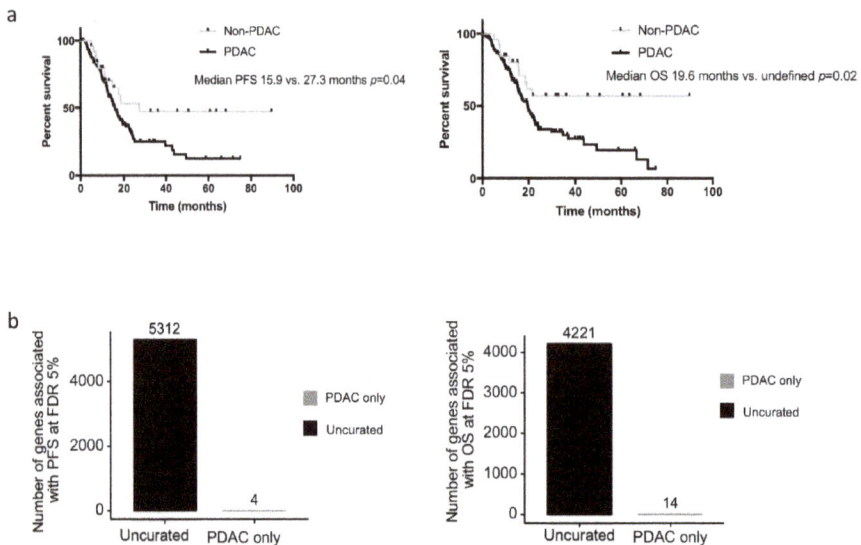

Figure 3. Progression-free and overall survival of the PDAC and non-PDAC cases. (**a**) Kaplan-Meier curves depicting the progression-free (left panel) and overall survival (right panel) of the PDAC cases ($n = 150$) and the non-PDAC cases ($n = 27$). (**b**) Number of genes associated significantly associated with the progression-free (left panel) and overall survival (right panel) in PDAC only cases and the uncurated cohort.

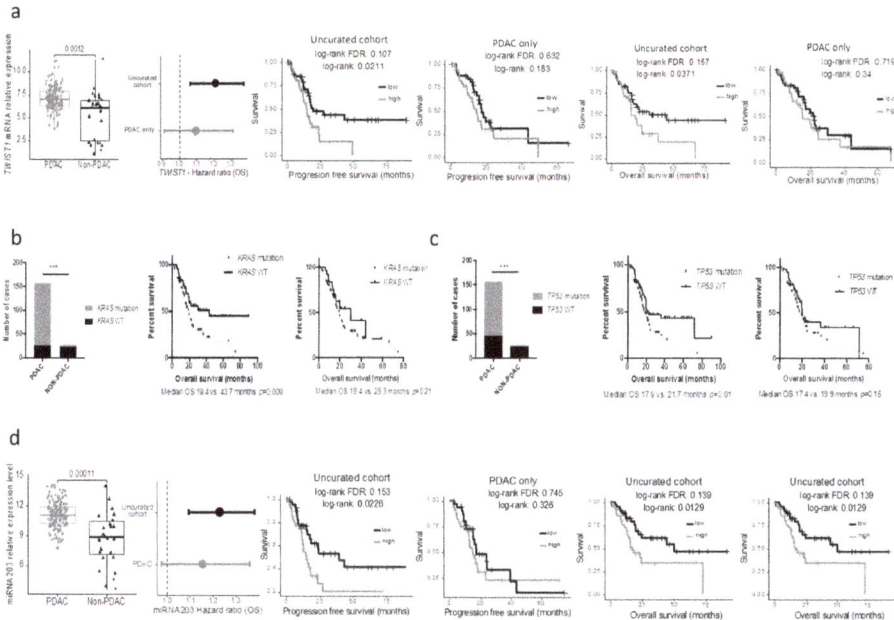

Figure 4. Bias in prognostic analysis when using the uncurated cohort. (**a**) *TWIST1* mRNA expression in PDAC and non-PDAC cases and prognostic impact (OS) in the uncurated and the PDAC only cohorts (left panels). Kaplan-Meier curves depicting the overall (middle panel) and progression-free survival (right panels) according to *TWIST1* expression in the uncurated cohort or the PDAC only cohort. (**b**) and (**c**) Distribution of the *KRAS* and *TP53* mutation in the PDAC and non-PDAC cases (left panels) and Kaplan-Meier curves depicting the overall survival according to the mutational status in the uncurated cohort (middle panels) or the PDAC-only cohort (right panels). (**d**) miR-203 mRNA expression in PDAC and non-PDAC cases and prognostic impact (OS) in the uncurated and the PDAC only cohorts (left panels). Kaplan-Meier curves depicting the overall (middle panel) and progression-free survival (right panels) according to miR-203 expression in the uncurated cohort or the PDAC only cohort.

Similar findings were observed when key mutations in PDAC were assessed. Here we included the seven PDAC cases with the DNA data available (but no RNAseq). The results were similar when using the minimal 150 PDAC cohort. While the mutational status of *KRAS* and *TP53* were strongly associated with the overall survival in the uncurated cohort, these mutations lost their prognostic significance in the pure PDAC cohort (Figure 3b,c). In a recent study, Shi et al. searched in silico miRNAs associated with the prognostic significance in the TCGA_PAAD cohort and reported that a five miRNA signature had a strong prognostic value [7]. Unfortunately, they used the uncurated cohort. As a consequence, when these miRNAs were assessed in the pure PDAC cohort, they lost their prognostic significance (mir-203 as an example, Figure 4d).

2.5. Web-Based Application to Query the Curated TCGA-PAAD Dataset

In order to quickly assess the prognostic significance of a gene in the curated TCGA_PPAD, we developed a web-based application [8]. The application requires a gene symbol and displays survival curves by splitting patients into groups depending on their level of expression of the selected gene, if it is available in the TCGA_PAAD RNAseq data. The patients are either separated in two groups, low versus high, or separated by a given percentile cut, 50% by default. In this splitting case, all 144 patients were used for the survival analysis. The patients could have also been divided by *interval* in which only the patients with the highest expression levels would be shown against the patients with the lowest levels of expression of the analyzed gene. By default, the upper quartile (>75%) was shown against the lower quartile (<25%). In both types of survival analysis, the *p*-value of a log-rank test was shown, as well as the median survival in each group. The log-rank test *p*-value and the Hazard Ratio of the continuous gene expression level were also shown.

3. Discussion

Clinical validation of their findings is often a bottleneck step for basic scientific laboratories. Consortium efforts such as those of the TCGA and the ICGC have been a tremendous help for this purpose. In addition, it facilitated alternative approaches based on in silico discovery completed by clinical validation. Here, we presented a thorough analysis of the TCGA dataset, which was dedicated to pancreatic neoplasms and highlighted the heterogeneity of the data sources and samples. In addition, we demonstrated that the curation of this dataset led to the exclusion of almost 20% of the cases but was a mandatory step, as it prevented false results on prognostic analyses.

TCGA data may be retrieved through numerous platforms. Confusion for researchers may arise from the fact that while data for a particular sample are homogeneous across all platforms, the list of available samples is heterogeneous with little to no information on the sample of most platforms. In addition, while the genomic data for a sample may be exploitable, the RNAseq data may not. The TCGA data portal provided the most comprehensive information on the nature of the samples, but it required a deeper exploration within the platform to find it. Due to most platforms providing the official clinical data, but not a detailed manifest of the samples analyzed, it is important to retrieve the final list of "good samples" and to only assess these, a function available on some platforms but not all.

In the TCGA_PAAD, there were three main reasons for sample exclusion. The first reason, valid across all the data (DNA, RNA, etc.) was the histology of the tumors. PDAC have a well-described biology (mutational and transcriptional patterns) and a clinical behavior, which is very distinct from other pancreatic neoplasm such as neuroendocrine neoplasms (NEN), acinar cell carcinomas or intraductal papillary neoplasm (IPMN). Well-differentiated NEN for instance, have a completely different mutational and transcriptional pattern from PDAC and a much longer survival rate. Therefore, any alteration specific to PDAC will artificially see its prognostic value increased. The second reason was that the sample analyzed was not a tumor. It was either a normal pancreas or from a PDAC-look alike histological lesion, often atrophic fibrosis with a stroma-like appearance. These patients had a prolonged survival compared to PDAC patients. As a result, the prognostic value was strongly biased in any alteration present in PDAC. Finally, for one sample, the single nucleotide variation data were not available (TCGA-L1-A7W4-01).

Peran et al. compared the clinical characteristics of the TCGA_PAAD cohort with that of the SEER and the national cancer database and reported that the TCGA_PAAD cohort had less locally advanced and metastatic tumors and therefore a much better chance of survival [5]. This highlights another potential bias in the cohorts required for this type of multi-omics analyses. As they require frozen tumor material, the cohorts usually include only surgical specimens. This is an important bias for PDAC as only 15% of patients present with a resectable tumor. In addition, only large tumors have frozen material set apart usually, leading to a nonconsecutive series. Yet, when comparing the pure-PDAC TCGA cohort with our large multicentric consecutive cohort, we have found few differences, except for the median tumor size and therefore a slightly worse overall survival. This confirmed the clinical validity of the curated cohort for prognostic studies.

The importance of the curation is also highlighted by the massive prognostic bias introduced by the samples (tumor or non-tumor) with a different molecular profile from the PDAC and a prolonged survival. We observed that many molecular alterations (gene mutation, mRNA or miRNA aberrant expression level) had a prognostic value only in the uncurated cohort. This is not surprising as most of these were absent from the good prognostic non-PDAC subgroup. Improper data curation led to the description of many PDAC prognostic factors that lost their value in the curated dataset [9,10].

This is in line with the study of Peran et al. that described on a limited number of genes how the use of a curated cohort led to the loss of their prognostic value.

We therefore developed a free web-based app to quickly assess the prognostic value (progression-free and overall survival) of the expression of any gene on the curated dataset. This is to our knowledge the only "click and play" tool to reliably assess the prognostic value of any gene using either a cut off based on the median expression value or any interval, and retrieve the survival and expression data.

4. Patients and Methods

4.1. Data Query from the Main Data Repository

The following data repository were queried to retrieve a sample list and biological annotations, whole normalized level 3 RNAseq and miRNA data, specific DNA mutation data (*KRAS*, *TP53*, *SMAD4*) and clinical data: TCGA (https://gdc.cancer.gov), the Broad Institute (https://gdac.broadinstitute.org), the University of California Santa Cruz (http://xena.ucsc.edu), cBioportal (http://www.cbioportal.org) and the Human Protein Atlas (https://www.proteinatlas.org). The sample list and the clinical data used in the TCGA group publication were also retrieved from the supplemental data [5].

4.2. Data from the Multicenter Ductal Adenocarcinoma Cohort

For comparison with the TCGA_PAAD cohort, we used a previously published cohort of 471 consecutive patients who underwent curative intent surgery for PDAC at 5 university centers between September 1996 and August 2009. Subjects were excluded if they had received preoperative treatment and macroscopically incomplete resection (R2) or if their tumor histology was not a ductal adenocarcinoma. Patients who died of postoperative complications within 30 days following surgery were also excluded.

4.3. Data Analysis

Survival analyses with gene expression were performed in R using the *survival* package. The gene expression or miRNA expression association to survival was evaluated by fitting a Cox proportional hazards regression model. The explanatory variable of the survival model fitted for each gene was either the continuous expression values or the discretized expression value (e.g., below versus over the median expression). The association to survival in the curated or uncurated cohorts was assessed for 17,302 genes. For each of them, the p-value of the log-rank test was retrieved and corrected using the Benjamini-Hochberg multiple comparison approach for controlling the false discovery rate. When defining the number of prognostic genes, the log-rank test was used and adjusted to obtain a False Discovery Rate of 5%.

Clinical characteristics of the two cohorts were compared using a Chi2-based test of equal proportions for discrete variables and a Student's t-test for continuous variables.

Survival curves were drawn using the *ggsurv* function from the *GGally* R package.

4.4. Web Based App

A web app to associate gene expression to overall and progression-free survival in the 144 TCGA patients (6 of the 150 curated sample/patient pair had missing clinical data for effective PFS analysis) is available at [8] (executable code available: [11]).

The TCGA data used for the application were obtained from the Broad's Institute firehose portal (https://gdac.broadinstitute.org, 20,160,128 release). The PDAC survival web application can be used to associate gene expression to overall and progression-free survival in three different ways: by splitting the series of patients into two subseries around a gene expression threshold (e.g., median), by separating the series of patients into two extremes intervals (e.g., upper quartile vs. lower quartile) or by directly associating the continuous gene expression values to the survival. For the splitting and interval analysis, the thresholds can be modified by the user which will update the results accordingly. Kaplan-Meier curves are used and the log-rank test p-values are shown. In addition, the raw survival and gene expression values are shown in order to let anyone reuse the curated data with any software.

5. Conclusions

In conclusion, we highlighted in this study the heterogeneity of the data available through the main repositories and the lack of a proper sample description leading to the inclusion in many studies dedicated to PDAC of non-PDAC tumor samples or even non-tumor samples. We confirmed that it introduced a major bias in biomarker prognostic value analysis and we provided a comprehensive list of the curated dataset together with a free web-based app to assess on the curated dataset the prognostic value of gene expression levels.

Supplementary Materials: The following are available online at http://www.mdpi.com/2072-6694/11/1/126/s1, Table S1: TCGA_PAAD sample list and biological nature of the samples, Table S2: Comparison of genes associated with PFS and OS in the uncurated and the curated TCGA_PAAD cohorts.

Author Contributions: Conceptualization, R.N. and J.C.; formal analysis, R.N. and Y.B.; funding acquisition, V.P. and A.C.; investigation, J.R.; methodology, R.N., V.P., A.d.R and Y.B.; resources, J.R. and A.C.; software, R.N.; supervision, J.C.; writing—original draft, J.C.; writing—review and editing, R.N., J.R., V.P., A.C., A.d.R., Y.B. and J.C.

Funding: J.R. was supported by the Nelia and Amadeo Foundation. J.C. was supported by the Soldati foundation.

Conflicts of Interest: The authors declare no conflicts of interest.

References

1. Bosman, F.T.; Carneiro, F.; Hruban, R.H.; Theise, N.D. World Health Organization Classification Tumors. In *Pathology and Genetics of Tumors of the Digestive System*, 4th ed.; IARC Press: Lyon, France, 2010.
2. Scarpa, A.; Chang, D.K.; Nones, K.; Corbo, V.; Patch, A.-M.; Bailey, P.; Lawlor, R.T.; Johns, A.L.; Miller, D.K.; Mafficini, A.; et al. Whole-genome landscape of pancreatic neuroendocrine tumours. *Nature* **2017**, *543*, 65–71. [CrossRef] [PubMed]
3. Jäkel, C.; Bergmann, F.; Toth, R.; Assenov, Y.; van der Duin, D.; Strobel, O.; Hank, T.; Klöppel, G.; Dorrell, C.; Grompe, M.; et al. Genome-wide genetic and epigenetic analyses of pancreatic acinar cell carcinomas reveal aberrations in genome stability. *Nat Commun.* **2017**, *8*, 1323. [CrossRef] [PubMed]
4. Cancer Genome Atlas Research Network. Integrated Genomic Characterization of Pancreatic Ductal Adenocarcinoma. *Cancer Cell* **2017**, *32*, 185–203.e13. [CrossRef] [PubMed]
5. Peran, I.; Madhavan, S.; Byers, S.W.; McCoy, M.D. Curation of the Pancreatic Ductal Adenocarcinoma Subset of the Cancer Genome Atlas Is Essential for Accurate Conclusions about Survival-Related Molecular Mechanisms. *Clin. Cancer Res.* **2018**, *24*, 3813–3819. [CrossRef] [PubMed]
6. Maréchal, R.; Bachet, J.-B.; Mackey, J.R.; Dalban, C.; Demetter, P.; Graham, K.; Couvelard, A.; Svrcek, M.; Bardier-Dupas, A.; Hammel, P.; et al. Levels of gemcitabine transport and metabolism proteins predict survival times of patients treated with gemcitabine for pancreatic adenocarcinoma. *Gastroenterology* **2012**, *143*, 664–674.e1-6. [CrossRef] [PubMed]
7. Shi, X.-H.; Li, X.; Zhang, H.; He, R.-Z.; Zhao, Y.; Zhou, M.; Pan, S.-T.; Zhao, C.-L.; Feng, Y.-C.; Wang, M.; et al. A Five-microRNA Signature for Survival Prognosis in Pancreatic Adenocarcinoma based on TCGA Data. *Sci. Rep.* **2018**, *8*, 7638. [CrossRef]
8. CIT—Gene Expression and Survival in the TCGA_PAAD Dataset. Available online: http://cit-apps.ligue-cancer.net/pancreatic_cancer/pdac.survival (accessed on 21 January 2019).
9. Hu, H.; Han, T.; Zhuo, M.; Wu, L.-L.; Yuan, C.; Wu, L.; Lei, W.; Jiao, F.; Wang, L.-W. Elevated COX-2 Expression Promotes Angiogenesis Through EGFR/p38-MAPK/Sp1-Dependent Signalling in Pancreatic Cancer. *Sci. Rep.* **2017**, *7*, 470. [CrossRef]

10. Li, H.; Wang, X.; Fang, Y.; Huo, Z.; Lu, X.; Zhan, X.; Deng, X.; Peng, C.; Shen, B. Integrated expression profiles analysis reveals novel predictive biomarker in pancreatic ductal adenocarcinoma. *Oncotarget* **2017**, *8*, 52571–52583. [CrossRef]

11. CIT—Gene Expression and Survival in the TCGA_PAAD Dataset (Executable Code). Available online: https://github.com/cit-bioinfo/TCGA_PAAD_survival (accessed on 21 January 2019).

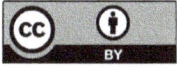

Article

Histopathological Imaging–Environment Interactions in Cancer Modeling

Yaqing Xu [1], Tingyan Zhong [2], Mengyun Wu [3,* and Shuangge Ma [1,*]

[1] Department of Biostatistics, Yale University, New Haven, CT 06520, USA; yaqing.xu@yale.edu
[2] SJTU-Yale Joint Center for Biostatistics, Department of Bioinformatics and Biostatistics,
    School of Life Sciences and Biotechnology, Shanghai Jiao Tong University,
    Shanghai 200240, China; tyzhong@sjtu.edu.cn
[3] School of Statistics and Management, Shanghai University of Finance and Economics,
    Shanghai 200433, China
* Correspondence: wu.mengyun@mail.shufe.edu.cn (M.W.); shuangge.ma@yale.edu (S.M.)

Received: 26 February 2019; Accepted: 19 April 2019; Published: 24 April 2019

Abstract: Histopathological imaging has been routinely conducted in cancer diagnosis and recently used for modeling other cancer outcomes/phenotypes such as prognosis. Clinical/environmental factors have long been extensively used in cancer modeling. However, there is still a lack of study exploring possible interactions of histopathological imaging features and clinical/environmental risk factors in cancer modeling. In this article, we explore such a possibility and conduct both marginal and joint interaction analysis. Novel statistical methods, which are "borrowed" from gene–environment interaction analysis, are employed. Analysis of The Cancer Genome Atlas (TCGA) lung adenocarcinoma (LUAD) data is conducted. More specifically, we examine a biomarker of lung function as well as overall survival. Possible interaction effects are identified. Overall, this study can suggest an alternative way of cancer modeling that innovatively combines histopathological imaging and clinical/environmental data.

Keywords: cancer modeling; interaction; histopathological imaging; clinical/environmental factors

---

1. Introduction

Cancer is extremely complex. Extensive statistical investigations have been conducted, modeling various cancer outcomes/phenotypes. A long array of measurements from different domains have been used in cancer modeling, including clinical/environmental factors, socioeconomic factors, omics (genetic, genomic, epigenetic, proteomic, etc.) measurements, histopathological imaging features, and others. However, none of the existing models is completely satisfactory, and it remains a challenging task to develop new ways of cancer modeling.

Imaging has been playing an irreplaceable role in cancer practice and research [1]. It is routine for radiologists to use Computed Tomography (CT), Magnetic Resonance Imaging (MRI), Positron Emission Computed Tomography (PET), and other techniques to generate radiological images, which can inform the size, location, and other "macro" features of tumors [2]. Biopsies are ordered, and pathologists review the slides of representative sections of tissues to make definitive diagnosis. This procedure generates histopathological (diagnostic) images [3]. Through microscopically examining small pieces of tissues, more "micro" features of tumors are obtained. Histopathological images have been used as the gold standard for diagnosis. More recently, histopathological imaging features have also been used to model other cancer outcomes/phenotypes. For example, in [4], they were used for predicting the prognosis of estrogen receptor-negative breast cancer, and a multivariate Cox regression was adopted. In [5], histopathological imaging features were used in a k-nearest neighbor classifier to assign images into different groups of Gleason tumor grading for prostate cancer patients.

With the complexity of cancer, a single domain of measurement is insufficient, and measurements from multiple sources are needed in modeling [6]. In the literature, histopathological imaging features and clinical/environmental risk factors have been combined in an additive manner for modeling cancer outcomes. In [7], for modeling lung cancer prognosis, clinical factors (including age, gender, cancer type, smoking history, and tumor stage) were combined with imaging features in a multivariate Cox regression model. This study and those alike have shown that combining the two sources of information are more informative than a single source. Our literature review suggests that most if not all of the existing studies have considered the additive effects of histopathological imaging features and clinical/environmental factors, and *studies that accommodate their interactions (referred to as "I–E" interactions, with "I" and "E" standing for imaging and clinical/environmental factors, in this study) are lacking*. Statistically, adding interactions when the main-effect models are not fully satisfactory is "normal". Biologically speaking, incorporating such interactions have been partly motivated by the success of gene–environment (G–E) interactions. Specifically, in the literature, the biological rationale and practical success of G–E interactions have been well established [8]. Cancer is a genetic disease. Histopathological images reflect essential information on the histological organization and morphological characteristics of tumor cells and their surrounding tumor microenvironment, which are heavily regulated by tumors' molecular features. As such, from G–E interactions, we may naturally derive I–E interactions. It is noted that I–E and G–E interaction analyses cannot replace each other. More specifically, not all genetic information is contained in imaging features, and histopathological features, as reflected in imaging data, are also affected by factors other than molecular changes.

This study has also been partly motivated by the ineffectiveness of techniques adopted in the existing studies. Histopathological images contain rich information, and the number of extracted features can be quite large, posing analytic challenges. This dimension problem is "brutally" handled in some studies. For example, in [9], the univariate Cox model was fit to each imaging feature, and those with the strongest marginal effects were selected. Such features were then used along with clinical characteristics, including age, gender, smoking status, and tumor stage, to construct the final prognostic model. When joint modeling is the ultimate goal, the aforementioned approach may miss truly important signals in the first step of screening. To accommodate the high dimensionality in joint modeling, penalization and other regularization techniques have been adopted. For example, in [10], the elastic net approach, which combines the Lasso and ridge penalties, was used along with Cox regression. With the differences between interactions and main effects, such methods cannot be directly applied to analysis that accommodates I–E interactions. There are also studies that use advanced deep learning techniques. For example, Bychkov and others [11] used the CNN (convolutional neural network) technique to predict colorectal cancer prognosis based on images of tumor tissue samples. Other examples also include [12,13]. Such deep learning techniques may excel in prediction, however, usually lack interpretations and also suffer from a lack of stability when sample size is small.

The main objective of this article is to explore accommodating I–E interactions in cancer modeling. Although the concept may seem simple, such an interaction analysis has not been conducted in the literature. The adopted statistical methods have been "borrowed" from G–E interaction analysis. With the connectedness between genetic and histopathological imaging features and parallelization of G–E and I–E interaction analysis, such a strategy is sensible. The proposed interaction analysis strategy and methods are demonstrated using the The Cancer Genome Atlas (TCGA) lung adenocarcinoma data. Overall, this study may suggest an alternative way of utilizing histopathological imaging data and modeling cancer more accurately.

2. Data

We demonstrate I–E interaction analysis using the TCGA lung cancer data. TCGA is a collective effort organized by lNational Cancer Institute (NCI) and has published comprehensive data, especially on outcomes/phenotypes, clinical/environmental measures, and histopathological images, for lung and other cancer types. Lung cancer is the leading cause of cancer death globally [14], and lung adenocarcinoma (LUAD) is the most common histological subtype and has posed increasing public concerns [15]. The TCGA LUAD data has been analyzed in multiple published studies, including [7,9], who analyzed histopathological images, and [16,17], who conducted analysis on clinical/environmental factors. Thus, it is of interest to "continue" these studies on main additive effects and further examine potential I–E interactions with the TCGA LUAD data. It also has the advantage of having a relatively larger sample size, which is critical to achieve meaningful findings. It is noted that the proposed analysis can be directly applied to data on other cancer types.

We acquire 541 whole slide histopathology images from the TCGA ldata portal [18]. To extract imaging features, we adopt the following pipeline developed by Luo and others [9]. First, as the size of the whole slide images, which is from 300 Mb up to 2 Gb with 110,000 × 70,000 pixels, is too huge to be analyzed directly, each image is cropped into sub-images with 500 × 500 pixels and saved as tiff image files using the Openslide Python library. Analyzing all the sub-images (more than 10 million image tiles in total) is still computationally unfeasible. Thus, twenty representative tiff sub-images that contain mostly (>50%) regions of interest are randomly selected as input for the following process. It is expected that the randomly selected sub-images are representative samples for the overall "population" of sub-images. Such cropping and random selection are common steps in whole slide image processing and widely adopted in published imaging studies [10,19–21]. It is noted that randomly selecting sub-images may lead to imaging features with very small differences (and so affect downstream analysis). However, as our main goal is cancer model building, as opposed to feature selection, such small differences may not be of major concern.

Second, we adopt *CellProfiler* [22], a platform designed for cell image processing and used in quite a few recent publications, to extract quantitative features from each sub-image. Specifically, image colors are separated based on hematoxylin and eosin staining, and converted to grayscale for extracting regional features. Next, cell nuclei are detected and segmented so that cell-level features can be specifically measured. Other features such as regional occupation, area fraction, and neighboring architecture are also captured. Irrelevant features such as file size and execution information are excluded from analysis. This procedure results in a total of 772 features which are categorized into the texture, geometry, and holistic groups. Specifically, the texture group contains Haralick, Gabor "wavelet", and Granularity features, which are classic image processing features, measure the texture properties of cells and tissues, and have been examined in a large number of imaging studies. The geometry group contains features that describe the geometry properties (such as area, perimeter, and so on), and those extracted by Zernike moments. The holistic group contains holistic statistics that describe overall information, such as the total area, perimeter and number of nuclei, and nuclear staining area fraction.

Third, for each patient, the features of images are normalized using sample mean at the patient level. Missing values (with a missing rate lower than 20%) are imputed using sample medians.

For clinical/environmental risk factors, we consider age, American Joint Committee on Cancer tumor pathologic stage, tobacco smoking history indicator, and sex. These variables have been suggested as associated with multiple lung cancer outcomes/phenotypes, including those analyzed in this article [23]. In particular, Nordquis and others [24] found that the mean age at diagnosis of lung adenocarcinoma among never-smokers was significantly higher than that among current smokers, and the never-smokers with lung adenocarcinoma were predominantly female. Studies have shown that tobacco smoking is responsible for 90% of lung cancer [25], and has been identified as a negative prognostic factor for lung adenocarcinoma [26]. In addition, these factors have also been considered in G–E interaction analysis [27].

Multiple outcome variables have been analyzed in the literature [7]. In this article, we consider two important response variables: (a) FEV1: the reference value for the pre-bronchodilator forced expiratory volume in one second in percent. It is an important biomarker for lung capacity. It is continuously distributed, with mean 80.28 and interquartile range [67.00, 96.25]. Data is available for 132 subjects; and (b) overall survival, which is subject to right censoring. Data is available for 271 subjects, among whom 102 died during follow-up. The mean observed time is 27.47 months, with interquartile range [14.06, 35.00].

The adopted feature extraction process follows [9], where the extracted imaging features were used to predict lung cancer prognosis. Similar processes have also been adopted in other publications [10,19]. Different from limited histopathological features recognized visually by pathologists, CellProfiler extracted features are morphological features of tissue texture, cells, nuclei, and neighboring architecture. These features are extracted and measured by comprehensive computer algorithms, and are impossible to be assessed by human eyes. As demonstrated in [9], quantitative imaging features provide objective and rich information contained in images that can reveal hidden information to decode tumor development and progression in lung cancer. Following the literature [9,20,21], we adopt feature names automatically assigned by CellProfiler, as can be partly seen in Tables 1–4. These names provide a brief description of the extracted information with the general form "Compartment_FeatureGroup_Feature_Channel_Parameters". For example, features "AreaShape_MedianRadius" and "AreaShape_MaximumRadius" measure the median and maximum radius of the identified tissue, respectively. As in some recent studies [9,20,21], in this study, our goal is not to identify specific imaging features as markers and make biological interpretations. Instead, we aim to conduct better cancer modeling by incorporating I–E interactions. As such, although they may not have simple, explicit biological interpretations, these features are sensible for our analysis.

3. Methods

In parallel to G–E interaction analysis [28], we conduct two types of I–E interaction analysis, namely marginal and joint analysis. The overall flowchart of analysis is provided in Figure 1. In marginal analysis, one imaging feature, one clinical/environmental variable (or multiple such variables), and their interaction are analyzed at a time. In joint analysis, all imaging features, all clinical/environmental variables, and their interactions are analyzed in a single model. The two types of analysis have their own pros and cons and cannot replace each other. We refer to the literature [29,30] for more detailed discussions on the two types of analysis.

First, consider a continuous cancer outcome, which matches the FEV1 analysis. Denote Y as the length N vector of outcome, where N is the sample size. Denote $\mathbf{E} = [E_1, \cdots, E_J]$ as the $N \times J$ matrix of clinical/environmental variables, and $\mathbf{X} = [X_1, \cdots, X_K]$ as the $N \times K$ matrix of imaging features. As represented by the LUAD data, usually clinical/environmental variables are pre-selected and low-dimensional, and imaging features are high-dimensional.

3.1. Marginal Analysis

Detailed discussions of marginal G–E interaction analysis are available in [31] and other recent literature. The marginal I–E interaction analysis proceeds as follows. First, assume that Y, $\mathbf{E}$, and $\mathbf{X}$ have been properly centered.

(a) For $j = 1, \ldots, J$ and $k = 1, \ldots, K$, consider the linear regression model

$$Y = \alpha_j E_j + \beta_k X_k + \gamma_{jk} E_j X_k + \epsilon, \tag{1}$$

where α_j and β_k respectively represent the main effects of the jth clinical/environmental factor and the kth imaging feature, γ_{jk} is the interactive effect, and ϵ is the random error. A total of $J \times K$ models are built.

(b) As each model has a low dimension, estimates can be obtained using standard likelihood based approaches and existing software. p-values can be obtained accordingly.

(c) Interactions (and main effects) with small *p*-values are identified as important. When more definitive conclusions are needed, the false discovery rate (FDR) or Bonferroni approach can be applied.

It is noted that, in Step (a), one clinical/environmental variable is analyzed in each model, which follows [31]. It is also possible to accommodate all clinical/environmental variables in each model. In Step (c), discoveries can be made on interactions only or interactions and main effects combined. Advantages of marginal analysis include its computational simplicity and stability. On the negative side, with the complexity of cancer, an outcome/phenotype is usually associated with multiple imaging features and clinical/environmental variables. As such, each marginal model can be "mis-specified" or "suboptimal". In addition, there is a lack of attention to the differences between interactions and main effects.

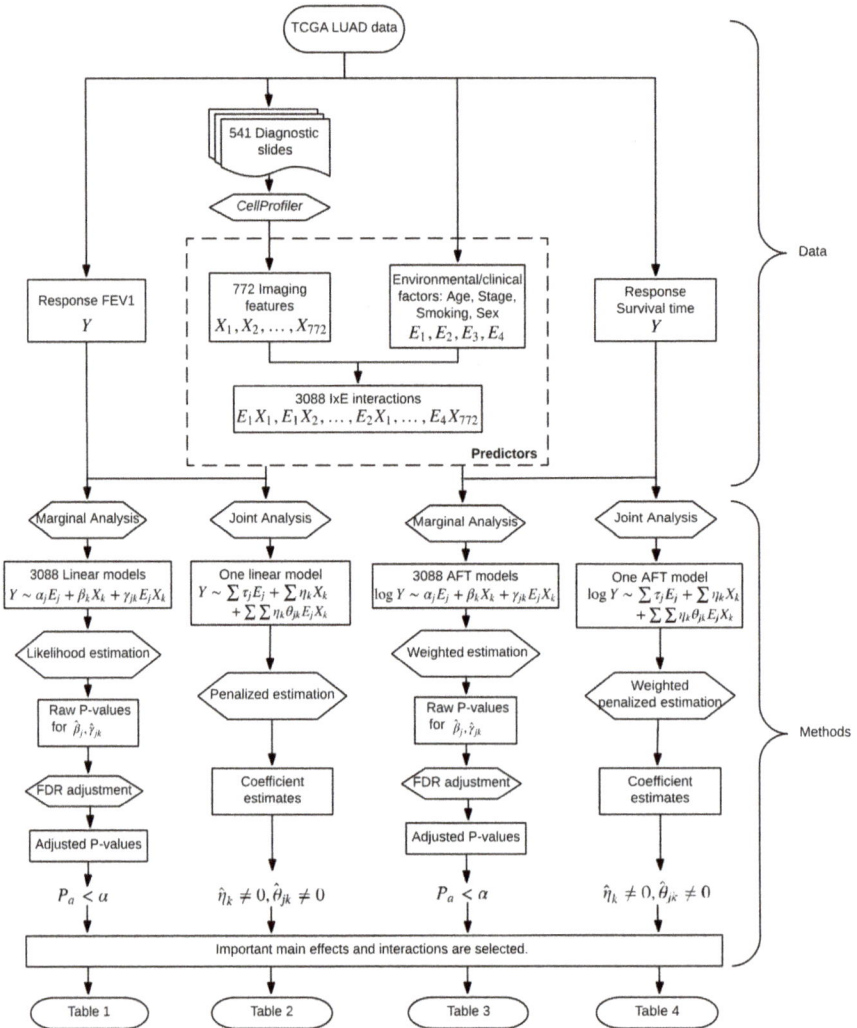

Figure 1. Flowchart of the I–E interaction analysis of The Cancer Genome Atlas (TCGA) lung adenocarcinoma (LUAD) data.

3.2. Joint Analysis

Joint analysis can tackle some limitations of marginal analysis, and is getting increasingly popular in statistical and bioinformatics literature. It proceeds as follows.

(a) Consider the joint model

$$Y = \sum_{j=1}^{J} \tau_j E_j + \sum_{k=1}^{K} \eta_k X_k + \sum_{j=1}^{J} \sum_{k=1}^{K} \eta_k \theta_{jk} E_j X_k + \epsilon, \tag{2}$$

where τ_j and η_k are the main effects of the jth environmental factor and the kth imaging feature, respectively, and the product of η_k and θ_{jk} corresponds to the interaction.

(b) For estimation, consider the Lasso penalization

$$\min_{\eta_k, \theta_{jk}} ||Y - f(\mathbf{E}, \mathbf{X})||^2 + \lambda_1 \sum_k |\eta_k| + \lambda_2 \sum_j \sum_k |\theta_{jk}|, \tag{3}$$

where $f(\mathbf{E}, \mathbf{X}) = \sum_j \tau_j E_j + \sum_k \eta_k X_k + \sum_j \sum_k \eta_k \theta_{jk} E_j X_k$, and $\lambda_1, \lambda_2 > 0$ are tuning parameters. In numerical study, we select the tuning parameters using the extended Bayesian information criterion [32].

(c) Interactions (and main effects) with nonzero estimates are identified as being associated with the outcome.

3.3. Accommodating Survival Outcomes

Consider cancer survival. Denote T as the N-vector of survival times. Below, we describe joint analysis, and marginal analysis can be conducted accordingly. We adopt the AFT (accelerated failure time) model, under which

$$\log(T) = \sum_{j=1}^{J} \tau_j E_j + \sum_{k=1}^{K} \eta_k X_k + \sum_{j=1}^{J} \sum_{k=1}^{K} \eta_k \theta_{jk} E_j X_k + \epsilon, \tag{4}$$

where notations have similar implications as in the above section. With high-dimensional data, the AFT model has been widely adopted because of its lucid interpretation and more importantly computational simplicity [33]. Under right censoring, denote C as the N-vector of censoring times, $Y = \log(\min(T, C))$, and $\delta = I(T \leq C)$, where operations are taken component-wise. To accommodate censoring, a weighted approach is adopted. Assume that data have been sorted according to Y_i's from the smallest to the largest. The Kaplan–Meier weights can be computed as $w_1 = \dfrac{\delta_1}{N}$, $w_i = \dfrac{\delta_i}{N-i+1} \prod_{j=1}^{i-1} \left(\dfrac{N-j}{N-j+1} \right)^{\delta_j}, i = 2, \ldots, N$. Similar to Equation (3), consider the penalized estimation

$$\min_{\eta_k, \theta_{jk}} ||\sqrt{w} \times (Y - f(\mathbf{E}, \mathbf{X}))||^2 + \lambda_1 \sum_k |\eta_k| + \lambda_2 \sum_j \sum_k |\theta_{jk}|, \tag{5}$$

where the square root and multiplication are taken component-wise. Interpretations and other operations are the same as for continuous outcomes.

In joint analysis, the most prominent challenge is the high dimensionality. Here, the penalization technique is adopted, which can simultaneously accommodate high dimensionality and identify relevant interactions/main effects. Another feature of this analysis that is worth highlighting is that it respects the "main effects, interactions" hierarchy. That is, if an I–E interaction is identified, the corresponding main imaging feature effect is automatically identified. It has been suggested that, statistically and biologically, it is critical to respect this hierarchy [34]. We refer to the literature [35,36] for alternative penalization and other joint interaction analysis methods. Compared to marginal analysis, joint analysis can be computationally more challenging, and well-developed software packages are still limited. In addition, the analysis results can be less stable.

The proposed analysis can be effectively realized. To facilitate data analysis within and beyond this study, we have developed R code and made it publicly available at www.github.com/shuanggema.

4. Results

4.1. Analysis of FEV1

4.1.1. Marginal Analysis

After the FDR adjustment, none of the main effects or interactions are statistically significant. In Table 1, we present the main effects and interactions with the smallest (unadjusted) p-values. The top ranked main effects are from the Geometry and Texture groups, and the top ranked interactions are from the Geometry group and with sex.

Based on the analysis results, we conduct a power calculation. First, assume the current levels of estimated effects and their variations. Then, with a sample size of 224, the top ranked I–E interactions can be identified as significant with target FDR 0.1. Second, consider the current sample size and levels of variations. Then, an effect of -0.35 can be identified as significant with target FDR 0.1.

For comparison, we conduct the analysis of main effects (without interactions). The top eight main effects (with the smallest p-values) have four overlaps with those in Table 1, suggesting that accommodating interactions can lead to different findings.

Table 1. Marginal analysis of the reference value for the pre-bronchodilator forced expiratory volume in one second in percent (FEV1): identified main effects and interactions, with raw p-values P_r.

Feature Group	Feature Name		Estimate	P_r
Geometry	AreaShape_Zernike_2_2	Main	0.270	0.002
Geometry	AreaShape_Zernike_5_3	Main	−0.319	0.001
Geometry	Mean_Identifyhemasub2_AreaShape_Zernike_9_9	Main	−0.259	0.004
Geometry	Median_Identifyhemasub2_AreaShape_Zernike_7_1	Main	−0.249	0.005
Geometry	Median_Identifyhemasub2_AreaShape_Zernike_8_6	Main	−0.272	0.003
Texture	StDev_Identifyeosinprimarycytoplasm_Texture_Correlation_maskosingray_3_01	Main	0.280	0.002
Geometry	StDev_Identifyhemasub2_AreaShape_Zernike_8_8	Main	−0.251	0.005
Geometry	StDev_Identifyhemasub2_AreaShape_Zernike_9_1	Main	−0.259	0.004
Geometry	StDev_Identifyhemasub2_AreaShape_Center_Y	Sex	0.291	0.002
Geometry	StDev_Identifyhemasub2_AreaShape_Zernike_8_2	Sex	0.304	0.001
Geometry	StDev_Identifyhemasub2_Location_Center_Y	Sex	0.294	0.002

4.1.2. Joint Analysis

The analysis results are provided in Table 2. A total of 11 imaging features are identified, representing the Geometry and Texture groups. A total of 11 interactions are identified, with all four clinical/environmental variables.

For comparison, we consider the joint model with all clinical/environmental variables and imaging features but no interactions. Lasso penalization is applied for selection and estimation. A total of eight imaging features are identified, with one overlapping with those in Table 2. We further compute the RV coefficient, which may more objectively quantify the amount of "overlapping information" between two analyses. Specifically, it measures the "correlation" between two data matrices of important effects identified by two different approaches, with a larger value indicating higher similarity. The RV coefficient is 0.24, suggesting a mild level of overlapping.

A significant advantage of joint analysis is that it can lead to a predictive model for the outcome variable. We conduct the evaluation of prediction based on a resampling procedure, which may provide support to the validity of analysis. Specifically, we split data into a training and a testing set, generate estimates using the training data, and make predictions for the testing set subjects. The PMSE (prediction mean squared error) is then computed. This procedure is repeated 100 times, and the mean PMSE is computed. The I–E interaction model has a mean PMSE of 0.84, whereas the main-effect-only model has a mean PMSE of 1.12. This significant improvement suggests the benefit of accommodating interactions.

Table 2. Joint analysis of FEV1: identified main effects and interactions.

Feature Group	Feature Name	Main	Age	Stage	Smoking	Sex
			−0.049	−0.052	−0.002	0.006
Geometry	AreaShape_Zernike_2_2	0.163	0.040	−0.014	−0.185	
Geometry	AreaShape_Zernike_5_3	−0.053				
Geometry	AreaShape_Zernike_6_0	−0.034				
Texture	Granularity_10_ImageAfterMath	0.137	0.110	−0.020		0.064
Geometry	Location_Center_X	0.002				
Geometry	Mean_Identifyeosinprimarycytoplasm_Location_Center_X	0.005				
Geometry	Median_Identifyhemasub2_AreaShape_Zernike_7_1	−0.127	−0.073		0.072	0.003
Geometry	StDev_Identifyhemasub2_AreaShape_Zernike_8_2	−0.170		−0.083		0.188
Texture	StDev_Identifyhemasub2_Granularity_6_ImageAfterMath	−0.029				
Texture	Texture_AngularSecondMoment_ImageAfterMath_3_00	−0.044				
Texture	Texture_AngularSecondMoment_ImageAfterMath_3_03	−0.010				

4.2. Analysis of Overall Survival

4.2.1. Marginal Analysis

The analysis results are provided in Table 3, where we present estimates, raw *p*-values, as well as the FDR adjusted *p*-values. Three imaging features from the Holistic group have the FDR adjusted *p*-values < 0.1. In addition, 36 imaging features from the Geometry group and 24 features from the Texture group are identified as having interactions with Smoking, the most important environmental factor for lung cancer. Compared to the above analysis, more "signals" are identified. Note that the effective sample size is smaller than that above. As such, the smaller *p*-values are likely to be caused by stronger signals.

For comparison, we conduct the analysis of main effects. One imaging feature is identified as having FDR adjusted *p*-value < 0.1, which is also identified in Table 3. With the complexity of lung cancer prognosis, the interaction analysis, which identifies more effects, can be more sensible.

4.2.2. Joint Analysis

The analysis results are provided in Table 4. A total of 31 imaging features are identified, representing the three feature groups. Two imaging features are identified as interacting with two and four clinical/environmental variables, respectively.

The analysis of main effects is conducted using the Lasso penalization. A total of two imaging features are identified, with one overlapping with those in Table 4. The RV coefficient is computed as 0.40, representing a moderate level of overlapping. As with FEV1, prediction evaluation is also conducted based on resampling. For the testing set, subjects are classified into low and high risk groups with equal sizes based on the predicted survival times, where subjects with predicted survival times larger than the median are classified into the low risk group. For one resampling of training and testing sets, in Figure 2, we plot the Kaplan–Meier curves estimated using the observed survival times for the predicted low and high risk groups, along with those generated under the additive main-effect model. Compared to the main-effect model, it is obvious that the two risk groups identified by the I–E interaction model have a much clearer separation of the survival functions, indicating better prediction performance. To be more rigorous, we further conduct a logrank test, which is a nonparametric test for comparing the survival distributions of two subject groups. With 100 resamplings, the average logrank statistics are 7.28 (I–E interaction model, *p*-value = 0.007) and 0.99 (main-effect model, *p*-value = 0.320), respectively. The superior prediction performance of the I–E interaction models suggests that incorporating interactions can lead to clinically more powerful models, justifying the value of the proposed analysis.

Table 3. Marginal analysis of overall survival: identified main effects and interactions, with raw *p*-values P_r and false discovery rate (FDR) adjusted *p*-values P_a.

Feature Group	Feature Name		Estimate	P_r	P_a
Holistic	Threshold_FinalThreshold_Identifyeosinprimarycytoplasm	Main	-0.301	0	0.095
Holistic	Threshold_OrigThreshold_Identifyeosinprimarycytoplasm	Main	-0.301	0	0.095
Holistic	Threshold_WeightedVariance_identifyhemaprimarynuclei	Main	-0.360	0	0.077
Geometry	AreaShape_Area	Smoking	0.253	0.004	0.078
Geometry	AreaShape_MaximumRadius	Smoking	0.266	0.004	0.074
Geometry	AreaShape_MeanRadius	Smoking	0.265	0.005	0.079
Geometry	AreaShape_MedianRadius	Smoking	0.266	0.005	0.079
Geometry	AreaShape_MinFeretDiameter	Smoking	0.257	0.003	0.073
Geometry	AreaShape_MinorAxisLength	Smoking	0.264	0.002	0.07
Geometry	AreaShape_Zernike_4_4	Smoking	-0.241	0.005	0.079
Geometry	AreaShape_Zernike_7_3	Smoking	-0.308	0	0.027
Geometry	AreaShape_Zernike_8_4	Smoking	-0.242	0.007	0.096
Geometry	AreaShape_Zernike_8_6	Smoking	-0.252	0.005	0.079
Geometry	AreaShape_Zernike_9_1	Smoking	-0.303	0	0.027
Texture	Granularity_13_ImageAfterMath.1	Smoking	-0.317	0.001	0.054
Texture	Mean_Identifyeosinprimarycytoplasm_Texture_Correlation_maskosingray_3_03	Smoking	0.232	0.005	0.079
Geometry	Mean_Identifyhemasub2_AreaShape_Area	Smoking	0.297	0.001	0.049
Geometry	Mean_Identifyhemasub2_AreaShape_MaximumRadius	Smoking	0.318	0.001	0.049
Geometry	Mean_Identifyhemasub2_AreaShape_MeanRadius	Smoking	0.318	0.001	0.049
Geometry	Mean_Identifyhemasub2_AreaShape_MedianRadius	Smoking	0.308	0.002	0.054
Geometry	Mean_Identifyhemasub2_AreaShape_MinFeretDiameter	Smoking	0.299	0.001	0.049
Geometry	Mean_Identifyhemasub2_AreaShape_MinorAxisLength	Smoking	0.310	0.001	0.045
Geometry	Mean_Identifyhemasub2_AreaShape_Zernike_4_4	Smoking	-0.263	0.003	0.07
Geometry	Mean_Identifyhemasub2_AreaShape_Zernike_5_1	Smoking	-0.268	0.002	0.07
Geometry	Mean_Identifyhemasub2_AreaShape_Zernike_8_2	Smoking	-0.277	0.003	0.073
Geometry	Mean_Identifyhemasub2_AreaShape_Zernike_8_8	Smoking	-0.290	0.003	0.073
Geometry	Mean_Identifyhemasub2_AreaShape_Zernike_9_1	Smoking	-0.226	0.004	0.074
Texture	Mean_Identifyhemasub2_Granularity_13_ImageAfterMath	Smoking	-0.325	0.001	0.054
Texture	Mean_Identifyhemasub2_Texture_Correlation_ImageAfterMath_3_01	Smoking	0.330	0	0.039
Texture	Mean_Identifyhemasub2_Texture_Correlation_ImageAfterMath_3_02	Smoking	0.297	0.002	0.07
Texture	Mean_Identifyhemasub2_Texture_Correlation_ImageAfterMath_3_03	Smoking	0.397	0	0.01
Texture	Mean_Identifyhemasub2_Texture_SumVariance_ImageAfterMath_3_02	Smoking	0.258	0.007	0.093
Texture	Median_Identifyeosinprimarycytoplasm_Texture_Correlation_maskosingray_3_03	Smoking	0.233	0.004	0.079
Geometry	Median_Identifyhemasub2_AreaShape_Area	Smoking	0.344	0	0.027
Geometry	Median_Identifyhemasub2_AreaShape_MaxFeretDiameter	Smoking	0.242	0.005	0.079
Geometry	Median_Identifyhemasub2_AreaShape_MaximumRadius	Smoking	0.323	0.001	0.049
Geometry	Median_Identifyhemasub2_AreaShape_MeanRadius	Smoking	0.323	0.001	0.049
Geometry	Median_Identifyhemasub2_AreaShape_MedianRadius	Smoking	0.266	0.005	0.079
Geometry	Median_Identifyhemasub2_AreaShape_MinFeretDiameter	Smoking	0.346	0	0.027
Geometry	Median_Identifyhemasub2_AreaShape_MinorAxisLength	Smoking	0.342	0	0.027
Geometry	Median_Identifyhemasub2_AreaShape_Perimeter	Smoking	0.247	0.006	0.085
Geometry	Median_Identifyhemasub2_AreaShape_Zernike_4_4	Smoking	-0.242	0.002	0.059
Geometry	Median_Identifyhemasub2_AreaShape_Zernike_5_1	Smoking	-0.256	0.003	0.073
Texture	Median_Identifyhemasub2_Granularity_13_ImageAfterMath	Smoking	-0.311	0.001	0.049
Texture	Median_Identifyhemasub2_Texture_Correlation_ImageAfterMath_3_01	Smoking	0.319	0.001	0.049
Texture	Median_Identifyhemasub2_Texture_Correlation_ImageAfterMath_3_02	Smoking	0.274	0.005	0.081
Texture	Median_Identifyhemasub2_Texture_Correlation_ImageAfterMath_3_03	Smoking	0.394	0	0.01
Texture	StDev_Identifyeosinprimarycytoplasm_Texture_SumAverage_maskosingray_3_00	Smoking	0.272	0.003	0.073
Texture	StDev_Identifyeosinprimarycytoplasm_Texture_SumAverage_maskosingray_3_01	Smoking	0.273	0.003	0.073
Texture	StDev_Identifyeosinprimarycytoplasm_Texture_SumAverage_maskosingray_3_02	Smoking	0.270	0.004	0.074
Texture	StDev_Identifyeosinprimarycytoplasm_Texture_SumAverage_maskosingray_3_03	Smoking	0.275	0.003	0.073
Geometry	StDev_identifyhemaprimarynuclei_Location_Center_Y	Smoking	-0.245	0.007	0.093
Geometry	StDev_Identifyhemasub2_AreaShape_Zernike_8_4	Smoking	-0.280	0.001	0.045
Geometry	StDev_Identifyhemasub2_AreaShape_Zernike_8_8	Smoking	-0.236	0.007	0.094
Texture	StDev_Identifyhemasub2_Texture_SumVariance_ImageAfterMath_3_01	Smoking	0.266	0.007	0.096
Texture	StDev_Identifyhemasub2_Texture_SumVariance_ImageAfterMath_3_02	Smoking	0.283	0.005	0.079
Texture	StDev_Identifyhemasub2_Texture_SumVariance_ImageAfterMath_3_03	Smoking	0.283	0.006	0.084
Geometry	StDev_identifytissueregion_Location_Center_Y	Smoking	-0.289	0.002	0.059
Texture	Texture_Correlation_ImageAfterMath_3_01	Smoking	0.252	0.004	0.078
Texture	Texture_Correlation_ImageAfterMath_3_03	Smoking	0.329	0	0.027
Texture	Texture_Correlation_maskosingray_3_03	Smoking	0.237	0.004	0.074
Texture	Texture_Entropy_ImageAfterMath_3_01	Smoking	0.220	0.007	0.093
Texture	Texture_Entropy_ImageAfterMath_3_03	Smoking	0.233	0.004	0.074

4.3. Simulation

Comparatively, joint analysis is newer and has been less conducted. To gain more insights into the validity of findings from our joint interaction analysis, we conduct a set of data-based simulation. Specifically, the observed imaging features and clinical/environmental factors are used. To generate variations across simulation replicates, we use resampling, with sample sizes set as 200. The "signals" and their levels are set as those in Tables 2 and 4, respectively. For both the continuous and (log) survival outcomes, we generate random errors from $N(0,1)$. For the survival setting, we generate the censoring times from randomly sampling the observed. The Lasso-based penalization approach is then applied, with tuning parameters selected using the extended Bayesian information criterion (BIC) approach. To evaluate identification, TP (true positive) and FP (false positive) values are computed.

Summary statistics are computed based on 100 replicates. Under the continuous outcome setting, there are 11 true main effects and 11 I–E interactions. For main effects, the TP and FP values are 9.75 (1.65) and 3.15 (1.39), respectively, where numbers in "()" are standard deviations. For interactions, the TP and FP values are 7.35 (0.99) and 0.05 (0.22), respectively. Under the censored survival outcome setting, there are 31 true main effects and 6 I–E interactions. For main effects, the TP and FP values are 24.41 (3.98) and 13.90 (2.47), respectively. For interactions, the TP and FP values are 3.24 (0.21) and 0.24 (0.12), respectively. Overall, at the estimated signal levels and with the observed feature distributions, the joint analysis is capable of identifying the majority of true interactions and main effects, with a moderate number of false discoveries. This provides a high level of confidence to the joint interaction analysis.

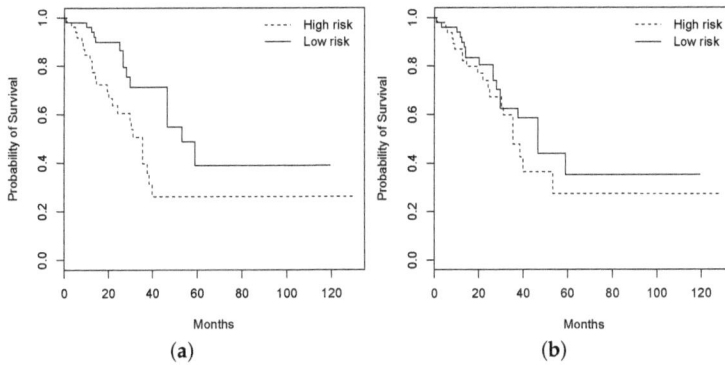

(a)   (b)

Figure 2. Kaplan–Meier curves of high and low risk groups identified by the approach that accommodates interactions ((**a**); logrank test *p*-value 0.007) and the one with main effects only ((**b**); logrank test *p*-value 0.320).

Table 4. Joint analysis of overall survival: identified main effects and interactions.

Feature Group	Feature Name	Main	Age	Stage	Smoking	Sex
			−0.024	−0.317	−0.038	−0.088
Geometry	AreaShape_Zernike_6_0	−0.038				
Geometry	AreaShape_Zernike_6_4	−0.019				
Geometry	AreaShape_Zernike_6_6	0.052				
Geometry	AreaShape_Zernike_9_3	0.027				
Geometry	AreaShape_Zernike_9_5	0.153				
Texture	Granularity_10_ImageAfterMath.1	−0.033				
Texture	Granularity_9_ImageAfterMath	0.081				
Geometry	Mean_Identifyhemasub2_AreaShape_Center_X	0.002				
Geometry	Mean_Identifyhemasub2_AreaShape_Zernike_5_1	0.013				
Geometry	Mean_Identifyhemasub2_AreaShape_Zernike_6_2	−0.002				
Geometry	Mean_Identifyhemasub2_AreaShape_Zernike_6_4	−0.010				
Geometry	Mean_Identifyhemasub2_AreaShape_Zernike_9_9	−0.146				
Geometry	Mean_Identifyhemasub2_Location_Center_X	0.002				
Geometry	Mean_identifytissueregion_Location_Center_X	0.056				
Geometry	Median_Identifyeosinprimarycytoplasm_Location_Center_X	−0.071				
Geometry	Median_Identifyhemasub2_AreaShape_Zernike_4_0	0.023				
Geometry	Median_Identifyhemasub2_AreaShape_Zernike_7_3	0.083				
Geometry	Median_Identifyhemasub2_AreaShape_Zernike_8_4	−0.120				
Geometry	Median_Identifyhemasub2_AreaShape_Zernike_8_6	−0.098				
Geometry	Median_Identifyhemasub2_AreaShape_Zernike_9_1	−0.044				
Geometry	Median_identifytissueregion_Location_Center_Y	−0.063				
Holistic	Neighbors_SecondClosestDistance_Adjacent	−0.170		−0.072	0.002	
Geometry	StDev_Identifyeosinprimarycytoplasm_Location_Center_Y	0.095				
Texture	StDev_Identifyeosinprimarycytoplasm_Texture _DifferenceVariance_maskosingray_3_00	0.036				
Geometry	StDev_Identifyhemasub2_AreaShape_Orientation	−0.159				
Geometry	StDev_Identifyhemasub2_AreaShape_Zernike_8_8	−0.146				
Texture	StDev_Identifyhemasub2_Granularity_12_ImageAfterMath	−0.101				
Texture	StDev_Identifyhemasub2_Granularity_13_ImageAfterMath	0.327	0.130	0.072	−0.189	0.174
Texture	StDev_Identifyhemasub2_Granularity_9_ImageAfterMath	0.003				
Texture	StDev_Identifyhemasub2_Texture_SumVariance _ImageAfterMath_3_01	−0.034				
Geometry	StDev_identifytissueregion_Location_Center_Y	0.016				

5. Discussion

Histopathological imaging analysis has been routine in cancer diagnosis, and recently, its application in the analysis of cancer biomarkers, outcomes, and phenotypes has been explored. This study has taken a natural next step and conducted the imaging-environment interaction analysis. Statistically and biologically speaking, the analysis has been partly motivated by G–E interaction analysis. It is noted that the statistical methods themselves have been almost fully "translated" from G–E interaction analysis. As I–E interaction analysis has not been conducted in published cancer modeling studies, it is sensible to first employ well-developed methods, and in the future, methods that are more tailored to imaging data may be developed. We also note that in cancer modeling and other biomedical fields, it is not uncommon to apply methods well developed in one field to other new fields. The proposed I–E interaction analysis, especially joint analysis, may seem considerably more complex than some cancer modeling approaches. With the complexity of cancer, models with a few variables and simple statistical analysis are getting increasingly insufficient. Published studies have suggested that advanced statistical techniques and complex models are needed. Recent developments for lung cancer, including the elastic net-Cox analysis [10], deep convolutional neural network [13], and deep network based on convolutional and recurrent architectures [11], have comparable or higher levels of complexity compared to the proposed analysis. Artificial intelligence (AI) techniques, which have been recently used for cancer modeling in particular including the radiomics analysis of non-small-cell lung cancer [37,38], have even higher levels of complexity. We conjecture that such complexity will also be needed for future developments in cancer modeling using imaging data. The increasing complexity in cancer modeling seems to be an inevitable trend, and domain specific expertise is a must for such analysis.

We have analyzed the TCGA LUAD data with a continuous and a censored survival outcome. This choice has been motivated by the clinical importance of lung adenocarcinoma as well as data availability (a larger sample size). It is noted that the proposed analysis and R program will be directly applicable to the analysis of data on other cancer types. I–E interactions have been identified in both marginal and joint analysis, for both FEV1 and overall survival. There is one prominent difference between imaging and genetic/clinical data. With extensive investigations and functional experiments, the biological and biomedical implications of most clinical/environmental factors and genes are at least partially known. It is thus possible to evaluate whether G–E interactions are biologically sensible. The circumstance is significantly different for histopathological imaging features. The rationale and algorithms for feature extraction have been made clear in the developments of CellProfiler and other software. However, the identified features do not have lucid biological interpretations. As such, we are not able to objectively assess the biological implications of the findings in Tables 1–4. It is noted that this limitation is also shared by recently published imaging studies [9,20,21], which have unambiguously demonstrated the great value of such imaging features in cancer modeling. It is also noted that imaging features derived from computer-aided pathological analysis have the unique advantage of being objective and comprehensive, and can reveal hidden information contained in histopathological images that cannot be recognized or assessed by pathologists. Our statistical evaluations, including the prediction evaluation and data-based simulation, can provide support to the analysis results to a great extent. In general, more investigations into the biological implications of the computer-program-extracted imaging features will be needed.

This study has suggested a new venue for cancer modeling. Although findings made on LUAD may not be applicable to other cancers, the analysis technique and R program will be broadly applicable. Following the flowchart in Figure 1 and detailed steps described in this article, and using the publicly available R program, cancer biostatisticians and clinicians should be able to carry out the proposed analysis with their own data. More specifically, with their own clinical/environmental and imaging data, they will be able to construct models for prognosis and other outcomes/phenotypes. Such models, as other cancer models (for example those using omics data), can be used to assist clinical decision making. Overall, this study may help advance the challenging field of cancer modeling.

6. Conclusions

Histopathological imaging data may harbor important information on cancer and has been recently used for modeling cancer clinical outcomes and phenotypes. This study has been the first to examine the interactions between imaging features and clinical/environmental risk factors in cancer modeling. Marginal and joint analysis approaches have been described. In the analysis of TCGA LUAD data, it has been shown that I–E interactions may be important for modeling FEV1 and overall survival. Overall, this study has suggested a new paradigm of cancer bioinformatics modeling.

Author Contributions: All authors contributed to conceptualization, methodology, and writing. T.Z. conducted data processing. Y.X. performed data analysis and simulation.

Funding: This work was supported by the NIH (R01CA204120, P50CA196530); the Yale Cancer Center Pilot Award; the National Natural Science Foundation of China (91546202, 71331006); and the Bureau of Statistics of China (2018LD02).

Acknowledgments: We thank the editor and reviewers for their careful review and insightful comments, which have led to a significant improvement of this article.

Conflicts of Interest: The authors declare no conflict of interest.

References

1. Fass, L. Imaging and cancer: A review. *Mol. Oncol.* **2008**, *2*, 115–152. [CrossRef]
2. Benzaquen, J.; Boutros, J.; Marquette, C.; Delingette, H.; Hofman, P. Lung cancer screening, towards a multidimensional approach: Why and how? *Cancers* **2019**, *11*, 212. [CrossRef]
3. Gurcan, M.N.; Boucheron, L.; Can, A.; Madabhushi, A.; Rajpoot, N.; Yener, B. Histopathological image analysis: A review. *IEEE Rev. Biomed. Eng.* **2009**, *2*, 147–171. [CrossRef] [PubMed]
4. Yuan, Y.; Failmezger, H.; Rueda, O.M.; Ali, H.R.; Gräf, S.; Chin, S.F.; Schwarz, R.F.; Curtis, C.; Dunning, M.J.; Bardwell, H.; et al. Quantitative image analysis of cellular heterogeneity in breast tumors complements genomic profiling. *Sci. Transl. Med.* **2012**, *4*, 157ra143. [CrossRef]
5. Tabesh, A.; Teverovskiy, M.; Pang, H.Y.; Kumar, V.P.; Verbel, D.; Kotsianti, A.; Saidi, O. Multifeature prostate cancer diagnosis and Gleason grading of histological images. *IEEE Trans. Med. Imaging* **2007**, *26*, 1366–1378. [CrossRef]
6. Zhong, T.; Wu, M.; Ma, S. Examination of independent prognostic power of gene expressions and histopathological imaging features in cancer. *Cancers* **2019**, *11*, 361. [CrossRef] [PubMed]
7. Wang, H.; Xing, F.; Su, H.; Stromberg, A.; Yang, L. Novel image markers for non-small cell lung cancer classification and survival prediction. *BMC Bioinform.* **2014**, *15*, 310. [CrossRef]
8. Hunter, D.J. Gene–environment interactions in human diseases. *Nat. Rev. Genet.* **2005**, *6*, 287–298. [CrossRef]
9. Luo, X.; Zang, X.; Yang, L.; Huang, J.; Liang, F.; Rodriguez-Canales, J.; Wistuba, I.I.; Gazdar, A.; Xie, Y.; Xiao, G. Comprehensive computational pathological image analysis predicts lung cancer prognosis. *J. Thorac. Oncol.* **2017**, *12*, 501–509. [CrossRef]
10. Yu, K.H.; Zhang, C.; Berry, G.J.; Altman, R.B.; Ré, C.; Rubin, D.L.; Snyder, M. Predicting non-small cell lung cancer prognosis by fully automated microscopic pathology image features. *Nat. Commun.* **2016**, *7*, 12474. [CrossRef] [PubMed]
11. Bychkov, D.; Linder, N.; Turkki, R.; Nordling, S.; Kovanen, P.E.; Verrill, C.; Walliander, M.; Lundin, M.; Haglund, C.; Lundin, J. Deep learning based tissue analysis predicts outcome in colorectal cancer. *Sci. Rep.* **2018**, *8*, 3395. [CrossRef] [PubMed]
12. Zhu, X.; Yao, J.; Zhu, F.; Huang, J. Wsisa: Making survival prediction from whole slide histopathological images. In Proceedings of the IEEE Conference on Computer Vision and Pattern Recognition, Honolulu, HI, USA, 21–26 July 2017; pp. 7234–7242.
13. Coudray, N.; Ocampo, P.S.; Sakellaropoulos, T.; Narula, N.; Snuderl, M.; Fenyö, D.; Moreira, A.L.; Razavian, N.; Tsirigos, A. Classification and mutation prediction from non–small cell lung cancer histopathology images using deep learning. *Nat. Med.* **2018**, *24*, 1559–1567. [CrossRef]
14. Boolell, V.; Alamgeer, M.; Watkins, D.; Ganju, V. The evolution of therapies in non-small cell lung cancer. *Cancers* **2015**, *7*, 1815–1846. [CrossRef] [PubMed]

15. Cancer Genome Atlas Research Network. Comprehensive molecular profiling of lung adenocarcinoma. *Nature* **2014**, *511*, 543–550. [CrossRef] [PubMed]

16. Karlsson, A.; Ringner, M.; Lauss, M.; Botling, J.; Micke, P.; Planck, M.; Staaf, J. Genomic and transcriptional alterations in lung adenocarcinoma in relation to smoking history. *Clin. Cancer Res.* **2014**, *20*, 4912–4924. [CrossRef]

17. Li, X.; Shi, Y.; Yin, Z.; Xue, X.; Zhou, B. An eight-miRNA signature as a potential biomarker for predicting survival in lung adenocarcinoma. *J. Transl. Med.* **2014**, *12*, 159. [CrossRef]

18. The Cancer Genome Atlas Data Portal Website. Available online: https://portal.gdc.cancer.gov/projects/TCGA-LUAD (accessed on 23 April 2019).

19. Yu, K.; Berry, G.J.; Rubin, D.L.; Re, C.; Altman, R.B.; Snyder, M. Association of omics features with histopathology patterns in lung adenocarcinoma. *Cell Syst.* **2017**, *5*, 620–627. [CrossRef] [PubMed]

20. Zhu, X.; Yao, J.; Luo, X.; Xiao, G.; Xie, Y.; Gazdar, A.F.; Huang, J. Lung cancer survival prediction from pathological images and genetic data-an integration study. In Proceedings of the 2016 IEEE 13th International Symposium on Biomedical Imaging, Prague, Czech Republic, 13–16 April 2016.

21. Sun, D.; Li, A.; Tang, B.; Wang, M. Integrating genomic data and pathological images to effectively predict breast cancer clinical outcome. *Comput. Methods Progr. Biomed.* **2018**, *161*, 45–53. [CrossRef] [PubMed]

22. Soliman, K. CellProfiler: Novel automated image segmentation procedure for super-resolution microscopy. *Biol. Proced. Online* **2015**, *17*, 11. [CrossRef]

23. Westcott, P.M.; Halliwill, K.D.; To, M.D.; Rashid, M.; Rust, A.G.; Keane, T.M.; Delrosario, R.; Jen, K.Y.; Gurley, K.E.; Kemp, C.J.; et al. The mutational landscapes of genetic and chemical models of Kras-driven lung cancer. *Nature* **2015**, *517*, 489–492. [CrossRef]

24. Nordquist, L.; Simon, G.; Cantor, A.; Alberts, W.; Bepler, G. Improved survival in never-smokers vs current smokers with primary adenocarcinoma of the lung. *Chest* **2004**, *126*, 347–351. [CrossRef]

25. Bryant, A.; Cerfolio, R. Differences in epidemiology, histology, and survival between cigarette smokers and never-smokers who develop non-small cell lung cancer. *Chest* **2008**, *132*, 185–192. [CrossRef]

26. Landi, M.; Dracheva, T.; Rotunno, M.; Figueroa, J.; Liu, H.; Dasgupta. A.; Mann, F.; Fukuoka, J.; Hames, M.; Bergen, A.; et al. Gene expression signature of cigarette smoking and its role in lung adenocarcinoma development and survival. *PLoS ONE* **2008**, *3*, e1651. [CrossRef]

27. Wu, M.; Zang, Y.; Zhang, S.; Huang, J.; Ma, S. Accommodating missingness in environmental measurements in gene–environment interaction analysis. *Genet. Epidemiol.* **2017**, *41*, 523–554. [CrossRef]

28. Wu, M.; Ma, S. Robust genetic interaction analysis. *Brief. Bioinform.* **2018**. [CrossRef]

29. Zhang, Y.; Dai, Y.; Zheng, T.; Ma, S. Risk factors of non-Hodgkin's lymphoma. *Expert Opin. Med. Diagn.* **2011**, *5*, 539–550. [CrossRef]

30. Witten, D.M.; Tibshirani, R. Survival analysis with high-dimensional covariates. *Stat. Methods Med. Res.* **2010**, *19*, 29–51. [CrossRef]

31. Xu, Y.; Wu, M.; Zhang, Q.; Ma, S. Robust identification of gene–environment interactions for prognosis using a quantile partial correlation approach. *Genomics* **2018**. [CrossRef]

32. Chen, J.; Chen, Z. Extended Bayesian information criteria for model selection with large model spaces. *Biometrika* **2008**, *95*, 759–771. [CrossRef]

33. Huang, J.; Ma, S.; Xie, H. Regularized estimation in the accelerated failure time model with high-dimensional covariates. *Biometrics* **2006**, *62*, 813–820. [CrossRef] [PubMed]

34. Choi, N.H.; Li, W.; Zhu, J. Variable selection with the strong heredity constraint and its oracle property. *J. Am. Stat. Assoc.* **2010**, *105*, 354–364. [CrossRef]

35. Bien, J.; Taylor, J.; Tibshirani, R. A lasso for hierarchical interactions. *Ann. Stat.* **2013**, *41*, 1111–1141. [CrossRef] [PubMed]

36. Liu, J.; Huang, J.; Zhang, Y.; Lan, Q.; Rothman, N.; Zheng, T.; Ma, S. Identification of gene–environment interactions in cancer studies using penalization. *Genomics* **2013**, *102*, 189–194. [CrossRef] [PubMed]

37. Hosny, A.; Parmar, C.; Quackenbush, J.; Schwartz, L.H.; Aerts, H. Artificial intelligence in radiology. *Nat. Rev. Cancer* **2018**, *18*, 500–510. [CrossRef] [PubMed]
38. Thrall, J.; Li, X.; Li, Q.; Cruz, C.; Do, S.; Dreyer, K.; Brink, J. Artificial intelligence and machine learning in radiology: Opportunities, challenges, pitfalls, and criteria for success. *J. Am. Coll. Radiol.* **2018**, *15*, 504–508. [CrossRef] [PubMed]

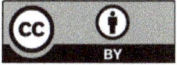

cancers

MDPI

Article

Examination of Independent Prognostic Power of Gene Expressions and Histopathological Imaging Features in Cancer

Tingyan Zhong [1], Mengyun Wu [2],* and Shuangge Ma [3],*

[1]   SJTU-Yale Joint Center for Biostatistics, Department of Bioinformatics and Biostatistics, School of Life
     Sciences and Biotechnology, Shanghai Jiao Tong University, Shanghai 200240, China; tyzhong@sjtu.edu.cn
[2]   School of Statistics and Management, Shanghai University of Finance and
     Economics, Shanghai 200433, China
[3]   Department of Biostatistics, Yale University, New Haven, CT 06520, USA
*   Correspondence: wu.mengyun@mail.shufe.edu.cn (M.W.); shuangge.ma@yale.edu (S.M.)

Received: 12 February 2019; Accepted: 10 March 2019; Published: 13 March 2019

Abstract: Cancer prognosis is of essential interest, and extensive research has been conducted searching for biomarkers with prognostic power. Recent studies have shown that both omics profiles and histopathological imaging features have prognostic power. There are also studies exploring integrating the two types of measurements for prognosis modeling. However, there is a lack of study rigorously examining whether omics measurements have independent prognostic power conditional on histopathological imaging features, and vice versa. In this article, we adopt a rigorous statistical testing framework and test whether an individual gene expression measurement can improve prognosis modeling conditional on high-dimensional imaging features, and a parallel analysis is conducted reversing the roles of gene expressions and imaging features. In the analysis of The Cancer Genome Atlas (TCGA) lung adenocarcinoma and liver hepatocellular carcinoma data, it is found that multiple individual genes, conditional on imaging features, can lead to significant improvement in prognosis modeling; however, individual imaging features, conditional on gene expressions, only offer limited prognostic power. Being among the first to examine the independent prognostic power, this study may assist better understanding the "connectedness" between omics profiles and histopathological imaging features and provide important insights for data integration in cancer modeling.

Keywords: cancer prognosis; independent prognostic power; omics profiles; histopathological imaging features

---

1. Introduction

In cancer research and practice, prognosis is of essential interest. Extensive statistical modeling has been conducted, and yet there is still much room for additional research [1,2]. Multiple families of biomarkers have been used in cancer prognosis modeling. In the past decades, with the development of profiling techniques, omics data have been extensively used and shown to be effective. For example, in [3], a signature composed of 21 gene expressions is used for modeling breast cancer prognosis. In [4], hsa-mir-155 and hsa-let-7a-2 microRNAs are found as prognostic for lung cancer. In [5], the prognostic power of methylated RASSF1A and/or APC serum DNA for breast cancer is identified. Such findings are biologically highly sensible as cancer is a genetic disease and the development and progression of cancer are strongly affected by molecular changes.

Imaging techniques have been extensively used in cancer practice. In particular, for definitive diagnosis, biopsies are usually ordered, and pathologists review the slides of representative sections of tissues. The histopathological imaging data generated in this process directly reflect the histological organization and morphological characteristics of tumor cells and their surrounding tumor microenvironment. More recently, beyond diagnosis, histopathological imaging data have also been used for modeling other cancer outcomes/phenotypes. For example, Harpole et al. [6] showed that the levels of tumor cell dedifferentiation are associated with survival outcomes. Automated histopathological imaging analysis systems have been shown to be effective in the prognostic determination of various malignancies, including breast cancer [7], neuroblastoma [8], lymphoma [9], nonsmall cell lung cancer [10], precancerous lesions in the esophagus [11], and others.

Omics profiles and histopathological images are biologically connected and contain overlapping information. In particular, properties of tumors and their microenvironment, as described in histopathological images, are highly regulated by molecular changes. Multiple statistical modelings have been conducted on their interconnections. For example, Yu et al. [10] found the correlation of quantitative histopathological features with TP53 mutation in lung adenocarcinoma. Cooper et al. [12] demonstrated that PDGFRA, EGFR, and MDM2 amplifications are associated with imaging features such as greater minor axis length, area, and circularity in glioblastoma.

On the other hand, it is also possible that omics profiles and histopathological images may contain independent information. Tissues used to generate omics measurements are usually heterogeneous and mixtures of different components, making the observed omics measurements represent an aggregation of distinct cells [12]. Histopathological images, with extremely high spatial resolutions, also contain information on tissue relationships and characteristics of the spatial organizations of tumor cells. Features of histopathological images, beyond regulated by molecular changes, may also be affected by personal immune system, microenvironment, and other factors. There are a few recent studies integrating omics measurements and imaging features and showing that such a data integration can lead to improved prognosis modeling for breast cancer [13], brain tumor [14], and nonsmall cell lung cancer [15]. Such studies seem to suggest that there is independent information in omics and histopathological imaging data.

Our literature review suggests that there is a lack of study rigorously quantifying whether omics profiles contain independent information, conditional on histopathological images, on cancer prognosis, and vice versa. It is noted that the aforementioned and other data integration studies do not suggest which type of measurement has independent information. In addition, they are mostly estimation-based and do not have a rigorous statistical inference framework. Some studies rely on prescreening to accommodate high data dimensionality and can be statistically limited. This study is conducted to directly tackle these problems. It can advance from the existing literature in multiple aspects. Specifically, it delivers an analysis pipeline which has a rigorous statistical inference framework and can show whether individuals of a type of measurement have additional prognostic power conditional on the other type of measurement. It can provide solid evidence on whether data integration is needed in modeling and clinical practice. In addition, data analysis may also provide further insights into two deadly cancers.

2. Data

The Cancer Genome Atlas (TCGA) is one of the largest and most comprehensive cancer projects, and is organized by the National Cancer Institute (NCI) and National Human Genome Research Institute (NHGRI) [16]. It has published high quality omics data and histopathological images for 33 types of cancer. In this study, we analyze data on lung adenocarcinoma (LUAD) and liver hepatocellular carcinoma (LIHC), both of which have high mortality rates and pose increasing public concerns. They also have relatively larger sample sizes, which is critical for making reliable findings. The proposed analysis can be extended to other cancer types straightforwardly. For omics measurements, we consider gene expressions, which have a central role in cancer prognosis modeling. The response of interest is overall survival time, which is right censored. It is noted that other types of omics measurements, for example protein expressions and microRNAs, and other prognosis outcomes can be analyzed in a similar manner.

2.1. mRNA Gene Expression Measurements

We download the mRNA gene expression data from cBioPortal (http://cbioportal.org), which have been measured using the Illumina Hiseq2000 RNA Sequencing Version 2 analysis platform, and processed and normalized using the RSEM software. We refer to the literature [17,18] and TCGA website for more detailed information on data collection and processing. Data are available on 25,031 gene expression measurements. As the number of cancer-related genes is not expected to be large, we conduct a simple prescreening to reduce the dimensionality and also improve the stability of estimation. Specifically, the top 5000 genes with the largest variances are selected for downstream analysis.

2.2. Histopathological Imaging Features

We download the whole-slide histopathology images directly from the TCGA website (https://portal.gdc.cancer.gov), which are in the svs format. These tissue slides are formalin-fixed, paraffin-embedded slides with which the cell morphology is well-preserved and thus appropriate for image feature recognition. They are captured at 20× or 40× magnification by the Aperio medical scanner. To extract imaging features, we conduct the following three-step preprocessing. The overall flowchart is provided in Figure 1.

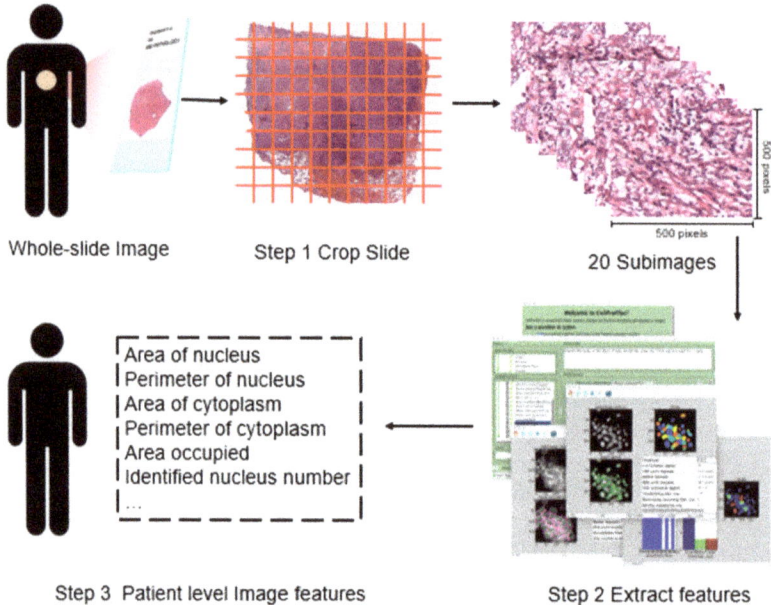

Figure 1. Flowchart of extracting imaging features. Step 1: whole-slide histopathology images are cropped into small subimages of 500 × 500 pixels, and 20 subimages are then randomly selected. Step 2: Imaging features are extracted using CellProfiler [19] for each subimage. Step 3: For each patient, features are averaged.

In the first step, we process the downloaded svs files using the Openslide Python library [20]. Specifically, to make data in an appropriate format for morphological feature extraction, each svs image is cropped into small subimages of 500 × 500 pixels, and each subimage is then saved in the tiff format. Among them, subimages that contain mostly (>50%) background white space are filtered out.

From the remaining subimages, twenty representative ones are randomly selected for each svs image to avoid potential subjective bias and reduce computational cost [21].

In the second step, we use CellProfiler [19] to extract features from each subimage. CellProfiler is an open source cell image analysis platform developed by the Broad Institute. Specifically, image colors are separated based on hematoxylin staining and eosin staining, and converted to grayscale to extract regional features, such as cell and tissue texture and granularity. These are "classic" image processing features, which have been examined in a large number of imaging studies. It is noted that they are not expected to be specific histopathological features, and cannot be recognized by pathologist. More specifically, texture describes a set of metrics calculated in CellProfiler to quantify the perceived texture of histopathological images, and includes information on the spatial arrangement of color or intensities in images. Granularity describes the size of how well the structure element fits in images. Then, cell nuclei are identified and segmented to collect the cell-level features, such as cell size, shape, distribution, and texture of nuclei. Other cell features such as regional occupation, area fraction, and neighboring architecture are also captured. The above process generates 832 features for each subimage. A further screening is conducted to exclude irrelevant features such as file size and execution information. Finally, for each subimage, a total of 772 features are available for analysis.

In the third step, for each slide, the average feature values over twenty representative subimages are computed. When a subject has multiple slides, the average values over multiple slides are further computed for downstream analysis.

The above preprocessing is applied to both LUAD and LIHC data. There are missing values in imaging feature data. Subjects with more than 25% missing imaging features are excluded. The remaining missing values are imputed using sample medians.

Remark 1. *We adopt CellProfiler to extract imaging features, which is a popular choice in recent literature. The feature names are automatically provided by CellProfiler. The extracted features represent objective attributes of histopathological images, including the area and perimeter of nucleus and cytoplasm, mean and standard deviation of these measures, and other general image attributes. For each patient, multiple slides and subimages may be available. To extract as much information as possible, we consider multiple slides and subimages simultaneously, and the average values are used to summarize information. A closer examination suggests that they are not explicitly associated with specific histopathological findings, such as cellularity, atypia, anaplasia, nuclear pleomorphism, and some others. However, these attributes have been shown to be associated with pathological stages [7,10] and prognosis [21], and also been used in multiple existing cancer modeling studies [13,15]. For example, Yu et al. [22] show that some of these features are associated with specific subtypes of lung cancer. In this study, our goal is to rigorously quantify independent information in omics profiles and histopathological images for cancer prognosis, as opposed to focusing on specific interpretation of imaging features. As such, these features are sensible for our analysis, although they may not have simple, explicit biological interpretations.*

2.3. Available Data

After data matching, we obtain records on 316 and 358 subjects for LUAD and LIHC, respectively, with 5000 gene expression measurements, 772 imaging features, and survival time. For LUAD, there are 103 deaths during follow-up, with survival times ranging from 0 to 214.77 months (median 6.03 months). For LIHC, there are 121 deaths during follow-up, with survival times ranging from 0 to 120.73 months (median 19.25 months). Summary information of the analyzed subjects is provided in Table 1.

Table 1. Sample characteristics.

Characteristic	LUAD	LIHC
Sample size	316	358
Age at diagnosis: median (range)	66 (39–88)	61 (16–90)
Follow-up: median (range)	6.03 (0–214.77)	19.25 (0–120.73)
Vital status: n (%)		
Alive	213 (67.4%)	233 (65.0%)
Deceased	103 (32.6%)	125 (35.0%)
Sex: n (%)		
Male	144 (45.6%)	242 (67.6%)
Female	172 (54.4%)	116 (32.4%)
Cancer stage: n (%)		
I	180 (57.0%)	166 (46.4%)
II	69 (18.7%)	82 (22.9%)
III	41 (13%)	83 (23.2%)
IV	21 (6.6%)	5 (1.4%)
NA	5 (1.6%)	22 (6.1%)

3. Methods

For describing cancer survival, we use the accelerated failure time (AFT) model. This model has been extensively adopted in cancer studies with high-dimensional variables because of its lucid interpretations and low computational cost [23]. For each gene expression, we consider the prognosis model with its effect along with all imaging features. A statistically rigorous test is then conducted on the gene expression's effect, which can suggest whether this particular gene has independent information for prognosis conditional on the imaging features. Then a parallel analysis is conducted, reversing the roles of gene expressions and imaging features. With a special emphasis on omics and imaging features, clinical factors are not included in the prognosis models.

Consider n independent subjects. For the ith subject, denote $x_i = (x_{i1}, x_{x2}, \ldots, x_{ip})$ and $z_i = (z_{i1}, z_{i2}, \ldots, z_{iq})$ as the p- and q-dimensional vectors of gene expressions and imaging features, T_i and C_i as the logarithm of the event and censoring times. With right censoring, we observe $(y_i = \min(T_i, C_i), \delta_i = I(T_i \leq C_i), x_i, z_i)$.

First consider the analysis with one gene expression and all imaging features. The analysis with one imaging feature and all gene expressions can be conducted in a similar manner and will not be reiterated. For the jth gene expression, consider the following AFT model:

$$T_i = \alpha + x_{ij}\beta_j + z_i\theta_j + \varepsilon_i \tag{1}$$

where α is the intercept, β_j and $\theta_j = (\theta_{j1}, \ldots, \theta_{jq})'$ are the unknown coefficients for the jth gene expression and all imaging features, and ε_i is the random error. A statistical test

$$H_0 : \beta_j = 0 \text{ vs. } H_1 : \beta_j \neq 0$$

can reveal whether x_{ij} is independently associated with T_i given z_i. Here, loosely speaking, a smaller p value can indicate a stronger association/more prognostic power. The analysis is challenging with the high dimensionality of imaging features, which makes the "standard" estimation and inference techniques not applicable. To tackle this problem, we consider a high-dimensional inference approach [24] recently developed under a related but simpler context. Specifically, for estimation, the weighted least squares approach is adopted. Assume that data have been sorted according to y_i's from the smallest to the largest. Then we have the Kaplan–Meier weights defined as

$$w_1 = \frac{\delta_1}{n}, \ w_i = \frac{y_i}{n-i+1} \prod_{j=1}^{i-1} \left(\frac{n-j}{n-j+1} \right)^{\delta_j}, i = 2, \ldots, n,$$

where a further normalization is conducted to make $\sum_{i=1}^{n} w_i = n$. Let $W = \text{diag}\{w_1, w_2, w_3, \ldots, w_n\}$, $x_{.j}$, $z_{.k}$, and y denote the vectors composed of x_{ij}'s, z_{ik}'s, and y_i's, which are weighted normalized such that $\mathbf{1}'Wx_{.j} = 0$, $\mathbf{1}'Wz_{.k} = 0$, and $\mathbf{1}'Wy = 0$, and $Z = (z_{.1}, \ldots, z_{.q})$. With the high data dimensionality, regularized estimation is needed. In addition, not all imaging features are expected to be associated with survival, posing a variable selection problem. Consider the weighted penalized estimation:

$$\begin{cases} \left(\widetilde{\beta}_j^*, \widetilde{\theta}_j \right) = \text{argmin}_{\beta_j, \theta \in R^{1+q}} \left\{ \frac{1}{2n} \| W^{\frac{1}{2}} \left(y - x_{.j}\beta_j - Z\theta_j \right) \|_2^2 + \lambda_0 \sum_{k=1}^{q} \left| \theta_{jk} \right| \right\} \\ \widetilde{b}_j = \text{argmin}_{b_j \in R^q} \left\{ \frac{1}{2n} \| W^{\frac{1}{2}} \left(x_{.j} - Zb_j \right) \|_2^2 + \lambda_1 \sum_{k=1}^{q} \left| b_{jk} \right| \right\} \end{cases}, \tag{2}$$

where $\|\cdot\|_2$ denotes the L_2 norm, $b_j = (b_{j1}, \ldots, b_{jq})'$ is the unknown coefficient vector, and $\lambda_0, \lambda_1 > 0$ are data-dependent tuning parameters for Lasso penalties.

With $\widetilde{\theta}_j$ and $\widetilde{b}_j$, the final estimate $\widetilde{\beta}_j$ of β_j is defined as

$$\widetilde{\beta}_j = \left(\widetilde{x}_{.j}'Wx_{.j} \right)^{-1} \widetilde{x}_{.j}'W\left(y - Z\widetilde{\theta}_j \right), \tag{3}$$

where $\widetilde{x}_{.j} = x_{.j} - Z\widetilde{b}_j$. It has been shown in [24] that $\sqrt{n}\left(\widetilde{\beta}_j - \beta_j \right)$ is asymptotically normal with variance defined as

$$\widetilde{\Sigma}\left(\widetilde{\beta}_j \right) = \frac{1}{n} \left(\widetilde{x}_{.j}'Wx_{.j} \right)^{-1} \widetilde{\Sigma}_1 \left(x_{.j}'W\widetilde{x}_{.j} \right)^{-1},$$

where $\widetilde{\Sigma}_1$ is the sample variance based on $\widetilde{x}_{ij}(y_i - x_{ij}\widetilde{\beta}_j + z_i\widetilde{\theta}_j)$. With this asymptotic normal distribution, the test statistic for $H_0 : \beta_j = 0$ can be defined as

$$\widetilde{\beta}_j / \sqrt{\widetilde{\Sigma}\left(\widetilde{\beta}_j \right)/n},$$

which follows Student's T distribution. The unadjusted p value can then be obtained. When all gene expressions are considered together, to accommodate multiple comparisons, p values are adjusted using the voxel-level false discovery rate approach [25].

An advantage of the above analysis is that it can be realized via simple coding. The most challenging step is the estimation in (2), which can be realized using the R function *glmnet*. The tuning parameters λ_0 and λ_1 are selected using the EBIC approach [26]. To facilitate data analysis in and beyond this study, we have developed R code implementing the proposed approach. To illustrate its usage, we have also provided an example R file with the LUAD data. The code and data are publicly available at http://www.github.com/shuanggema/TestLDHD as well as in Supplementary Materials.

Remark 2. *The effectiveness of the AFT model for cancer prognosis modeling has been well tested. Penalization has been shown effective for screening out irrelevant variables and accommodating high dimensionality. As shown in [24], the estimation (2) can effectively "single out" the effect of the one gene expression. It is noted that, as the gene expression effect is of particular interest, its coefficient is not subject to penalization in estimation. A "byproduct" of penalized estimation is that imaging features associated with prognosis, conditional on the one gene expression effect, are identified, which may assist understanding the associations between imaging features and prognosis as well as the associations between imaging features and gene expressions. The statistical distribution result for the test statistic has been rigorously proved in [24]. The T distribution makes inference very easy.*

4. Results

4.1. Identification of Gene Expressions with Independent Prognostic Power Conditional on Imaging Features

We first apply the analysis approach described above to identify individual gene expressions that have independent prognostic power conditional on the high dimensional histopathological imaging features. With significance level 0.05 as cutoff, 85 genes are identified as significantly associated with prognosis for LUAD. Detailed estimation results are provided in the Table S1. A quick literature search of PubMed suggests that many of the findings have sound biological basis. For top ten representative genes, we provide brief information and references on their associations with lung cancer prognosis in Table 2. For LIHC, we identify 386 genes as significantly associated with prognosis conditional on imaging features. Again, it is found that many of those genes have established evidences of being associated with liver cancer prognosis. Brief information on the representative genes is provided in Table 3. The solid evidences from existing studies provide support to the validity of analysis. To more comprehensively comprehend the identified genes, we examine the genes' functional and biological connections by conducting Gene Ontology (GO) and KEGG pathway enrichment analysis. The processes with the smallest *p* values are presented in Figure 2. It is observed that both LUAD and LIHC have enriched processes associated with cell adhesion. This may result from high-dimensional imaging features capturing more information on cell interaction. The identified genes are also enriched in traditional cancer hallmarks, such as the positive regulation of mitotic cell cycle, proteoglycans in cancer, and extracellular matrix regulation. It is interesting that some immune response-related pathways, such as MHC assembly, are also identified, considering that there are promising developments in immunotherapy for cancer treatment recently.

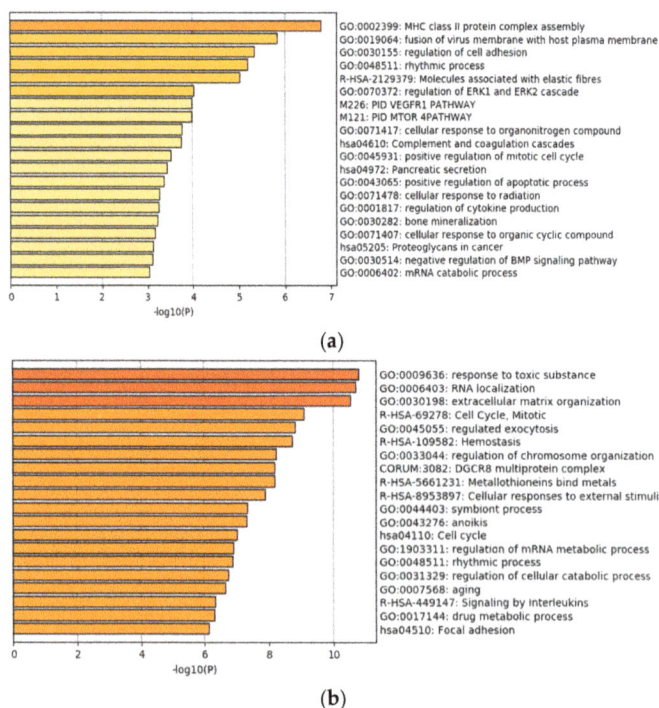

Figure 2. Gene ontology (GO) and pathway enrichment analysis of the identified genes. (**a**) lung adenocarcinoma (LUAD), (**b**) liver hepatocellular carcinoma (LIHC).

It is also noted that the proposed analysis takes an angle different from the literature. As such, there are also new findings. For example, the top ranked genes (with the smallest *p* values) also include DCAF6 and LITAF for LUAD and IARS and LRPPRC for LIHC. Gene DCAF6 is a transcriptional cofactor that enhances androgen receptor (AR)-mediated transcriptional activity. Chen et al. [27] have found that the expression of DCAF6 is upregulated in prostate cancer patient and may be a candidate tumor promoter for prostate cancer, indicating its important role in cancer etiology. For gene LITAF, Zhou et al. [28] have established the regulatory axis of AMPK–LITAF–TNFSF15, where AMPK activation upregulates the transcription of LITAF and consequently upregulates the expression of TNFSF15. TNFSF15 inhibits the growth of prostate cancer cells and bovine aortic endothelial cells in vitro, supporting that LITAF may function as a tumor suppressor. Gene IARS is the coding gene of isoleucyl-tRNA synthetase (ARSs). ARSs has been shown to catalyze the amino acylation of tRNAs by their cognate amino acid, linking amino acids with the correct nucleotide triplets and ensuring the correct transformation of the genetic code to the protein level. Kopajtich et al. [29] have reported that biallelic IARS mutations can cause infantile hepatopathy, suggesting its potential association with liver function. LRPPRC is another interesting gene, which regulates the expression of all mitochondrial DNA-encoded mRNAs, and thus has important contributions to mitochondrial function. Tian et al. [30] have examined the expression of LRPPRC in six types of cancer and observed that LRPPRC plays an important role in tumorigenesis through the resistance to apoptosis and high invasive activity. Other newly identified genes, such as FLS353 [31], IPO7 [32], PDS5A [33], and MPP-2 [34], have also been demonstrated to be related to tumorigenesis. This brief literature search suggests that the implications of these new findings in lung and liver cancer prognosis have not been well established, however, they have been observed to have important contributions to cancer etiology. The new findings are also not surprising. It is conceptually sensible that the strongest "signals" are perhaps reflected in both omics profiles and histopathological images. The proposed analysis seeks for additional "signals" in gene expressions that are not reflected in images. As such, the findings may complement those in the literature.

Table 2. Analysis of LUAD data: representative identified genes.

Gene	Evidence	PMID
HYAL2	Real-time PCR studies showed that HYAL2 genes were down regulated in non-small cell lung cancer [35].	19140316
MAPK1IP1L	MAPK1IP1L gene was found to be related with acquired resistance to MET inhibitors in lung cancer cells [36].	28396363
HLA-DRA	Lack of surface class II expression was found to be associated with a specific defect in HLA-DRA induction in non-small cell lung carcinoma cells [37].	8786310
HNRNPK	Higher levels of hnRNP mRNAs were found in SCLC as compared to NSCLC. hnRNP K protein localization varied with cellular confluence [38].	12871776
GPNMB	Osteoactivin (GPNMB) ectodomain protein was shown to promote growth and invasive behavior of human lung cancer cells [39].	26883195
BMP2	Positive correlation was found between gene expressions of two angiogenic factors, VEGF and BMP-2, in lung cancer patients [40].	19324447
COMMD6	COMMD9 was demonstrated to promote TFDP1/E2F1 transcriptional activity via interaction with TFDP1 in non-small cell lung cancer [41].	27871936
HLA-DRB1	Lung cancer patients in Japan showed an increased frequency of HLA-DRB1*0901 and a decreased frequency of HLA-DRB1*1302 and DRB1*14-related alleles when compared to the other subjects [42].	9808426
LARP1	LARP1 post-transcriptionally regulates mTOR and contributes to cancer progression [43].	25531318
ZAK	ZAK inhibits human lung cancer cell growth via ERK and JNK activation in an AP-1-dependent manner [44].	20331627

* The star is a sign indicating the location of the mutated allel.

Table 3. Analysis of LIHC data: representative identified genes.

Gene	Evidence	PMID
LAPTM4B	LAPTM4B is a potential proto-oncogene, whose overexpression is involved in carcinogenesis and progression of HCC [45].	12902989
CAPZA1	CAPZA1 expression levels were negatively correlated with the biological characteristics of primary HCC and patient prognosis [46].	28093067
PLOD2	PLOD2 expression was identified as a significant, independent factor of poor prognosis for HCC patients [47].	22098155
STIP1	STIP1 was upregulated in HCC and associated with poor clinical prognosis [48].	28887036
IGF1	Inhibition of IGF-1R tyrosine kinase (IGF-1R-TK) by NVP-AEW541 induces growth inhibition, apoptosis and cell cycle arrest in human HCC cell lines without accompanying cytotoxicity [49].	16530734
HTATIP2	HepG2 cells that expressed transgenic HTATIP2 formed more invasive tumors in mice following administration of sorafenib. Sorafenib therapy prolonged recurrence-free survival in patients who expressed lower levels of HTATIP2 compared with higher levels [50].	22922424
GNAI3	GNAI3 inhibits tumor cell migration and invasion and is post-transcriptionally regulated by miR-222 in hepatocellular carcinoma [51].	25444921
XPO1	Exportin-1 (XPO1, CRM1) mediates the nuclear export of several key growth regulatory and tumor suppressor proteins [52].	25030088
PLVAP	PLVAP was identified as a gene specifically expressed in vascular endothelial cells of HCC but not in non-tumorous liver tissues [53].	25376302
EPAS1	HIF-2alpha/EPAS1 expression may play an important role in tumor progression and prognosis of HCC [54].	17589895

Analysis is further conducted to better comprehend the additional prognostic information in gene expressions. Specifically, for each identified gene expression, two AFT models are considered. The first model, referred to as A1, contains the single gene expression as well as selected imaging features; in contrast, the second model, referred to as A2, contains only the selected imaging features. Comparing the two models can straightforwardly describe the contribution of the gene expression to prognosis. To facilitate the comparison, subjects are classified into low and high risk groups with equal sizes based on the survival times predicted using A1 and A2, and the log rank test is conducted to compare survival of the two groups. p values from the log rank tests are provided in the Table S1. For LUAD, it is observed that 56 out of the 85 A1 type models can effectively separate the high and low risk groups (with the adjusted log rank test p values < 0.05); In contrast, 47 of the A2 type models have significant adjusted log rank p values. In addition, 51 A1 type models have p values smaller than their A2 counterparts. In the analysis of LIHC data, the numbers of significant adjusted p values for the A1 and A2 type of models are 237 and 66, respectively. In addition, 286 genes have p values smaller under the A1 type models than their A2 counterparts. These results suggest that gene expressions can significantly improve prognosis modeling beyond histopathological imaging features. For a more intuitive presentation, we present the Kaplan–Meier curves for two representative genes in Figure 3. Specifically, we show the survival functions of the low and high risk groups under the A1 and A2 models. The A1 models have a much clearer and more significant separation. Such results suggest that, for clinical practice, it may be necessary to integrate gene expression data beyond histopathological imaging data.

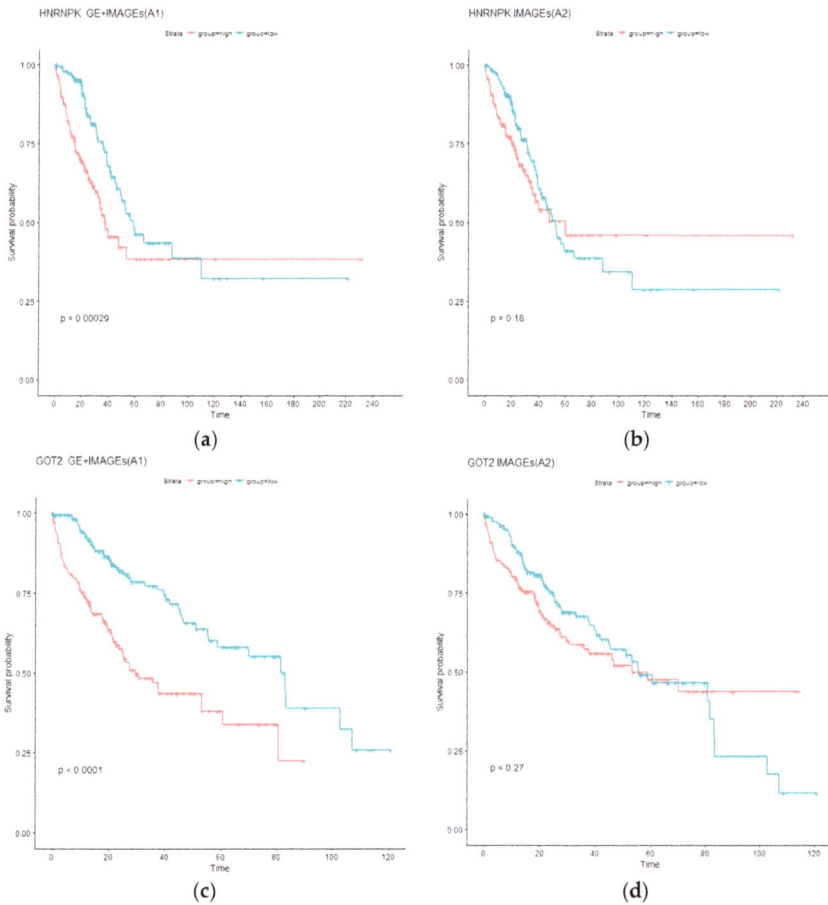

Figure 3. Kaplan–Meier (KM) curves for low (blue) and high (red) risk groups under models A1 and A2. (**a**,**b**) for LUAD: Gene HNRNPK as well as selected imaging features (A1), and only selected imaging features (A2). (**c**,**d**) for LIHC: Gene GOT2 as well as selected imaging features (A1), and only selected imaging features (A2). *p* values are computed from log rank tests.

4.2. Identification of Imaging Features with Independent Prognostic Power Conditional on Gene Expressions

Analysis parallel to the above is conducted, reversing the roles of gene expressions and imaging features. With significance level 0.05, the identified imaging features along with their *p* values are shown in Table 4. Detailed estimation results are provided in the Table S1. In the LUAD data analysis, 11 imaging features are found as significantly associated with prognosis conditional on the selected gene expressions. Among them, six are texture related, which is consistent with the literature [21]. In the analysis of LIHC data, nine imaging features are found as significantly associated with prognosis conditional on gene expressions, among which eight belong to the morphological category of nuclei texture. There is one notable difference between gene expression and histopathological imaging measurements. With extensive functional studies accumulated over years, the biological functions of many genes are known; In contrast, the biological interpretations of imaging features mostly remain unclear. As such, interpretations as in Table 2; Table 3 cannot be pursued.

Table 4. Identified histopathological features.

LUAD		LIHC	
Feature Name	Adjusted p Value	Feature Name	Adjusted p Value
Mean_Identifyeosinprimarycytoplasm_Texture_Correlation_maskosingray_3_00	1.16×10^{-4}	StDev_Identifyhemasub2_Texture_DifferenceEntropy_ImageAfterMath_3_02	9.46×10^{-6}
Median_Identifyeosinprimarycytoplasm_Texture_Correlation_maskosingray_3_00	1.59×10^{-4}	StDev_Identifyhemasub2_Texture_SumEntropy_ImageAfterMath_3_00	9.46×10^{-6}
StDev_Identifyeosinprimarycytoplasm_Texture_Correlation_maskosingray_3_00	1.59×10^{-4}	StDev_Identifyhemasub2_Texture_SumEntropy_ImageAfterMath_3_02	1.85×10^{-5}
StDev_Identifyhemasub2_AreaShape_Orientation	1.59×10^{-4}	StDev_Identifyhemasub2_Texture_DifferenceEntropy_ImageAfterMath_3_00	2.92×10^{-5}
StDev_Identifyhemasub2_AreaShape_Zernike_6_6	1.05×10^{-4}	StDev_Identifyhemasub2_Texture_SumEntropy_ImageAfterMath_3_01	3.64×10^{-5}
StDev_Identifyhemasub2_AreaShape_Zernike_9_1	1.59×10^{-4}	StDev_Identifyhemasub2_Texture_DifferenceEntropy_ImageAfterMath_3_01	4.08×10^{-5}
StDev_Identifyhemasub2_AreaShape_Zernike_9_9	1.59×10^{-4}	StDev_Identifyhemasub2_Texture_DifferenceEntropy_ImageAfterMath_3_03	4.82×10^{-5}
StDev_Identifyhemasub2_Texture_DifferenceEntropy_ImageAfterMath_3_03	1.64×10^{-4}	StDev_Identifyhemasub2_Texture_SumEntropy_ImageAfterMath_3_03	9.24×10^{-5}
StDev_Identifyhemasub2_Texture_SumEntropy_ImageAfterMath_3_01	1.64×10^{-4}	Granularity_2_ImageAfterMath	1.07×10^{-4}
Texture_Correlation_maskosingray_3_00	1.59×10^{-4}		
Granularity_15_ImageAfterMath	7.66×10^{-4}		

As in the above section, additional analysis is conducted. Specifically, two types of AFT models are considered. The first type, referred to as B1, is based on an individual imaging feature and selected gene expressions; whereas the second type, referred to as B2, is only based on selected gene expressions. Detailed results are provided in the Table S1. For LUAD, it is observed that ten out of the 11 B1 type models can effectively separate the high and low risk groups, whereas 11 of the B2 type models have significant adjusted log rank p values. For the identified imaging feature Granularity_15_ImageAfterMath, the B1 model is not significant, however, the corresponding B2 model is significant. This can be explained by the larger degrees of freedom of the B1 model and possible correlation between the two types of measurements. It is also found that six imaging features have p values smaller under the B1 type models than their B2 counterparts. In the LIHC data analysis, the overall findings are similar. Specifically, all tests under both B1 and B2 types of models have adjusted p values smaller than 0.05. All tests under B1 have p values larger than those under B2. Again, this can be possibly explained by the larger numbers of parameters under B1 and correlations. The KM curves for two representative imaging features are examined in Figure 4. The differences between the left and right panels are much less distinct compared to Figure 3. Overall, the analysis suggests that, conditional on the presence of gene expression measurements, histopathological imaging features have limited independent prognostic power.

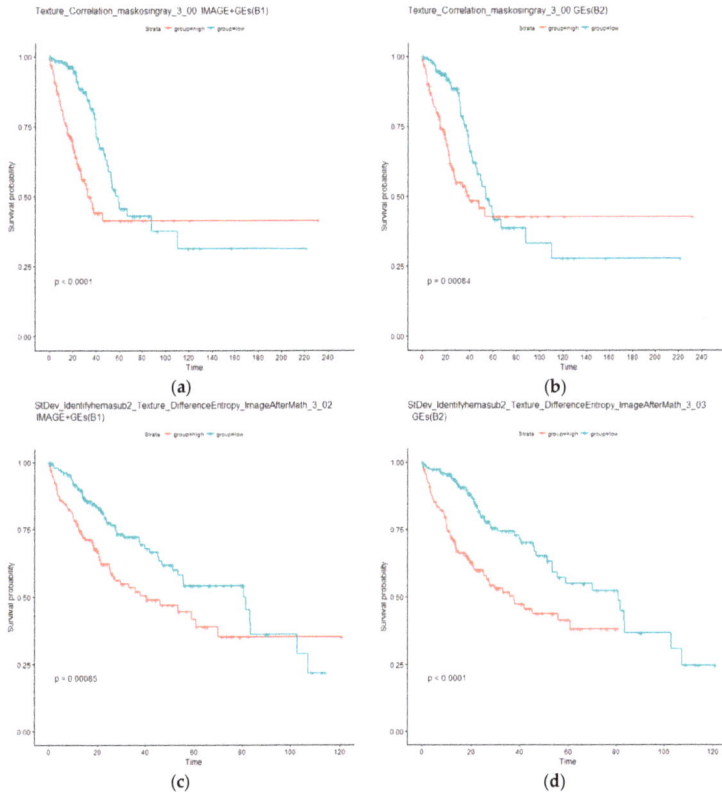

Figure 4. KM curves for low (blue) and high (red) risk groups under models B1 and B2. (**a**,**b**) for LUAD: Imaging feature Texture_Correlation_maskosingray_3_00 as well as selected gene expressions (B1), and only selected gene expressions (B2). (**c**,**d**) for LIHC: Imaging feature StDev_Identifyhemasub2_Texture_DifferenceEntropy_ImageAfterMath_3_00 as well as selected gene expressions (B1), and only selected gene expressions (B2). p values are computed from log rank tests.

5. Discussion

In the literature, the separate and integrated analyses of omics and histopathological imaging data have been conducted. This study has taken a different perspective and tried to answer the fundamental question of whether a type of measurement has independent prognostic power conditional on the collective effect of the other type. A rigorous statistical testing approach, developed under simpler settings, has been adopted and extended. In the analysis of TCGA data on two cancer types, it has been found that, conditional on imaging features, individual gene expressions may still have significant prognostic power; however, conditional on gene expressions, individual imaging features may have limited prognostic power. As such, at least for the analyzed datasets, gene expressions and histopathological imaging features have an irreversible independent relationship in modeling prognosis. Such findings, to the best of our knowledge, are the first in the literature. They may have important implications for cancer practice. Specifically, in cancer clinical practice, gene expression profiling is becoming routine. Our analysis suggests that, for modeling prognosis, when gene expression data are available, clinicians may not need to order histopathological imaging. However, this is not true the other way around. For a more accurate prognosis modeling, with imaging data, clinicians may still want to order gene expression profiling, and use integrated analysis techniques (developed in published and future literature) to integrate gene expression and imaging data. The biological implications of the findings, pertinent to the associations between gene expressions and imaging features, are worth further investigation.

This study can be extended in multiple directions. Specifically, other types of omics measurements, such as DNA mutations, miRNA expressions, methylation, and copy number variations, can be analyzed similarly. It is noted that the findings are not necessarily the same as in this article. In our analysis, we have considered high dimensional imaging features, which may include more information but do not have simple biological interpretations. It is possible to conduct a similar analysis using low dimensional imaging features such as vascular invasion and lymphocyte cells—this is postponed to future research. It is noted that in the literature [55], techniques have already been developed to identify cancer regions, extract such low dimensional imaging features, and use them in analysis. The analysis has been focused on gene expression and imaging data. We acknowledge the importance of clinical, environmental, and other factors in cancer prognosis. These factors are not included in analysis with the following concerns. First, the most important objective of this study is to evaluate the overlapping/independent information in omics and histopathological imaging data. As such, we focus on these two types of measurements. Second, to the best of our knowledge, techniques for making inference with the "one gene expression + low dimensional clinical factors + high dimensional imaging features" model are not available. This analysis can be more complex than that in this article with the significant differences between clinical factors and imaging features. Table 1 has been provided so that researchers can comprehend properties of the TCGA cohorts. Extending the proposed analysis and accommodating clinical factors will be postponed to future research. It is also of interest to conduct similar analysis for other types of cancer outcomes. For a continuous cancer marker, the described analysis technique can be directly applied. New developments will be needed for other types of outcomes/phenotypes. It is also noted that the detailed results can be data and model dependent. It is impossible to conduct analysis with all cancer types and models. However, the "spirit" of the proposed analysis will be broadly applicable. Although with certain limitations, being the first of its kind, this study may still provide important insights into cancer modeling and characteristics of cancer as reflected in omics profiles and histopathological images.

6. Conclusions

Omics and histopathological imaging data have been co-collected in cancer practice and analyzed in recent integrated analysis. In this study, we have presented a pipeline for analyzing their independent prognostic power conditional on the other type of data. The adopted statistical inference technique has a solid ground and can be broadly applied. The "asymmetric" finding is interesting, has not been observed in the literature, and has sound interpretations. It is reasonable to expect that the proposed analysis and its downstream integrated analysis will gain popularity fast and have a deep impact on cancer practice.

Supplementary Materials: The following are available online at http://www.mdpi.com/2072-6694/11/3/361/s1, Table S1: Detailed estimation results referred to in Section 4, TestLDHD: R code and example data.

Author Contributions: T.Z., M.W., and S.M. contributed to conceptualization, methodology, and writing. T.Z. conducted programming and numerical study.

Funding: This research was funded by National Institutes of Health, grant number CA216017, CA204120, CA196530; National Natural Science Foundation of China, grant number 91546202, 71331006; Bureau of Statistics of China, grant number 2018LD02.

Acknowledgments: We thank the editor and reviewers for their careful review and insightful comments, which have led to a significant improvement of this article.

Conflicts of Interest: The authors declare no conflict of interest.

References

1. Mallett, S.; Royston, P.; Dutton, S.; Waters, R.; Altman, D.G. Reporting methods in studies developing prognostic models in cancer: A review. *BMC Med.* **2010**, *8*, 20. [CrossRef] [PubMed]
2. Kourou, K.; Exarchos, T.P.; Exarchos, K.P.; Karamouzis, M.V.; Fotiadis, D.I. Machine learning applications in cancer prognosis and prediction. *Comput. Struct. Biotechnol. J.* **2015**, *13*, 8–17. [CrossRef] [PubMed]
3. Rath, M.G.; Uhlmann, L.; Fiedler, M.; Heil, J.; Golatta, M.; Dinkic, C.; Hennigs, A.; Schott, S.; Ernst, V.; Koch, T.; et al. Oncotype DX((R)) in breast cancer patients: Clinical experience, outcome and follow-up-a case-control study. *Arch. Gynecol. Obstet.* **2018**, *297*, 443–447. [CrossRef] [PubMed]
4. Yanaihara, N.; Caplen, N.; Bowman, E.; Seike, M.; Kumamoto, K.; Yi, M.; Stephens, R.M.; Okamoto, A.; Yokota, J.; Tanaka, T.; et al. Unique microRNA molecular profiles in lung cancer diagnosis and prognosis. *Cancer Cell* **2006**, *9*, 189–198. [CrossRef] [PubMed]
5. Muller, H.M.; Widschwendter, A.; Fiegl, H.; Ivarsson, L.; Goebel, G.; Perkmann, E.; Marth, C.; Widschwendter, M. DNA methylation in serum of breast cancer patients: An independent prognostic marker. *Cancer Res.* **2003**, *63*, 7641–7645. [PubMed]
6. Harpole, D.H., Jr.; Herndon, J.E., 2nd; Wolfe, W.G.; Iglehart, J.D.; Marks, J.R. A prognostic model of recurrence and death in stage I non-small cell lung cancer utilizing presentation, histopathology, and oncoprotein expression. *Cancer Res.* **1995**, *55*, 51–56. [PubMed]
7. Romo-Bucheli, D.; Janowczyk, A.; Gilmore, H.; Romero, E.; Madabhushi, A. Automated tubulenuclei quantification and correlation with Oncotype DX risk categories in ER+ breast cancer whole slide Images. *Sci. Rep.* **2016**, *6*, 32706. [CrossRef] [PubMed]
8. Sertel, O.; Kong, J.; Shimada, H.; Catalyurek, U.V.; Saltz, J.H.; Gurcan, M.N. Computer-aided prognosis of neuroblastoma on whole-slide images: Classification of stromal development. *Pattern Recognit.* **2009**, *42*, 1093–1103. [CrossRef]
9. Sertel, O.; Kong, J.; Catalyurek, U.V.; Lozanski, G.; Saltz, J.H.; Gurcan, M.N. Histopathological Image Analysis Using Model-Based Intermediate Representations and Color Texture: Follicular Lymphoma Grading. *J. Signal Process. Syst.* **2009**, *55*, 169–183. [CrossRef]
10. Yu, K.H.; Berry, G.J.; Rubin, D.L.; Re, C.; Altman, R.B.; Snyder, M. Association of omics features with histopathology patterns in lung adenocarcinoma. *Cell Syst.* **2017**, *5*, 620–627.e3. [CrossRef]
11. Sabo, E.; Beck, A.H.; Montgomery, E.A.; Bhattacharya, B.; Meitner, P.; Wang, J.Y.; Resnick, M.B. Computerized morphometry as an aid in determining the grade of dysplasia and progression to adenocarcinoma in Barrett's esophagus. *Lab. Investig.* **2006**, *86*, 1261–1271. [CrossRef]
12. Cooper, L.A.; Kong, J.; Gutman, D.A.; Dunn, W.D.; Nalisnik, M.; Brat, D.J. Novel genotype-phenotype associations in human cancers enabled by advanced molecular platforms and computational analysis of whole slide images. *Lab. Investig.* **2015**, *95*, 366–376. [CrossRef] [PubMed]
13. Sun, D.; Li, A.; Tang, B.; Wang, M. Integrating genomic data and pathological images to effectively predict breast cancer clinical outcome. *Comput. Methods Programs Biomed.* **2018**, *161*, 45–53. [CrossRef] [PubMed]

14. Mobadersany, P.; Yousefi, S.; Amgad, M.; Gutman, D.A.; Barnholtz-Sloan, J.S.; Vega, J.V.; Brat, D.J.; Cooper, L.A. Predicting cancer outcomes from histology and genomics using convolutional networks. *Proc. Natl. Acad. Sci. USA* **2018**, *115*, E2970–E2979. [CrossRef] [PubMed]

15. Zhu, X.L.; Yao, J.W.; Luo, X.; Xiao, G.H.; Xie, Y.; Gazdar, A.; Huang, J.Z. Lung cancer survival prediction from pathological images and genetic data—An integration study. In Proceedings of the 2016 IEEE 13th International Symposium on Biomedical Imaging (ISBI), Prague, Czech Republic, 13–16 April 2016; pp. 1173–1176.

16. Hutter, C.; Zenklusen, J.C. The Cancer Genome Atlas: Creating Lasting Value beyond Its Data. *Cell* **2018**, *173*, 283–285. [CrossRef] [PubMed]

17. Cerami, E.; Gao, J.; Dogrusoz, U.; Gross, B.E.; Sumer, S.O.; Aksoy, B.A.; Jacobsen, A.; Byrne, C.J.; Heuer, M.L.; Larsson, E.; et al. The cBio cancer genomics portal: An open platform for exploring multidimensional cancer genomics data. *Cancer Discov.* **2012**, *2*, 401–404. [CrossRef] [PubMed]

18. Gao, J.; Aksoy, B.A.; Dogrusoz, U.; Dresdner, G.; Gross, B.; Sumer, S.O.; Sun, Y.; Jacobsen, A.; Sinha, R.; Larsson, E.; et al. Integrative analysis of complex cancer genomics and clinical profiles using the cBioPortal. *Sci. Signal.* **2013**, *6*, pl1. [CrossRef] [PubMed]

19. Soliman, K. CellProfiler: Novel Automated Image Segmentation Procedure for Super-Resolution Microscopy. *Biol. Proced. Online* **2015**, *17*, 11. [CrossRef]

20. Goode, A.; Gilbert, B.; Harkes, J.; Jukic, D.; Satyanarayanan, M. OpenSlide: A vendor-neutral software foundation for digital pathology. *J. Pathol. Inform.* **2013**, *4*, 27. [CrossRef] [PubMed]

21. Luo, X.; Zang, X.; Yang, L.; Huang, J.; Liang, F.; Rodriguez-Canales, J.; Wistuba, I.I.; Gazdar, A.; Xie, Y.; Xiao, G. Comprehensive Computational Pathological Image Analysis Predicts Lung Cancer Prognosis. *J. Thorac. Oncol.* **2017**, *12*, 501–509. [CrossRef] [PubMed]

22. Yu, K.H.; Zhang, C.; Berry, G.J.; Altman, R.B.; Re, C.; Rubin, D.L.; Snyder, M. Predicting non-small cell lung cancer prognosis by fully automated microscopic pathology image features. *Nat. Commun.* **2016**, *7*, 12474. [CrossRef] [PubMed]

23. Buckley, J.; James, I. Linear regression with censored data. *Biometrika* **1979**, *66*, 429–436. [CrossRef]

24. Chai, H.; Zhang, Q.Z.; Huang, J.; Ma, S.G. Inference for low-dimensional covariates in a high-dimensional accelerated failure time model. *Stat. Sin.* **2019**. [CrossRef]

25. Benjamini, Y.; Yekutieli, D. The control of the false discovery rate in multiple testing under dependency. *Ann. Stat.* **2001**, *29*, 1165–1188.

26. Chen, J.H.; Chen, Z.H. Extended Bayesian information criteria for model selection with large model spaces. *Biometrika* **2008**, *95*, 759–771. [CrossRef]

27. Chen, H.H.; Fan, P.; Chang, S.W.; Tsao, Y.P.; Huang, H.P.; Chen, S.L. NRIP/DCAF6 stabilizes the androgen receptor protein by displacing DDB2 from the CUL4A-DDB1 E3 ligase complex in prostate cancer. *Oncotarget* **2017**, *8*, 21501–21515. [CrossRef] [PubMed]

28. Zhou, J.; Yang, Z.; Tsuji, T.; Gong, J.; Xie, J.; Chen, C.; Li, W.; Amar, S.; Luo, Z. LITAF and TNFSF15, two downstream targets of AMPK, exert inhibitory effects on tumor growth. *Oncogene* **2011**, *30*, 1892–1900. [CrossRef]

29. Kopajtich, R.; Murayama, K.; Janecke, A.R.; Haack, T.B.; Breuer, M.; Knisely, A.S.; Harting, I.; Ohashi, T.; Okazaki, Y.; Watanabe, D.; et al. Biallelic IARS Mutations Cause Growth Retardation with Prenatal Onset, Intellectual Disability, Muscular Hypotonia, and Infantile Hepatopathy. *Am. J. Hum. Genet.* **2016**, *99*, 414–422. [CrossRef]

30. Tian, T.; Ikeda, J.; Wang, Y.; Mamat, S.; Luo, W.; Aozasa, K.; Morii, E. Role of leucine-rich pentatricopeptide repeat motif-containing protein (LRPPRC) for anti-apoptosis and tumourigenesis in cancers. *Eur. J. Cancer* **2012**, *48*, 2462–2473. [CrossRef]

31. Van Beijnum, J.R.; Moerkerk, P.T.M.; Gerbers, A.J.; de Brune, A.P.; Arends, J.W.; Hoogenboom, H.R.; Hufton, S.E. Target validation for genomics using peptide-specific phage antibodies: A study of five gene products overexpressed in colorectal cancer. *Int. J. Cancer* **2002**, *101*, 118–127. [CrossRef]

32. Szczyrba, J.; Nolte, E.; Hart, M.; Doll, C.; Wach, S.; Taubert, H.; Keck, B.; Kremmer, E.; Stohr, R.; Hartmann, A.; et al. Identification of ZNF217, hnRNP-K, VEGF-A and IPO7 as targets for microRNAs that are downregulated in prostate carcinoma. *Int. J. Cancer* **2013**, *132*, 775–784. [CrossRef] [PubMed]

33. Losada, A. Cohesin in cancer: Chromosome segregation and beyond. *Nat. Rev. Cancer* **2014**, *14*, 389–393. [CrossRef] [PubMed]

34. Sivula, A.; Talvensaari-Mattila, A.; Lundin, J.; Joensuu, H.; Haglund, C.; Ristimaki, A.; Turpeenniemi-Hujanen, T. Association of cyclooxygenase-2 and matrix metalloproteinase-2 expression in human breast cancer. *Breast Cancer Res. Treat.* **2005**, *89*, 215–220. [CrossRef] [PubMed]

35. Anedchenko, E.A.; Dmitriev, A.A.; Krasnov, G.S.; Kondrat'eva, T.T.; Kopantsev, E.P.; Vinogradova, T.V.; Zinov'eva, M.V.; Zborovskaia, I.B.; Polotskii, B.E.; Sakharova, O.V.; et al. Down-regulation of RBSP3/CTDSPL, NPRL2/G21, RASSF1A, ITGA9, HYAL1 and HYAL2 genes in non-small cell lung cancer. *Mol. Biol. (Mosk)* **2008**, *42*, 965–976. [CrossRef] [PubMed]

36. Gimenez-Xavier, P.; Pros, E.; Bonastre, E.; Moran, S.; Aza, A.; Grana, O.; Gomez-Lopez, G.; Derdak, S.; Dabad, M.; Esteve-Codina, A.; et al. Genomic and Molecular Screenings Identify Different Mechanisms for Acquired Resistance to MET Inhibitors in Lung Cancer Cells. *Mol. Cancer Ther.* **2017**, *16*, 1366–1376. [CrossRef] [PubMed]

37. Lu, Y.; Boss, J.M.; Hu, S.X.; Xu, H.J.; Blanck, G. Apoptosis-independent retinoblastoma protein rescue of HLA class II messenger RNA IFN-gamma inducibility in non-small cell lung carcinoma cells. Lack of surface class II expression associated with a specific defect in HLA-DRA induction. *J. Immunol.* **1996**, *156*, 2495–2502. [PubMed]

38. Pino, I.; Pio, R.; Toledo, G.; Zabalegui, N.; Vicent, S.; Rey, N.; Lozano, M.D.; Torre, W.; Garcia-Foncillas, J.; Montuenga, L.M. Altered patterns of expression of members of the heterogeneous nuclear ribonucleoprotein (hnRNP) family in lung cancer. *Lung Cancer* **2003**, *41*, 131–143. [CrossRef]

39. Oyewumi, M.O.; Manickavasagam, D.; Novak, K.; Wehrung, D.; Paulic, N.; Moussa, F.M.; Sondag, G.R.; Safadi, F.F. Osteoactivin (GPNMB) ectodomain protein promotes growth and invasive behavior of human lung cancer cells. *Oncotarget* **2016**, *7*, 13932–13944. [CrossRef] [PubMed]

40. Bieniasz, M.; Oszajca, K.; Eusebio, M.; Kordiak, J.; Bartkowiak, J.; Szemraj, J. The positive correlation between gene expression of the two angiogenic factors: VEGF and BMP-2 in lung cancer patients. *Lung Cancer* **2009**, *66*, 319–326. [CrossRef]

41. Zhan, W.; Wang, W.; Han, T.; Xie, C.; Zhang, T.; Gan, M.; Wang, J.B. COMMD9 promotes TFDP1/E2F1 transcriptional activity via interaction with TFDP1 in non-small cell lung cancer. *Cell Signal.* **2017**, *30*, 59–66. [CrossRef] [PubMed]

42. Tokumoto, H. Analysis of HLA-DRB1-related alleles in Japanese patients with lung cancer—relationship to genetic susceptibility and resistance to lung cancer. *J. Cancer Res. Clin. Oncol.* **1998**, *124*, 511–516. [CrossRef] [PubMed]

43. Mura, M.; Hopkins, T.G.; Michael, T.; Abd-Latip, N.; Weir, J.; Aboagye, E.; Mauri, F.; Jameson, C.; Sturge, J.; Gabra, H.; et al. LARP1 post-transcriptionally regulates mTOR and contributes to cancer progression. *Oncogene* **2015**, *34*, 5025–5036. [CrossRef] [PubMed]

44. Yang, J.J.; Lee, Y.J.; Hung, H.H.; Tseng, W.P.; Tu, C.C.; Lee, H.; Wu, W.J. ZAK inhibits human lung cancer cell growth via ERK and JNK activation in an AP-1-dependent manner. *Cancer Sci.* **2010**, *101*, 1374–1381. [CrossRef] [PubMed]

45. Shao, G.Z.; Zhou, R.L.; Zhang, Q.Y.; Zhang, Y.; Liu, J.J.; Rui, J.A.; Wei, X.; Ye, D.X. Molecular cloning and characterization of LAPTM4B, a novel gene upregulated in hepatocellular carcinoma. *Oncogene* **2003**, *22*, 5060–5069. [CrossRef]

46. Huang, D.; Cao, L.; Zheng, S. CAPZA1 modulates EMT by regulating actin cytoskeleton remodelling in hepatocellular carcinoma. *J. Exp. Clin. Cancer Res.* **2017**, *36*, 13. [CrossRef] [PubMed]

47. Noda, T.; Yamamoto, H.; Takemasa, I.; Yamada, D.; Uemura, M.; Wada, H.; Kobayashi, S.; Marubashi, S.; Eguchi, H.; Tanemura, M.; et al. PLOD2 induced under hypoxia is a novel prognostic factor for hepatocellular carcinoma after curative resection. *Liver Int.* **2012**, *32*, 110–118. [CrossRef] [PubMed]

48. Chen, Z.; Xu, L.; Su, T.; Ke, Z.; Peng, Z.; Zhang, N.; Peng, S.; Zhang, Q.; Liu, G.; Wei, G.; et al. Autocrine STIP1 signaling promotes tumor growth and is associated with disease outcome in hepatocellular carcinoma. *Biochem. Biophys. Res. Commun.* **2017**, *493*, 365–372. [CrossRef] [PubMed]

49. Hopfner, M.; Huether, A.; Sutter, A.P.; Baradari, V.; Schuppan, D.; Scherubl, H. Blockade of IGF-1 receptor tyrosine kinase has antineoplastic effects in hepatocellular carcinoma cells. *Biochem. Pharmacol.* **2006**, *71*, 1435–1448. [CrossRef] [PubMed]

50. Zhang, W.; Sun, H.C.; Wang, W.Q.; Zhang, Q.B.; Zhuang, P.Y.; Xiong, Y.Q.; Zhu, X.D.; Xu, H.X.; Kong, L.Q.; Wu, W.Z.; et al. Sorafenib down-regulates expression of HTATIP2 to promote invasiveness and metastasis of orthotopic hepatocellular carcinoma tumors in mice. *Gastroenterology* **2012**, *143*, 1641–1649. [CrossRef]

51. Zhang, Y.; Yao, J.; Huan, L.; Lian, J.; Bao, C.; Li, Y.; Ge, C.; Li, J.; Yao, M.; Liang, L.; et al. GNAI3 inhibits tumor cell migration and invasion and is post-transcriptionally regulated by miR-222 in hepatocellular carcinoma. *Cancer Lett.* **2015**, *356*, 978–984. [CrossRef]

52. Zheng, Y.; Gery, S.; Sun, H.; Shacham, S.; Kauffman, M.; Koeffler, H.P. KPT-330 inhibitor of XPO1-mediated nuclear export has anti-proliferative activity in hepatocellular carcinoma. *Cancer Chemother. Pharmacol.* **2014**, *74*, 487–495. [CrossRef] [PubMed]

53. Wang, Y.H.; Cheng, T.Y.; Chen, T.Y.; Chang, K.M.; Chuang, V.P.; Kao, K.J. Plasmalemmal Vesicle Associated Protein (PLVAP) as a therapeutic target for treatment of hepatocellular carcinoma. *BMC Cancer* **2014**, *14*, 815. [CrossRef] [PubMed]

54. Bangoura, G.; Liu, Z.S.; Qian, Q.; Jiang, C.Q.; Yang, G.F.; Jing, S. Prognostic significance of HIF-2alpha/EPAS1 expression in hepatocellular carcinoma. *World J. Gastroenterol.* **2007**, *13*, 3176–3182. [CrossRef] [PubMed]

55. Bejnordi, B.E.; Veta, M.; van Diest, P.J.; van Ginneken, B.; Karssemeijer, N.; Litjens, G.; van der Laak, J.; the CAMELYON16 Consortium; Hermsen, M.; Manson, Q.F.; et al. Diagnostic Assessment of Deep Learning Algorithms for Detection of Lymph Node Metastases in Women With Breast Cancer. *JAMA* **2017**, *318*, 2199–2210. [CrossRef] [PubMed]

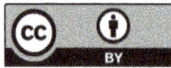

cancers

MDPI

Article

Developing a Prognostic Gene Panel of Epithelial Ovarian Cancer Patients by a Machine Learning Model

Tzu-Pin Lu [1], Kuan-Ting Kuo [2], Ching-Hsuan Chen [1], Ming-Cheng Chang [3,4], Hsiu-Ping Lin [3], Yu-Hao Hu [3], Ying-Cheng Chiang [3,5,*], Wen-Fang Cheng [3,6,7] and Chi-An Chen [3]

[1] Institute of Epidemiology and Preventive Medicine, Department of Public Health, National Taiwan University, Taipei 10055, Taiwan; tplu@ntu.edu.tw (T.-P.L.); ponponmiao@gmail.com (C.-H.C.)

[2] Department of Pathology, College of Medicine, National Taiwan University, Taipei 10002, Taiwan; pathologykimo@gmail.com

[3] Department of Obstetrics and Gynecology, College of Medicine, National Taiwan University, Taipei 10041, Taiwan; mcchang@iner.gov.tw (M.-C.C.); wfc5166@gmail.com (H.-P.L.); jinmaw@gmail.com (Y.-H.H.); wenfangcheng@yahoo.com (W.-F.C.); chianchen@ntu.edu.tw (C.-A.C.)

[4] Institute of Nuclear Energy Research, Atomic Energy Council, Executive Yuan, Taoyuan 32546, Taiwan

[5] Department of Obstetrics and Gynecology, National Taiwan University Hospital Yunlin branch, Yunlin 64041, Taiwan

[6] Graduate Institute of Clinical Medicine, College of Medicine, National Taiwan University, Taipei 10002, Taiwan

[7] Graduate Institute of Oncology, College of Medicine, National Taiwan University, Taipei 10002, Taiwan

* Correspondence: ycchiang@ntuh.gov.tw; Tel.: +886-2-2312-3456 (ext. 71964); Fax: +886-2-2311-4965

Received: 11 January 2019; Accepted: 22 February 2019; Published: 25 February 2019

Abstract: Epithelial ovarian cancer patients usually relapse after primary management. We utilized the support vector machine algorithm to develop a model for the chemo-response using the Cancer Cell Line Encyclopedia (CCLE) and validated the model in The Cancer Genome Atlas (TCGA) and the GSE9891 dataset. Finally, we evaluated the feasibility of the model using ovarian cancer patients from our institute. The 10-gene predictive model demonstrated that the high response group had a longer recurrence-free survival (RFS) (log-rank test, $p = 0.015$ for TCGA, $p = 0.013$ for GSE9891 and $p = 0.039$ for NTUH) and overall survival (OS) (log-rank test, $p = 0.002$ for TCGA and $p = 0.016$ for NTUH). In a multivariate Cox hazard regression model, the predictive model (HR: 0.644, 95% CI: 0.436–0.952, $p = 0.027$) and residual tumor size < 1 cm (HR: 0.312, 95% CI: 0.170–0.573, $p < 0.001$) were significant factors for recurrence. The predictive model (HR: 0.511, 95% CI: 0.334–0.783, $p = 0.002$) and residual tumor size < 1 cm (HR: 0.252, 95% CI: 0.128–0.496, $p < 0.001$) were still significant factors for death. In conclusion, the patients of high response group stratified by the model had good response and favourable prognosis, whereas for the patients of medium to low response groups, introduction of other drugs or clinical trials might be beneficial.

Keywords: chemotherapy; microarray; ovarian cancer; predictive model; machine learning

---

1. Introduction

Ovarian carcinoma is a major cause of cancer death in women [1,2]. Due to the lack of initial symptoms and effective screening tools, most patients are diagnosed at an advanced stage with a 5-year survival of less than 50% [3,4]. The clinical prognostic factors include cancer stage, histological subtypes, tumor grade, the residual tumor size after debulking surgery and the response to chemotherapy. Despite good initial response, most ovarian cancer patients experience tumor recurrence and eventually are resistant to salvage treatments [3,5]. The serum CA-125 level is the current biomarker, but it is not ideal due to its limited specificity. Many potential biomarkers have been evaluated alone or in combination with CA-125, but the majority show disappointing results [6].

Precision medicine is the direction for cancer treatments, and the strategy of management depends on the distinct molecular features among these subtypes of ovarian carcinoma. However, the clinical benefits of targeted therapies are limited even though there are marked abnormalities in genetic or molecular pathways in ovarian cancer [7]. To date, the most promising agents are only anti-angiogenesis and poly ADP-ribose polymerase inhibitors. Bevacizumab, in combination with chemotherapy, demonstrates an improved progression-free survival, but a benefit on overall survival is only observed in high-risk patients [8,9]. Olaparib is approved for maintenance therapy in platinum-sensitive *BRCA*-mutated serous ovarian cancer patients [10]. The progression-free survival is significantly longer in platinum-sensitive recurrent ovarian cancer patients receiving niraparib, regardless of the *BRCA* mutation status [11]. In fact, the clinical dilemma is that these targeted drugs are expensive and benefit only a small subpopulation of ovarian cancer patients.

With the advancement in high-throughput genomic technology in recent years, many large-scale genomic and genetic studies have been performed to investigate cancer cell lines and patients [12,13]. For examples, the Cancer Cell Line Encyclopedia (CCLE) project analyzed more than 1000 cancer cell lines and reported their drug responses to more than 20 drugs and The Cancer Genome Atlas (TCGA) studied different kinds of genetic changes in real patients from more than 30 major cancer types. Due to the limitations from research ethnics and the difficulties in performing many clinical trials in real patients, these materials can serve as a good starting point to develop a machine learning model by using the cell lines first. Subsequently, the developed model can be validated in other large-scale studies, and such big data mining approach has been demonstrated its effectiveness in several studies [14,15].

Currently, cytotoxic chemotherapy still plays a key role in managing ovarian cancer. Determining how to predict the response of chemotherapy and identify which patients benefit from chemotherapy is important [16]. In this study, we initially developed a predictive model of chemo-response using CCLE and then selected for the optimal combination of predictors in TCGA and the GSE9891 dataset. Finally, we validated the model using clinical ovarian cancer tissue samples. We analysed the expression of the 10 predictive genes and correlated the clinical outcomes of the ovarian cancer patients to confirm the utility of the model.

2. Results

2.1. Development of A Predictive Model from Cancer Cell Line Encyclopaedia (CCLE)

After preprocessing, we utilized the Kruskal-Wallis test to identify the genes showing significant differences among the cell lines divided into three groups with an unequal drug efficacy in GSE36133 (Figure 1). The expression levels of 575 probes with a uniquely mapped gene name were significantly associated with the response ($p < 0.01$), and thus, they served as the original gene pool that might be possible predictive biomarkers. To identify a set of genes that could be used to develop a predictive model, we used the genetic algorithm (GA) shown in Figure S1 to select the best combination of 10 genes from the 575 significant genes. A predictive model composed of the 10 selected genes was developed using the SVM algorithm, and its performance was evaluated based on the leave one out cross-validation strategy. Notably, the prediction accuracy gradually increased through the GA processes and became stable before 10 generations that were set as the last generation in the GA. The best combination of the 10 genes selected by the GA is summarized in Table S1, and the corresponding SVM predictive model showed an accuracy of 100% for classifying the cell lines into three groups with different efficacies.

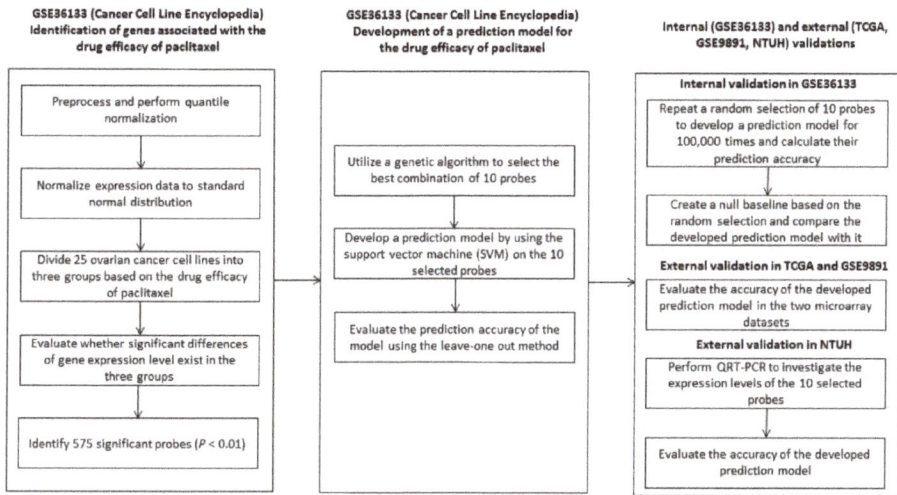

Figure 1. The overall protocol utilized in this study to develop the predictive model.

2.2. Evaluation of The Performance of The Developed Predictive Model

Even though the developed predictive model perfectly classified the cell lines into distinct groups corresponding to the efficacy, we still cannot exclude the possibility that the predictive model was identified purely based on a random chance. To address this issue, a permutation test was repeated 100,000 times to evaluate the probability of identifying a model with the same prediction accuracy. The details of the permutation test are described in the Methods section, and the results demonstrated that only 570 combinations out of the 100,000 trials showed 100% accuracy. Thus, the random chance of identifying a set of 10 genes showing 100% accuracy was only 0.0057. With such a low probability, the permutation test suggested that our proposed GA efficiently identified a set of genes with good prediction performances, and thus, the probability of identifying the developed predictive model is low.

2.3. Validation of The Predictive Model in Two Independent Datasets: TCGA and GSE9891

To validate the predictive model, two microarray datasets from patients with ovarian cancer were downloaded. One was from the TCGA, and another one was from the GEO (GSE9891). Because this study focused on the drug efficacy, only those patients receiving chemotherapy were used for the analyses. After preprocessing, the two microarray datasets were analysed using the developed SVM model. Therefore, each patient in the two datasets was classified into one of the three groups according to the predictive model. As shown in Figure S2A,B, the high response group showed a better survival outcome, and no obvious differences were observed between the low response and medium response groups. To reduce the ambiguity, only the two groups with high and low responses are illustrated in Figure 2A,B. Significant differences in the RFS between the two groups were shown in the two datasets (log-rank test, $p = 0.015$ for TCGA and $p = 0.013$ for GSE9891), suggesting the effectiveness of the predictive model in predicting the chemo-response. Intriguingly, the proportion of patients showing a good response was 14.5% in TCGA and 19.3% in GSE9891, which concurred with the finding of less than 30% of a good response in the ovarian cancer patients receiving chemotherapy [17]. In addition to the RFS, we evaluated whether the developed SVM model was predictive for the OS. In general, the pattern of the three groups for the OS was similar to the RFS (Figure S3). Notably, a significant difference was observed in the TCGA dataset (log-rank test, $p = 0.002$, Figure 3A), whereas the OS was not significantly different in GSE9891 (Figure 3B). In addition, the proportion of patients showing a longer OS (>5 years) and RFS (>2 years) are summarized in Table S2, and the proportion from the high response group was higher than that in the other two groups. The results showed that the SVM model we developed identified patients with a high response to chemotherapy, and a significant difference in the RFS was observed between the high and low response groups.

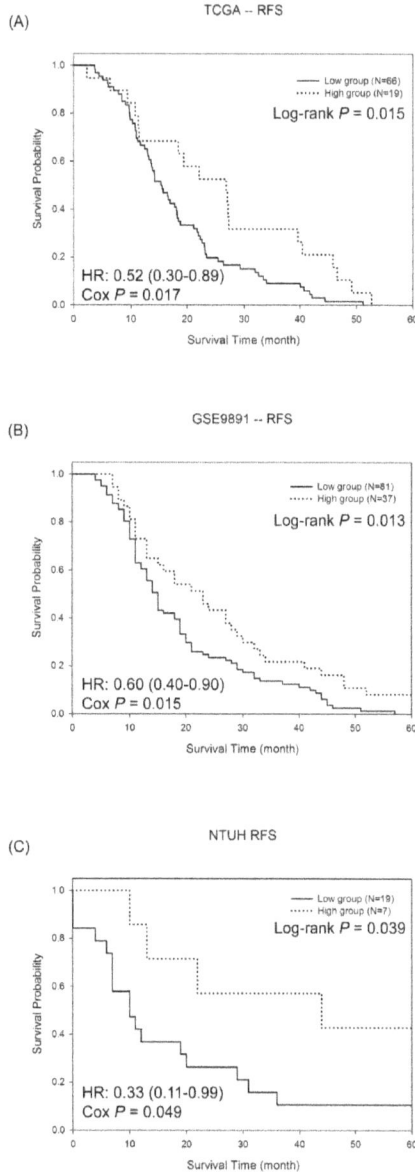

(A)

(B)

(C)

Figure 2. The Kaplan-Meier survival curves of the recurrence free survival (RFS) in the high and low response groups in the (**A**) TCGA dataset, (**B**) GSE9891 dataset and (**C**) NTUH patients. Patients of high response group had longer RFS than low response group in the three cohorts. The hazard ratio (HR) was estimated by the Cox hazard regression model.

(A)

(B)

(C)

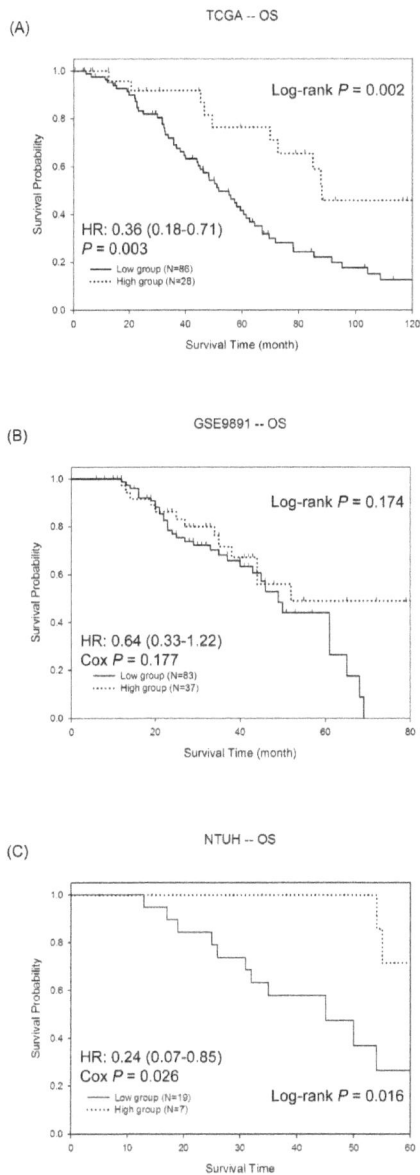

Figure 3. The Kaplan-Meier survival curves of the overall survival (OS) in the high and low response groups in the (**A**) TCGA dataset, (**B**) GSE9891 dataset and (**C**) NTUH patients. Patients of high response group had longer OS than low response group in the three cohorts. The hazard ratio (HR) was estimated by the Cox hazard regression model.

2.4. Validation of The Predictive Model by QRT-PCR in Ovarian Cancer Tissue of NTUH

In addition to the microarray datasets, we validated the prediction performance of the developed SVM model in another cohort of ovarian cancer patients. The study subjects were recruited from the NTUH, and the gene expression values of the 10 selected genes were measured using QRT-PCR. The clinical characteristics of this cohort are shown in Table 1. Similar to the previous validation in the microarrays, the patients were classified into three groups based on the developed SVM model after standardization. The survival curves for RFS and OS in the three groups from the NTUH patients were similar to the TCGA and GSE9891 datasets (Figures S2 and S3). As shown in Figures 2C and 3C, significant differences were observed between the high and low response groups for both the RFS (log-rank test, $p = 0.039$) and the OS (log-rank test, $p = 0.016$), suggesting the effectiveness of the developed SVM model even if the experimental technology is different.

Table 1. Clinical characteristics of the epithelial ovarian cancer patients at NTUH.

Feature	Number (Proportion)
Total patients	84
Age (years)	54.94 ± 11.25
Histological subtype	
Serous	59 (0.7)
Endometrioid	12 (0.14)
Clear cell	13 (0.16)
Tumor grade	
1	4 (0.05)
2	10 (0.12)
3	57 (0.68)
Not available	13 (0.15)
FIGO_stage	
Early (I + II)	11 (0.13)
Advanced (III + IV)	73 (0.87)
Debulking surgery	
Residual tumor size < 1 cm	42 (0.5)
Residual tumor size $\geq$ 1 cm	42 (0.5)

Lastly, we evaluated whether the developed SVM model was an independent predictor to known clinical factors (Table 2). A Cox hazard regression model was utilized to compare the predictive model with several clinical features, including residual tumor size < 1 cm, FIGO stage, tumor grade and histological subtypes. In univariate Cox regression, the predictive model (HR: 0.643, 95% CI: 0.415–0.998, $p = 0.049$), residual tumor size < 1 cm (HR: 0.273, 95% CI: 0.160–0.468, $p < 0.001$), advanced FIGO stage (HR: 7.954, 95% CI: 1.934–32.71, $p = 0.004$) and high tumor grade (HR: 2.289, 95% CI: 1.156–4.530, $p = 0.018$) were significant factors for recurrence. For death, the predictive model (HR: 0.559, 95% CI: 0.351–0.890, $p = 0.014$), residual tumor size < 1 cm (HR: 0.198, 95% CI: 0.107–0.365, $p < 0.001$), advanced FIGO stage (HR: 6.13, 95% CI: 1.489–25.24, $p = 0.012$) and clear cell carcinoma (HR: 0.284, 95% CI: 0.102–0.793, $p = 0.016$) were significant factors in univariate Cox regression. In multivariate Cox regression analysis, the predictive model (HR: 0.644, 95% CI: 0.436–0.952, $p = 0.027$) and residual tumor size < 1 cm (HR: 0.312, 95% CI: 0.170–0.573, $p < 0.001$) were significant factors for recurrence. For death, the predictive model (HR: 0.511, 95% CI: 0.334–0.783, $p = 0.002$) and residual tumor size < 1 cm (HR: 0.252, 95% CI: 0.128–0.496, $p < 0.001$) were still significant factors. As shown in Table 2, the developed SVM model was an independent and significant predictor after adjusting with these clinical factors. Therefore, the results indicated that the developed SVM model further improved the prediction of the patients' chemo-response.

Table 2. Cox regression model for the clinical features and predictive model in recurrence and death of NTUH patients.

Feature	Numbers	Recurrence				Death			
		Univariate		Multivariate		Univariate		Multivariate	
		HR (95% CI)	*p* Value	HR (95% CI)	*p* Value	HR (95% CI)	*p* Value	HR (95% CI)	*p* Value
Predictive model									
Low	19	1.00		1.00		1.00		1.00	
Medium + High	65	0.643 (0.415–0.998)	0.049	0.644 (0.436–0.952)	0.027	0.559 (0.351–0.890)	0.014	0.511 (0.334–0.783)	0.002
Residual tumor size <1 cm									
No	42	1.00		1.00		1.00		1.00	
Yes	42	0.273 (0.160–0.468)	<0.001	0.312 (0.170–0.573)	<0.001	0.198 (0.107–0.365)	<0.001	0.252 (0.128–0.496)	<0.001
FIGO stage									
Early (I + II)	11	1.00		1.00		1.00		1.00	
Advanced (III + IV)	73	7.954 (1.934–32.71)	0.004	2.149 (0.257–17.93)	0.480	6.13 (1.489–25.24)	0.012	1.732 (0.201–14.90)	0.617
Tumor grade									
1	4	1.00		1.00		1.00		1.00	
2 + 3	67	2.289 (1.156–4.530)	0.018	2.125 (0.992–4.552)	0.053	1.756 (0.953–3.234)	0.071	1.533 (0.761–3.09)	0.232
Histological subtype									
Serous	59	1.00		1.00		1.00		1.00	
Endometrioid	12	0.454 (0.193–1.067)	0.070	1.023 (0.422–2.475)	0.960	0.562 (0.239–1.323)	0.187	1.077 (0.443–2.618)	0.870
Clear cell	13	0.531 (0.239–1.180)	0.120	NA	NA	0.284 (0.102–0.793)	0.016	NA	NA

3. Discussion

Our model predicted the chemo-response in ovarian carcinoma patients. Several types of chemotherapy sensitivity and resistance assays (CSRAs) have been reported, such as the adenosine triphosphate assay, the human tumor cloning assay, the methylthiazolyldiphenyltetrazolium bromide assay, and the extreme drug resistance assay, as well as the drug-induced apoptosis assay, but the role of CSRAs remains controversial [18]. Other platforms, including proteomics [19], exosomes [20], next generation sequencing [21] and in vivo ovarian cancer patient-derived xenografts [22], also have weaknesses of inconsistent results, expensive costs and time-consuming processes. With the advancement of high-throughput technologies, researchers are now able to measure the gene expression profiles of one patient at a low cost. Therefore, considering the genetic features in one single individual may shed light on how to achieve the concept of providing precision medicine. However, it is difficult to develop a predictive model of one specific drug by investigating and manipulating the samples directly from real patients. Han et al. developed multiple gene predictive models for the platinum/paclitaxel response from the TCGA gene expression dataset [23]. Murakami et al. developed a multiple-gene scoring system for predicting a platinum or taxane response in ovarian cancer from the TCGA and GSE datasets [24]. However, both studies were not validated in ovarian cancer tissue samples by evaluating the clinical feasibility of the predictive models. To address this issue, we used cell lines as the identification set and validated the results in clinical samples [25].

In this study, we demonstrated the usefulness of the model in predicting the chemo-response, and survival benefits were observed in three independent datasets, including ovarian cancer tissue samples from our institute. Notably, relatively few samples from the NTUH cohort have been classified into "high" or "low" response groups. It can be mainly attributed to that we tried to classify the samples into three groups, which may result in some false positive classifications. However, as shown in Figures S1 and S2, the curves from the "medium" response group showed no significant differences to the curves from the "low" response group. This suggests that only the patients classified into "high" response group have definite benefits from receiving the drug treatment. For the other two groups, we should be more cautious while designing the treatment plan and selecting the appropriate drugs. In clinical practice, the cancer tissue of ovarian cancer patients could be tested by our 10 gene model before chemotherapy. For the patients of high response group, they have the best response to the paclitaxel-platinum chemotherapy which could be the standard treatment. However, in the patients of medium to low response groups, the response to the paclitaxel-platinum chemotherapy is not good enough, and early introduction or combination of other drugs should be considered.

The reason why we utilized a GA to select 10 possible predictors from 575 genes is its low computational complexity and good classification accuracy. Notably, the number of possible combinations of the original 575 genes is $C_{10}^{575} = 1.01 \times 10^{21}$, which cannot be analysed in a practical amount of time. The GA is a greedy approach that randomly selects and tests possible combinations through many generations. By doing so, the GA avoids calculating all the combinations and still can identify useful predictors in a reasonable amount of time [14]. Furthermore, in order to reduce the cost and simplify the experimental processes, we wished to minimize the number of predictors in the predictive model. However, the prediction accuracy was poor when the number of predictors was <10; thus, we defined it as 10.

Several studies demonstrated that the genes of our predictive model were involved in the growth, proliferation, and drug response of cancer cells [26–31]. We utilized the Ingenuity Pathway Analysis website to explore the possible interaction network among the 10 genes. As shown in Figure S4, five out of the 10 genes are summarized into one network centering on *TGFB1* and *E2F1* which are important regulators in the cell cycle. The results indicated that the genes of our predictive model have an important functional impact in ovarian cancer cells relating to chemo-response.

The study had some limitations. Notably, the standard regimen of chemotherapy for epithelial ovarian cancer is combination of platinum and paclitaxel. In this study, we only used the drug response efficacy of paclitaxel in the CCLE dataset to identify possible biomarkers, which might result in some biases and neglect the combination effects after treated with two different drugs. This was certain a potential limitation in our approach. However, the large-scale gene expression data along with the drug efficacy after treatment with these two drugs was not available currently. Therefore, it was not feasible to develop a prediction model by performing an integrated analysis of these two drugs simultaneously. In our identification set, the CCLE dataset, those studied ovarian cancer cell lines included both platinum-sensitive and platinum-resistant, such as ES-2, NIH:OVCAR-3, and SKOV-3. Therefore, those identified genes reflected the effect which was not solely from paclitaxel. Validation of this prediction model in three datasets in real clinical patients also showed a good performance, suggesting that although the approach in this study was not a perfect one, the resulted prediction model still had a good utility in daily clinical practice. The other limitation was the different definition of RFS in TCGA, GSE9891 and our set. RFS was calculated from the completion of adjuvant chemotherapy and we used the definition in our own NTUH dataset. However, in the data from the public domains including GSE9891 and the TCGA dataset, we used those provided RFS information along with their microarray data. However, this might result in some potential biases from different definitions of the RFS. Lastly, it was a limitation that the NTUH cohort did not include the tissue samples of the non-ovarian cancer group, which may help to provide more detailed information of our gene model about the chemo-response of ovarian cancer.

4. Materials and Methods

4.1. Identification of The Genes Associated with The Drug Response

The protocol used to identify the probes associated with the drug efficacy and develop the predictive model is illustrated in Figure 1. The details about selecting predictive biomarkers from GSE36133 (Table S3) were described in the supplementary data. Briefly, after pre-processing, we analysed the 25 ovarian cancer cell lines (Table S4) to identify the genes associated with the efficacy of paclitaxel treatment. The 25 ovarian cancer cell lines were classified into three groups based on their sensitivity, which was the activity area provided by the GSE36133 dataset. Furthermore, a quantile normalization algorithm was performed and a Kruskal-Wallis test was utilized to identify the probes showing significantly different expression levels in the three groups ($p < 0.01$). Only the probes mapped to a unique gene symbol remained for further analyses. When multiple probes were annotated to the same gene, their coefficients of variation (CVs) were calculated, and only the probe possessing the largest CV was kept. In order to reduce systematic biases resulted from different technological platforms, the expression value of each gene was normalized to Z-value based on its mean and standard deviation, respectively.

4.2. Development of a Predictive Model Using a Genetic Algorithm

Among the probes showing a significant association with the response of paclitaxel, a genetic algorithm (GA) was designed to select the best combination of 10 probes to classify the 25 cell lines into the three groups, corresponding to the drug efficacy (Figure S1). The detailed procedures in the GA were described in the supplementary data. In general, the GA algorithm mimics the concept of the "survival of the fittest," which indicates that a combination showing a better prediction performance has a higher probability of being selected in the next generation. Therefore, the model showing the highest accuracy for predicting the paclitaxel response was developed in the last generation. We also performed a permutation test to evaluate the random chance of identifying 10 probes with the same prediction accuracy.

The definitions of response groups were based on the activity area of the drug efficacy provided in the CCLE dataset. We sorted the values ascendingly and divided them into three groups accordingly. That is after being sorted, the first nine cell lines with lower activity area values from the 25 ovarian cancer cell lines were classified into "low" response group (i.e., activity area less than 4 in Table S4).

Subsequently, the eight cell lines with medium activity values were classified into "medium" response group and the last eight cell lines with higher activity values were classified into "high" response group (i.e., activity area higher than 5.29 in Table S4).

4.3. Validation of the Predictive Model in Two Independent Datasets

In addition to the internal validations using permutation and cross-validation in the CCLE dataset, two ovarian cancer microarray datasets from TCGA [13] and GSE9891 [32], composed of real clinical samples, were analysed (Table S3). To focus on the chemo-response, only those patients who received the drug treatment and survived longer than 30 days were analysed. All the analysis procedures followed the same steps previously described, and all the patients were classified into distinct groups using the predictive model. The gene expression data from the microarray datasets were normalized to the standard normal distribution, and the drug response of one patient was predicted by the developed SVM model that was composed of the 10 selected probes. For the patient groups with different drug efficacies, the log-rank test was utilized to evaluate whether significant differences existed in the overall survival (OS) and/or recurrence-free survival (RFS).

4.4. Validation of the Predictive Model by a Quantitative Real-Time Polymerase Chain Reaction (QRT-PCR) Using Ovarian Cancer Tissue

Lastly, we validated the predictive model using the QRT-PCR method in patients recruited from the National Taiwan University Hospital (NTUH). The study protocol was approved by the National Taiwan University Hospital Research Ethics Committee. Informed consents were obtained and the methods were performed in accordance with the guidelines and regulations. From January 2012 to March 2014, 84 women diagnosed with ovarian carcinoma who received debulking surgery and adjuvant chemotherapy were enrolled. Part of cancerous tissue specimen collected in debulking surgery was immediately frozen in liquid nitrogen and stored at −70 °C. The remaining tissue specimens were sent for frozen section and pathology examinations to confirm the diagnosis and ensure sufficient tumor tissue in the specimens collected for the following experiments. The medical records of the patients were reviewed until June 2017 to obtain clinical data, including the age, cancer stage, surgical findings during debulking, treatment courses, recurrence and survival. Residual tumor size was recorded as <1 cm or ≥1 cm after debulking surgery. The tumor grading was based on the International Union Against Cancer criteria, and the staging was based on the criteria of the International Federation of Gynecology and Obstetrics (FIGO) [33]. The patients received regular follow-ups every 3 months after the primary treatment. Abnormal results from imaging studies (including computerized tomography or magnetic resonance imaging), elevated CA-125 (more than 2 times the upper normal limit) for two consecutive tests in 2-week intervals, or biopsy-proven disease were defined as recurrence. The RFS was calculated as the period from the date of chemotherapy completion to the date of confirmed recurrence, disease progression, or the last follow-up. The OS was calculated as the period from the surgery to the date of death associated with the disease or the date of the last follow-up. To evaluate the required the sample size for the validation, we utilized the estimated hazard ratio from the TCGA data (HR = 0.52). Therefore, using the parameters (type 1 error: 0.05, power: 70%, overall probability of event: close to 1, and the proportion of samples in "low" risk group: 0.776, the estimated sample size is 84.

Total RNA of the cancerous tissue was isolated with TRIzol reagent (Invitrogen Corporation, Carlsbad, CA, USA) according to the manufacturer's instructions. The samples were subsequently passed over a Qiagen RNeasy column (Qiagen, Valencia, CA, USA) to remove the small fragments that affect the RT reaction and hybridization quality. After RNA recovery, double-stranded cDNA was synthesized by a chimeric oligonucleotide with an oligo-dT and a T7 RNA polymerase promoter at a concentration of 100 pmol/μL. The protocol for the quantitative real-time polymerase chain reaction is briefly described. First-strand cDNA was synthesized with a RevertAid first strand cDNA synthesis kit (Fermentas, Burlington, ON, Canada; Vilnius, Lithuania). Quantitative PCR was performed using the LightCycler Real-Time detection system (Roche Diagnostics, Mannheim, Germany). The relative abundance of the mRNA level was calculated by using the comparative method with glyceraldehyde-3-phosphate dehydrogenase (*GAPDH*) as the internal control. The quantitative PCR primers for the TaqMan probes are listed in Table S1. The detection of *GAPDH* was carried out by the LightCycler h-*GAPDH* housekeeping gene set (Roche Applied Science, Indianapolis, IN, USA) for 50 cycles of 10 s at 95 °C, 15 s at 55 °C, and 15 s at 72 °C.

The expression levels of the 10 probes were normalized to the standard normal distribution. Following the prediction procedures previously described, each patient was classified into a different group based on the SVM predictive model. The differences in the OS and RFS in the predicted groups were compared using the log-rank test, and a Cox hazard regression model was utilized to evaluate the prediction performance.

5. Conclusions

The epithelial ovarian cancer patients of high response group stratified by our 10 gene model had good response to the paclitaxel-platinum chemotherapy which could be the standard treatment. However, for the patients of medium to low response groups, introduction of other drugs or clinical trials might be beneficial.

Supplementary Materials: The following are available online at http://www.mdpi.com/2072-6694/11/2/270/s1, Figure S1: The proposed genetic algorithm (GA) to identify the best combinations of predictors for the SVM model, Figure S2: The Kaplan Meier survival curves of the RFS in the three response groups in the (A) TCGA, (B) GSE9891 and (C) NTUH datasets, Figure S3: The Kaplan Meier survival curves of the OS in the three response groups in the (A) TCGA, (B) GSE9891 and (C) NTUH datasets, Figure S4: The gene-gene interaction network of the 10 genes analyzed using the Ingenuity Pathway Analysis website, Table S1: The quantitative PCR primers of TaqMan probes, Table S2: Distribution of OS and RFS in the patients classified into three groups, Table S3: Characteristics of the three microarray datasets, Table S4: The 25 ovarian cancer lines in GSE36133 utilized as the training set.

Author Contributions: Conception and design: T.-P.L., K.-T.K. and Y.-C.C.; Development of methodology: T.-P.L., K.-T.K. and Y.-C.C.; Acquisition of data (provided animals, acquired and managed patients, provided facilities, etc.): T.-P.L., M.-C.C., H.-P.L., Y.-H.H., Y.-C.C., W.-F.C. and C.-A.C.; Analysis and interpretation of data (e.g., statistical analysis, biostatistics, computational analysis): T.-P.L., K.-T.K., C.-H.C. and Y.-C.C.; Writing, review, and/or revision of the manuscript: T.-P.L., K.-T.K., C.-H.C. and Y.-C.C.; Administrative, technical, or material support (i.e., reporting or organizing data, constructing databases): T.-P.L., M.-C.C. and Y.-C.C.; Study supervision: T.-P.L., K.-T.K., Y.-C.C., W.-F.C. and C.-A.C.

Funding: This research was funded by the Ministry of Science and Technology, Taipei, Taiwan, MOST 104-2314-B-002-108-MY2 and MOST 106-2314-B-002 -194 -MY2, and National Taiwan University Hospital, NTUH. 104-S2711 and NTUH. 105-M3347.

Acknowledgments: This work was supported in part by the 7th Core Laboratory Facility of the Department of Medical Research of National Taiwan University Hospital.

Conflicts of Interest: The authors declare no conflict of interest.

References

1. Siegel, R.L.; Miller, K.D.; Jemal, A. Cancer Statistics, 2017. *CA Cancer J. Clin.* **2017**, *67*, 7–30. [CrossRef] [PubMed]

2. Chiang, Y.-C.; Chen, C.-A.; Chiang, C.-J.; Hsu, T.-H.; Lin, M.-C.; You, S.-L.; Cheng, W.-F.; Lai, M.-S. Trends in incidence and survival outcome of epithelial ovarian cancer: 30-year national population-based registry in Taiwan. *J. Gynecol. Oncol.* **2013**, *24*, 342–351. [CrossRef] [PubMed]

3. Jayson, G.C.; Kohn, E.C.; Kitchener, H.C.; Ledermann, J.A. Ovarian cancer. *Lancet* **2014**, *384*, 1376–1388. [CrossRef]

4. Vaughan, S.; Coward, J.I.; Bast, R.C., Jr.; Berchuck, A.; Berek, J.S.; Brenton, J.D.; Coukos, G.; Crum, C.C.; Drapkin, R.; Etemadmoghadam, D.; et al. Rethinking ovarian cancer: Recommendations for improving outcomes. *Nat. Rev. Cancer* **2011**, *11*, 719–725. [CrossRef] [PubMed]

5. Coleman, R.L.; Monk, B.J.; Sood, A.K.; Herzog, T.J. Latest research and treatment of advanced-stage epithelial ovarian cancer. *Nat. Rev. Clin. Oncol.* **2013**, *10*, 211–224. [CrossRef] [PubMed]

6. Bottoni, P.; Scatena, R. The Role of CA 125 as Tumor Marker: Biochemical and Clinical Aspects. *Adv. Exp. Med. Biol.* **2015**, *867*, 229–244. [PubMed]
7. Liu, J.; Westin, S.N. Rational selection of biomarker driven therapies for gynecologic cancers: The more we know, the more we know we don't know. *Gynecol. Oncol.* **2016**, *141*, 65–71. [CrossRef] [PubMed]
8. Perren, T.J.; Swart, A.M.; Pfisterer, J.; Ledermann, J.A.; Pujade-Lauraine, E.; Kristensen, G.; Carey, M.S.; Beale, P.; Cervantes, A.; Kurzeder, C.; et al. A phase 3 trial of bevacizumab in ovarian cancer. *N. Engl. J. Med.* **2011**, *365*, 2484–2496. [CrossRef] [PubMed]
9. Burger, R.A.; Brady, M.F.; Bookman, M.A.; Fleming, G.F.; Monk, B.J.; Huang, H.; Mannel, R.S.; Homesley, H.D.; Fowler, J.; Greer, B.E.; et al. Incorporation of bevacizumab in the primary treatment of ovarian cancer. *N. Engl. J. Med.* **2011**, *365*, 2473–2483. [CrossRef] [PubMed]
10. Ledermann, J.; Harter, P.; Gourley, C.; Friedlander, M.; Vergote, I.; Rustin, G.; Scott, C.; Meier, W.; Shapira-Frommer, R.; Safra, T.; et al. Olaparib maintenance therapy in platinum-sensitive relapsed ovarian cancer. *N. Engl. J. Med.* **2012**, *366*, 1382–1392. [CrossRef] [PubMed]
11. Mirza, M.R.; Monk, B.J.; Herrstedt, J.; Oza, A.M.; Mahner, S.; Redondo, A.; Fabbro, M.; Ledermann, J.A.; Lorusso, D.; Vergote, I.; et al. Niraparib Maintenance Therapy in Platinum-Sensitive, Recurrent Ovarian Cancer. *N. Engl. J. Med.* **2016**, *375*, 2154–2164. [CrossRef] [PubMed]
12. Barretina, J.; Caponigro, G.; Stransky, N.; Venkatesan, K.; Margolin, A.A.; Kim, S.; Wilson, C.J.; Lehár, J.; Kryukov, G.V.; Sonkin, D.; et al. The Cancer Cell Line Encyclopedia enables predictive modelling of anticancer drug sensitivity. *Nature* **2012**, *483*, 603–607. [CrossRef] [PubMed]
13. Cancer Genome Atlas Research Network. Integrated genomic analyses of ovarian carcinoma. *Nature* **2011**, *474*, 609–615. [CrossRef] [PubMed]
14. Wang, W.A.; Lai, L.C.; Tsai, M.H.; Lu, T.P.; Chuang, E.Y. Development of a prediction model for radiosensitivity using the expression values of genes and long non-coding RNAs. *Oncotarget* **2016**, *7*, 26739–26750. [CrossRef] [PubMed]
15. Chuang, M.K.; Chiu, Y.C.; Chou, W.C.; Hou, H.A.; Chuang, E.Y.; Tien, H.F. A 3-microRNA scoring system for prognostication in de novo acute myeloid leukemia patients. *Leukemia* **2015**, *29*, 1051–1059. [CrossRef] [PubMed]
16. Marchetti, C.; Ledermann, J.A.; Benedetti Panici, P. An overview of early investigational therapies for chemoresistant ovarian cancer. *Expert Opin. Investig. Drugs* **2015**, *24*, 1163–1183. [CrossRef] [PubMed]
17. Kumar, S.; Mahdi, H.; Bryant, C.; Shah, J.P.; Garg, G.; Munkarah, A. Clinical trials and progress with paclitaxel in ovarian cancer. *Int. J. Womens Health* **2010**, *2*, 411–427. [CrossRef] [PubMed]
18. Grendys, E.C., Jr.; Fiorica, J.V.; Orr, J.W., Jr.; Holloway, R.; Wang, D.; Tian, C.; Chan, J.K.; Herzog, T.J. Overview of a chemoresponse assay in ovarian cancer. *Clin. Transl. Oncol.* **2014**, *16*, 761–769. [CrossRef] [PubMed]
19. Au, K.K.; Josahkian, J.A.; Francis, J.A.; Squire, J.A.; Koti, M. Current state of biomarkers in ovarian cancer prognosis. *Future Oncol.* **2015**, *11*, 3187–3195. [CrossRef] [PubMed]
20. Dorayappan, K.D.; Wallbillich, J.J.; Cohn, D.E.; Selvendiran, K. The biological significance and clinical applications of exosomes in ovarian cancer. *Gynecol. Oncol.* **2016**, *142*, 199–205. [CrossRef] [PubMed]
21. Davidson, B. Recently identified drug resistance biomarkers in ovarian cancer. *Expert Rev. Mol. Diagn.* **2016**, *16*, 569–578. [CrossRef] [PubMed]
22. Alkema, N.G.; Wisman, G.B.; van der Zee, A.G.; van Vugt, M.A.; de Jong, S. Studying platinum sensitivity and resistance in high-grade serous ovarian cancer: Different models for different questions. *Drug Resist. Updat.* **2016**, *24*, 55–69. [CrossRef] [PubMed]
23. Han, Y.; Huang, H.; Xiao, Z.; Zhang, W.; Cao, Y.; Qu, L.; Shou, C. Integrated analysis of gene expression profiles associated with response of platinum/paclitaxel-based treatment in epithelial ovarian cancer. *PLoS ONE* **2012**, *7*, e52745. [CrossRef] [PubMed]
24. Murakami, R.; Matsumura, N.; Brown, J.B.; Wang, Z.; Yamaguchi, K.; Abiko, K.; Yoshioka, Y.; Hamanishi, J.; Baba, T.; Koshiyama, M.; et al. Prediction of taxane and platinum sensitivity in ovarian cancer based on gene expression profiles. *Gynecol. Oncol.* **2016**, *141*, 49–56. [CrossRef] [PubMed]
25. Wang, L.P.; Chuang, E.Y.; Lu, T.P. Identification of predictive biomarkers for ZD-6474 in lung cancer. *Transl. Cancer Res.* **2015**, *4*, 324–331.

26. Kim, S.W.; Kim, S.; Nam, E.J.; Jeong, Y.W.; Lee, S.H.; Paek, J.H.; Kim, J.H.; Kim, J.W.; Kim, Y.T. Comparative proteomic analysis of advanced serous epithelial ovarian carcinoma: Possible predictors of chemoresistant disease. *OMICS* **2011**, *15*, 281–292. [CrossRef] [PubMed]

27. Arner, E.; Forrest, A.R.; Ehrlund, A.; Mejhert, N.; Itoh, M.; Kawaji, H.; Lassmann, T.; Laurencikiene, J.; Rydén, M.; Arner, P.; et al. Ceruloplasmin is a novel adipokine which is overexpressed in adipose tissue of obese subjects and in obesity-associated cancer cells. *PLoS ONE* **2014**, *9*, e80274. [CrossRef] [PubMed]

28. Dentice, M.; Ambrosio, R.; Salvatore, D. Role of type 3 deiodinase in cancer. *Expert Opin. Ther. Targets* **2009**, *13*, 1363–1373. [CrossRef] [PubMed]

29. Ciavardelli, D.; Bellomo, M.; Crescimanno, C.; Vella, V. Type 3 deiodinase: Role in cancer growth, stemness, and metabolism. *Front. Endocrinol.* **2014**, *5*, 215. [CrossRef] [PubMed]

30. Galluzzi, L.; Goubar, A.; Olaussen, K.A.; Vitale, I.; Senovilla, L.; Michels, J.; Robin, A.; Dorvault, N.; Besse, B.; Validire, P.; et al. Prognostic value of LIPC in non-small cell lung carcinoma. *Cell Cycle* **2013**, *12*, 647–654. [CrossRef] [PubMed]

31. Fang, Y.; Qin, Y.; Zhang, N.; Wang, J.; Wang, H.; Zheng, X. DISIS: Prediction of drug response through an iterative sure independence screening. *PLoS ONE* **2015**, *10*, e0120408. [CrossRef] [PubMed]

32. Tothill, R.W.; Tinker, A.V.; George, J.; Brown, R.; Fox, S.B.; Lade, S.; Johnson, D.S.; Trivett, M.K.; Etemadmoghadam, D.; Locandro, B.; et al. Novel molecular subtypes of serous and endometrioid ovarian cancer linked to clinical outcome. *Clin. Cancer Res.* **2008**, *14*, 5198–5208. [CrossRef] [PubMed]

33. Prat, J. Staging classification for cancer of the ovary, fallopian tube, and peritoneum. *Int. J. Gynaecol. Obstet.* **2014**, *124*, 1–5. [CrossRef] [PubMed]

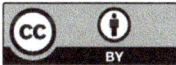

Article

The Potential Mechanism of Bufadienolide-Like Chemicals on Breast Cancer via Bioinformatics Analysis

Yingbo Zhang [1,2,†], Xiaomin Tang [3,†], Yuxin Pang [3,4,*], Luqi Huang [4,*], Dan Wang [1,2], Chao Yuan [1,2], Xuan Hu [1,2] and Liping Qu [5]

[1] Tropical Crops Genetic Resources Institute, Chinese Academy of Tropical Agricultural Sciences, Danzhou 571737, China; zhangyingbo1984@catas.cn or zhangyingbo1984@163.com (Y.Z.); wang_dan1414@163.com (D.W.); yuanchao79@126.com (C.Y.); mchuxuan@163.com (X.H.)
[2] Hainan Provincial Engineering Research Center for Blumea Balsamifera, Danzhou 571737, China
[3] School of Traditional Chinese Medicine, Guangdong Pharmaceutical University, Guangzhou 510006, China; txm1209@163.com
[4] National Resource Center for Chinese Materia Medica, China Academy of Chinese Medical Sciences, Beijing 100700, China
[5] College of Pharmacy, Chengdu University of Traditional Chinese Medicine, Chengdu 611137, China; quliping2018@163.com
* Correspondence: pyxmarx@126.com (Y.P.); huangluqi01@126.com (L.H.); Tel.: +86-898-2330-0268 (Y.P.)
† The author had the same contribution to this work.

Received: 28 November 2018; Accepted: 8 January 2019; Published: 14 January 2019

Abstract: Bufadienolide-like chemicals are mostly composed of the active ingredient of Chansu and they have anti-inflammatory, tumor-suppressing, and anti-pain activities; however, their mechanism is unclear. This work used bioinformatics analysis to study this mechanism via gene expression profiles of bufadienolide-like chemicals: (1) Differentially expressed gene identification combined with gene set variation analysis, (2) similar small -molecule detection, (3) tissue-specific co-expression network construction, (4) differentially regulated sub-networks related to breast cancer phenome, (5) differentially regulated sub-networks with potential cardiotoxicity, and (6) hub gene selection and their relation to survival probability. The results indicated that bufadienolide-like chemicals usually had the same target as valproic acid and estradiol, etc. They could disturb the pathways in RNA splicing, the apoptotic process, cell migration, extracellular matrix organization, adherens junction organization, synaptic transmission, Wnt signaling, AK-STAT signaling, BMP signaling pathway, and protein folding. We also investigated the potential cardiotoxicity and found a dysregulated subnetwork related to membrane depolarization during action potential, retinoic acid receptor binding, GABA receptor binding, positive regulation of nuclear division, negative regulation of viral genome replication, and negative regulation of the viral life cycle. These may play important roles in the cardiotoxicity of bufadienolide-like chemicals. The results may highlight the potential anticancer mechanism and cardiotoxicity of Chansu, and could also explain the ability of bufadienolide-like chemicals to be used as hormones and anticancer and vasoprotectives agents.

Keywords: Bufadienolide-like chemicals; molecular mechanism; anti-cancer; bioinformatics

---

1. Introduction

Despite considerable efforts on early diagnosis and treatment in the last decade, breast cancer remains the most common malignancies for women worldwide, representing ~22% of female malignancies [1–4]. In addition to early diagnosis, new chemotherapeutic agents and more effective therapies are needed to reduce mortality. Traditional Chinese medicine has existed for thousands of years and can treat cancer. Chansu is one of the most famous traditional Chinese medicines. It has been used for centuries in various aspects, such as anaesthesia for anesthesia, antitumor, anti-inflammation, and anti-arrhythmia conditions [5–8]. Chansu is mostly from the glandular secretion and dried product of *Bufo* bufo gargarizans Cantor or *Bufo* melanostictus Schneider [8]. It includes resibufogenin, bufalin, arenobufagin, cinobufagin, bufotoxin, telocinobufagin, bufotaline, and cinobufotalin [5,6,8] (Figure 1).

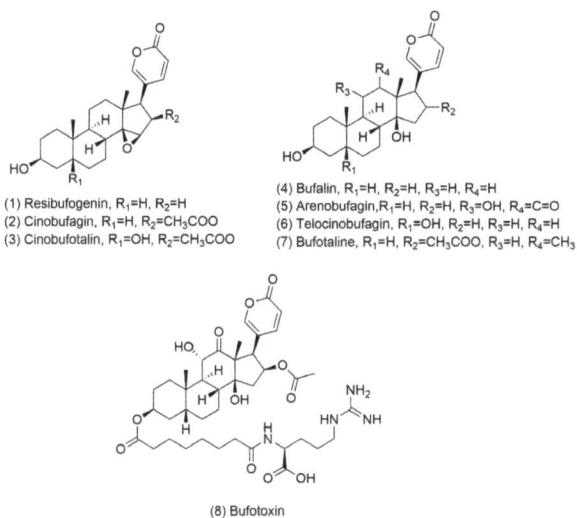

(1) Resibufogenin, R_1=H, R_2=H
(2) Cinobufagin, R_1=H, R_2=CH$_3$COO
(3) Cinobufotalin, R_1=OH, R_2=CH$_3$COO

(4) Bufalin, R_1=H, R_2=H, R_3=H, R_4=H
(5) Arenobufagin, R_1=H, R_2=H, R_3=OH, R_4=C=O
(6) Telocinobufagin, R_1=OH, R_2=H, R_3=H, R_4=H
(7) Bufotaline, R_1=H, R_2=CH$_3$COO, R_3=H, R_4=CH$_3$

(8) Bufotoxin

Figure 1. The structural formula of the eight bufadienolide-like chemicals.

Over the last decade, many groups have studied the pharmacological activities and antitumor activity of bufadienolide-like chemicals. For example, Li et al. [9] reported that cinobufagin has significant cancer-killing capacity for a range of cancers, including HCT116 cells, HT29 cells, A431 cells, PC3 cells, A549 cells, and MCF-7 cells. Mechanistic studies showed that cinobufagin can induce tumor cells apoptosis and modulate hypoxia-inducing factor-1 alpha subunit (HIF-1α). Yeh et al. [10] and Yu et al. [11] reported that bufalin and cinobufagin have a potent inhibiting effect on androgen-dependent and -independent prostate cancer cells, similar to Dong et al. [12], Wang et al. [13], and Ko et al. [14] via HepG2 cells, T24 cells, and HeLa cells.

Immunotherapy, an evolving approach for the management of triple negative breast cancer: Converting non-responders to responders. These results demonstrate that Chansu is a potent anticancer agent for a range of cancers, but its potential anticancer mechanisms are unclear. Here, the gene set variation analysis (GSVA) algorithm [15] was first used to identify differentially expressed genes (DEGs) and relative enrichment pathways underlying eight bufadienolide-like chemicals. A series of bioinformatics analyses, including gene enrichment analysis, tissue-specific co-expression network construction, and differentially-regulated sub-network detection, can relate the findings to the breast cancer phenome and hub gene selection. The relation to survival probability and similar small-molecule detection used the DEGs with relative enrichment pathways (Figure 2). This work shows the potential mechanism of bufadienolide-like chemicals on breast cancer, especially differentially regulated sub-networks that relate to breast cancer and hub genes disturbed by bufadienolide-like chemicals. This work highlights the potential application of bufadienolide-like chemicals on breast cancer, especially as a novel agent for cancer therapy.

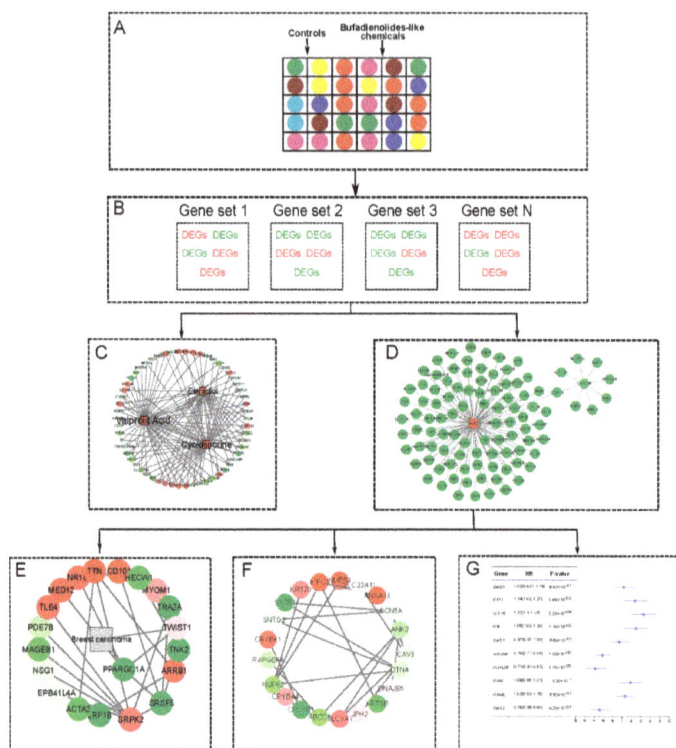

Figure 2. The workflow to study the potential mechanism of bufadienolides-like chemicals on breast cancer via bioinformatics analysis. (**A**) The experimental design and basic information of this analysis. (**B**) The DEGs'(Differentially expressed genes) identification with the GSVA (Gene set variation analysis) algorithm [15]. (**C**) Similar small-molecule detection with the Comparative Toxicogenomics Database (CTD) [16] and connectivity map (CMAP2) [17,18] database. (**D**) The tissue-specific co-expression network constructed with the TCSBN (Tissue and cancer specific biological networks) database [19]. (**E**) The differentially expressed subnetworks detected with the UberPheno database and PhenomeScape plug [20]. (**F**) The arrhythmia-related subnetworks detected with the UberPheno database and PhenomeScape plug [20]. (**G**) The expression and survival relation of hub genes validated by TCGA (The Cancer Genome Atlas) [21] and the Kaplan-Meier (KM) plotter databases [22].

2. Results

2.1. Identification of DEGs

Based on the differentially expressed genes analysis associated with the gene sets enrichment variation analysis strategy, a total of 80 differentially expressed genes (DEGs) involved in the 44 MSigDB C2 curated gene sets were identified (Figure 3A,B), and the top 20 DEGs' expression heatmap is shown in Figure 3C. Of which, 38 genes involved in the Singh NFE2L2 targets gene sets, Chang dominant negative gene sets immortalized by HPV31 and Lin silenced gene sets by tumor microenvironment were up-regulated (Tables S1 and S2), including IF16 (interferon-inducible protein 6), IRF9 (interferon regulatory factor 9), IFIT1 (IFN-induced protein 1 with tetratricopeptide repeats), ISG15 (Interferon-stimulated gene 15), BST2 (bone marrow stromal cell antigen 2), OAS3 ($2'$-$5'$-oligoadenylate synthetase 3), OAS1 ($2'$-$5'$-oligoadenylate synthetase 1), DDX60 (DEAD box polypeptide 60), CYP1A1 (cytochrome P450 1A1), CEACAM6 (carcinoembryonic antigen-related cell adhesion molecule 6), keratin genes KRT81, and so on.

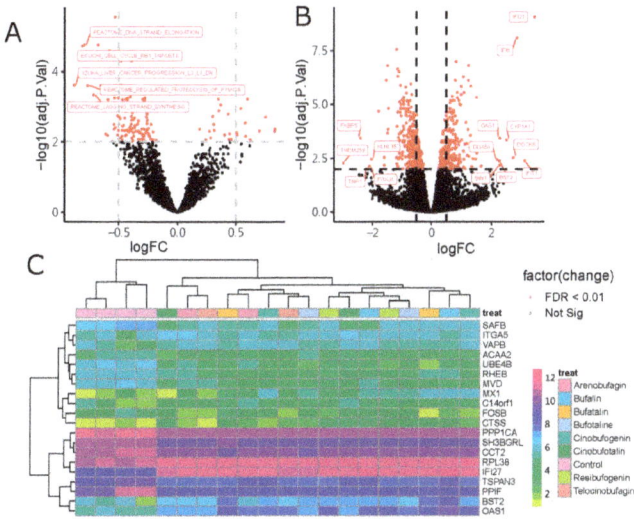

Figure 3. The differentially expressed genes (DEGs) disturbed by bufadienolide-like chemicals through the gene set variation analysis (GSVA) algorithm. (**A**) The differentially expressed gene sets disturbed by bufadienolide-like chemicals (| logFC | ≥ log2(2) and adjPvalue < 0.001). (**B**) The DEGs relate to differentially expressed gene sets (| logFC | ≥ log2(2) and adjPvalue < 0.001). (**C**) The heatmap of the top 20 DEGs disturbed by bufadienolide-like chemicals.

Among the differentially expressed genes associated with enrichment gene sets, 42 genes involved in the 41 gene sets were down-regulated (Tables S1 and S2), such as the genes involved in the Iizuka (Table S1) liver cancer progression pathway, including PPIF (peptidylprolyl isomerase F), TMED2 (transmembrane trafficking protein 2 with emp24 domain), SAFB (scaffold attachment factor B), SQLE (squalene epoxidase), PICALM (phosphatidylinositol binding clathrin assembly protein), STIP1 (stress-induced phosphoprotein 1), CYB561 (cytochromes b561), CCT2 (chaperonin 2β with TCP1 domain); the genes sets involved Thum systolic heart failure pathway, including CCNG2 (cyclin G2), TMED2 (transmembrane emp24 domain trafficking protein 2), FH (fumarate hydratase), TAF9B (ATA-box binding protein associated factor 9b), CCT2 (chaperonin-containing t-complex polypeptide 1 beta), transmembrane receptor NOTCH2, PICALM (subfamily A (MS4A), and CCNL2 (cyclin L2); and also Reactome DNA strand elongation, Reactome regulated proteolysis of P75NTR, and other gene sets were downregulated, with logFC form −0.89~−0.27.

In order to obtain a biological interpretation of those genes in the GO and KEGG pathway functional groups, GO and KEGG enrichment analysis were performed with the clueGO plug [23] in Cystoscape [24]. Results indicated that those genes that were up-regulated were rich in terms of type I interferon signaling response to virus, defense to other organisms, regulation of viral genome replication, and 2′-5′-oligoadenylate synthetase activity, and those activated may be because of the up-regulation of IRF9, IFI6, IFI27, ISG15, IFIT1, OAS1, and OAS3 (Figure 4A). Further investigation with the KEGG pathway enrichment analysis showed those up-regulated genes could cause the activation of the IFN-induced pathway, type II interferon signaling pathway, and regulation of protein ISGylation by the ISG15 deconjugating enzyme USP18 pathway (Figure 4B). The genes that were down-regulated were rich in terms of protein kinase complex, transcription factor TFTC complex-1, the SAGA-complex, and cargo loading into vesicle (Figure 4A). Further investigation with KEGG pathway enrichment analysis showed those genes could negatively affect the transport of fringe-modified NOTCH to the plasma membrane pathway (Figure 4B).

A

B

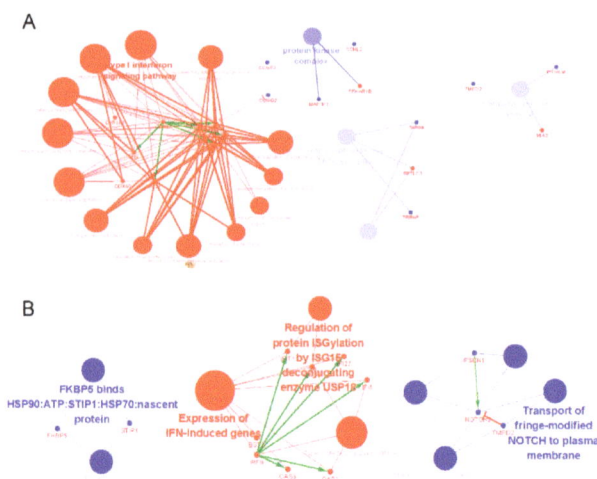

Figure 4. The GO and KEGG enrichment result of DEGs disturbed by bufadienolide-like chemicals. (**A**) Representative biomolecular network of GO enrichment terms. The bigger red nodes imply enrichment of GO terms with up-regulated genes. The bigger blue nodes suggest enrichment of GO terms with down-regulated genes. The small red nodes imply up-regulated genes. The small blue nodes are down-regulated genes. Undirected edges imply enrichment, green directed edges are activated according to the string database. The red directed edges implies suppression from the evidence generated by the String database. (**B**) Representative biomolecular network of KEGG enrichment term, the nodes, and edges also had the same means with Figure 4A.

2.2. Similar Small Molecule Detection

Detection of the similar small molecule with the Comparative Toxicogenomics Database (CTD) (http://ctdbase.org/) [16] and connectivity map (CMAP2) (https://portals.broadinstitute.org/cmap/) [17,18] database provides a better understanding the molecular mechanism of bufadienolide-like chemicals, and its potential value as a novel agent for cancer therapy. Based on the results with detecting the CTD Database, valproic acid, cyclosporine, and estradiol had the most similar target with bufadienolide-like chemicals (Figure 5). Valproic acid, a histone deacetylase inhibitor, which once was widely used as an antiepileptic, has recently also shown anti-cancer activity in an vitro/vivo model [25]. Estradiol is a sex hormone with anticancer activity, and is also widely used for the treatment of breast cancer, especially for postmenopausal women [26–28].

Based on the results from the CMAP2 database (https://portals.broadinstitute.org/cmap/) [17,18], V03AF, G03GB, C05AX, and C05CX were the top matching drugs with bufadienolide-like chemicals (Table 1). V03AF, a type of detoxifying agent for antineoplastic treatment, had an opposing effect on the expression of bufadienolide-like chemicals. This result provided evidence for bufadienolide-like chemicals' potential value as a novel agent for cancer therapy. G03GB, one type of sex hormone and a modulator of the genial system, had the most similar expression profile with bufadienolide-like chemicals. This means the bufadienolide-like chemicals also use estradiol, epimestrol and cyclofenil in breast cancer. C05AX and C05CX are two types of vasoprotectives agents, indicating that bufadienolide-like chemicals also have a potential use as vasoprotectives-like drugs.

From the evidence from detecting the similar small molecules with the CTD database and CMAP2 database, it was indicated that bufadienolide-like chemicals were one kind of steroid with the same physiological activity as estradiol and G03GB (ATC code), with potential value for use in cancer, especially breast cancer.

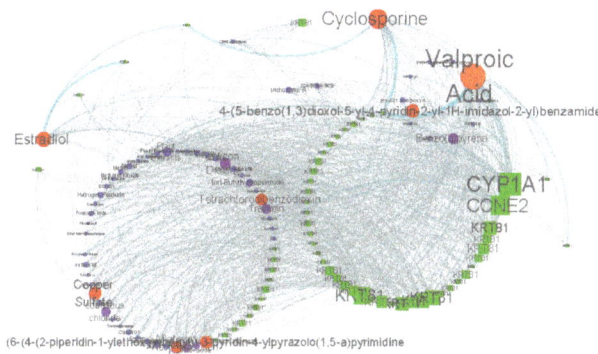

Figure 5. Chemicals-gene interaction network for the DEGs disturbed by bufadienolide-like chemicals. Square nodes represent the DEGs. Circle nodes represent the chemicals predicted by the CTD Database. The size of the nodes represents the degree. Circle nodes with red represent the similar small molecule predicted by degree (degree $\geq$ 30).

Table 1. Top 20 CMAP2 (connectivity map, https://portals.broadinstitute.org/cmap/) hits correlated with bufadienolide-like chemicals' treatment.

Rank	ATC Code	Mean Score	Enrichment	p-Value	Specificity
1	V03AF	−0.471	−0.71	4.45×10^{-3}	3.82×10^{-2}
2	G03GB	0.449	0.655	3.29×10^{-2}	7.47×10^{-2}
3	C05AX	0.41	0.689	1.95×10^{-2}	4.76×10^{-2}
4	C05CX	0.41	0.689	1.95×10^{-2}	4.76×10^{-2}
5	D07XC	−0.372	−0.661	1.44×10^{-3}	8.10×10^{-3}
6	N05BE	−0.359	−0.719	1.26×10^{-2}	1.22×10^{-2}
7	C08EA	0.292	0.539	1.87×10^{-2}	1.45×10^{-1}
8	N05AC	0.259	0.365	2.32×10^{-3}	3.90×10^{-1}
9	D06BB	−0.252	−0.405	9.39×10^{-3}	1.44×10^{-1}
10	D06BX	−0.249	−0.72	3.74×10^{-3}	1.38×10^{-2}
11	N02BB	0.244	0.404	2.71×10^{-3}	1.75×10^{-2}
12	N02CX	0.189	0.481	3.16×10^{-2}	4.43×10^{-2}
13	A07EA	−0.186	−0.343	6.96×10^{-3}	2.55×10^{-2}
14	S02BA	−0.167	−0.383	5.03×10^{-3}	1.31×10^{-2}
15	B01AC	0.152	0.243	2.71×10^{-2}	1.19×10^{-1}
16	S03BA	−0.144	−0.366	2.02×10^{-2}	4.80×10^{-2}
17	R03BA	−0.141	−0.29	1.19×10^{-2}	4.00×10^{-2}
18	S01CB	−0.136	−0.326	1.21×10^{-2}	2.61×10^{-2}
19	R01AD	−0.113	−0.266	4.30×10^{-3}	4.83×10^{-2}
20	C07AA	−0.109	−0.262	1.14×10^{-2}	2.22×10^{-1}

2.3. The Tissue Specific Co-Expression Network and Breast Cancer Associated Subnetwork Regulated by Bufadienolide-Like Chemicals

It is clear that most of the genes exert their function by collaborating with other genes in the network, which represent rigid molecular machines, cellular structures, or dynamic signaling pathways [29]. Here, a breast tissue specific co-expression network with DEGs was generated with the TCSBN database (http://inetmodels.com/) [19] through the NetworkAnalyst web server (https://www.networkanalyst.ca/) [18]. Results indicated that the co-expression networks consisted of 743 nodes and 876 edges (Figure 6 and Table 2).

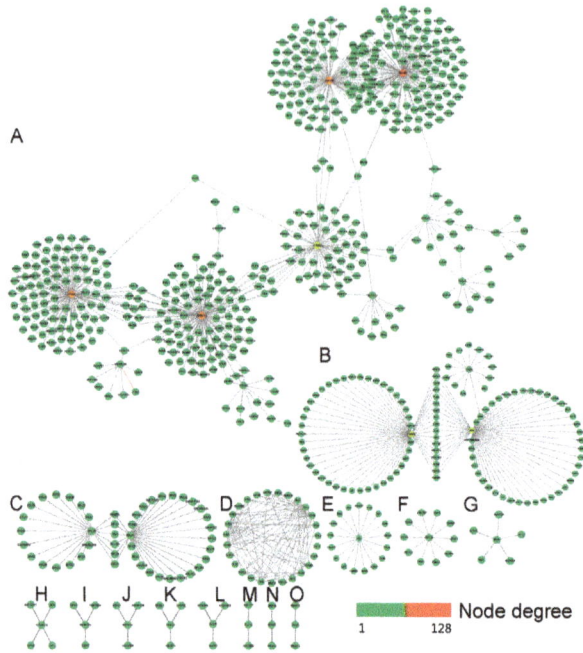

Figure 6. The breast tissue specific co-expression network with DEGs generated by the TCSBN (Tissue and cancer specific biological networks) database (http://inetmodels.com/) through the NetworkAnalyst (https://www.networkanalyst.ca/) web server. (**A–O**), the subnetworks of co-expression network origin from the seeds of DEGs.

Table 2. The tissue specific co-expression network regulated by bufadienolide-like chemicals and their enrichment with GO and KEGG.

Subnetwork Number	Nodes	Edges	Seeds	KEGG Enrichment		GO Enrichment	
				KEGG Pathway	*p*-Value	BP Term	*p*-Value
A	492	558	13	Tight junction	4.19×10^{-4}	Establishment or maintenance of cell polarity	2.83×10^{-4}
B	113	128	3	PPAR signaling pathway	7.75×10^{-6}	Triglyceride metabolic process	1.25×10^{-7}
C	46	50	2	mTOR signaling pathway	9.62×10^{-3}	Protein targeting to membrane	4.93×10^{-67}
D	27	86	6	Influenza A	3.04×10^{-10}	Defense response to virus	1.24×10^{-22}
E	18	17	1	Tuberculosis	2.01×10^{-4}	Tuberculosis	2.01×10^{-4}
F	11	10	1	N-Glycan biosynthesis	9.19×10^{-3}	Post-translational protein modification	6.33×10^{-3}
G	6	5	1	Terpenoid backbone biosynthesis	1.72×10^{-4}	Coenzyme biosynthetic process	1.55×10^{-5}
H	5	4	1	Notch signaling pathway	2.98×10^{-2}	Gamete generation	1.34×10^{-2}
I	4	3	1	Null	Null	Transcription, DNA-dependent	1.31×10^{-2}
J	4	3	1	Null	Null	Positive regulation of translation	1.17×10^{-2}
K	4	3	1	Null	Null	Endoplasmic reticulum unfolded protein response	6.51×10^{-3}
L	4	3	1	Regulation of cyclin-dependent protein kinase activity	1.24×10^{-2}	Regulation of cyclin-dependent protein kinase activity	1.24×10^{-2}
M	3	2	1	Steroid biosynthesis	7.68×10^{-3}	Steroid biosynthetic process	2.07×10^{-6}
N	3	2	1	Null	Null	Regulation of transcription, DNA-dependent	1.84×10^{-2}
O	3	2	1	Null	Null	Intra-Golgi vesicle-mediated transport	4.47×10^{-3}

Furthermore, a functional enrichment analysis with KEGG pathways revealed that the co-expression networks with DEGs were enriched in pathways related to tight junction, PPAR signaling pathway, mTOR signaling pathway, influenza A, tuberculosis, N-Glycan biosynthesis, terpenoid backbone biosynthesis, Notch signaling pathway, regulation of cyclin-dependent protein kinase activity, and steroid biosynthesis (Table 2). The GO BP term enrichment analysis showed those genes mostly involved in the establishment or maintenance of cell polarity, triglyceride metabolic process, protein targeting to membrane, defense response to virus, tuberculosis, post-translational protein modification, coenzyme biosynthetic process, gamete generation, transcription, DNA-dependent, positive regulation of translation, endoplasmic reticulum unfolded protein response, regulation of cyclin-dependent protein kinase activity, steroid biosynthetic process, regulation of the transcription of DNA-dependent, intra-Golgi vesicle-mediated transport term, and other rigid molecular machines in the biological process.

Based on the novel differentially regulated sub-networks detection tool, PhenomeScape [20], which could combine the fold changes of genes into the knowledge of networks and disease phenotypes, a series of differentially regulated sub-networks associated with phenotypes were identified with the random walk algorithm. In this research, seven phenotypes related to breast cancer were selected as the seed phenotypes (Table 5); subsequently, a total of 19 differentially regulated sub-networks enriched in the breast cancer phenotype related subnetwork were identified (Table 3). The sub-networks distributed by bufadienolide-like chemicals included RNA splicing (p-value = 2.00×10^{-3}), apoptotic process (p-value = 2.00×10^{-3}), extracellular matrix organization (p-value = 1.00×10^{-3}), canonical Wnt signaling pathway (p-value = 2.20×10^{-2}), synaptic transmission (p-value = 1.40×10^{-2}), negative regulation of the JAK-STAT cascade (p-value = 4.20×10^{-2}), adherens junction organization (p-value = 3.80×10^{-2}), BMP signaling pathway (p-value = 4.10×10^{-2}), negative regulation of cell migration (p-value = 1.30×10^{-2}), and activation of signaling protein activity involved in the unfolded protein response (p-value = 1.90×10^{-2}) (Figure 7).

Table 3. Summary of differentially regulated sub-networks disturbed by bufadienolide-like chemicals.

Subnetwork Number	No. of Nodes	GO-BP	Empirical *p*-Value
A	21	RNA splicing	2.00×10^{-3}
B	73	apoptotic process	2.00×10^{-3}
C	11	extracellular matrix organization	1.00×10^{-3}
D	6	canonical Wnt signaling pathway	2.20×10^{-2}
E	7	synaptic transmission	1.40×10^{-2}
F	11	negative regulation of JAK-STAT cascade	4.20×10^{-2}
G	9	adherens junction organization	3.80×10^{-2}
H	9	BMP signaling pathway	4.10×10^{-2}
I	6	negative regulation of cell migration	1.30×10^{-2}
J	4	activation of signaling protein activity involved in unfolded protein response	1.90×10^{-2}
K	12	drug metabolic process	1.20×10^{-2}
L	6	negative regulation of lipid storage	4.50×10^{-2}
M	6	xenobiotic metabolic process	1.70×10^{-2}
N	8	relaxation of cardiac muscle	4.80×10^{-2}
O	5	very long-chain fatty acid metabolic process	1.70×10^{-2}
P	4	oligosaccharide metabolic process	3.10×10^{-2}
Q	4	collagen catabolic process	2.50×10^{-2}
R	4	response to cocaine	2.70×10^{-2}
S	4	behavioral response to nicotine	4.20×10^{-2}

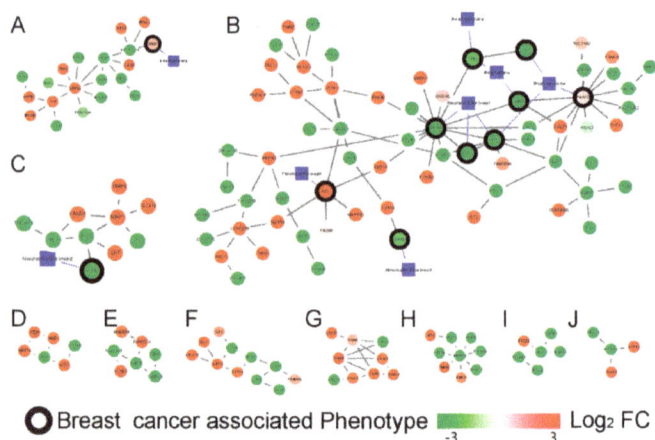

Figure 7. The differentially expressed networks regulated by bufadienolide-like chemicals, and generated by the PhenomeScape plug. Sub-networks linked to breast cancer, RNA splicing (2.00×10^{-3}) (**A**), apoptotic process (2.00×10^{-3}) (**B**), extracellular matrix organization (1.00×10^{-3}) (**C**), canonical Wnt signaling pathway (2.20×10^{-2}) (**D**), synaptic transmission (1.40×10^{-2}) (**E**), negative regulation of JAK-STAT (Janus kinase/signal transducers and activators of transcription) cascade (4.20×10^{-2}) (**F**), adherens junction organization (3.80×10^{-2}) (**G**), BMP signaling pathway (4.10×10^{-2}) (**H**), negative regulation of cell migration (1.30×10^{-2}) (**I**), and activation of signaling protein activity involved in the unfolded protein response (1.90×10^{-2}) (**J**). The fold change of the proteins is shown by the node color, and breast cancer-associated phenotype annotated proteins were used to generate the sub-networks and are shown with a black border.

The subnetwork A (Figure 7A), related to the RNA splicing function, was the first identified dysregulation subnetwork. It showed the genes involved in the mRNA splicing spliceosome were down-regulated, including the serine- and arginine- rich splicing factor members, SRSF4, SRSF5, and SRSF6, and peroxisome proliferator activated receptor gamma coactivator (PPARGC1A). The apoptotic process (Figure 7B) could have been dysregulated by bufadienolide-like chemicals, and this dysregulation was performed with the increased expression of SYT11, PARK2, PYHIN1, APC, RNF40, SERPINB3, TIAM2, ITSN1, SH3GL2, CASP1, GATA4, ITSN2, and PDE4DIP. Several cancer signaling pathways, including the Wnt signaling pathway, the JAK-STAT signaling pathway, and the BMP signaling pathway, also could had been dysregulated by bufadienolide-like chemicals (Figure 7D,F,H). This suggests that bufadienolide-like chemicals could increase the apoptotic process through a series of pathways or regulation networks. The subnetwork C (Figure 7C) was mostly related to the extracellular matrix organization being upregulated, including the genes, TIMP4, MMP3, SPARC, DPT, and ACAN. Also in this subnetwork, those genes that referred to the regulation of cell migration were downregulated, including the genes, TNFAIP6, DCN, SPARC, THBS1, and CCL8. This means the increase of the extracellular matrix may have hindered the migration of the tumor. Also, negative synaptic transmission, adherens junction organization, and regulation of cell migration was found in subnetwork E, G, and I (Figure 7E,G,I). Several metabolic processes were also discovered, including the drug metabolic process, xenobiotic metabolic process, oligosaccharide metabolic process, etc. All other PhenomeScape networks can be found in Supplementary Figure S1.

Although, there is no evidence to prove the bufadienolide-like chemicals having obvious toxicity with the CEBS database (https://manticore.niehs.nih.gov/cebssearch/) [30]. In this research, in order to identify the potential cardiotoxicity of bufadienolide-like chemicals, 11 cardiotoxicity relation phenotypes (Table 6), including arrhythmia (HP:0011675), atrial fibrillation (HP:0005110), atrial flutter (HP:0004749), and other phenotypes, were chosen as seed phenotypes of cardiotoxicity with the aim of searching for the potential dysregulation subnetworks with cardiotoxicity. Results indicated six subnetwork related to membrane depolarization during the action potential (*p*-value = 3.70×10^{-3}, Figure 8A), retinoic acid receptor binding (*p*-value = 2.00×10^{-3}, Figure 8B), GABA receptor binding ((*p*-value = 3.00×10^{-3}, Figure 8C), positive regulation of nuclear division (*p*-value = 5.00×10^{-3}, Figure 8D), negative regulation of viral genome replication (*p*-value = 3.00×10^{-3}, Figure 8E), and negative regulation of viral life cycle (*p*-value = 1.00×10^{-3}), which were identified as potential cardiotoxicity subnetworks disturbed by bufadienolide-like chemicals (Table 4 and Figure 8). The subnetwork related to membrane depolarization may be the key potential cardiotoxic target of bufadienolide-like chemicals. These were also be observed by several widely used anticancer drugs with cardiotoxicity. For example, Adriamycin, Gleevec, and Herceptin were observed with a membrane depolarization appearance during clinical research [31,32].

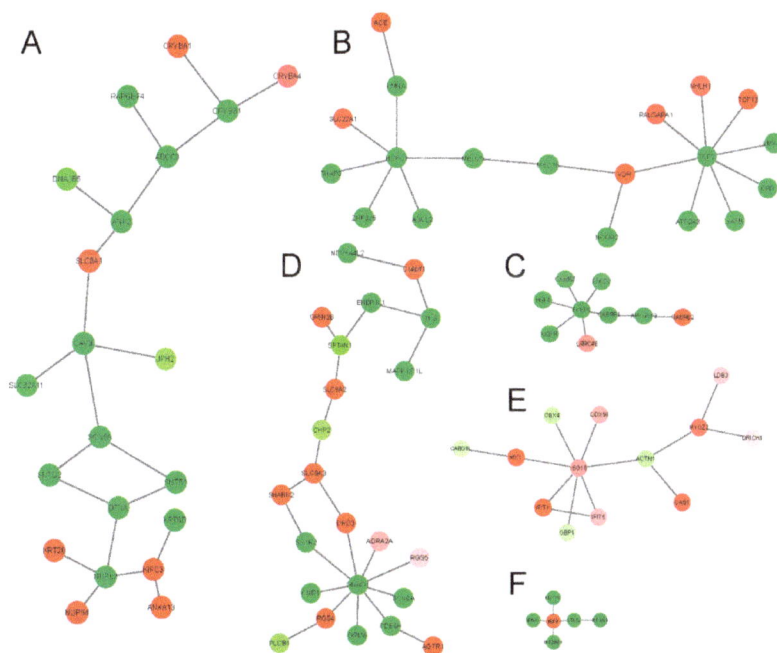

Figure 8. The differentially regulated sub-networks with potential cardiotoxicity disturbed by bufadienolide-like chemicals, generated by the PhenomeScape plug with seeds of 11 cardiotoxicity phenotypes. (**A**) Subnetwork related to membrane depolarization during action potential (3.70×10^{-2}), (**B**) Subnetwork related to retinoic acid receptor binding (2.00×10^{-3}), (**C**) Subnetwork related to GABA receptor binding (3.00×10^{-3}), (**D**) Subnetwork related to positive regulation of nuclear division (5.00×10^{-3}), (**E**) subnetwork related to negative regulation of viral genome replication (3.00×10^{-3}), and (**F**) subnetwork related to negative regulation of viral life cycle (1.00×10^{-3}).

Table 4. Summary of differentially regulated sub-networks with potential cardiotoxicity disturbed by bufadienolide-like chemicals.

Subnetwork Number	No. of Nodes	GO-BP	Empirical *p*-Value
A	21	Membrane depolarization during action potential	3.70×10^{-2}
B	19	Retinoic acid receptor binding	2.00×10^{-3}
C	9	GABA receptor binding	3.00×10^{-3}
D	23	Positive regulation of nuclear division	5.00×10^{-3}
E	13	Negative regulation of viral genome replication	3.00×10^{-3}
F	6	Negative regulation of viral life cycle	1.00×10^{-3}

Hub genes, mostly the highly connected nodes in the network, were identified by node degree and the MCC (Maximal clique centrality) algorithm with the Cytoscape plugin, cytoHubba [33]. Based on the threshold of the degree (degree > 5) and the MCC algorithm, 10 genes with MCC scores ranging from 126 to 953 were identified as hub genes (Figure 9A,B). Ten hub genes, including three 2′-5′-oligoadenylate synthetase genes, OAS1, OAS2, and OAS3; five interferon-induced genes, ISG15, IFIT1, IFI6, IFI44, and IFIL44L; and two other genes, including the kelch-like family member 35 (KLHL35) and Golgi Membrane Protein 1 (GOLM1) were identified. These were selected as the hub genes. Further investigation with TCGA [21] and the Kaplan-Meier databases [22] indicated that the 10 hub genes except KLHL35 were increased both in the treatment with bufadienolide-like chemicals and the TCGA breast cancer sample (Figure 9C). Six hub genes, including IFIT1, ISG15, IFI6, GOLM5, KLHL35, and OAS2, were associated with the total survival probability in breast cancer patients (Figure 9D). Further analysis of the correlation between the hub genes and the total survival time in breast cancer indicated that the high expression of GOLM5, KLHL35, and OAS2 was associated with a better survival probability.

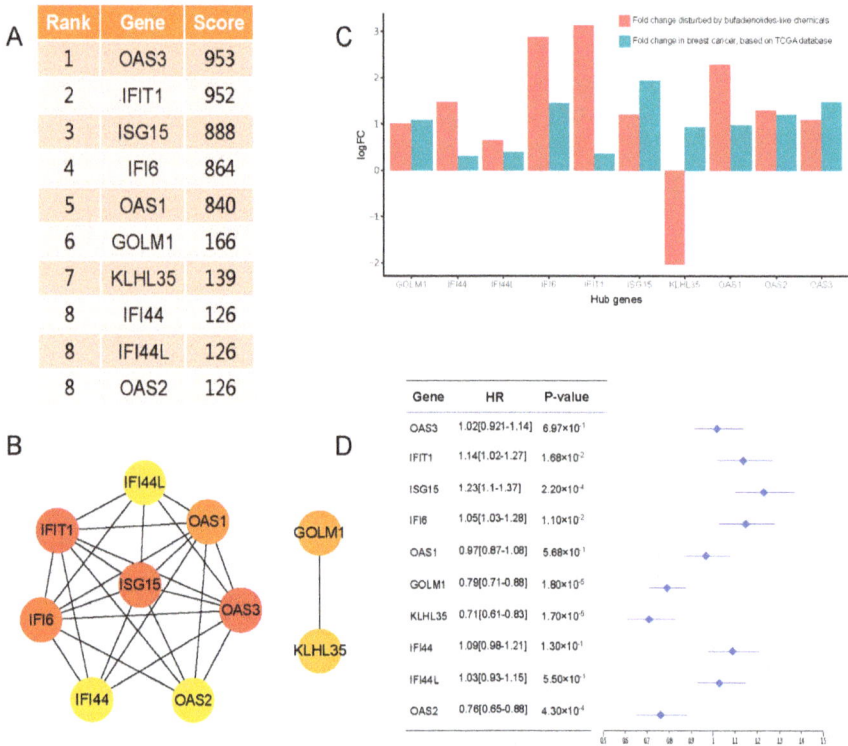

Figure 9. The 10 hub genes and their correlation with the total survival probability in breast cancer. (**A**) The 10 hub genes and their MCC (Maximal clique centrality) score. (**B**) The network of hub genes. (**C**) The expression correlation with breast cancer, validated by the TCGA database. (**D**) The total survival probability correlation with breast cancer, validated by the Kaplan-Meier (KM) plotter database.

3. Discussion

Recently, gene expression profile technology, including the microarray and RNA-seq, has been widely used to detect the potential mechanism of chemicals, however, a central problem still perplexes researchers on pharmacology and biology; that is, how chemicals disturb pathways and phenotypes through genes and their co-expression networks. In this research, with the use of bioinformatics tools, especially the differentially regulated sub-networks detection tools, PhenomeScape [20], CTD (http://ctdbase.org/) [16], and CMAP2 (https://portals.broadinstitute.org/cmap/) [17,18] databases, several dysregulated sub-networks related to the potential anticancer mechanism and cardiotoxicity were revealed, which was also further verified by the expression correlation and survival probability correlation with other databases. These results may highlight the potential molecular mechanism and application of bufadienolide-like chemicals on cancer, especially as a novel agent for breast cancer.

First, during the process of differentially expressed gene identification, in contrast to using the conventional method of differentially expressed gene selection with significance in statistics, a non-parametric unsupervised method of gene set variation analysis was used for differentially expressed gene identification. The results indicated a total of 80 DEGs involved in the 44 MSigDB C2 curated gene sets were identified (Figure 3A,B). After further analysis with the enrichment of the GO and KEGG pathway, we found genes that were up-regulated were most rich in their interferon signaling response to virus, defense to other organisms, regulation of viral genome replication, and 2′-5′-oligoadenylate synthetase activity. KEGG pathway enrichment analysis showed those genes could activate the IFN-induced pathway, type II interferon signaling pathway, and regulate the protein ISGylation pathway. However, the genes that were down-regulated were rich in protein kinase complex, transcription factor TFTC complex-1, SAGA- complex, and cargo loading into vesicle. KEGG pathway enrichment analysis showed those genes may be involved in negative transport of fringe-modified NOTCH to the plasma membrane pathway. By comparing the DEGs identification method with the statistical significance strategy, the number of DEGs enriched in MSigDB C2 curated gene sets may be much less compared to those DEGS with enrichment in the same biology function or similar pathway. Also, the same results were proven by the examples of the GSVA package [15].

Second, during the process of similar small molecule detection, CTD (http://ctdbase.org/) [16] and CMAP2 (http://www.broadinstitute.org/cMAP/) [17,18] databases were used. The results indicated that the bufadienolide-like chemicals had the same effect as valproic acid and estradiol. Valproic acid is a histone deacetylase inhibitor, and it was shown to inhibit proliferation via Wnt/β catenin signaling activation. Estradiol was also proven to have anticancer activity, especially in postmenopausal women. Also, the evidence from the CTD database (http://ctdbase.org/) indicated bufadienolide-like chemicals have the potential ability to be used as hormones and anticancer and vasoprotectives agents.

Third, during the process of co-expression network reconstruction and dysregulated sub-networks detection, a novel plug of PhenomeScape was used, which could combine the data of gene expression into the knowledge of protein–protein interaction networks and disease phenotype [20]. During the analysis with the damaged osteoarthritic cartilage gene expression profile, several significant sub-networks related to damaged osteoarthritic cartilage were identified: Mitotic cell cycle, Wnt signaling, apoptosis, and matrix organisation [34,35]. In this research, with the PhenomeScape tool [20], a total of 19 differentially regulated sub-networks were identified, and 10 sub-networks were proven to relate to breast cancer by evidence, including RNA splicing, apoptotic process, cell migration, extracellular matrix organization, adherens junction organization, synaptic transmission, and so on. Also, with the PhenomeScape tool [20], six dysregulated subnetworks, including the subnetwork related to membrane depolarization during the action potential, retinoic acid receptor binding, GABA receptor binding, positive regulation of nuclear division, negative regulation of viral genome replication, and negative regulation of viral life cycle, were identified. Those dysregulated subnetworks may play important roles in the cardiotoxicity of bufadienolide-like chemicals.

Hub gene selection and its relation to survival probability indicated that 10 hub genes (except KLHL35) were increased in both breast cancer and samples treated with bufadienolide-like chemicals. Further analysis in relation to the total survival probability showed six hub genes, including IFIT1, ISG15, IFI6, GOLM5, KLHL35, and OAS2, were associated the total survival time and high expression of GOLM5, KLHL35, and OAS2 was associated with better survival probability.

4. Materials and Methods

4.1. Microarray Data Information

The gene expression profiles of GSE85871 (https://www.ncbi.nlm.nih.gov/gds/), which is a gene expression profile treated with 102 chemicals from Chinese traditional medicine, and is based on the Affymetrix GPL571 platform (Affymetrix Human Genome U133A 2.0 Array, Santa Clara, CA, USA), was submitted by Lv et al. [36].

In this study, the raw data of 4 controls and 14 samples treated with bufadienolide-like chemicals (1 μM and treatment with 12 h), including resibufogenin, bufalin, arenobufagin, cinobufagin, bufotoxin, telocinobufagin, bufotaline, and cinobufotali, were downloaded from the GEO database via GEOquery [37] packages in the R3.5.1 [38] environment.

4.2. Identification of DEGs Associated with Relative Enrichment Pathways

In order to obtain a series of differentially expressed genes (DEGs) with biological interpretation, a novel R package, GSVA [15], was employed, which allowed the assessment of the DEGs underlying pathway activity variation by transforming the gene expression profile into the prior knowledge of the gene set. In accordance with MIAME (Minimum Information About a Microarray Experiment) standards [39,40], the DEGs disturbed by bufadienolide-like chemicals were identified by a series of standard flow with the R environment. First, the quality assessments, background correction, and normalization were preprocessed and normalized with the affy [41] and gcrma [42] packages. Then, the batch effects were examined and removed with the combat and sva functions in the SVA (Surrogate Variable Analysis) package [43]. Subsequently, a non-specific probes filtering step was performed with the nsFilter function in the genefilter package [44], the quality control probes of Affymetrix, probe sets without Entrez ID annotation, probesets whose associated Entrez ID was duplicated in the annotation, and the top 20% with smaller variability were first removed. Finally, the GSVA [43], GSEABase [45], limma [46] package, and c2BroadSets from Molecular Signatures Database (MSigDB) [47,48] were used to select the DEGs enriched in the relative enrichment pathways.

During the process of DEGs selection with relative enrichment sets, the gene expression profile was first transformed into the prior knowledge gene sets of c2BroadSets and the enriched gene sets were selected with the screening criteria of FDR < 0.01. Then, the DEGs enriched in the c2BroadSets gene sets were selected with the limma [46] package, and the screening criteria were set with FDR < 0.01 and | logFC | > 1. The DEGs associated with relative enrichment pathways were used for further analysis.

During the process of DEGs identification, the Biobase [49] package and GSVAdata [50] package were also applied. The results were visualized with the ggplot2 [51], ggpubr [52], pheatmap [53], and cowplot [54] packages.

4.3. Gene Enrichment Analysis

In order to obtain a comprehensive understanding of those genes involved in the prior knowledge of gene sets, GO and KEGG enrichment analysis were performed with the clueGO plug [23] in Cystoscape [24]. The significantly enriched GO terms and KEGG pathways were calculated by the hypergeometric test [55], and cut-off criteria were set as FDR < 0.05. Another statistical parameter of the Kappa Score were set as middle stringency, which means the terms in the network were merged with the middle related terms based on their overlapping genes. The minimum percentage and minimum genes enriched in GO terms or KEGG pathways were set as 1.0% and 2; also, the term fusion parameter was also chosen. Other options, including the statistical options, reference options, grouping options, and visual options, were set with the default setting.

4.4. Similar Small Molecule Detection

In order to detect the similar small molecules with bufadienolide-like chemicals, the DEGs with up or down were respectively submitted to the CTD (http://ctdbase.org/) [16] and CMAP2 (http://www.broadinstitute.org/cMAP/) database [16,17]. During the process of detection of similar small molecules with the CTD database, the threshold of degree in the degree filter network was set as 10. During the process of detection of similar small molecules with the connectivity map database, the enrichment score and *p*-value were chosen as the similarity index between the gene expression profile of the query signature and that of chemicals in the CMAP2 database.

Also, the potential toxicity the same as bufadienolide-like chemicals were also detected with the CEBS database (https://manticore.niehs.nih.gov/cebssearch/) [30], but there was no evidence to prove the bufadienolide-like chemicals had obvious toxicity.

4.5. Gene Co-Expression Network Analysis and Disease Phenotype Association

To obtain a comprehensive understanding of the potential mechanism of DEGs involved in breast cancer, co-expression network analysis, phenome association, and survival correlation analysis were investigated with the NetworkAnalyst database (https://www.networkanalyst.ca/) [56] and PhenomeScape plug [20] in Cystoscape [24]. Also, other plugs and databases, including the cytoHubba [33], TCSBN database (http://inetmodels.com/) [19], TCGA database [21] and Kaplan-Meier (KM) plotter database (http://kmplot.com/) [22], and the Phenomiser (http://compbio. charite.de/phenomizer/) [57] web tool, were also used for hub gene selection and survival correlation analysis. First, the breast mammary tissue-specific co-expression networks were investigated with the TCSBN database (http://inetmodels.com/) through the NetworkAnalyst web server (https://www. networkanalyst.ca/). The GO and KEGG enrichment terms of networks were also investigated with the NetworkAnalyst web server (https://www.networkanalyst.ca/). Subsequently, the differentially regulated sub-networks enriched in genes associated with the breast cancer phenotype were identified by random sampling (10,000 sub-networks) methods with the PhenomeScape plug and Phenomiser (http://compbio.charite.de/phenomizer/) web tool. First, through the search with Phenomiser web tool and the manual of UberPheno ontology [57], 6 breast carcionma phenotypes (Table 5) and 11 cardiotoxicity relation phenotypes (Table 6) were chosen as the potential anticancer mechanism or potential cardiotoxicity association phenotype. Parameters of the maximum initial sub-network size of 7 and an empirical *p*-value threshold of 0.05 were used for filtering the differentially regulated sub-networks enriched in genes associated with breast cancer or the cardiotoxicity phenotype.

Hub genes, highly interconnected with nodes in the network, are considered functionally significant in the network. In our study, the top 10 hub genes were defined by the node degree and MCC algorithm in the Cytoscape plugin, cytoHubba [33]. We used the previously described workflow that selected the essential proteins from the yeast protein interaction network with the MCC algorithm [33]. First, the degrees of nodes were computed by the NetworkAnalyzer [58] in Cytoscape. Then, the nodes with a degree greater than a threshold were selected as potential candidate hub genes, and the threshold was the maximum integer as $2 \times \sum\limits_{v \in V,\ Deg(v) > t} Deg(v) > \sum\limits_{v \in V,} Deg(v)$, where *v* is the collection of nodes within the network *V*, *Deg(v)* is the degree of node *v*. Last, the top 10 hub genes were ranked by the MCC algorithm in the cytoHubba plugin. The hub genes common in breast tissue co-expression networks were chosen as the candidates for further validation with TCGA [21] and the Kaplan-Meier (KM) plotter database (http://kmplot.com/analysis/) [22].

Table 5. UberPheno phenotype terms selected for identification of the differentially regulated sub-network with the potential anticancer mechanism of bufadienolide-like chemicals.

Phenotype ID	Phenotype Description
HP:0100783	Breast aplasia
HP:0100013	Neoplasm of the breast
HP:0003002	Breast carcionma
HP:0003187	Breast hypoplasia
HP:0000769	Abnormality of the breast
HP:0010619	Fibroma of the breast

Table 6. UberPheno phenotype terms selected for identification of the differentially regulated sub-network with potential cardiotoxicity of bufadienolide-like chemicals.

Phenotype ID	Phenotype Description
HP:0011675	Arrhythmia
HP:0005110	Atrial fibrillation
HP:0004749	atrial flutter
HP:0011215	Hemihypsarrhythmia
HP:0002521	Hypsarrhythmia
HP:0040182	Inappropriate sinus tachycardia
HP:0001962	Palpitations
HP:0005115	Supraventricular arrhythmia
HP:0004755	Surpraventricular tachycardia
HP:0004308	Ventricular arrhythmia
HP:0011841	Ventricular flutter

5. Conclusions

In this research, with a serious of bioinformatics analysis, we noticed that the bufadienolide-like chemicals may perform anticancer activity through RNA splicing, apoptotic process, cell migration, extracellular matrix organization, adherens junction organization, synaptic transmission, Wnt signaling, AK-STAT signaling, BMP signaling pathway, and the unfolded protein response (Figure 10A). Also, further investigation of the potential cardiotoxicity of bufadienolide-like chemicals indicated the dysregulated subnetwork related to membrane depolarization during the action potential, retinoic acid receptor binding, GABA receptor binding, positive regulation of nuclear division, negative regulation of viral genome replication, and negative regulation of viral life cycle may play important roles in cardiotoxicity (Figure 10B). Additionally, those may highlight the potential molecular mechanism of bufadienolide-like chemicals on breast cancer, but still, there are several problems with no better solution, including the renal toxicity of bufadienolide-like chemicals, and the difference of potential molecular mechanisms among different stem nuclei in bufadienolide-like chemicals was also clearly illuminated in this research.

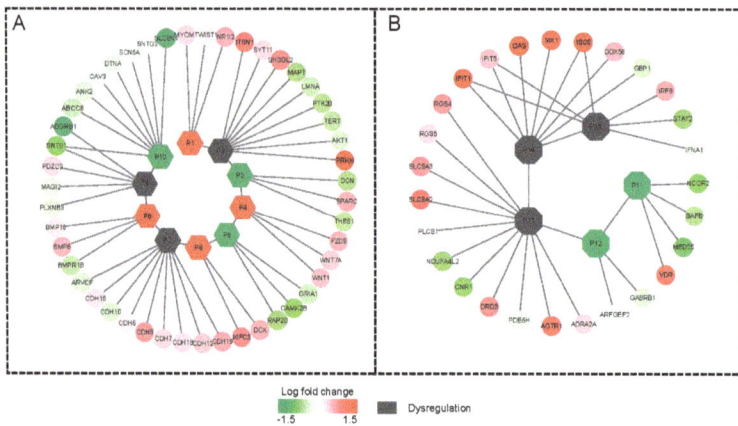

Figure 10. The potential anticancer mechanism and cardiotoxicity of bufadienolide-like chemicals. (**A**) The potential anticancer mechanism of bufadienolide-like chemicals. Nodes p1–p10 means the 10 differentially regulated sub-networks in Figure 7. (**B**) The potential cardiotoxicity of bufadienolide-like chemicals: Node p11–p15 means the five differentially regulated sub-networks in Figure 8.

Cancers **2019**, *11*, 91

Supplementary Materials: The following are available online at http://www.mdpi.com/2072-6694/11/1/91/s1, Figure S1: Other differentially expressed networks regulated by bufadienolide-like chemic, Table S1: The DEGs disturbed by bufadienolide-like chemicals, Table S2: The different gene sets disturbed by bufadienolide-like chemicals.

Author Contributions: Conceptualization, Y.P. and L.H.; methodology, Y.P. and L.H.; software, D.W. and X.H.; validation, C.Y., Y.Z. and X.H.; formal analysis, Y.Z. and X.T.; investigation, D.W. and X.H.; resources, D.W.; data curation, Y.Z. and X.T.; writing—original draft preparation, Y.Z. and X.T.; writing—review and editing, Y.Z., X.T. and L.Q.; visualization, Y.Z. and L.Q.; supervision, Y.P. and L.H.; project administration, Y.P. and L.H.; funding acquisition, Y.P. and L.H.

Funding: This work was supported by grants from National Natural Science Foundation of China (No. 81374065 and No. 81403035), and Basal Research Fund of Central Public-interest Scientific Institution (No. 1630032015039).

Acknowledgments: We thank Fulai Yu and Xiaolu Chen, for the advice and review of the manuscript.

Conflicts of Interest: The following authors report no conflicts of interest.

References

1. Zhou, H.; Li, J.; Zhang, Z.; Ye, R.; Shao, N.; Cheang, T.; Wang, S. RING1 and YY1 binding protein suppresses breast cancer growth and metastasis. *Int. J. Oncol.* **2016**, *49*, 2442–2452. [CrossRef] [PubMed]

2. Xu, H.; Wu, K.; Tian, Y.; Liu, Q.; Han, N.; Yuan, X.; Zhang, L.; Wu, G.S.; Wu, K. CD44 correlates with clinicopathological characteristics and is upregulated by EGFR in breast cancer. *Int. J. Oncol.* **2016**, *49*, 1343–1350. [CrossRef] [PubMed]

3. Pan, Z.; Jing, W.; He, K.; Zhang, L.; Long, X. SATB1 is Correlated with Progression and Metastasis of Breast Cancers: A Meta-Analysis. *Cell. Physiol. Biochem.* **2016**, *38*, 1975–1983. [CrossRef] [PubMed]

4. Mai, F.T.; Omar, H.A. Immunotherapy, an evolving approach for the management of triple negative breast cancer: Converting non-responders to responders. *Crit. Rev. Oncol. Hematol.* **2018**, *122*, 202–207.

5. Akiko, E.; Mun-Chual, R.; Kanki, K.; Masahiko, H. Inhibitory effects of bufadienolides on interleukin-6 in MH-60 cells. *J. Nat. Prod.* **2004**, *67*, 2070–2072.

6. Qin, T.-J.; Zhao, X.-H.; Yun, J.; Zhang, L.-X.; Ruan, Z.-P. Efficacy and safety of gemcitabine-oxaliplatin combined with huachansu in patients with advanced gallbladder carcinoma. *World J. Gastroenterol.* **2008**, *14*, 5210–5216. [CrossRef]

7. Wang, J.; Jin, Y.; Xu, Z.; Zheng, Z.; Wan, S. Involvement of caspase-3 activity and survivin downregulation in cinobufocini-induced apoptosis in A 549 cells. *Exp. Boil. Med.* **2009**, *234*, 566–572. [CrossRef]

8. Hong, Z.; Chan, K.; Yeung, H.W. Simultaneous determination of bufadienolides in the traditional Chinese medicine preparation, liu-shen-wan, by liquid chromatography. *J. Pharm. Pharmacol.* **2011**, *44*, 1023–1026. [CrossRef]

9. Chun, L.; Hashimi, S.M.; Siyu, C.; Mellick, A.S.; Wei, D.; David, G.; Wei, M.Q. The mechanisms of chansu in inducing efficient apoptosis in colon cancer cells. *Evid. Based Complement. Altern. Med.* **2013**, *2013*, 849054. [CrossRef]

10. Yeh, J.-Y.; Huang, W.J.; Kan, S.-F.; Wang, P.S. Effects of bufalin and cinobufagin on the proliferation of androgen dependent and independent prostate cancer cells. *Prostate* **2010**, *54*, 112–124. [CrossRef]

11. Yu, C.H.; Kan, S.F.; Pu, H.F.; Chien, E.J.; Wang, P.S. Apoptotic signaling in bufalin- and cinobufagin-treated androgen-dependent and -independent human prostate cancer cells. *Cancer Sci.* **2010**, *99*, 2467–2476. [CrossRef]

12. Dong, Y.Q.; Ma, W.L.; Gu, J.B.; Zheng, W.L. Effect of cinobufagin on nuclear factor-kappa B pathway in HepG2 cells. *J. South. Med. Univ.* **2010**, *30*, 137–139.

13. Wang, L.; Jun, W.U.; Min, L.I.; Yang, X.W. Pilot study on the mechanisms of growth inhibitory effect of cinobufagin on HeLa cells. *Chin. J. Oncol.* **2005**, *27*, 717–720.

14. Ko, W.S.; Park, T.Y.; Park, C.; Kim, Y.H.; Yoon, H.J.; Lee, S.Y.; Hong, S.H.; Choi, B.T.; Lee, Y.T.; Choi, Y.H. Induction of apoptosis by Chansu, a traditional Chinese medicine, in human bladder carcinoma T24 cells. *Oncol. Rep.* **2005**, *14*, 475–480. [PubMed]

15. Hänzelmann, S.; Castelo, R.; Guinney, J. GSVA: Gene set variation analysis for microarray and RNA-Seq data. *BMC Bioinform.* **2013**, *14*, 7. [CrossRef] [PubMed]

16. Davis, A.P.; Grondin, C.J.; Johnson, R.J.; Sciaky, D.; King, B.L.; McMorran, R.; Wiegers, J.; Wiegers, T.C.; Mattingly, C.J. The Comparative Toxicogenomics Database: Update 2017. *Nucleic Acids Res.* **2017**, *45*, D972–D978. [CrossRef] [PubMed]

17. Justin, L.; Crawford, E.D.; David, P.; Modell, J.W.; Blat, I.C.; Wrobel, M.J.; Jim, L.; Jean-Philippe, B.; Aravind, S.; Ross, K.N. The Connectivity Map: Using gene-expression signatures to connect small molecules, genes, and disease. *Science* **2006**, *313*, 1929–1935.

18. Subramanian, A.; Narayan, R.; Corsello, S.M.; Peck, D.D.; Natoli, T.E.; Lu, X.; Gould, J.; Davis, J.F.; Tubelli, A.A.; Asiedu, J.K. A Next Generation Connectivity Map: L1000 Platform and the First 1,000,000 Profiles. *Cell* **2017**, *171*, 1437–1452. [CrossRef]

19. Lee, S.; Zhang, C.; Arif, M.; Liu, Z.; Benfeitas, R.; Bidkhori, G.; Deshmukh, S.; Al, S.M.; Lovric, A.; Boren, J. TCSBN: A database of tissue and cancer specific biological networks. *Nucleic Acids Res.* **2018**, *46*, D595–D600. [CrossRef]

20. Soul, J.; Dunn, S.L.; Hardingham, T.E.; Boothandford, R.P.; Schwartz, J.M. PhenomeScape: A cytoscape app to identify differentially regulated sub-networks using known disease associations. *Bioinformatics* **2016**, *32*, 3847–3849. [CrossRef]

21. Kosinski, M.; Biecek, P. *RTCGA: The Cancer Genome Atlas Data Integration*, R package version 1.12.0 [Software]; 2018. Available online: https://rdrr.io/bioc/RTCGA/ (accessed on 28 November 2018).

22. Balazs, G.; Andras, L.; Eklund, A.C.; Carsten, D.; Jan, B.; Qiyuan, L.; Zoltan, S. An online survival analysis tool to rapidly assess the effect of 22,277 genes on breast cancer prognosis using microarray data of 1,809 patients. *Breast Cancer Res. Treat* **2010**, *123*, 725–731.

23. Bindea, G.; Mlecnik, B.H.; Charoentong, P.; Tosolini, M.; Kirilovsky, A.; Fridman, W.H.; Pages, F.; Trajanoski, Z.; Galon, J. ClueGO: A Cytoscape plug-in to decipher functionally grouped gene ontology and pathway annotation networks. *Bioinformatics* **2009**, *25*, 1091–1093. [CrossRef] [PubMed]

24. Su, G.; Morris, J.H.; Demchak, B.; Bader, G.D. Biological network exploration with cytoscape 3. *Curr. Protoc. Bioinform.* **2014**, *47*, 8.13.1–8.13.24. [CrossRef] [PubMed]

25. Minegaki, T.S.A.; Mori, M.; Tsuji, S.; Yamamoto, S.; Watanabe, A.; Tsuzuki, T.; Tsunoda, T.; Yamamoto, A.; Tsujimoto, M.; Nishiguchi, K. Histone deacetylase inhibitors sensitize 5-fluorouracil-resistant MDA-MB-468 breast cancer cells to 5-fluorouracil. *Oncol. Lett.* **2018**, *16*, 6202–6208. [CrossRef] [PubMed]

26. Hankinson, S.E.; Willett, W.C.; Manson, J.E.; Colditz, G.A.; Hunter, D.J.; Spiegelman, D.; Barbieri, R.L.; Speizer, F.E. Plasma sex steroid hormone levels and risk of breast cancer in postmenopausal women. *J. Natl. Cancer Inst.* **1998**, *91*, 1292–1299. [CrossRef]

27. Barros-Oliveira, M.d.C.; Costa-Silva, D.R.; Andrade, D.B.d.; Borges, U.S.; Tavares, C.B.; Borges, R.S.; Silva, J.d.M.; Silva, B.B.d. Use of anastrozole in the chemoprevention and treatment of breast cancer: A literature review. *Rev. Assoc. Medica Bras.* **2017**, *63*. [CrossRef] [PubMed]

28. Bennink, H.J.T.C.; Verhoeven, C.; Dutman, A.E.; Thijssen, J. The use of high-dose estrogens for the treatment of breast cancer. *Maturitas* **2017**, *95*, 11–23. [CrossRef]

29. Barabási, A.L.; Oltvai, Z.N. Network biology: Understanding the cell's functional organization. *Nat. Rev. Genet.* **2004**, *5*, 101–113. [CrossRef]

30. Lea, I.A.; Gong, H.; Paleja, A.; Rashid, A.; Fostel, J. CEBS: A comprehensive annotated database of toxicological data. *Nucleic Acids Res.* **2017**, *45*, D964–D971. [CrossRef]

31. Pecoraro, M.; Sorrentino, R.; Franceschelli, S.; Pizzo, M.D.; Pinto, A.; Popolo, A. Doxorubicin-Mediated Cardiotoxicity: Role of Mitochondrial Connexin 43. *Cardiovasc. Toxicol.* **2015**, *15*, 1–11. [CrossRef] [PubMed]

32. Varga, Z.V.; Peter, F.; Lucas, L.; Pál, P. Drug-induced mitochondrial dysfunction and cardiotoxicity. *Am. J. Physiol. Heart Circ. Physiol.* **2015**, *309*, 1453–1467. [CrossRef] [PubMed]

33. Chin, C.H.; Chen, S.H.; Wu, H.H.; Ho, C.W.; Ko, M.T.; Lin, C.Y. cytoHubba: Identifying hub objects and sub-networks from complex interactome. *BMC Syst. Boil.* **2014**, *8* (Suppl. 4), S11. [CrossRef] [PubMed]

34. Soul, J.; Hardingham, T.E.; Boot-Hanford, R.P.; Schwartz, J.M. PhenomeExpress: A refined network analysis of expression datasets by inclusion of known disease phenotype. *Sci. Rep.* **2015**, *5*, 8117. [CrossRef] [PubMed]

35. Dunn, S.L.; Soul, J.; Anand, S.; Schwartz, J.M.; Boot-Handford, R.P.; Hardingham, T.E. Gene expression changes in damaged osteoarthritic cartilage identify a signature of non-chondrogenic and mechanical responses. *Osteoarthr. Cartil.* **2016**, *24*, 1431–1440. [CrossRef] [PubMed]

36. Chao, L.; Wu, X.; Xia, W.; Su, J.; Zeng, H.; Jing, Z.; Shan, L.; Liu, R.; Li, H.; Xuan, L. The gene expression profiles in response to 102 traditional Chinese medicine (TCM) components: A general template for research on TCMs. *Sci. Rep.* **2017**, *7*, 352. [CrossRef]

37. Sean, D.; Meltzer, P.S. GEOquery: A bridge between the Gene Expression Omnibus (GEO) and BioConductor. *Bioinformatics* **2007**, *23*, 1846–1847.

38. Team, R.C. *R: A Language and Environment for Statistical Computing*; R Foundation for Statistical Computing: Vienna, Austria, 2018.

39. Brazma, A. Minimum Information About a Microarray Experiment (MIAME)—Successes, failures, challenges. *Sci. World J.* **2009**, *9*, 420–423. [CrossRef]

40. Dondrup, M.; Albaum, S.P.; Griebel, T.; Henckel, K.; Jünemann, S.; Kahlke, T.; Kleindt, C.K.; Küster, H.; Linke, B.; Mertens, D. EMMA 2—A MAGE-compliant system for the collaborative analysis and integration of microarray data. *BMC Bioinform.* **2009**, *10*, 50. [CrossRef]

41. Gautier, L.; Cope LBolstad, B.M.; Irizarry, R.A. Affy—Analysis of Affymetrix GeneChip data at the probe level. *Bioinformatics* **2004**, *20*, 307–315. [CrossRef]

42. Gharaibeh, R.Z.; Fodor, A.A.; Gibas, C.J. Background correction using dinucleotide affinities improves the performance of GCRMA. *BMC Bioinform.* **2008**, *9*, 452. [CrossRef]

43. Leek, J.T.; Johnson, W.E.; Parker, H.S.; Jaffe, A.E.; Storey, J.D. The sva package for removing batch effects and other unwanted variation in high-throughput experiments. *Bioinformatics* **2012**, *28*, 882–883. [CrossRef] [PubMed]

44. Gentleman, R.C.V.; Huber, W.; Hahne, F. *Genefilter: Genefilter: Methods for Filtering Genes from High-throughput Experiments*, R package version 1.64.0 [Software]; 2018. Available online: https://rdrr.io/bioc/genefilter/ (accessed on 28 November 2018).

45. Morgan, M.; Falcon, S.; Gentleman, R. *GSEABase: Gene Set Enrichment Data Structures and Methods*, R package version 1.44.0 [Software]; 2018. Available online: https://rdrr.io/bioc/GSEABase/ (accessed on 28 November 2018).

46. Ritchie, M.E.; Belinda, P.; Wu, D.; Hu, Y.; Law, C.W.; Shi, W.; Smyth, G.K. limma powers differential expression analyses for RNA-sequencing and microarray studies. *Nucleic Acids Res.* **2015**, *43*, e47. [CrossRef] [PubMed]

47. Arthur, L.; Aravind, S.; Reid, P.; Helga, T.; Pablo, T.; Mesirov, J.P. Molecular signatures database (MSigDB) 3.0. *Bioinformatics* **2011**, *27*, 1739–1740.

48. Liberzon, A.; Birger, C.; Thorvaldsdóttir, H.; Ghandi, M.; Mesirov, J.P.; Tamayo, P. The Molecular Signatures Database (MSigDB) hallmark gene set collection. *Cell Syst.* **2015**, *1*, 417–425. [CrossRef]

49. Wolfgang, H.; Carey, V.J.; Robert, G.; Simon, A.; Marc, C.; Carvalho, B.S.; Hector Corrada, B.; Sean, D.; Laurent, G.; Thomas, G. Orchestrating high-throughput genomic analysis with Bioconductor. *Nat. Methods* **2015**, *12*, 115–121.

50. Castelo, R. *GSVAdata: Data Employed in the Vignette of the GSVA Package*, R package version 1.18.0 [Software]; 2018. Available online: https://www.bioconductor.org/packages/release/data/experiment/html/GSVAdata.html (accessed on 28 November 2018).

51. Wickham, H. *ggplot2: Elegant Graphics for Data Analysis*; Springer: New York, NY, USA, 2016.

52. Kassambara, A. *ggpubr: 'ggplot2' Based Publication Ready Plots*, R package version 0.2 [Software]; 2018. Available online: https://rdrr.io/cran/ggpubr/ (accessed on 28 November 2018).

53. Kolde, R. *pheatmap: Pretty Heatmaps*, R package version 1.0.12 [Software]; 2018. Available online: https://rdrr.io/cran/pheatmap/ (accessed on 28 November 2018).

54. Wilke, C.O. *cowplot: Streamlined Plot Theme and Plot Annotations for 'ggplot2'*, R package version 0.9.4 [Software]; 2018. Available online: https://rdrr.io/cran/cowplot/ (accessed on 28 November 2018).

55. Berkopec, A. HyperQuick algorithm for discrete hypergeometric distribution. *J. Discret. Algorithms* **2007**, *5*, 341–347. [CrossRef]

56. Xia, J.; Gill, E.E.; Hancock, R.E.W. NetworkAnalyst for statistical, visual and network-based meta-analysis of gene expression data. *Nat. Protoc.* **2015**, *10*, 823–844. [CrossRef]

57. Sebastian, K.H.; Schulz, M.H.; Peter, K.; Sebastian, B.; Sandra, D.L.; Ott, C.E.; Christine, M.; Denise, H.; Stefan, M.; Robinson, P.N. Clinical diagnostics in human genetics with semantic similarity searches in ontologies. *Am. J. Hum. Genet.* **2009**, *85*, 457–464.

58. Yassen, A.; Fidel, R.; Sven-Eric, S.; Thomas, L.; Mario, A. Computing topological parameters of biological networks. *Bioinformatics* **2008**, *24*, 282–284.

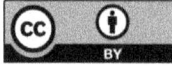

cancers

MDPI

Article

Personalized Prediction of Acquired Resistance to EGFR-Targeted Inhibitors Using a Pathway-Based Machine Learning Approach

Young Rae Kim [1], Yong Wan Kim [1], Suh Eun Lee [1], Hye Won Yang [2] and Sung Young Kim [1,*]

[1] Department of Biochemistry, School of Medicine, Konkuk University, 120, Neungdong-ro, Gwangjin-gu, Seoul 05029, Korea; youngrae@gmail.com (Y.R.K.); yongwankim87@gmail.com (Y.W.K.); sephinlee@gmail.com (S.E.L.)

[2] School of Medicine, Trinity Biomedical Sciences Institute, Trinity College Dublin, 152-160 Pearse Street, D02 R590 Dublin, Ireland; hyewonheidi@hotmail.com

* Correspondence: palelamp@kku.ac.kr; Tel.: +82-2-2049-6060

Received: 7 December 2018; Accepted: 26 December 2018; Published: 4 January 2019

Abstract: Epidermal growth factor receptor (EGFR) inhibitors have benefitted cancer patients worldwide, but resistance inevitably develops over time, resulting in treatment failures. An accurate prediction model for acquired resistance (AR) to EGFR inhibitors is critical for early diagnosis and according intervention, but is not yet available due to personal variations and the complex mechanisms of AR. Here, we have developed a novel pipeline to build a meta-analysis-based, multivariate model for personalized pathways in AR to EGFR inhibitors, using sophisticated machine learning algorithms. Surprisingly, the model achieved excellent predictive performance, with a cross-study validation area under curve (AUC) of over 0.9, and generalization performance on independent cohorts of samples, with a perfect AUC score of 1. Furthermore, the model showed excellent transferability across different cancer cell lines and EGFR inhibitors, including gefitinib, erlotinib, afatinib, and cetuximab. In conclusion, our model achieved high predictive accuracy through robust cross study validation, and enabled individualized prediction on newly introduced data. We also discovered common pathway alteration signatures for AR to EGFR inhibitors, which can provide directions for other follow-up studies.

Keywords: drug resistance; gefitinib; erlotinib; biostatistics; bioinformatics

1. Introduction

Despite the initial benefits of EGFR inhibitors in cancer patients harboring EGFR mutations, the rapid development of acquired resistance (AR) is a major obstacle in clinical practice and often leads to therapeutic failure and disease recurrence. A broad range of mechanisms of AR to EGFR inhibitors have been proposed, from mutational to non-mutation-based mechanisms. However, the exact mechanisms still remain unclear due to the multifactorial natures of cancer and intracellular signaling networks. Inherent crosstalk and redundancy of signaling pathways introduces huge complexity [1,2]. Therefore, inhibiting a single signaling network via drugs may trigger other survival pathways and limit efficacy. These complex dynamics make it more difficult to understand the underlying causes of AR and predict potential EGFR inhibitor sensitivity.

With the recent growth of publically available genomic data, meta-analysis and computational modeling have emerged as key tools to overcome the limitations of insufficient statistical power in individual studies. Conventional meta-analysis methods are often univariate, performing statistical analysis on each feature independently. As conventional classification algorithms tend to overfit high-throughput datasets, also known as high dimension low sample size (HDLSS) datasets, analyses are practically infeasible, resulting in lower accuracy rates when the model is applied to blind data [3,4]. In recent years, regularized regression classifiers such as lasso and elastic net have emerged as more effective ways to perform feature selection and prediction in high dimensional data [4]. These methods modify the conventional ordinary least squares model, using a sparsity penalty that shrinks regression coefficients by imposing a constraint on their size. While this penalty function pushes some coefficients towards zero and introduces some bias, the decrease in variance can potentially improve predictive performance on new, unseen data. These techniques are more interpretable than alternative state-of-the-art algorithms such as support vector machines (SVM), artificial neural networks (ANN), and random forests, which are often considered to be black box models [5]. It is hard to interpret these alternative models, since their inner workings are incomprehensible. Model interpretability and parsimony are especially important in medical field, where numbers of predictors are much larger than sample sizes. In this aspect, regularized regression classifier is regarded as the most optimal model, since it has both more interpretability and similar or superior predicting performance compared with the alternative algorithms. Another possible strategy that reduces model complexity and increases interpretability is the pathway-based approach, which has the potential to better reflect the heterogeneous nature of cancer pathophysiology, compared to classical single gene- or molecule-based methods.

Early detection of acquired EGFR inhibitors resistance is critical, and can help physicians establish a treatment plan by predicting the outcome of a disease. However, previous prediction models are often only applicable to specific types of EGFR tyrosine kinase inhibitors (TKIs), provide insufficient sensitivity or specificity for other types of EGFR inhibitors, and fail to detect generalized predictors.

In this study, using a sophisticated penalized machine learning technique, we built a meta-analysis-based, multivariate model for personalized pathways in acquired EGFR inhibitor resistance. This resulted in a more interpretable and robust model with high generalized predictive performance throughout various EGFR inhibitors and cancer types.

2. Results

To build a robust and generalized prediction model based on individualized pathway information, we developed a novel pipeline that integrates meta-analysis-based regularized regression with pathway-level measurement of abnormality (Figure 1). A total of 8 studies, all of which followed the strict AR criteria mentioned in the methods section, were used for model building. The study cohort was very heterogeneous in terms of the types of EGFR inhibitors, platforms, and cancer cell lines (Table S1). We merged 8 studies through an empirical Bayes algorithm [6] to create an internal training and validation set, after reserving 30% of the samples in GSE34228 and GSE10696 for an external validation set with the createDataPartition function from R package Caret. This function performs a stratified random split of the data by sampling within each class to preserve the overall class distribution [7]. These studies were selected because they were the only cohorts with large enough sample sizes for this purpose.

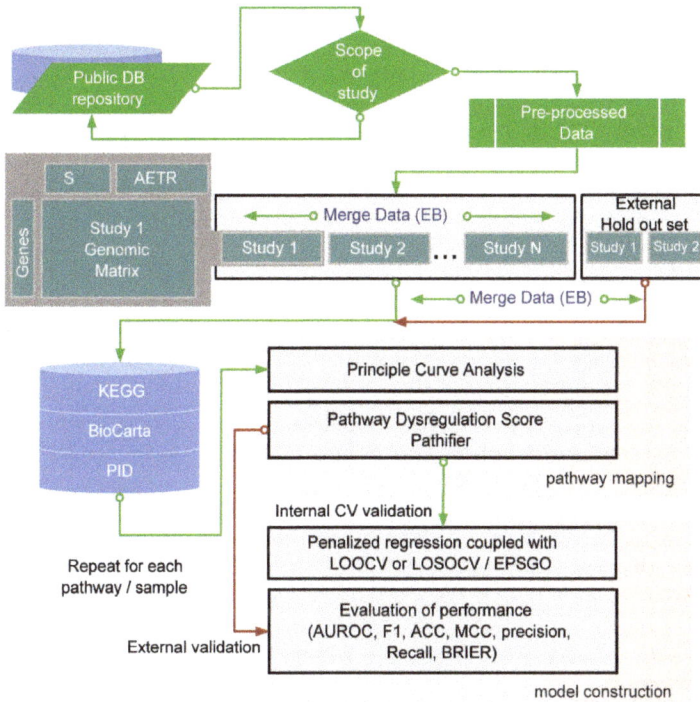

Figure 1. Pipeline for performing a meta-analysis-derived, multivariate model for personalized pathways in acquired epidermal growth factor inhibitor tyrosine kinase inhibitor (EGFR TKI) resistance (AETR). The pipeline consists of three main parts: cross study normalization, pathway mapping, and prediction model construction. The study cohort was preprocessed and categorized into an internal training/validation study set (N) and an external validation study set (M). For cross-study normalization, an empirical Bayes (EB) method was used. Pathway mapping for each individual sample was conducted using a Pathifier algorithm and public pathway databases (KEGG, BioCarta, and PID). The regularized regression model was built using elastic net. The optimal values of the hyper-parameters α and λ for elastic net regression were obtained from robust cross validation (leave-one-study-out cross validation (LOSOCV) or leave-one-out cross validation (LOOCV)) with Efficient Parameter Selection via Global Optimization (EPSGO) algorithm. S, sensitive.

We then used the Pathifier algorithm to convert the transcriptomics-level data matrix to a pathway-based matrix containing pathway dysregulation scores (PDS) [8]. Recently developed, the Pathifier algorithm is viewed as the best functional class scoring relevant algorithm currently available for deducing pathway level scores. This method finds a principal curve, which nonparametrically and nonlinearly generalizes the first principal component for dimension reduction, using the algorithm by Hastie and Stuetzle [9]. Pathifier produces a one-dimensional principal curve from a cluster of data points in a high-dimensional space. The PDS is a metric that represents the extent of pathway abnormality per sample, and can be calculated using the distance from the starting point of the principal curve to the point projected by a particular individualized pathway. In our study, the initial point was the centroid of the control group, sensitive to EGFR inhibitors. A PDS can range from 0 to 1, with a score closer to 1 indicating a more abnormal pathway. Using this method, it is possible to represent samples using fewer, but more informative variables, based on prior biological pathway knowledge [8]. Applying pathway information from curated databases, including the Kyoto Encyclopedia of Genes and Genomes (KEGG) [10], BioCarta [11], and the National Cancer

Institute–Nature Pathway Interaction Database [12], we obtained principal curves for each pathway, and a PDS matrix with 752 rows (pathway features) and 90 columns (samples) (Figure 2A,B). With this PDS matrix, we then used a meta-analysis-based penalized regression method to construct a prediction model for AR to EGFR inhibitors. Penalized regression approaches such as lasso, ridge, and elastic net have been developed to address the challenges caused by high dimensionality of the feature space [4,13,14]. These methods have recently been used to successfully analyze high dimensional human genetic data [4,15,16]. Regression coefficients are shrunk by adding a penalty function to the loss function, which potentially introduces bias but also reduces model variance. Elastic net is a linear combination of lasso and ridge penalties. Two hyperparameters (α and λ) are calibrated for an optimal elastic net penalty function. The α hyperparameter adjusts the levels of contributions from the ridge (L2-norm penalty) and lasso penalties (L1-norm penalty), while λ controls the overall degree of penalization [14]. We used a meta-heuristic algorithm called efficient parameter selection via global optimization (EPSGO) [17], rather than the commonly used fixed grid search methods which are highly arbitrary (see Materials and Methods section for details). Elastic net showed excellent performance on leave-one-out cross-validation (LOOCV), compared to ridge or lasso regression, and EPSGO-tuned elastic net further increased the discrimination power of the classifier (Figures S1 and S2, Table S2). Consequently, EPSGO tuning was employed to find the optimal values of α and λ with minimum binomial deviance (Figure 3A). These optimal parameter values were used for feature selection (Figure 3B,C, Figure S2). At the value for which the penalization parameter gave the lowest cross validation error, the overall area under curve of receiver operating characteristic (AUROC) of the classifier was 0.91 and 1 for the LOSOCV and LOOCV settings, respectively (Figure 4A,C and Figure S3). The results were quite surprising, because all eight studies in the cohort came from different types of cancer cell lines, EGFR inhibitors, and technology platforms (Figure 2A and Table S1). This suggests that pathway-based features have high transferability and generalizability. In addition, other performance metrics (F1, precision, recall, Brier score, accuracy, and Matthews correlation coefficient (MCC)) that examine prediction error further support the predictive power of this model (Figure 4B,D, Figure S3 and Table S5).

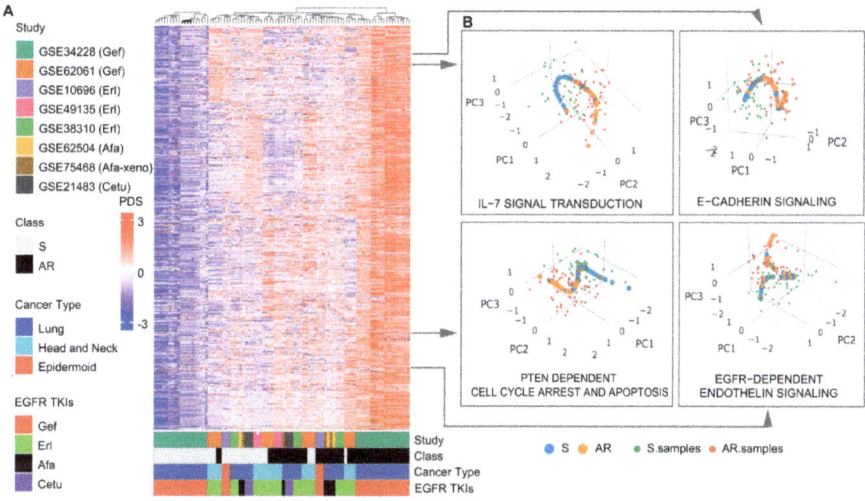

Figure 2. Meta-analysis-derived pathway deregulation analysis. (**A**) Pathway dysregulation score (PDS) matrix for the 8 internal training/validation study sets. Each row represents the z-score-normalized PDS for each individual sample in each cohort. The color-bars in the bottom indicate the following from top to bottom: (1) the study cohort. (2) The resistance status of samples. (3) The cancer subtype of the samples. (4) The type of EGFR-TKI. (**B**) Principal curves of selected pathways. The principal curve learned for the pathways on the 8 study cohort. The data points and the principal curve are projected onto the three principal components (PCs; PC1 to PC3). The principal curve goes through the cloud of samples and is directed so that EGFR-TKI-sensitive samples are near the beginning of the curve. The acquired EGFR-TKI-resistant samples are projected onto the curve. AR, acquired resistance; S, sensitive; Gef, Gefitinib; Erl, Erlotinib; Afa, Afatinib; Cetu, Cetuximab.

The leave-one-study-out strategy gave a more parsimonious model with 21 non-zero pathway coefficients, compared to 55 features by the leave-one-out strategy, suggesting that this model is more interpretable and has less risk of overfitting (Figure 3A and Figure S2C). The detailed results are given in Tables S3 and S4. Next, we further validated our model using an independent blind test set (Gef-GSE34228 and Erl-GSE10696) that was not used in model discovery. The resulting pathway-based predictive model still achieved very high performance on the independent test sets, with perfect AUCs of 1 for both the Gef and Erl sets (Figure 4A,C). Moreover, the additional evaluation metrics also confirmed the robustness and generality of our meta-analysis-based pathway-based learning model (Figure 4B,D and Table S5).

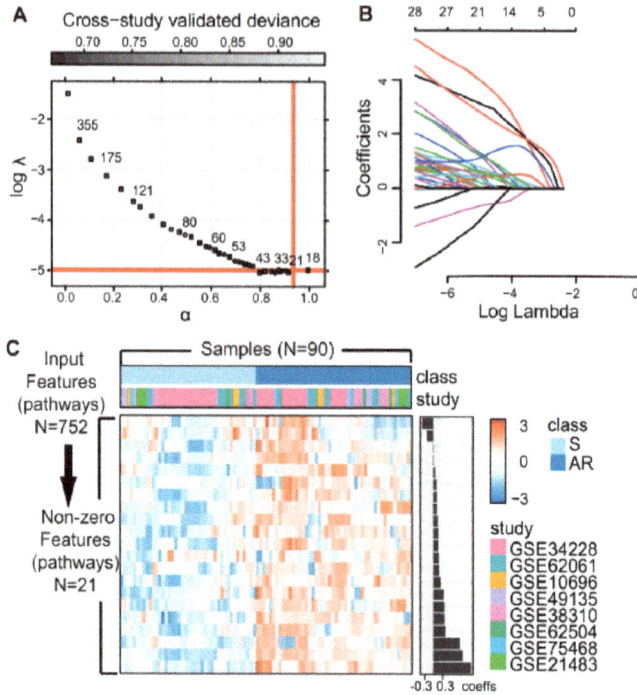

Figure 3. Optimizing meta-analysis-derived elastic net using LOSOCV. (**A**) Hyperparameter optimization for elastic net with EPSGO. Cross validation deviance as a function of both tuning hyperparameters α and log λ. The number of selected features in minimum deviance is shown next to the symbol. The solid lines highlight the final EPSGO solution where the deviance is within 1SE of the minimum. The initial points are plotted as rectangles and iteration points as circles. The optimal parameter values with minimal deviance were found for α = 0.96 and log λ = −4.99, and are highlighted as a solid line. (**B**) Coefficient paths for elastic net penalized regression models applied to the 8 study cohort. The solution path is scaled to reflect log λ on the x-axis. (**C**) Heatmap of the pathways with non-zero coefficients. Sensitive or acquired resistance condition for EGFR-TKIs is indicated above the heatmap. The pathway features are listed in descending order with regard to their coefficient. The optimal hyperparameter values were determined by LOSOCV. AR, acquired resistance; S, sensitive.

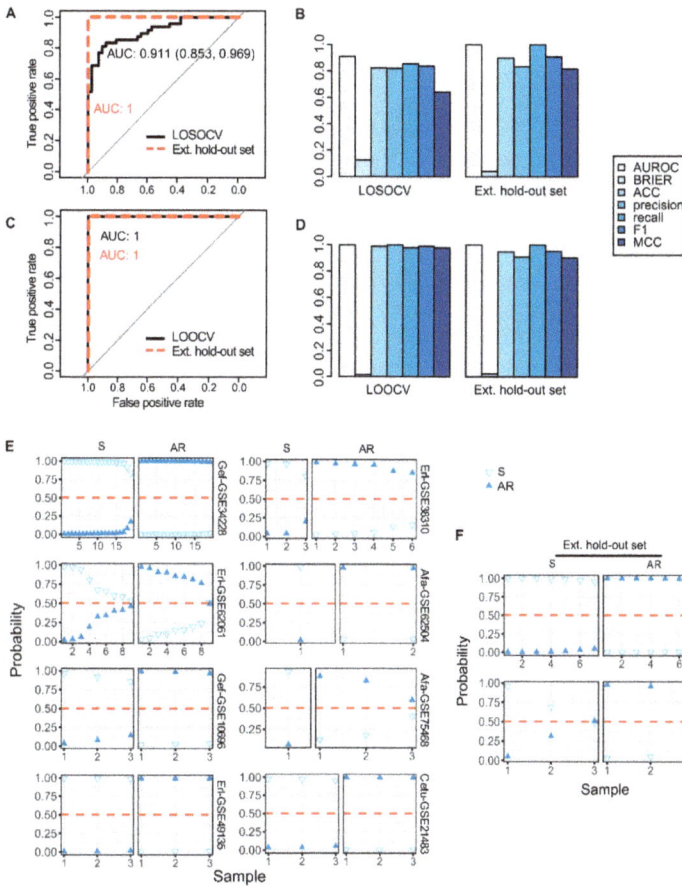

Figure 4. Internal and external evaluation of model performance to distinguish sensitive and acquired resistance to EGFR TKIs. (**A**) Receiver operating characteristic (ROC) curves for the binary classifier in the leave-one-study-out cross validation (LOSOCV). The black line indicates the cross-validation curve, and the dotted red line indicates the external test set. The curve shows sensitivity versus specificity, based on probabilities computed through elastic net regression. (**B**) Different performance metrics (Brier, ACC, precision, recall, F1, and MCC) for the evaluation of classification in LOSOCV. (**C**) Receiver operating characteristic (ROC) curves for the binary classifier in the leave-one-out cross validation (LOOCV). (**D**) Different performance metrics (Brier, ACC, precision, recall, F1, and MCC) for the evaluation of classification in LOOCV. (**E**) Estimated probabilities for samples in cross-study validation. Within study set and subgroup, samples are sorted by the probability of the true group. (**F**) Estimated probabilities for samples in external independent validation. AR, acquired resistance; S, sensitive; ACC, accuracy; MCC, Matthews correlation coefficient.

3. Discussion

Most EGFR inhibitor resistance predictive models use genomic predictors such as gene signatures, filtered with arbitrary cutoff values and often hard to interpret. The use of a meta-analytic approach and pathway features offers a more robust and comprehensive look into underlying biological processes than individual genes. The novelty and strength of our approach is that we considered all dimensions and applied pathway mapping to a multi-study model to build a generalized predictive model for

AR to EGFR inhibitors. Through this, we achieved excellent predictive performance for both the cross study validation set and the independent blind test set.

Our study employed a two-step approach to dimensionality reduction: cross-study pathway-level representation and penalized regression with a global-tuning algorithm. The first step of complexity reduction is to convert individual gene-level information into pathway-level information. A growing body of evidence suggests that pathway-based features can provide more insight into the biological aspects of disease prediction [8,18]. In our study, although the cohort was highly heterogeneous, the model performed remarkably well, which suggests that pathway-based features are good representatives of the true phenotypes. The second step of complexity reduction is regularization. Due to the intrinsic nature of high dimensionality, the low sample size, and heterogeneity of the studies we employed, a regularized regression approach was paired with a fine-tuning algorithm to build a generalized classifier for EGFR inhibitor resistance. This regularization regression is comprised of a loss function with a penalty function, with the latter function placing a heavier penalty on more complex models. The severity of the penalty is tuned empirically using cross-study validation in addition to the more traditional cross validation approach, and is then further optimized using the state-of-the-art EPSGO algorithm to find the global optimization parameter. This process provides additional reduction in model complexity and increases model interpretability.

From the 752 pathways used for the analysis, LOSOCV selected 21 non-zero pathway coefficients for the final model, reflecting much more sparsity than the final model by LOOCV, which contains 55 non-zero features (Table S3). The common genes shared in more than 10 pathways were PI3K, AKT1, MAPK1, SRC, SHC1, FYN, and GRB2. All of them are known to play a central role in EGFR-mediated signaling pathways (Table S4 and Figure S4B). The majority of the pathways are closely related to previously identified potential EGFR inhibitor drug resistance pathways (NCI's 'Regulation of p38-alpha and p38-beta' [19]; NCI's 'E−Cadherin signaling' pathway' [19]; 'Hedgehog signaling events mediated by Gli proteins' [20]; 'Atypical NF-kb pathway' [21]; BioCarta's 'PTEN dependent cell cycle arrest and apoptosis' [22]; 'CXCR4 signaling pathway' [23]; 'Hypoxia-inducible factor in the cardiovascular system' [23]). The associations between the rest of the pathways and acquired resistance are relatively unexplored and require follow-up functional studies. One of them is BioCarta's ER associated degradation (ERAD) pathway, which had the highest non-zero coefficient (Table S3). Traditionally, EGFR proteins are known as cell surface receptors activated by ligand binding, which results in tyrosine kinase activation and downstream signaling. These downstream signaling pathways are crucial for aggressiveness and resistance development of cancers. Recent evidence has indicated that EGFR receptors are transported from the cell surface to the nucleus, and transmit signals to influence a variety of biological functions. It has been hypothesized that EGFR receptors are shuttled to the cytoplasm through the ERAD pathway, and to the nucleus through the nuclear pore complex (NPC) and importin-β [24]. Nuclear EGFR has been reported in various tumors, and was associated with poor outcomes [25,26]. One previous study indicated nuclear EGFR is accountable for cetuximab acquired resistance [27]. Further investigation into the ERAD pathway and nuclear EGFR is urgently needed, as it may provide invaluable knowledge into acquired resistance. Some of the others are directly involved in growth factor signaling, among them the NCI's 'EGFR-dependent Endothelin signaling events' and 'Ephrin a reverse signaling pathway'. Nectins and DeltaNp63 signaling pathways are known to be implicated in the tumor progression and anticancer drug resistance [28,29], but their potential roles in EGFR inhibitors resistance have not yet been studied. Three out of 21 non-zero pathways are metabolic pathways. Two of them are associated with the biosynthesis of fatty acids, and the other with phenylalanine metabolism (Table S3 and Figure S4A). Glycosylated sphingolipids are involved in the formation of lipid rafts, which have long been suggested to play an important role in the development of multidrug resistance (MDR) [30]. It has been reported that EGFR is commonly localized to lipid rafts, most prominently in the EGFR TKI resistant cell lines [31]. Phenylalanine has been shown to have the potential to suppress the MDR phenotype [32]. However, whether phenylalanine metabolism is involved in EGFR TKI resistance had not been reported. A better understanding of these pathway features could potentially serve as a basis for discovering the mechanism of resistance development.

Having parsimony and transferability without losing predictive capacity is very important in models, especially for medical applications. This is the first study of its kind to report such high validation accuracy and transferability over different types of cancer cell lines and EGFR inhibitors. In this study, using a state-of-the art machine learning technique, we successfully developed a meta-analysis-derived, multivariate model for personalized pathways in acquired EGFR inhibitor resistance that is able to accurately identify general predictors.

4. Materials and Methods

4.1. Data Set Configurations

Eight publicly available study cohorts (GSE34228, GSE10696, GSE62061, GSE49135, GSE38310, GSE62504, GSE75468, GSE21483) [33–38] only included samples that were stepwise selected for acquired resistant cell lines and encompassed 4 different types of EGFR inhibitors (gefitinib, erlotinib, afatinib and cetuximab), 3 types of cancer (lung, head and neck, and epidermoid cancer), and 4 types of array platforms (Table S1). GSE75468 included acquired afatinib-resistant non-small cell lung cancer cell lines derived from a tumor xenograft model. We excluded studies with insufficient information on the type of drug resistance (innate or acquired). Animal studies and studies with extremely small sample sizes or an inadequate control conditions were also ruled out. The selection process resulted in a total of eight studies to be included in the study cohort. Of these, the gefininb (GSE34228) and erlotinib (GSE62061) studies had large enough sample sizes to be partially used to construct an external test set. Stratified random sampling was used to select 30% of the samples from each study for external use. The other six studies were solely used for model training and cross-study validation due to the smaller sample sizes. Detailed information of the study subjects is given in Table S1.

4.2. Data Processing

All data used in this paper is publicly available from the Gene Expression Omnibus (GEO). Normalization and log-transformation of expression values from each dataset were performed as previously described in detail [15]. If raw data from Affymetrix platforms were available, they were pre-processed by robust multi-array average (RMA) [15]. Otherwise, we used pre-processed data from the authors. For gene level summarization, we employed an interquartile range (IQR) method, in which we selected the probe set ID with the largest IQR of expression values among all multiple probe set IDs to represent the gene. Cross-study normalization to correct batch effect was performed using the ComBat function in the sva R package [39]. ComBat uses an empirical Bayes method, which tunes data to remove batch effects and is very effective for datasets with small sample sizes [6]. Blind sets for external validation were not used in internal cross-study normalization to prevent any effects in model building, which established the model's generalizability to predict from any unknown data [15]. In external validation, we used ComBat for cross-study normalization for each addition of a blind set using the same protocol. Next, as biological pathways are the aggregate of gene activities and generally much more robust than gene markers, we converted gene-wise information to pathway-wise information to detect the common features for acquired drug resistance, regardless of EGFR inhibitors and cancer cell lines [40,41].

4.3. Pathway Mapping

Pathway dysregulation scores (PDS) for each individual sample were calculated using a pipeline that employed the Pathifier algorithm as previously described [7]. Pathifier is a non-linear method for quantifying degree of pathway abnormality. The algorithm learns the standard pathway flow from control samples and utilizes this to construct a principal curve. Every sample is projected onto this principal curve, and the PDS is calculated from the normalized projection distance for each sample's pathway. Pathway information used to form PDS matrix was extracted from ConsensusPathDB (CPDB) (http://consensuspathdb.org/) [42], which comprises curated information from BioCarta, Kyoto Encyclopedia of Genes and Genomes (KEGG), and the National Cancer Institute—Nature Pathway Interaction Database. We used the R package pathifier [8] to calculate PDS.

4.4. Model Building

We built the prediction model using elastic net regularization using the R package glmnet [13]. Friedman et al. [13,14] describe the elastic net algorithm in detail. To construct the meta-analysis-derived classifier, we referred to and modified the function from R package C060 and a pre-published script by Sill et al. [43], which is available online. We built additional wrapper functions for the glmnet algorithm to fit and tune the model. We used leave-one-study-out cross validation (LOSOCV) and leave-one-out cross validation (LOOCV) to find the optimal value of the regularization parameter with both minimum deviance and minimum deviance + 1SE. In LOSOCV, one study was then taken as the validation set for testing the model, and the remaining studies were used as training data. The cross-validation procedure was repeated for the number of studies to estimate the average standard error and find the optimal parameter values. The efficient parameter selection via global optimization (EPSGO) algorithm was then used to further fine-tune the parameter [17]. EPSGO is a meta-heuristic algorithm which bases its learning an online Gaussian process, and its parameters are chosen by maximum likelihood. Compared to the grid search method, this algorithm is computationally efficient and robust against local minima. LOOCV followed the same process, except for using a sample in place of a study. The optimal parameter values were then used for variable selection.

4.5. Evaluation Strategies

We mainly used area under receiver operation characteristic curve (AUROC) to assess the model's performance. In the context of binary classification, the classifier can produce four possible outcomes: true positive (TP), true negative (TN), false positive (FP), and false negative (FN). The ratio of true positives over the sum of ground truth positives is called the true positive rate (TPR, also known as sensitivity or recall), and is expressed as TP/(TP + FN). The ratio of false positives over the sum of ground truth negatives is called the false positive rate (FPR or 1-specificity), and is expressed as FP/(FP + TN). AUROC is the true positive rate as a function of the false positive rate, and measures the aggregated classification performance with its value ranging between 0.5 and 1. A value of 0.5 corresponds to a random guess, while 1 means a perfect prediction. Precision is the ratio of true positives over the sum of predicted positives, and is expressed as TP/(TP + FP). Precision recall curve summarizes the model performance in terms of precision and recall. F-score is the harmonic mean of precision and recall, expressed as 2*recall*precision/(recall + precision). Brier score is the mean squared error between predicted probabilities and the actual outcome. MCC, taking all four outcomes (TP, TN, FP, and FN) into account and expressed as (TP*TN) − (FP*FN)/square root((TP + FP)*(TP + FN)*(TN + FP)*(TN + FN)), is a geometric mean corrected for chance agreement and generally regarded as a balanced measure. All statistic measures except the Brier score are directly proportional to predictive performance. For the Brier score, higher values denote worse performances. MCC has a range from −1 (completely incorrect) to 1 (completely correct). All other metrics mentioned above have a range of (0, 1). All statistical evaluation and visualization were performed in the R software environment.

5. Conclusions

Accurate prediction of chemotherapy resistance is clinically crucial for the management of cancers. Using pathway mapping and machine learning algorithms, we developed a pipeline to build a meta-analysis-based, multivariate model for personalized prediction. Our model achieved high prediction accuracy with generalizability and transferability through robust internal cross-study validation and external validation, enabling personalized prediction for resistance over different types of cancer cell lines and EGFR inhibitors, including gefitinib, erlotinib, afatinib, and cetuximab. From 752 pieces of pathway information, LOSOCV selected 21 pathway coefficients, which was sparser than LOOCV. The highest non-zero coefficient for a pathway was BioCarta's ER associated degradation (ERAD) pathway, which is implicated in the shuttling of nuclear EGFR into the cytoplasm before its eventual translocation into the nucleus. Further molecular and clinical confirmations are urgently needed, as the associations of nuclear EGFR with various cancers and resistance to cetuximab have been previously described.

Supplementary Materials: The following are available online at http://www.mdpi.com/2072-6694/11/1/45/s1, Figure S1: Performance comparison of the four classifiers including ridge, lasso, elastic net, and EPSGO-elastic net on the merged cohort. (A) Receiver operating characteristic (ROC) and Precision-Recall curves of four classifiers. (B) Different performance metrics for the evaluation of classification. EPSGO, Efficient Parameter Selection via Global Optimization; AUROC, area under curve of receiver operating characteristic; ACC, accuracy; MCC, Matthews correlation coefficient. Figure S2: Log loss as a function of the regularization hyper-parameter λ for LOSOCV (A) and LOOCV (B) on the merged cohort. Points and, error bars correspond to the mean and the standard deviation, respectively. The dashed lines indicate the final λ solution where the minimum deviance + 1SE was recorded. (C) meta-analysis-derived elastic net with LOOCV. The heatmap shows the pathways with non-zero coefficents. AR, acquired resistance; S, sensitive; LOSOCV, leave-one-study-out cross validation; LOOCV, leave-one-out cross validation. Figure S3: Precision-Recall curves for the binary classifiers ability to distinguish sensitive and acquired resistance to EGFR TKIs in the internal leave-one-study-out (left) or leave-one-sample-out (right) CV (green) and external test set (red). Figure S4: (A) additional principal curves of selected pathways. (B) overlapping gene count in the 752 pathways listed (left) and genes shared in more than 5 pathways (right). Table S1: Characteristics of individual studies. Table S2: The performances of four penalized regression models. Table S3: Pathways with non-zero coefficients using LOOCV and LOSOCV. Table S4: The genes that overlaps between pathways (overlap counts $\geq$ 3). Table S5: Performance scores for internal and validation.

Author Contributions: Conceptualization, S.Y.K.; Data curation, S.Y.K. and Y.R.K.; Formal analysis, S.Y.K. and Y.R.K.; Investigation, S.Y.K., Y.R.K., Y.W.K., S.E.L. and H.W.Y.; Methodology, S.Y.K. and Y.R.K.; Supervision, S.Y.K.; Validation, S.Y.K. and Y.R.K.; Writing—original draft, S.Y.K., Y.R.K., Y.W.K., S.E.L. and H.W.Y.

Funding: This research received no external funding.

Acknowledgments: This paper was supported by the National Research Foundation (NRF)-2016R1A1A1A05921984.

Conflicts of Interest: The authors declare no conflict of interest.

References

1. Sun, X.; Bao, J.; You, Z.; Chen, X.; Cui, J. Modeling of signaling crosstalk-mediated drug resistance and its implications on drug combination. *Oncotarget* **2016**, *7*, 63995–64006. [CrossRef]
2. Eberlein, C.A.; Stetson, D.; Markovets, A.A.; Al-Kadhimi, K.J.; Lai, Z.; Fisher, P.R.; Meador, C.B.; Spitzler, P.; Ichihara, E.; Ross, S.J.; et al. Acquired Resistance to the Mutant-Selective EGFR Inhibitor AZD9291 Is Associated with Increased Dependence on RAS Signaling in Preclinical Models. *Cancer Res.* **2015**, *75*, 2489–2500. [CrossRef] [PubMed]
3. Clarke, R.; Ressom, H.W.; Wang, A.; Xuan, J.; Liu, M.C.; Gehan, E.A.; Wang, Y. The properties of high-dimensional data spaces: Implications for exploring gene and protein expression data. *Nat. Rev. Cancer* **2008**, *8*, 37–49. [CrossRef] [PubMed]
4. Lever, J.; Krzywinski, M.; Altman, N. Points of Significance: Regularization. *Nat. Methods* **2016**, *13*, 803–804. [CrossRef]
5. Bibal, A.; Frénay, B. Interpretability of Machine Learning Models and Representations: An Introduction. In Proceedings of the ESANN 2016 Proceedings, European Symposium on Artificial Neural Networks, Computational Intelligence and Machine Learning, Bruges, Belgium, 27–29 April 2016.
6. Johnson, W.E.; Li, C.; Rabinovic, A. Adjusting batch effects in microarray expression data using empirical Bayes methods. *Biostatistics* **2007**, *8*, 118–127. [CrossRef] [PubMed]
7. Kuhn, M. Building Predictive Models in R Using the caret Package. *J. Stat. Softw.* **2008**, *28*. [CrossRef]
8. Drier, Y.; Sheffer, M.; Domany, E. Pathway-based personalized analysis of cancer. *Proc. Natl. Acad. Sci. USA* **2013**, *110*, 6388–6393. [CrossRef] [PubMed]
9. Hastie, T.; Stuetzl, W. Principal curves. *J. Am. Stat. Assoc.* **1989**, *406*, 501–516. [CrossRef]

10. Kanehisa, M.; Goto, S. KEGG: Kyoto encyclopedia of genes and genomes. *Nucleic Acids Res.* **2000**, *28*, 27–30. [CrossRef]

11. Nishimura, D. BioCarta. *Biotech Softw. Internet Rep.* **2001**, *2*, 117–120. [CrossRef]

12. Schaefer, C.F.; Anthony, K.; Krupa, S.; Buchoff, J.; Day, M.; Hannay, T.; Buetow, K.H. PID: The pathway interaction database. *Nucleic Acids Res.* **2009**, *37*, D674–D679. [CrossRef] [PubMed]

13. Friedman, J.; Hastie, T.; Tibshirani, R. Regularization Paths for Generalized Linear Models via Coordinate Descent. *J. Stat. Softw.* **2010**, *33*, 1–22. [CrossRef]

14. Zou, H.; Hastie, T. Regularization and variable selection via the elastic net. *J. R. Stat. Soc. B* **2005**, *67*, 301–320. [CrossRef]

15. Hughey, J.J.; Butte, A.J. Robust meta-analysis of gene expression using the elastic net. *Nucleic Acids Res.* **2015**, *43*, e79. [CrossRef]

16. Cancer Cell Line Encyclopedia Consortium. Genomics of Drug Sensitivity in Cancer Consortium Pharmacogenomic agreement between two cancer cell line data sets. *Nature* **2015**, *528*, 84–87.

17. Froehlich, H.; Zell, A. Efficient Parameter Selection for Support Vector Machines in Classification and Regression via Model-Based Global Optimization. In Proceedings of the IEEE International Joint Conference of Neural Networks, Montreal, QC, Canada, 31 July–4 August 2005; pp. 1431–1438.

18. Glaab, E. Using prior knowledge from cellular pathways and molecular networks for diagnostic specimen classification. *Brief. Bioinform.* **2016**, *17*, 440–452. [CrossRef] [PubMed]

19. Fernando, R.I.; Hamilton, D.H.; Dominguez, C.; David, J.M.; McCampbell, K.K.; Palena, C. IL-8 signaling is involved in resistance of lung carcinoma cells to erlotinib. *Oncotarget* **2016**, *7*, 42031–42044. [CrossRef]

20. Bai, X.-Y.; Zhang, X.-C.; Yang, S.-Q.; An, S.-J.; Chen, Z.-H.; Su, J.; Xie, Z.; Gou, L.-Y.; Wu, Y.-L. Blockade of Hedgehog Signaling Synergistically Increases Sensitivity to Epidermal Growth Factor Receptor Tyrosine Kinase Inhibitors in Non-Small-Cell Lung Cancer Cell Lines. *PLoS ONE* **2016**, *11*, e0149370. [CrossRef] [PubMed]

21. Galvani, E.; Sun, J.; Leon, L.G.; Sciarrillo, R.; Narayan, R.S.; Sjin, R.T.T.; Lee, K.; Ohashi, K.; Heideman, D.A.M.; Alfieri, R.R.; et al. NF-κB drives acquired resistance to a novel mutant-selective EGFR inhibitor. *Oncotarget* **2015**, *6*, 42717–42732. [CrossRef]

22. Huang, L.; Fu, L. Mechanisms of resistance to EGFR tyrosine kinase inhibitors. *Acta Pharm. Sin. B* **2015**, *5*, 390–401. [CrossRef]

23. Murakami, A.; Takahashi, F.; Nurwidya, F.; Kobayashi, I.; Minakata, K.; Hashimoto, M.; Nara, T.; Kato, M.; Tajima, K.; Shimada, N.; et al. Hypoxia increases gefitinib-resistant lung cancer stem cells through the activation of insulin-like growth factor 1 receptor. *PLoS ONE* **2014**, *9*, e86459. [CrossRef] [PubMed]

24. Wang, Y.N.; Yamaguchi, H.; Hsu, J.M.; Hung, M.C. Nuclear trafficking of the epidermal growth factor receptor family membrane proteins. *Oncogene* **2010**, *29*, 3997. [CrossRef]

25. Xia, W.; Wei, Y.; Du, Y.; Liu, J.; Chang, B.; Yu, Y.L.; Huo, L.F.; Miller, S.; Hung, M.C. Nuclear expression of epidermal growth factor receptor is a novel prognostic value in patients with ovarian cancer. *Mol. Carcinog.* **2009**, *48*, 610–617. [CrossRef] [PubMed]

26. Hoshino, M.; Fukui, H.; Ono, Y.; Sekikawa, A.; Ichikawa, K.; Tomita, S.; Imai, Y.; Imura, K.; Hiraishi, H.; Fujimori, T. Nuclear expression of phosphorylated EGFR is associated with poor prognosis of patients with esophageal squamous cell carcinoma. *Pathobiology* **2007**, *74*, 15–21. [CrossRef] [PubMed]

27. Li, C.; Iida, M.; Dunn, E.F.; Ghia, A.J.; Wheeler, D.L. Nuclear EGFR contributes to acquired resistance to cetuximab. *Oncogene* **2009**, *28*, 3801–3813. [CrossRef] [PubMed]

28. Ghidouche, A.; Lopez, M.; Olive, D. P8.08 * Roles of Nectin-4 in tumor progression. *Ann. Oncol.* **2015**, *26*, ii34. [CrossRef]

29. Das, D.; Satapathy, S.R.; Siddharth, S.; Nayak, A.; Kundu, C.N. NECTIN-4 increased the 5-FU resistance in colon cancer cells by inducing the PI3K-AKT cascade. *Cancer Chemother. Pharmacol.* **2015**, *76*, 471–479. [CrossRef]

30. Gouaze-Andersson, V.; Cabot, M.C. Glycosphingolipids and drug resistance. *Biochim. Biophys. Acta* **2006**, *1758*, 2096–2103. [CrossRef]

31. Irwin, M.E.; Mueller, K.L.; Bohin, N.; Ge, Y.; Boerner, J.L. Lipid raft localization of EGFR alters the response of cancer cells to the EGFR tyrosine kinase inhibitor gefitinib. *J. Cell. Physiol.* **2011**, *226*, 2316–2328. [CrossRef]

32. Elstad, C.A.; Thrall, B.D.; Raha, G.; Meadows, G.G. Tyrosine and phenylalanine restriction sensitizes adriamycin-resistant P388 leukemia cells to adriamycin. *Nutr. Cancer* **1996**, *25*, 47–60. [CrossRef]

33. Yamauchi, M.; Yamaguchi, R.; Nakata, A.; Kohno, T.; Nagasaki, M.; Shimamura, T.; Imoto, S.; Saito, A.; Ueno, K.; Hatanaka, Y.; et al. Epidermal growth factor receptor tyrosine kinase defines critical prognostic genes of stage I lung adenocarcinoma. *PLoS ONE* **2012**, *7*, e43923. [CrossRef] [PubMed]

34. Guix, M.; Faber, A.C.; Wang, S.E.; Olivares, M.G.; Song, Y.; Qu, S.; Rinehart, C.; Seidel, B.; Yee, D.; Arteaga, C.L.; et al. Acquired resistance to EGFR tyrosine kinase inhibitors in cancer cells is mediated by loss of IGF-binding proteins. *J. Clin. Investig.* **2008**, *118*, 2609–2619. [CrossRef] [PubMed]

35. Stanam, A.; Love-Homan, L.; Joseph, T.S.; Espinosa-Cotton, M.; Simons, A.L. Upregulated interleukin-6 expression contributes to erlotinib resistance in head and neck squamous cell carcinoma. *Mol. Oncol.* **2015**, *9*, 1371–1383. [CrossRef] [PubMed]

36. Giles, K.M.; Kalinowski, F.C.; Candy, P.A.; Epis, M.R.; Zhang, P.M.; Redfern, A.D.; Stuart, L.M.; Goodall, G.J.; Leedman, P.J. Axl mediates acquired resistance of head and neck cancer cells to the epidermal growth factor receptor inhibitor erlotinib. *Mol. Cancer Ther.* **2013**, *12*, 2541–2558. [CrossRef] [PubMed]

37. Zhang, Z.; Lee, J.C.; Lin, L.; Olivas, V.; Au, V.; LaFramboise, T.; Abdel-Rahman, M.; Wang, X.; Levine, A.D.; Rho, J.K.; et al. Activation of the AXL kinase causes resistance to EGFR-targeted therapy in lung cancer. *Nat. Genet.* **2012**, *44*, 852–860. [CrossRef] [PubMed]

38. Hatakeyama, H.; Cheng, H.; Wirth, P.; Counsell, A.; Marcrom, S.R.; Wood, C.B.; Pohlmann, P.R.; Gilbert, J.; Murphy, B.; Yarbrough, W.G.; et al. Regulation of heparin-binding EGF-like growth factor by miR-212 and acquired cetuximab-resistance in head and neck squamous cell carcinoma. *PLoS ONE* **2010**, *5*, e12702. [CrossRef]

39. Leek, J.T.; Johnson, W.E.; Parker, H.S.; Jaffe, A.E.; Storey, J.D. The sva package for removing batch effects and other unwanted variation in high-throughput experiments. *Bioinformatics* **2012**, *28*, 882–883. [CrossRef] [PubMed]

40. Khunlertgit, N.; Yoon, B. Identification of Robust Pathway Markers for Cancer through Rank-Based Pathway Activity Inference. *Adv. Bioinform.* **2013**, *2013*, 618461.

41. Tian, L.; Greenberg, S.A.; Kong, S.W.; Altschuler, J.; Kohane, I.S.; Park, P.J. Discovering statistically significant pathways in expression profiling studies. *Proc. Natl. Acad. Sci. USA* **2005**, *102*, 13544–13549. [CrossRef] [PubMed]

42. Kamburov, A.; Stelzl, U.; Lehrach, H.; Herwig, R. The ConsensusPathDB interaction database: 2013 update. *Nucleic Acids Res.* **2013**, *41*, D793–D800. [CrossRef]

43. Sill, M.; Hielscher, T.; Becker, N.; Zucknick, M. c060: Extended Inference with Lasso and Elastic-Net Regularized Cox and Generalized Linear Models. *J. Stat. Softw.* **2014**, *62*, 1–22. [CrossRef]

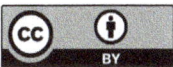

Article

Network Pharmacology to Unveil the Biological Basis of Health-Strengthening Herbal Medicine in Cancer Treatment

Jiahui Zheng [1], Min Wu [1], Haiyan Wang [2], Shasha Li [2], Xin Wang [1], Yan Li [3], Dong Wang [2] and Shao Li [1,*]

[1]   MOE Key Laboratory of Bioinformatics; Bioinformatics Division Biology/Center for TCM-X, BNRist, TFIDT/Department of Automation, Tsinghua University, 100084 Beijing, China; zjh1228@yeah.net (J.Z.); minwu8@foxmail.com (M.W.); roymaleo@163.com (X.W.)

[2]   Department of Basic Medicine, School of Medicine, Tsinghua University, 100084 Beijing, China; wanghaiyan0917@sina.com (H.W.); ss-li14@tsinghua.org.cn (S.L.); dwang@biomed.tsinghua.edu.cn (D.W.)

[3]   State Key Laboratory of Bioactive Substances and Functions of Nature Medicines, Institute of Materia Medica, Chinese Academy of Medical Sciences & Peking Union Medical College, 100730 Beijing, China; lyhzytt@163.com

*   Correspondence: shaoli@mail.tsinghua.edu.cn; Tel.: +86-10-6279-7035

Received: 12 September 2018; Accepted: 16 November 2018; Published: 21 November 2018

Abstract: Health-strengthening (*Fu-Zheng*) herbs is a representative type of traditional Chinese medicine (TCM) widely used for cancer treatment in China, which is in contrast to pathogen eliminating (*Qu-Xie*) herbs. However, the commonness in the biological basis of health-strengthening herbs remains to be holistically elucidated. In this study, an innovative high-throughput research strategy integrating computational and experimental methods of network pharmacology was proposed, and 22 health-strengthening herbs were selected for the investigation. Additionally, 25 pathogen-eliminating herbs were included for comparison. First, based on network-based, large-scale target prediction, we analyzed the target profiles of 1446 TCM compounds. Next, the actions of 166 compounds on 420 antitumor or immune-related genes were measured using a unique high-throughput screening strategy by high-throughput sequencing, referred to as HTS^2. Furthermore, the structural information and the antitumor activity of the compounds in health-strengthening and pathogen-eliminating herbs were compared. Using network pharmacology analysis, we discovered that: (1) Functionally, the predicted targets of compounds from health strengthening herbs were enriched in both immune-related and antitumor pathways, similar to those of pathogen eliminating herbs. As a case study, galloylpaeoniflorin, a compound in a health strengthening herb *Radix Paeoniae Alba* (*Bai Shao*), was found to exert antitumor effects both in vivo and in vitro. Yet the inhibitory effects of the compounds from pathogen eliminating herbs on tumor cells proliferation as a whole were significantly stronger than those in health-strengthening herbs ($p < 0.001$). Moreover, the percentage of assay compounds in health-strengthening herbs with the predicted targets enriched in the immune-related pathways (e.g., natural killer cell mediated cytotoxicity and antigen processing and presentation) were significantly higher than that in pathogen-eliminating herbs ($p < 0.05$). This finding was supported by the immune-enhancing effects of a group of compounds from health-strengthening herbs indicated by differentially expressed genes in the HTS^2 results. (2) Compounds in the same herb may exhibit the same or distinguished mechanisms in cancer treatment, which was demonstrated as the compounds influence pathway gene expressions in the same or opposite directions. For example, acetyl ursolic acid and specnuezhenide in a health-strengthening herb *Fructus Ligustri lucidi* (*Nv Zhen Zi*) both upregulated gene expressions in T cell receptor signaling pathway. Together, this study suggested greater potentials in tumor immune microenvironment regulation and tumor prevention than in direct killing tumor cells of health-strengthening herbs generally, and provided a systematic strategy for unveiling the commonness in the biological basis of health-strengthening herbs in cancer treatment.

Keywords: traditional Chinese medicine; health strengthening herb; cancer treatment; network pharmacology; network target; high-throughput analysis

1. Introduction

China has a long history of using traditional Chinese medicine (TCM) for treating cancer [1]. A large amount of medication experience and clinical cases have been accumulated by TCM practitioners, which makes TCM contribute greatly to the development of China's national health status. According to an urban basic medical insurance survey of inpatient use of health services in China from 2008 to 2010, 42.4% of oncology patients have used antineoplastic TCMs in the Chinese national medical insurance catalogue [2]. With increasing scientific evidence in biological, chemical, and medical research, as well as clinical trials, the use of traditional Chinese medicine in cancer treatment is gradually being recognized as a complementary and alternative therapy all over the world [3–6].

Traditionally, TCM adopts a relative and holistic point of view in cancer treatment. The clinical treatment strategy by strengthening health reflects the characteristics of focusing on regulatory effects instead of the antagonistic effects of TCM, and embodies the classical therapeutic theory that "pathogenic-qi cannot invade the body if health-qi remains strong" in the Canon of Internal Medicine (*Huangdi Neijing*). Therefore, an in-depth exploration on the antitumor effects exerted by health- strengthening herbs is meaningful and urgently needed. TCMs in the Chinese national medical insurance catalogue (2017) for oncology treatment are officially divided into two categories, including antitumor TCM and adjuvant TCM for tumors, which contain 40 TCM prescriptions in total [7]. Additionally, some health-strengthening prescriptions are widely applied in cancer treatment, such as *Sijunzi* decoction in colorectal cancer [8], *Shenqi Fuzheng* injection in colorectal cancer and breast cancer [9,10], *Shenling Baizhu San* in gastric cancer [11], and *Buzhong Yiqi* decoction in colorectal and lung cancer [12,13]. The wide application and the distinctive therapeutic strategy of health-strengthening herbs have given rise to the growing research interests in the investigation on the effects and the underlying mechanisms of health-strengthening herbs in cancer treatment. A large amount of research effort has been put into the studies on the biological basis of health-strengthening TCM from a variety of perspectives, such as their immune and metabolic regulatory effects. For example, previous studies on various health strengthening formulae (e.g., *Shenqi Fuzheng* injection, *Danggui Buxue* decoction, *Huangqi Jianzhong* decoction, and *Liu-wei-di-huang* pill) revealed their protective effect on immune functions in cancer therapy [14–17]. Metabolic regulatory function is also involved in the antitumor effects of health-strengthening formulae, suggested by the pharmacological studies on the *Liu-wei-di-huang* pill, *Jianpi Yiqi* decoction, and *Yishen Gukang* decoction [17–19]. Considering the situation that more studies emphasize the immune regulatory effects of health strengthening herbs, in this study, we took the immunological effects of health strengthening herbs as an example to explore the commonness in their biological basis of in cancer treatment. Despite the great efforts in the research field, the understanding of the antitumor mechanism of health-strengthening medicine is not clear enough [20,21]. The solution is constrained by the following three interrelated factors: the complex composition of TCM, the lack of target information of TCM, and the complex biological system involved in cancer development. To further promote the application of TCM in the treatment of cancer, proposing a comprehensive analysis strategy for exploring the impact of TCM from a holistic point of view is urgently needed.

An increasing amount of evidence indicates that TCM may exert therapeutic effects by targeting a variety of biomolecules [22]. However, due to the complexity of the ingredients and the limitations in the application of experimental methods, the targets of many TCM compounds are still unclear [23]. It has been proposed that TCM formulae and herbs impact the network of targets in complex diseases, such as cancer [24–27], and researchers may investigate the systemic effects of drugs on biological networks. The systematic concept is consistent with the multitarget characteristic of TCM and makes it suitable for studying the complex mechanism of TCM [28,29]. The advent of the big data era, the continuous accumulation of omics data, and the progress of bioinformatics methods provide strong support for the development of network pharmacology [30]. As a core concept in network pharmacology, network targets have changed the current research mode of "single target" and provided a potential research strategy for analyzing the biological basis of TCM from the perspective of networks and guiding the discovery of new active ingredients in TCM [31].

The development of high-throughput transcriptional assay technologies provides researchers with a comprehensive viewpoint for exploring the effect of compounds on gene expression. High-throughput methods are an integral part of pharmacological studies and have led to many achievements in biomedical fields [32]. High-throughput experimental methods, together with other genomic technologies, enables a comprehensive and systematic approach to the biological basis of medicine. TCM is widely recognized as a holistic treatment to diseases [13] and the mechanisms of TCM in cancer treatment are still unclear. Hopefully, the development of high-throughput methods will shed light on deciphering the comprehensive mechanism of TCM in cancer treatment. Here, a unique high-throughput screening strategy by high-throughput sequencing, referred to as HTS^2 [33], was adopted for investigating the biological basis of 166 TCM compounds in cancer simultaneously. In the HTS^2 assay, we added the compound library to the cell line and obtained a large-scale and quantitative transcriptional profiling in cells by detecting the signals of the designed gene probes.

To approach the systematic mechanisms of TCM compounds for cancer treatment, we combined network pharmacology prediction methods with HTS^2 assay methods in our data analysis process. In this research, the Kyoto Encyclopedia of Genes and Genomes (KEGG) pathways involved in the antitumor or immunological activities of the TCM compounds are identified [34]. Taking advantage of the prediction and assay results, we conducted a systematic investigation on the antitumor mechanism of compounds in the two types of herbs (health-strengthening and pathogen-eliminating herbs), compounds in the same herb, and compounds that regulate the same pathway. Our study also revealed a potential bioactive compound, galloylpaeoniflorin, for cancer therapy, which may exhibit its efficacy via both regulating immune-related and antitumor pathways.

Together, by combining target prediction and high-throughput assay, this study proposed a systematic overview on the biological basis underlying the pharmacological effects of health strengthening herbs in cancer treatment. Despite the need for further investigation, it was indicated that health-strengthening herbs may provide researchers with a valuable candidate library for tumor immune regulatory and tumor preventive drug development.

2. Results

2.1. The Prediction and Examination of Potential Targets of by Literature Mining and the HTS^2 Assay

Due to the complex composition of TCM and the lack of corresponding target records, the potential target lists of TCM compounds were obtained by using a computational prediction method, drugCIPHER-CS [12]. Literature mining based on text searching was conducted to verify the reliability of the target prediction results. The co-occurrence of the compound and target appearing in one or more abstracts was used to define the association between them. For each investigated TCM compound, we searched the PubMed database by its name in the abstracts and counted the total item number of the search results. Since the numbers of the related reports of the different TCM compounds varied greatly, which would influence the following analysis results (e.g., the percentage of predicted targets verified by literature), we only selected the compounds with adequate related reports (total item number ranging from 500 to 1000) for the verification of target prediction results. All the related abstracts of the selected compounds were downloaded, and text-processing codes were programed for extracting the biomolecules mentioned in the abstracts. The results from literature mining were then verified via manual examination by deleting the false positive responses.

After literature mining, we obtained the biomolecules mentioned in the abstracts related to the compounds in Figure 1A. Additionally, the differentially expressed genes (DEGs) after treatment with these TCM compounds in the cell line were achieved using the HTS^2 assay. We examined whether a predicted target was directly or indirectly related with the biomolecules in the literature or DEGs in the HTS^2 assay. The indirect relationship was established if the predicted target was in the upstream in a KEGG pathway of the biomolecules in the abstracts or DEGs, or if they were related by protein–protein interaction (PPI) in the HPRD, BIND, IntAct, MINT, or OPHID database [35–39]. The cover rate demonstrated in Figure 1A stands for the percentage of the predicted targets supported by literature or the HTS^2 assay. The cover rate was calculated as $\frac{|\text{The predicted targets related to the reported targets (or DEGs)}|}{|\text{The predicted targets}|} \times$ 100%. The results (Figure 1A) indicated that the predicted target lists of TCM compounds for cancer basically covered 75%–90% of the biomolecules in the literature and had a relatively strong reliability. In addition, some potential targets were verified by the HTS^2 experimental results, which demonstrated that the HTS^2 assay may be an alternative method for exploring the novel biological functions of TCM compounds.

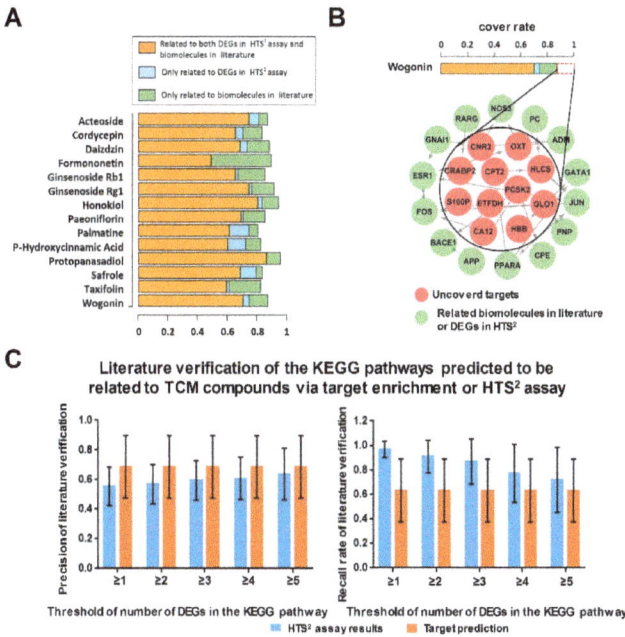

Figure 1. Evaluation of the target prediction results based on the literature and the HTS^2 assay results. (**A**) The ratio of the predicted targets of the TCM compounds covered by the literature and the assay results. The cover rate was calculated as $\frac{|\text{The predicted targets related to the reported targets (or DEGs)}|}{|\text{The predicted targets}|} \times 100\%$. (**B**) Some targets of wogonin, which were not related to biomolecules in the literature or the DEGs in the HTS^2 assay, were in the same pathway or connected via the protein–protein interaction (PPI) in STRING with the biomolecules in the literature or the DEGs in the HTS^2 assay for wogonin. (**C**) Literature verification of the KEGG pathways related to the TCM compounds for cancer treatment with target enrichment and HTS^2 evidence. Error bars represent the precision and recall rates of different TCM compounds. The precision was $\frac{|\text{The predicted relevant pathways related to the reported relevant pathways}|}{|\text{The predicted relevant pathways}|} \times$ 100%. The recall rate was $\frac{|\text{The predicted relevant pathways related to the reported relevant pathways}|}{|\text{The reported relevant pathways}|} \times 100\%$. Data represent mean $\pm$ SD.

In Figure 1A, we found that 87% of the predicted targets of wogonin, a representative compound from *Radix Scutellariae* (*Huang Qin*), were supported with literature or assay evidence. As for the other

13% of the potential targets of wogonin predicted by drugCIPHER-CS, some of them were connected to the biomolecules in the literature or the DEGs in the HTS^2 assay by an additional indirect mapping, as shown in Figure 1B. The indirect mapping in Figure 1B represented protein–protein interaction (PPI) in the STRING database [40] or relations via pathways in KEGG.

Next, to further analyze the mechanism of the action of the compounds, we performed KEGG pathway enrichment analysis based on the target prediction results. We checked the enrichment *p*-values of the targets in 26 cancer hallmarks (immune-excluded) and immune-related KEGG pathways. The literature verification of the pathways with HTS^2 or enrichment evidence was conducted manually by reading the papers in the PubMed database. If a significantly enriched pathway was related to the bioactivity records in the published papers in the PubMed database [41] or included enough DEGs (the cut-off value was set as between one to five DEGs and the robustness of the threshold was measured in Figure 1C) in the HTS^2 assay results, then it would be considered as a predicted related pathway with supports from literature records or HTS^2 assay results. As shown in Figure 1C, a series of cut-off values (from one to five DEGs in a pathway in the HTS^2 assay) was set to examine the robustness of the literature verification results. Our results indicated that the cut-off values had little influence on the precision rate for the related pathways determined using an HTS^2 assay, and the recall rate scaled from 97% to 72% as the cut-off changed. The precision and recall rate of the significantly enriched KEGG pathways ($p < 0.05$, false discovery rate (fdr) adjusted) were approximately 60% and 70%, respectively, which indicated the reliability of the pathway prediction results. By comprehensively considering both the precision and recall results, we selected the pathways with three or more DEGs in the HTS^2 assay as the ones with support from the assay data for further investigation.

2.2. Target Prediction and Assay Results Indicate that the Two Types of TCM Herbs May Regulate Several Key Biological Processes in Cancer Treatment, Including Antitumor and Immune Modulation

Historically, TCM encompasses a two-way philosophy in cancer treatment in that it is involved in both health strengthening and pathogen elimination. TCMs applied in curing cancer are classified as health-strengthening or pathogen-eliminating herbs according to their therapeutic effects. However, the biological functions of the two types of anti-cancer TCMs have not yet been elucidated. Therefore, we hoped to identify the regulated pathways of both types of TCM herbs by taking advantage of network pharmacology prediction and the HTS^2 assay. As shown in Figure 2A, 1446 compounds were selected for target prediction, including 655 compounds in health-strengthening herbs, 667 compounds in pathogen-eliminating herbs, and 124 compounds in both types of herbs. In Figure 2B, the structural similarities among the compounds were measured by applying a principle component analysis (PCA) method to the compound 2-D structure information from the ChEMBL database [42]. A total of 881-dimensional CADD Group Chemoinformatics Tools and User Services (CACTVS) substructures in PubChem [43] were adopted to encode the structures of the investigated TCM compounds into binary vectors. The PCA analysis was conducted by using the princomp function in the R packages stats v3.2.2 (RStudio, Boston, MA, USA) under the environment of RStudio v1.1.447 [44]. As demonstrated in Figure 2B, the compounds in health-strengthening and pathogen-eliminating herbs may contain similar substructures. This result was consistent with the fact that health-strengthening and pathogen-eliminating herbs contained multiple compounds with common herbal chemical types, such as saponins, flavonoids, and alkaloids. For further unveiling the structural basis of the two clouds of compounds in Figure 2B, we examined the 10 CACTVS substructures that contributed the most to the first and the second feature vectors in the PCA analysis. The selection of the feature vectors was consistent with the two dimensions depicted in Figure 2B. The contributions were determined by the absolute values of the coefficients of the first two feature vectors. C:CC=C, C=C-C:C, O-C-C:C, C:C-C:C, and O-C-C:C-C were the five strongest positive features, and ≥ 3 any ring size 6, ≥ 4 any ring size 6, C(-C)(-C)(-H)(-O), C(-C)(-H)(-O), and [#1]-C-O-[#1] were the five strongest negative features. Therefore, the left cloud of compounds was more likely to contain the substructures among the negative features and the right cloud of compounds was more likely to contain the substructures among the positive features in Figure 2B. As shown in Figure 2C, it was found that the average structure similarity score of the specific compounds in the two types of herbs was significantly higher than that between the TCM compounds and antineoplastic Western drugs ($p < 0.001$). The structure similarity analysis was conducted by calculating Tanimoto coefficients [45] between the 881-dimensional CACTVS substructures of the compounds.

Among the 1446 TCM compounds applied in target prediction, 166 compounds were used in the HTS^2 assay, including 67 compounds in health-strengthening herbs, 66 compounds in pathogen-eliminating herbs, and 33 compounds in both types of herbs (Figure 2D). In the HTS^2 assay, approximately 3000 HCT116 colorectal cancer cells were seeded in each well of a 384-well plate for 24 h. Then the TCM compound library were added to the cells for 24 h to achieve a transcriptional profile after compounds treatment. Eight dimethyl sulfoxide (DMSO) replicates were also added in the wells as controls. After obtaining the gene probe reads, we performed gene expression normalization by using 18 stable genes in in colorectal cancer (GSE44076, GSE44861, GSE53295, and GSE53965 in the Gene Expression Omnibus (GEO) database [46]). The normalized expression of a gene was defined as the reads of the gene probe divided by the median number of the reads of 18 housekeeping genes. The fold change was calculated as the normalized gene expression after the drug treatment divided by the median number of normalized gene expression after the eight DMSO replicates treatment. For each TCM compound, genes with a fold change > 2 were considered DEGs.

To explore the inhibitory effects on proliferation in the different cell lines of compounds from health-strengthening and pathogen-eliminating herbs, we analyzed the half-maximal inhibitory concentration (IC50) and the half-maximal inhibitory concentration on cell growth (GI50) data of the TCM compounds collected from the ChEMBL database or literature. The median IC50 (or GI50) was calculated as the median number of all the human cell line specific experiments in ChEMBL and literature records after the TCM compound treatment. These two metrics were considered as the same and were merged in the analysis. Even though the compounds from pathogen-eliminating herbs exhibited the lower median IC50s (or GI50s) than compounds from health-strengthening herbs in Figure 2E, the results indicated that compounds in health-strengthening herbs might be anti-proliferative to tumor cells. The IC50 and GI50 data were also adopted as reference concentrations in the (3-(4,5-dimethylthiazol-2-yl)-5-(3-carboxymethoxyphenyl)-2-(4-sulfophenyl)-2H-tetrazolium (MTS) assay, a cell survival rate measurement assay, and these bioactivity data were then applied in setting the concentrations of the TCM compounds in the HTS^2 assay after the manual adjustment.

In Figure 2F, target prediction and HTS^2 assay suggested that some compounds may regulate immune and cancer hallmarks (immune-excluded) pathways simultaneously. As shown in Figure 2G, in the cell cycle pathway, the expression of the CDK4, CDK6, and CCND1 genes in the HTS^2 assay were reduced after treatment with several compounds in the two types of herbs, while the gene expressions in T cell receptor signaling pathways were upregulated after treatment with several TCM compounds from the two types of herbs. The percentage of the experimental compounds in health-strengthening herbs with predicted targets enriched in the immune-related pathways was significantly higher than that in pathogen eliminating herbs (e.g., 37.3% and 22.7%, respectively, in antigen processing and presentation, and 65.7% and 47.0%, respectively, in natural killer cell mediated cytotoxicity) (Fisher exact test, $p < 0.05$). In Table 1, the regulated pathways of several compounds from health-strengthening and pathogen-eliminating herbs predicted using target enrichment and the HTS^2 assay results were listed. These results indicated that TCM herbs, no matter their therapeutic classification, may exhibit therapeutic effects in cancer treatment via both immune regulation and other antitumor functions.

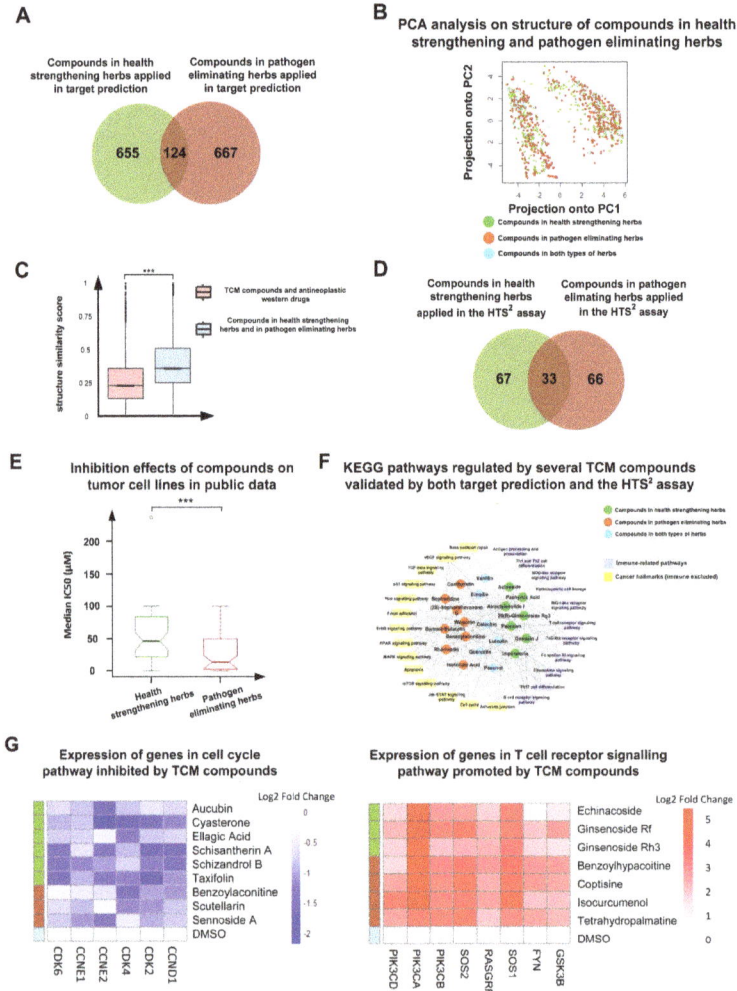

Figure 2. An overview of types of TCM applied in the research on their structures, inhibitory effects on tumor cells, and regulated bioactivities, based on public data, target prediction, and the HTS^2 assay. (**A**) The number of compounds in the two types of TCM herbs in cancer treatment applied in the target prediction. (**B**) PCA analysis on structure of compounds in the two types of herbs in cancer treatment. (**C**) The structure similarity comparison between the compounds from health-strengthening herbs and pathogen-eliminating herbs and that between the TCM compounds and antineoplastic Western drugs via Tanimoto coefficients. Data represent median ± interquartile range. Statistical analysis was performed using a Kolmogorov–Smirnov (KS) test. *** $p < 0.001$. (**D**) The number of compounds from the two types of TCM herbs applied in the HTS^2. (**E**) The inhibitory effects of compounds in the two types of herbs on proliferation of tumor cell lines in public bioactivity databases. Data represent median ± interquartile range. Statistical analysis was performed using a Wilcoxon rank sum test. *** $p < 0.001$. (**F**) The regulated immune and cancer hallmarks (immune-excluded) pathways of several TCM compounds supported using target prediction and the HTS^2 assay. (**G**) Expression data of several genes in the cell cycle and T cell receptor signaling pathways after TCM compound treatments.

Table 1. Several KEGG pathways predicted to be regulated by compounds from health-strengthening and pathogen-eliminating herbs using target enrichment and the HTS^2 assay.

KEGG Pathway	Herb Type	Herb	Compounds	Enrichment p-value	DEG Number
Apoptosis	Fu-Zheng	*Radix Angelicae sinensis* (*Shan Yao*)	Batatasin IV	2.1×10^{-4}	13
			Dioscin	1.1×10^{-2}	23
	Qu-Xie	*Rhizoma Curcumae* (*E Zhu*)	Curcumin	1.7×10^{-3}	11
			Isocurcumenol	1.7×10^{-3}	31
vascular endothelial growth factor (VEGF) signaling pathway	Fu-Zheng	*Fructus Schisandrae* (*Wu Wei Zi*)	Schisanhenol	3.2×10^{-3}	14
			Gomisin J	3.2×10^{-3}	7
	Qu-Xie	*Radix et Rhizoma Rhei* (*Da Huang*)	Chrysaron	2.3×10^{-6}	9
			Rhein	3.2×10^{-3}	5
Cell cycle	Fu-Zheng	*Fructus Ligustri lucidi* (*Nv Zhen Zi*)	Ligustroflavone	2.4×10^{-3}	4
			Specnuezhenide	1.5×10^{-3}	10
	Qu-Xie	*Cortex Moutan* (*Gan Chan Pi*)	Cinobufagin	1.5×10^{-3}	20
			Telocinobufagin	2.3×10^{-4}	26
T cell receptor signaling pathway	Fu-Zheng	*Poria* (*Fu Ling*)	Pachymic Acid	8.7×10^{-7}	5
			Poricoic Acid B	7.8×10^{-5}	8
	Qu-Xie	*Cortex Magnoliae officinali* (*Huang Qin*)	Baicalein	7.8×10^{-5}	18
			Wogonin	3.8×10^{-3}	15
Toll-like receptor signaling pathway	Fu-Zheng	*Radix Astragali* (*Huang Qi*)	Astragaloside A	4.1×10^{-3}	5
			Formononetin	4.1×10^{-3}	3
	Qu Xie	*Venenum Bufonis* (*Chan Su*)	Bufarenogin	4.1×10^{-3}	15
			Cinobufagin	4.1×10^{-3}	20
Nucleotide-binding oligomerization domain (NOD)-like receptor signaling pathway	Fu-Zheng	*Radix Ginseng* (*Ren Shen*)	Ginsenoside Rh3	4.9×10^{-5}	23
			Protopanaxadiol	4.9×10^{-5}	15
	Qu-Xie	*Fructus Bruceae* (*Ya Dan Zi*)	Bruceantin	1.6×10^{-3}	7
			Bruceine D	3.0×10^{-4}	14

2.3. HTS^2 Assay Results Show that Health-Strengthening Medicine May Regulate Tumor Immunity Via Promoting NK Cell Activity and Tumor Cell Antigen Presentation

NK cells recognize and kill tumor cells containing the mutated gene fragments [47]. In the tumor environment, the NK cell activity is inhibited by the biological function of the tumor cells [48]. In Figure 3A, some TCM compounds from health-strengthening herbs with the potential biological functions of promoting NK cell activity were listed at the top, as indicated by the HTS^2 assay results. For instance, ginsenoside Re, a compound in *Radix Ginseng (Ren Shen)*, was suggested to exert an NK cell activation effect by upregulating the expression of genes involved in degranulation and NK cell-related cytokines release.

Antigen processing and presentation plays an important role in tumor immunity [49]. In the tumor environment, the antigen presentation functions of tumor cells are relatively suppressed [50]. Therefore, the immune system may not fully recognize and kill tumor cells. The analysis of the HTS^2 assay results revealed that several health strengthening herbs may comprehensively increase the level of antigen presentation in tumor cells by promoting intracellular synthesis of main histocompatibility complex class I (MHC-I) molecules, improving antigen processing efficiency, and combining tumor cell biopeptides with MHC-I molecules (Figure 3B). For example, sinnamaldehyde, a compound in *Cortex Cinnamomi (Rou Gui)*, was indicated to upregulate antigen processing and MHC biosynthesis related genes, as shown in Figure 3B. Additionally, as demonstrated in Figure 3B, some compounds that may enhance the NK cell activities may also improve the levels of antigen processing and presentation in tumor cells.

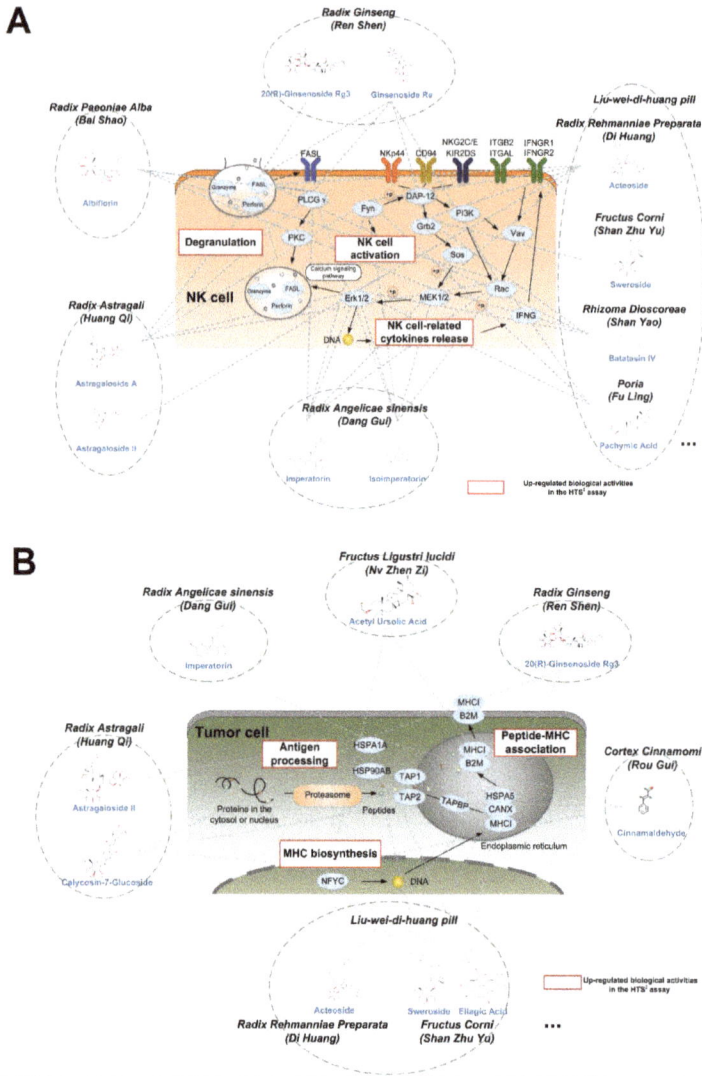

Figure 3. The regulatory effects on immune-related pathways induced by a group of compounds from health-strengthening herbs. The dotted lines linked the TCM compounds and the DEGs after compound treatment in the HTS[2] assay. (**A**) The HTS[2] assay results showed that compounds from health strengthening herbs upregulated the biomolecules in the NK cell mediated cytotoxic pathway. (**B**) The HTS[2] assay results showed that compounds from health strengthening herbs upregulated the biomolecules involved in the MHC-I antigen processing and presentation pathway.

2.4. Target Prediction and HTS[2] Assay Results Show that Compounds in the Same Herb May Exhibit Different Patterns in Modulating Antitumor or Immune Processes

To further identify how the combinations of the TCM compounds in the same herb may regulate the same biological process, we extracted the HTS[2] results of the TCM compounds that were predicted to regulate the same pathway. Next, we examined the expression data of the genes in the predicted regulated pathways. After the integration of the HTS[2] results from the TCM compounds and the gene information in the KEGG pathways, we concluded that the TCM compounds in the same herb may have interactions in several patterns in regulating the same KEGG pathway. As shown in Figure 4, the selected TCM compounds may regulate the same pathway in the same or opposite directions to induce the final effects, as indicated by the HTS^2 assay results. For instance, kaempferol and kaempferide are two compounds from the health-strengthening herb *Fructus Corni* (*Shan Zhu Yu*). After analyzing the HTS^2 assay results of kaempferol and kaempferide, we discovered that they have similar molecular patterns for inhibiting cell cycles, as shown in Figure 4B. Additionally, paeonol and galloylpaeoniflorin, two compounds in *Radix Paeoniae Alba* (*Bai shao*), were indicated to influence gene expression in the mitogen-activated protein kinase (MAPK) signaling pathway in the opposite directions (Figure 4C). These results suggested that compounds in the same herb may exhibit similar or distinguished mechanisms in cancer treatment. The compounds with different mechanisms may have the potential bioactivities in treating different types of tumors.

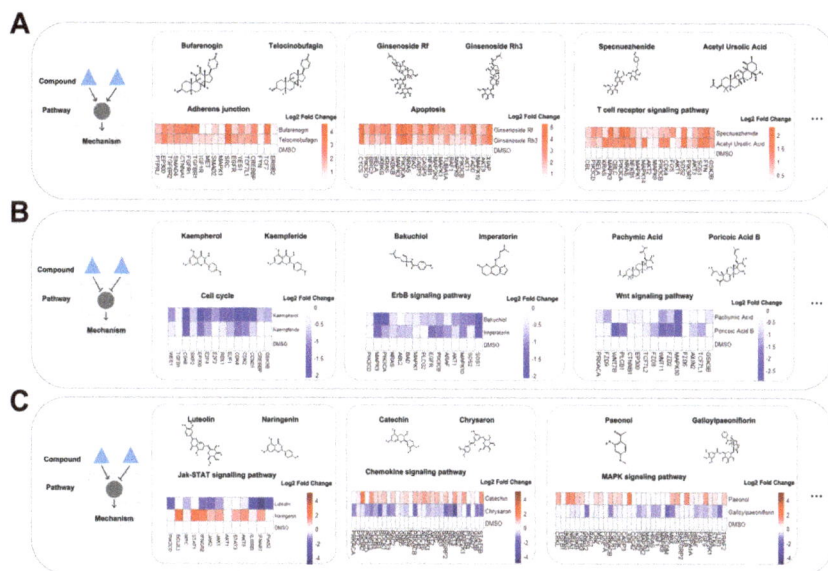

Figure 4. The HTS^2 assay results indicated that within the same pathway, compounds from the same herb may influence gene expression in the same cancer hallmarks (immune-excluded) or immune-related KEGG pathway in the same or opposite directions, as shown in the three boxes. (**A**) Compounds from the same herb may simultaneously upregulate the gene expression in the same pathway. (**B**) Compounds in the same herb may simultaneously downregulate the gene expression in the same pathway. (**C**) Compounds from the same herb may regulate the gene expression in the same pathway in opposite directions.

2.5. Prediction and Assay Results Imply that Compounds in One Health-Strengthening Herb or a Single Compound May Exert Antitumor and Immune-Related Functions Simultaneously for Cancer Therapy

Considering the multicompound characteristics of TCM herbs, it is necessary to examine the biological functions of different compounds from one herb in treating cancer. As we know, *Radix Paeoniae Alba* (*Bai Shao*) and *Radix Sophorae flavescentis* (*Ku Shen*) are two typical health-strengthening and pathogen-eliminating herbs that are widely used for cancer treatment [2]. After target prediction and KEGG pathway enrichment, we extracted the mRNA expression induced by the compounds from *Radix Paeoniae Alba* and *Radix Sophorae flavescentis* in the HTS^2 assay. The target enrichment results of the pathways with the assay evidence are shown in Figures 5 and 5. T cell receptor signaling pathway, B cell receptor signaling pathway, Th17 cell differentiation, MAPK signaling pathway, mTOR signaling pathway, and some other pathways were regulated by several compounds from *Radix Paeoniae Alba*, including 1,2,3,4,6-pentagalloylglucose, albiflorin, coumarin, galloylpaeoniflorin, paeoniflorin, and paeonol (Figure 5A). The target enrichment and HTS^2 assay results suggested that all the compounds in Figure 5A might regulate both immune-related and other antitumor pathways. The similar pattern was found in the target enrichment results of the compounds from *Radix Sophorae flavescentis*. As shown in Figure 5B, nine compounds from *Radix Sophorae flavescentis* were selected for the HTS^2 assay, and all of them may influence at least one immune-related pathway and one other antitumor pathway.

One of the compounds from *Radix Paeoniae Alba*, galloylpaeoniflorin, had no relevant antitumor records or any other biological activity records. The target prediction and HTS^2 assay results indicated that galloylpaeoniflorin might regulate several immune-related pathways (i.e., T cell receptor signaling pathway, Th17 cell differentiation, and B cell receptor signaling pathway), and cancer hallmarks pathways (i.e., MAPK signaling pathway, cell cycle, and mTOR signaling pathway) (Figure 5C). For instance, the relative expression of genes in the cell cycle in the HTS^2 assay was shown in the right part of Figure 5C, and the expression of the biomolecules listed in the subnetwork were reduced by galloylpaeoniflorin. Moreover, we examined the antitumor effects of galloylpaeoniflorin both in vitro and in vivo (Figure 5D,E). As shown in Figure 5D, galloylpaeoniflorin effectively inhibited the proliferation of several cell lines (IC50 < 40µg/mL), including HCT116 (a colorectal cancer cell line), B16F10 (a melanoma cell line), MCF-7 (a breast cancer cell line), and NCI-H460 (a lung cancer cell line) cells. Different solvents were applied (DMSO and ethanol) in the top and the bottom of Figure 5D and the results demonstrated robust inhibitory effects on the tumor cell lines induced by galloylpaeoniflorin. The in vitro inhibitory effects of galloylpaeoniflorin in Figure 5D on not only the HTC116 cells, which was adopted in the HTS^2 assay, but also several cell lines of varied cancer types indicated its antineoplastic potentials in treating different tumors. The experiment in Figure 5D was done once in triplicate. Our in vivo results confirmed that the tumor weight of the H22 liver tumor mice was significantly reduced after the treatment with galloylpaeoniflorin (Figure 5E). Twenty-one BALB/c/nu nude female mice injected with H22 tumor were utilized for the in vivo assay.

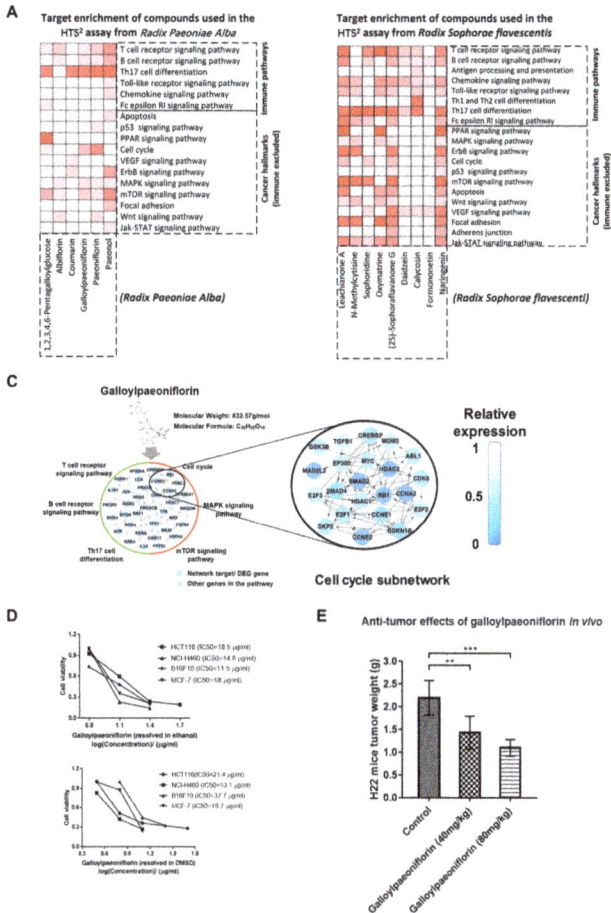

Figure 5. Identification of the immune regulatory and other antitumor biological functions of compounds from *Radix Paeoniae Alba* (*Bai Shao*) and *Radix Sophorae flavescentis* (*Ku Shen*). (**A,B**) The comprehensive functional characterization of the compounds in *Radix Paeoniae Alba* (A) or *Radix Sophorae flavescentis* (B) using the pathway enrichment analysis based on target prediction results. The white blanks represent pathways not regulated by the compounds according to HTS^2 assay results. (**C**) The pathway regulation effects of galloylpaeoniflorin, a compound in *Radix Paeoniae Alba* (*Bai Shao*) using the target enrichment and HTS^2 assay. A subnetwork representing the expression of the predicted targets of galloylpaeoniflorin in the cell cycle pathway was shown. (**D**) Inhibitory effects of galloylpaeoniflorin on tumor cell proliferation using the cell lines of several tumor types, as assessed using an MTT assay. The experiment was done once in triplicate. (**E**) Inhibitory effects of galloylpaeoniflorin on tumor growth in H22 mice. The assay was performed on seven BALB/c/nu nude female mice injected with the H22 tumor for each group. ** $p < 0.01$, *** $p < 0.001$, compared with the solvent control group. Statistical analysis was performed using multiple t tests. Data represent mean $\pm$ SD.

3. Discussion

Health-strengthening medicine is seen as a representative application of the classical philosophy of TCM in cancer therapy. It is reported that, unlike Western medicine, which may exhibit direct killing effects on tumor cells, health-strengthening medicine is developed to treat cancer by systematically regulating the tumor microenvironment [51–54]. According to the traditional efficacy of TCM, health-strengthening herbs can be classified into different categories, such as yin-nourishing (*Zi-Yin*) herbs and qi-tonifying (*Yi-Qi*) herbs. In this research, as a first step, we treated health-strengthening herbs as a whole rather than the subcategories for the following network pharmacological analysis. Several biological processes may be involved in the regulatory effects of health-strengthening medicine, including some immune-related bioactivities. This finding is in accord with the previous studies on the comprehensive anti-tumor mechanisms of nuciferine, a compound from a yin-nourishing health-strengthening herb, *Nelumbo nucifera Gaertn* (*He Ye*) [55]. Additionally, some classical TCM formulae with the health-strengthening efficacy are clinically proven to enhance the innate immunological function (e.g., the killing abilities of NK cells) and the sensitivity of immune system to tumor cells [56,57]. These results were consistent with our findings that health-strengthening medicine might regulate the immune function in multiple aspects, including NK-cell-mediated cytotoxicity and antigen processing and presentation. However, the biological activities of health strengthening medicine have not been fully elucidated.

Here, based on the target prediction and the HTS^2 assay results, we analyzed the potential bioactivities of compounds from health-strengthening herbs. Several pathogen-eliminating herbs were also included in the research paradigm for comparison. Our prediction and assay results suggested that compounds from both types of TCMs may regulate both immune and cancer hallmarks (immune-excluded) pathways. This finding was consistent with the multitarget characteristic of TCM compounds. We further investigated the differences between these two types of TCMs and discovered that the overall inhibitory effects of the compounds in pathogen-eliminating herbs on tumor cells were significantly stronger than those in health-strengthening herbs. The results were consistent with the traditional understanding that pathogen-eliminating herbs tend to target the tumor directly. However, the traditional therapeutic advantages of health-strengthening herbs on the immune system need to be further explored by adopting immunological experimental results, and our high-throughput assay was conducted on tumor cells. Additionally, we revealed a group of compounds from the same herb that influences pathway gene expression in the same or different directions. The compounds with opposite influences on pathway gene expression may be explained by the different underlying mechanisms in cancer treatment. Therefore, it was suggested that they may be applied for treating different types of tumors.

In addition, galloylpaeoniflorin, a compound from a health-strengthening herb *Radix Paeoniae Alba* (*Bai Shao*) was predicted to impact several pathways that are significant in tumor development, including T cell receptor signaling pathway, B cell receptor signaling pathway, cell cycle, and mTOR signaling pathway. The regulatory effects were further supported by the HTS^2 gene expression profile of the related genes in the pathways after the treatment with galloylpaeoniflorin. In fact, the antitumor effects of *Radix Paeoniae Alba* and its total glucosides were found in recent research, and the mechanism may be related to the inhibitory effects on the cell cycle of tumor cells [58,59]. Notably, to the best of our knowledge, there is no activity record of galloylpaeoniflorin. Therefore, we examined and initially validated the antitumor effects of galloylpaeoniflorin both in vitro and in vivo. More work should be conducted for further evaluating the antitumor ability as well as unveiling the potential mechanism of galloylpaeoniflorin.

In this work, we divided cancer-related pathways into two categories: immune pathways and other cancer hallmarks for separate investigations. The distinction was made for the following reason: in the aspect of clinical treatment, immunotherapy and other approaches (e.g., targeted approaches and cytotoxic agents) are distinguished treatment options available in cancer treatment [60]. That was because the mechanisms that cancer immunotherapy are based on differ greatly from those of other approaches in cancer therapy [61]. Even though immune evasion is one of cancer's hallmarks, it characterizes the responses using the immune system [62]. Also, this distinction was consistent with the Anatomical Therapeutic Chemical (ATC) drug classification, a drug classification system based on pharmacological and anatomical properties by WHO, in which antineoplastic (L01) and immunomodulating (L03 and L04) agents are independent drug catalogues [63].

To be mentioned, previous studies indicated that health-strengthening herbs may exert their therapeutic effects in cancer treatment in multiple aspects (e.g., immunity and metabolism) [14–19]. In this study, the immunological efficacy was selected as an example and more work is needed for a comprehensive understanding of their efficacy in other aspects, such as the metabolic regulation effects. Moreover, TCM syndrome (Zheng) is an essential concept in the TCM theory [64]. It is reported that TCM syndromes correlates with treatment response to TCM in cancer therapy [65]. Therefore, future studies on the therapeutic effects of health strengthening herbs cancers with different TCM syndromes would further promote the understanding of the biological basis of health-strengthening herbs.

According to the analysis results in this study, health-strengthening herbs may exhibit both immune-regulatory and antitumor effects. Taking into consideration the generally weaker antitumor effects (IC50 or GI50) in vitro of compounds in health strengthening herbs than that in pathogen-eliminating herbs in public records, the high percentage of selected compounds in health-strengthening herbs related to immune-related pathways, and the good safety of health-strengthening herbs, it was indicated that health-strengthening herbs may have more pharmacological potential in preventing tumors and improving a tumor-immune microenvironment, compared to directly killing tumor cells.

In contrast to previous studies, our study features the usage of high-throughput computational and experimental methods for a more comprehensive understanding of underlying mechanism of health-strengthening herbs. HTS^2 may significantly promote the parallel processing of candidate compounds and genes, and has been applied in drug screening [66]. However, this study only provided in vitro large-scale experimental results of the HTS^2 assay on one cell line, HCT116, and it does not represent cells of the immune system. Therefore, most of the results in this manuscript are hypothesis-generating and more experimental studies are needed to further explore the bioactivities regulated by TCM compounds. Still, the research strategy in this study does provided avenues for large-scale experimentation. Hopefully, our study may help reveal the biological basis of health-strengthening herbs, a characteristic herb type which has been used for a long period by TCM practitioners, and shed light on the future researches on anti-tumor drugs by unveiling the wisdom of TCM.

4. Materials and Methods

4.1. TCM Compounds Data Preparation

We collected compound information of 47 TCM herbs (including 22 health-strengthening herbs and 25 pathogen-eliminating herbs for comparison) that are widely used in cancer therapy from the Chinese national medical insurance catalogue and commonly used prescriptions (e.g., Liu-wei-di-huang pill, *Buzhong Yiqi* decoction, and *Sijunzi* decoction) (Supplementary Table S1). The 22 health-strengthening herbs include different categories, such as yin-nourishing (*Zi-Yin*) herbs and qi-tonifying (*Yi-Qi*) herbs, and the 25 pathogen-eliminating herbs include categories, such as heat clearing and detoxifying (*Qing-Re-Jie-Du*) herbs, and blood activating and stasis dissolving (*Huo-Xue-Hua-Yu*) herbs, according to the traditional classification based on TCM efficacy. Together, 1446 TCM compounds with PubChem records were collected, including 655 compounds from health-strengthening herbs, 667 compounds from pathogen-eliminating herbs, and 124 compounds from both types of herbs.

4.2. Analysis Workflow Based on Network Pharmacology

In this study, we proposed an approach based on network pharmacology to study the antitumor mechanisms of health-strengthening medicine. The network pharmacology approach was applied for predicting the potential targets of the TCM compounds and to visualize the analysis results as networks in this manuscript. After the TCM compounds data preparation, we predicted the potential targets of the TCM compounds by utilizing an algorithm based on the correlation between the pharmacological network and genomic network. The prediction results were analyzed via literature mining, the HTS^2 assay, public assay data, and in vitro and in vivo experiments. Taking advantage of the prediction and analysis results, we analyzed the molecular functional patterns of health-strengthening herbs (Figure 6).

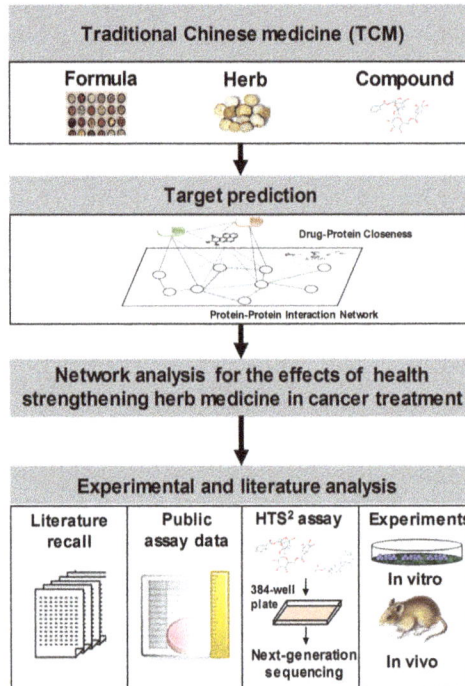

Figure 6. The network analysis workflow for understanding the effects of health-strengthening medicine compounds in cancer treatment.

4.3. Literature Mining

The literature mining was performed via text searching and no algorithm was applied in the process. By literature mining, we aimed to obtain the related biomolecules for each TCM compound and to compare the results with the predicted targets. The co-occurrence of compound and target appearing in one or more abstracts was used to define the association of them.

We searched the PubMed database using the name of each TCM compound in the abstracts and recorded the number of returned search results. In this study, we selected the compounds with an adequate number of search results (between 500 to 1000) for further analysis. The interval was necessary because the number of the related literature varied greatly, and this would have impacts on the following analysis (e.g., the percentage of predicted targets verified by literature records). All the related abstracts of the selected compounds were downloaded, and text-processing codes were programed for extracting the biomolecules mentioned in the abstracts. If a biomolecule co-occurred in the abstract with the compound name, then we considered that the biomolecule was related to the compound.

The results from the literature mining were then verified via a manual examination by deleting the false positive responses. Then, the results were used as the verification set for target prediction and HTS[2] assay results.

4.4. Target Prediction for the TCM Compounds Applied in Cancer Treatment

The potential targets of the TCM compounds were predicted by drugCIPHER-CS [24] using Matlab 2016a (MathWorks, Natick, MA, USA) [67], a network-based target prediction method. Using a liner regression model, this method correlates pharmacological and genomic spaces for predicting the drug targets. In this method, the likelihood of a candidate compound targeting a specific protein can be described as a concordance score between the structural similarity vector of the candidate compound and drugs in DrugBank [68] and the drug-protein closeness vector based on PPI. According the article on drugCIPHER-CS, the accuracy of target prediction is 77.3% when the top 100 biomolecules were chosen to form a potential target profile, as measured using cross-validation. Therefore, in this study, the top 100 biomolecules in the prediction result list were selected as the potential target list of each TCM compound. The PPI network was constructed by combining the PPI information recorded in HPRD, BIND, IntAct, MINT, and OPHID in May 2011 [35–39], and it contained 137,037 PPIs for 13,388 human proteins. Drug–protein interactions were retrieved from DrugBank associated to the PubChem database in May 2015 [43]. Drug structural similarity vectors were the Tanimoto coefficients [45] based on 881-dimensional CACTVS substructures in PubChem.

Moreover, to measure the reliability of target prediction results, biomolecules mentioned in the literature and DEGs in HTS[2] results were collected. If a predicted target is directly or indirectly related to a biomolecule which co-occurred with the compound in the literature or to a DEG in the HTS[2] assay after treatment with the compound, it is considered to be supported by the literature mining and HTS[2] assay. The indirect relationship was established if the predicted target in in the upstream in a KEGG pathway of the biomolecules in the abstracts or DEGs, or if they are related via PPI. The cover rate was calculated as $\frac{|\text{The predicted targets related to the reported targets (or DEGs)}|}{|\text{The predicted targets}|} \times 100\%$.

4.5. KEGG Pathway Enrichment Analysis

We performed the KEGG pathway enrichment analysis for the predicted targets of the TCM compounds applied in cancer therapy in order to identify their biological functions. We used a hypergeometric test for enrichment analysis. We performed target enrichment under the background of 13388 human proteins and checked the p-values of the pathways to see if they were significantly enriched. The enrichment p-values of 26 pathways from cancer hallmarks and immune-related pathways in the KEGG database were examined. The enrichment analysis was performed using RStudio v1.1.447 and an open source programming language, Ruby 2.3.0. The significantly enriched KEGG pathways ($p < 0.05$, fdr adjusted) were retained for further research.

4.6. Chemical Space Analysis

CACTVS substructures in PubChem were adopted in the chemical space analysis. In the analysis, we used 881-dimensional substructure binary vectors to encode the investigated TCM compounds. A PCA analysis was conducted using the princomp function in the R packages stats v3.2.2 under the environment of RStudio v1.1.447 [44]. The Tanimoto coefficients of the binary vectors of the TCM compounds in the two types of herbs and antineoplastic Western drugs were calculated.

4.7. Network Visualization

Network visualization was performed using Cytoscape v3.6.0 (National Resource for Network Biology, Bethesda, MD, USA) [69]. For visualization, the KEGG, HPRD, BIND, IntAct, MINT, and OPHID databases were used for providing pathway and PPI information.

4.8. Cell Culture

HCT116 (a colorectal cancer cell line), B16F10 (a melanoma cell line), MCF-7 (a breast cancer cell line), and NCI-H460 (a lung cancer cell line) cells were obtained from the cell center of Chinese Academy of Medical Sciences and Peking Union Medical College (CAMS and PUMC). The cells were cultured in an incubator with 5% CO_2 at 37 °C. Dulbecco's modified eagle medium (DMEM) containing 10% fetal bovine serum, 100 U/mL penicillin and 100 g/mL streptomycin were applied for the incubation.

4.9. The HTS² Assay

The HTS² assay is a high-throughput screening strategy that enables a large-scale and quantitative analysis of gene transcriptional profiles in cells [33]. In the HTS² assay, approximately 3000 HCT116 colorectal cancer cells were seeded in each well of a 384-well plate for 24 h. After that, the TCM compounds library was added to the cells for another 24 h, including eight DMSO replicates as negative controls. The HTS² assay was then conducted to obtain the transcriptional profiles of the designed gene probes. The cells were lysed in GentLys buffer (Nanopure, Beijing, China). The instrumentation of the HTS² assay was an automated liquid handling system, which contained the Agilent Bravo automated liquid handling platform (Agilent, Santa Clara, CA, USA) and the Agilent bench robot (Agilent, Santa Clara, CA, USA). By RNA annealing, selection and ligation, the instrumentation automatically performed the HTS² assay. Pooled pairs of oligonucleotides targeting selected gene probes by streptavidin-magnetic beads and the biotinylated oligo-dT were used. Then, the paired oligonucleotides were ligated using T4 DNA ligase and were amplified using Polymerase Chain Reaction (PCR). Using unique bar-coded primer in Illumina flowcells, the HTS² assay allowed a high-throughput transcriptional profiling of up to 1400 genes from 2000 samples.

4.9.1. Selection and Preparation of the TCM Compounds for HTS²

The selection of the TCM compounds for the HTS² assay were performed considering their recorded biological activity data and the offer lists provided by the suppliers. The bioactivity data (IC50 and GI50) of the TCM compounds were collected from ChEMBL or via manual literature searching. The median IC50 and GI50 of a compound were achieved via calculating the median number in all human cell line specific experiments in ChEMBL and literature records. The two metrics, IC50 and GI50 were used as the same metrics in the analysis. Then, we chose the compounds with an adequate antitumor activity (median IC50 or GI50 < 100 μM) as candidate compounds for the HTS² assay. The candidate compounds were further selected considering the product availability of the suppliers.

The TCM compounds were dissolved in DMSO. The concentrations were preliminarily set as the median IC50 and were adjusted afterwards based on the cell survival rate using MTS assay for the HCT116 cells to meet the standard for the HTS² assay (cell survival rate > 70%). Detailed information about the compounds applied in the HTS² assay (e.g., PubChem Compound Identifier (CID), supplier, and purity) was presented in Table S2.

4.9.2. The Gene Selection and Probe Design of the HTS² Assay

A total of 420 genes were selected to form a gene set for the HTS² assay. The gene set contained immune-related and other antitumor-related genes. The selection of the 420 genes were achieved in three steps. First, the genes were selected from databases and by predictions to form a cancer-related gene lists, including genes in pathways in cancer (hsa05200) in KEGG, genes in colorectal cancer (hsa05210) in KEGG, the colorectal cancer related genes in OMIM (MIM Number: 114500) [70], the targets of antineoplastic drugs in DrugBank, and the colorectal cancer related genes predicted using CIPHER, a phenotype-gene network based algorithm [71,72]. The reason why we selected some genes related to colorectal cancer was that the HCT116 cell line applied in the following HTS^2 assay was a colorectal cancer cell line.

Then, we referred to the public gene expression profiles in the GEO database for selecting a reliable set of genes with adequate expression levels. Here, we selected two profiles of samples from patients with colorectal cancer (GSE44076 and GSE44861) and two profiles of the HCT116 cell line (GSE53295 and GSE53965) for measuring the gene expression. A gene was selected if it had at least three of the above profiles in its expression data and if the expression ranked 10% to 60% in the detected gene set in at least one profile. Additionally, we selected 30 housekeeping genes that meet the following standards: (1) it was not in the cancer-related gene lists achieved in the first step; (2) the expression of the gene was detected in the four gene expression profiles (GSE44076, GSE44861, GSE53295, and GSE53965), and was not a DEG in any one of these profiles; and (3) the expression of the gene ranked 10% to 60% in the gene sets of at least one profile. The moderate ranking was to ensure that the gene expression was neither too high or too low, which may impair the credibility of the HTS^2 assay results.

At last, the probes for the genes were designed, and 420 genes with efficient probes, were selected for the HTS^2 assay, including 18 housekeeping genes. Sequences of 10 probes used in the HTS^2 assay were provided in Table S3.

4.9.3. HTS^2 Data Processing

First, the reads were mapped to the probe sequences, and three mismatches for each were permitted. The raw experimental data of HTS^2 assay after treatment with DMSO and several TCM compounds were provided in Table S4. The numbers in Table S4 were the reads of gene probes using the HTS^2 assay, which represent the abundance of genes. The HTS^2 data was normalized by the expression of 18 stable housekeeping genes. The normalized gene expression was computed with raw reads of the gene after the drug treatment and the median number of raw reads of 18 housekeeping genes after the drug treatment.

Second, to identify the DEGs for each TCM compound, we calculated the fold change of the tested genes as the normalized gene expression after the drug treatment divided by the median number of normalized gene expression after the eight DMSO replicates treatments. For each TCM compound, genes with fold change > 2 were considered DEGs.

Third, to evaluate the reliability of the transcriptional profile, we calculated the Pearson correlations among the normalized transcriptional data after treatment with the eight DMSO replicates. The results are demonstrated in Figure S1. The correlations ranged from 0.84 to 0.99, which indicated the reliability of the assay results.

4.10. Cell Viability Assay

For exploring the antitumor effects of galloylpaeoniflorin, we further performed an MTT cell viability assay on different tumor cells. The HCT116, B16F10, MCF-7, and NCI-H460 cell lines were seeded in a 96-well plate before the drug treatment. Various concentrations of galloylpaeoniflorin dissolved in DMSO and ethanol respectively were added to the cells after incubation for 24 h. To assess the IC50s of the cell lines, the MTT cell viability assay was conducted after incubation for another 120 h. The IC50s were achieved by fitting the dose-response curve. The MTT assay was done once in triplicate.

4.11. Animal Studies

Twenty-one six-weeks-old BALB/c/nu nude female mice obtained from the Vital River Laboratories (Vital River Laboratories, Beijing, China) and were used for the xenograft experiments. H22 cells were injected into the left flank of the mice. When the tumor volume reached the size of 100–250 mm^3, the mice were randomly separated into three groups and were administered an oral dose of galloylpaeoniflorin (40 mg/kg/day or 80 mg/kg/day) or vehicle control (1 × solution with cremophor EL/ethanol/water (12.5:12.5:75)). The mice were sacrificed at the end of the treatment period. The tumor volume was measured and weighted for the analysis.

The animal experiments were conducted in accordance with the guidelines for the care and use of laboratory animals. The work was approved by the Animal Care Committee of Chinese Academy of Medical Sciences and Peking Union Medical Colleges (Beijing, China) (Permit Number: SYXK 2015-0025).

4.12. Statistical Analysis

Data are shown as the means $\pm$ standard deviation (SD) (Figures 1 and 5) and median $\pm$ interquartile range (Figures 2 and 2). Multiple types of data were used in the manuscript and various statistical analysis methods were applied. Statistical analysis was performed using Kolmogorov-Smirnov (KS) test in Figure 2C, Wilcoxon rank sum test in Figure 2E and Student *t*-tests in Figure 5E. The significance levels were set at * $p < 0.05$, ** $p < 0.01$, and *** $p < 0.001$.

5. Conclusions

In conclusion, in this study, we performed a network-based analysis of health-strengthening medicine by integrating a series of methods, including target prediction, literature mining, the HTS^2 experiment, and some low-throughput assays. The expression levels of 420 genes, associated with tumor growth and immune functions, were detected after a parallel treatment of 166 TCM compounds. By combining evidence from different sources, we helped further uncover the biological basis of health-strengthening medicine. We concluded that health-strengthening herbs, might regulate both immune-related and antitumor pathways, similar to pathogen-eliminating herbs. A typical case was demonstrated by *Radix Paeoniae Alba (Bai Shao)*, a health-strengthening herb widely used in TCM cancer treatment. Galloylpaeoniflorin, a compound from *Radix Paeoniae Alba*, was predicted to regulate several essential biological processes in cancer development, and its antitumor effect was preliminarily proven both in vivo and in vitro. Additionally, some TCM compounds in the same herb were indicated to regulate pathway gene expression with similar or different patterns, suggesting the urgent need for further in-depth studies on TCM prescriptions. For instance, acetyl ursolic acid and specnuezhenide, two compounds in a health strengthening herb *Fructus Ligustri lucidi (Nv Zhen Zi)*, both upregulated gene expressions in T cell signaling pathway in HTS^2 assay. In summary, this study provided a new research strategy for explaining the biological basis of health-strengthening herbs, and further suggested the tumor immune regulatory and tumor preventive potentials of health-strengthening herbs.

Supplementary Materials: The following are available online at http://www.mdpi.com/2072-6694/10/11/461/s1. Table S1: The basic information of the herbs applied in the research. Table S2: The resources of the compounds used in the HTS^2 assay. Table S3: Sequences of 10 probes used in the HTS^2 assay. Table S4: The raw experimental data of HTS^2 assay after treatment with DMSO or TCM compounds in Figures 3 and 4. The numbers are the reads of gene probes by HTS^2 assay, which represent the abundance of genes. Figure S1: Transcriptional profile correlations of the DMSO replicates.

Author Contributions: Conceptualization, S.L.; Methodology, J.Z., S.L., and D.W.; Software, J.Z. and X.W.; Validation, J.Z., M.W., Y.L., H.W., and S.L.; Formal Analysis, J.Z., M.W., and X.W.; Investigation, J.Z. and H.W.; Data Curation, J.Z and S.L.; Writing—Original Draft Preparation, J.Z.; Writing—Review and Editing, S.L. and D.W.; Visualization, J.Z and X.W.; Supervision, S.L.; Project Administration, S.L. and D.W.; Funding Acquisition, S.L.

Funding: This study was supported by the National Natural Science Foundation of China (81630103, 91729301, and 81225025) and the Project of Tsinghua-Fuzhou Institute for Data Technology (TFIDT2018001).

Acknowledgments: Not applicable.

Conflicts of Interest: The authors declare no conflict of interest.

References

1. Liu, J.; Wang, S.; Zhang, Y.; Fan, H.T.; Lin, H.S. Traditional Chinese medicine and cancer: History, present situation, and development. *Thorac. Cancer* **2015**, *6*, 561–569. [CrossRef] [PubMed]

2. Min, W.; Peng, L.; Shi, L.; Li, S. Traditional Chinese patent medicines for cancer treatment in China: A nationwide medical insurance data analysis. *Oncotarget* **2015**, *6*, 38283–38295.

3. Qi, F.; Zhao, L.; Zhou, A.; Zhang, B.; Li, A.; Wang, Z.; Han, J. The advantages of using traditional Chinese medicine as an adjunctive therapy in the whole course of cancer treatment instead of only terminal stage of cancer. *Biosci. Trends* **2015**, *9*, 16–34. [CrossRef] [PubMed]

4. Chien, T.J.; Liu, C.Y.; Lu, R.H.; Kuo, C.W.; Lin, Y.C.; Hsu, C.H. Therapeutic efficacy of Traditional Chinese medicine, "Kuan-Sin-Yin", in patients undergoing chemotherapy for advanced colon cancer—A controlled trial. *Complement. Ther. Med.* **2016**, *29*, 204–212. [CrossRef] [PubMed]

5. Parekh, H.S.; Liu, G.; Wei, M.Q. A new dawn for the use of traditional Chinese medicine in cancer therapy. *Mol. Cancer* **2009**, *8*, 21. [CrossRef] [PubMed]

6. Wang, C.Y.; Bai, X.Y.; Wang, C.H. Traditional Chinese medicine: A treasured natural resource of anticancer drug research and development. *Am. J. Chin. Med.* **2014**, *42*, 543–559. [CrossRef] [PubMed]

7. Ministry of Human Resources and Social Security of the People's Republic of China. *China's National Basic Medical Insurance, Work Injury Insurance and Maternity Insurance Drugs Catalog*; (2017 Edition); China Labour and Social Security Publishing House: Beijing, China, 2017.

8. Xiao, H.; Yang, J. Immune Enhancing Effect of Modified Sijunzi Decoction on Patients with Colorectal Cancer Undergoing Chemotherapy. *Chin. J. Integr. Tradit. West. Med.* **2011**, *31*, 164–167.

9. Zhang, Y.; Guo, L.L.; Zhao, S.P. Effect of Shenqi Fuzheng Injection combined with chemotherapy in treating colorectal cancer. *Zhongguo Zhong XI Yi Jie He Za Zhi* **2010**, *30*, 280–282. [PubMed]

10. Chen, Y.; Gan, L.; Zheng, W.; Wang, C.H.; Cheng, D.H. Effect of Shenqi Fuzheng Injection Combined with Chemotherapy in Treating Cancer Breast Cancer. *Clin. J. Tradit. Chin. Med.* **2016**, *08*, 1120–1122.

11. Zhang, H.; Zhi-Xin, S.U. Curative effect of Shenling Baizhu powder on chemotherapy-induced toxicity in advanced gastric cancer. *J. Tradit. Chin. Med. Univ. Hunan* **2008**. [CrossRef]

12. Zhang, C.; Yang, W.J. Clinical Observation the Recurrence of Colon Cancer after Treating with BuZhong YiQiTang Combined with Chemotherapy. *West. J. Trad. Chin. Med.* **2011**, *24*, 73–74. [CrossRef]

13. Hu, Q.; Wang, H. Buzhong Yiqi Decoction Relieve Toxic and Adverse Reactions of Advanced Lung Cancer Taking Chemotherapy. *J. Zhejiang Univ. Tradit. Chin. Med.* **2008**, *32*, 220–221.

14. Zhu, X.; Chen, Y.; Zhong, X.; Zhang, X.Z.; Liu, J.H.; He, M. The protective effect of Shenqi Fuzheng Injection on immune function of BALB/c mice after chemo—therapy. *Chin. J. Immunol.* **2006**, *22*, 925–928.

15. Fan, Y.; Dechuan, L.I.; Xinya, X.U. Study on Effect of Danggui Buxue Decoction Combined with Chemotherapy for Advanced Colorectal Cancer Patients with Immune Function. *Chin. Arch. Tradit. Chin. Med.* **2013**. [CrossRef]

16. Bao, S.Z.; Zhang, A.Q.; Sun, Z.D. Effect of Huangqijianzhong Decoction on Immune Function and Cyclin D1 Gene Expression in Mice with Lung Cancer of Spleen Qi Deficiency Syndrome. *J. Emerg. Tradit. Chin. Med.* **2012**, *7*, 032.

17. Liang, X.; Li, H.; Li, S. A novel network pharmacology approach to analyse traditional herbal formulae: The Liu-Wei-Di-Huang pill as a case study. *Mol. BioSyst.* **2014**, *10*, 1014–1022. [CrossRef] [PubMed]

18. Zhuo, S.Y.; Fang, Z.Q.; Guan, D.Y.; Wu, Z.H.; Gao, B.F. Study on the Mechanism of JianpiYiqi Decoction Regulating DEN- induced Hepatocarcinogenesis in Rats by Bioinformatic Analysis. *Lishizhen Med. Mater. Med. Res.* **2014**, *25*, 1765–1768.

19. Yin, Y.; Feng, L.; Zhou, L.; Li, J.; Gao, Y.; Wang, N.J.; Yu, J.H.; Jiang, Z.L.; He, S.Q.; Lu, D.R.; et al. Effects of Yishengukang decoction on expression of bone-specific alkaline phosphatase, carboxyterminal propeptide of type I. procollagen, and carboxyterminal cross-linked telepeptide of type collagen in malignant tumor patients with bone metastasis. *West. J. Trad. Chin. Med.* **2017**, *37*, 30–34.

20. Hsiao, W.L.; Liu, L. The role of traditional Chinese herbal medicines in cancer therapy—from TCM theory to mechanistic insights. *Plant. Med.* **2010**, *76*, 1118. [CrossRef] [PubMed]

21. Lao, Y.; Wang, X.; Xu, N.; Zhang, H.M.; Xu, H.X. Application of proteomics to determine the mechanism of action of traditional Chinese medicine remedies. *J. Ethnopharmacol.* **2014**, *155*, 1–8. [CrossRef] [PubMed]

22. Hao, D.C.; Xiao, P.G. Network pharmacology: A Rosetta Stone for traditional Chinese medicine. *Drug Dev. Res.* **2014**, *75*, 299. [CrossRef] [PubMed]

23. Zhao, M.; Zhou, Q.; Ma, W.; Wei, D.Q. Exploring the Ligand-Protein Networks in Traditional Chinese Medicine: Current Databases, Methods, and Applications. *Evid. Based Complement. Altern. Med.* **2013**, *2013*, 227–257. [CrossRef] [PubMed]

24. Zhao, S.; Li, S. Network-Based Relating Pharmacological and Genomic Spaces for Drug Target Identification. *PLoS ONE* **2010**, *5*, e11764. [CrossRef] [PubMed]

25. Li, S.; Zhang, B. Traditional Chinese medicine network pharmacology: Theory, methodology and application. *Chin. J. Nat. Med.* **2013**, *11*, 110. [CrossRef] [PubMed]

26. Guo, Y.; Nie, Q.; MacLean, A.; Li, Y.; Lei, J.; Li, S. Multiscale modeling of inflammation-induced tumorigenesis reveals competing oncogenic and onco-protective roles for inflammation. *Cancer Research* **2017**, *77*, 6429–6441. [CrossRef] [PubMed]

27. Liang, X.; Li, H.; Tian, G.; Li, S. Dynamic microbe and molecule networks in a mouse model of colitis-associated colorectal cancer. *Sci. Rep.* **2014**, *4*, 4985. [CrossRef] [PubMed]

28. Li, R.; Ma, T.; Gu, J.; Liang, X.; Li, S. Imbalanced network biomarkers for traditional Chinese medicine Syndrome in gastritis patients. *Sci. Rep.* **2013**, *3*, 1543. [CrossRef] [PubMed]

29. Li, S. Mapping ancient remedies: Applying a network approach to traditional Chinese medicine. *Science* **2015**, *350*, S72–S74.

30. Hopkins, A.L. Network pharmacology:the next paradigm in drug discovery. *Nat. Chem. Biol.* **2008**, *4*, 682. [CrossRef] [PubMed]

31. Zhang, B.; Wang, X.; Li, Y.; Wu, M.; Wang, S.; Li, S. Matrine is identified as a novel macropinocytosis inducer by a network target approach. *Front. Pharmacol.* **2018**, *9*, 10. [CrossRef] [PubMed]

32. Macarron, R.; Banks, M.N.; Bojanic, D.; Burns, D.J.; Cirovic, D.A.; Garyantes, T.; Green, D.V.S.; Hertzberg, R.P.; Janzen, W.P.; Paslay, J.W.; et al. Impact of high-throughput screening in biomedical research. *Nat. Rev. Drug Discov.* **2011**, *10*, 188. [CrossRef] [PubMed]

33. Li, H.; Zhou, H.; Wang, D.; Qiu, J.S.; Zhou, Y.; Li, X.Q.; Rosenfeld, M.G.; Ding, S.; Fu, S.D. Versatile pathway-centric approach based on high-throughput sequencing to anticancer drug discovery. *Proc. Nat. Acad. Sci. USA* **2012**, *109*, 4609–4614. [CrossRef] [PubMed]

34. Kanehisa, M.; Furumichi, M.; Tanabe, M.; Sato, Y.; Morishima, K. KEGG: New perspectives on genomes pathways diseases drugs. *Nucleic Acids Res.* **2017**, *45*, D353–D361. [CrossRef] [PubMed]

35. Keshava Prasad, T.S.; Goel, R.; Kandasamy, K.; Keerthikumar, S.; Kumar, S.; Mathivanan, S.; Telikicherla, D.; Raju, R.; Shafreen, B.; Venugopal, A.; et al. Human Protein Reference Database—2009 update. *Nucleic Acids Res.* **2009**, *37*, 767–772. [CrossRef] [PubMed]

36. Bader, G.D.; Betel, D.; Hogue, C.W.V. BIND: The biomolecular interaction network database. *Nucleic Acids Res.* **2003**, *31*, 248–250. [CrossRef] [PubMed]

37. Kerrien, S.; Aranda, B.; Breuza, L.; Bridge, A.; Broackes-Carter, F.; Chen, C.; Duesbury, M.; Dumousseau, M.; Feuermann, M.; Hinz, U.; et al. The IntAct molecular interaction database in 2012. *Nucleic Acids Res.* **2011**, *40*, D841–D846. [CrossRef] [PubMed]

38. Licata, L.; Briganti, L.; Peluso, D.; Perfetto, L.; Iannuccelli, M.; Galeota, E.; Sacco, F.; Palma, A.; Nardozza, A.P.; Santonico, E.; et al. MINT, the molecular interaction database: 2012 update. *Nucleic Acids Res.* **2011**, *40*, D857–D861. [CrossRef] [PubMed]

39. Brown, K.R.; Jurisica, I. Online predicted human interaction database. *Bioinformatics* **2005**, *21*, 2076–2082. [CrossRef] [PubMed]

40. Szklarczyk, D.; Morris, J.H.; Cook, H.; Kuhn, M.; Wyder, S.; Simonovic, M.; Santos, A.; Doncheva, N.T.; Roth, A.; Bork, P.; et al. The STRING database in 2017: Quality-controlled protein–protein association networks made broadly accessible. *Nucleic Acids Res.* **2017**, *45*, D362–D368. [CrossRef] [PubMed]

41. Coordinators, N.R. Database resources of the national center for biotechnology information. *Nucleic Acids Res.* **2013**, *41*, D8. [CrossRef] [PubMed]

42. Gaulton, A.; Bellis, L.J.; Bento, A.P.; Chambers, J.; Davies, M.; Hersey, A.; Light, Y.; McGlinchey, S.; Michalovich, D.; Al-Lazikani, B.; Overington, J.P. ChEMBL: A large-scale bioactivity database for drug discovery. *Nucleic Acids Res.* **2011**, *40*, D1100–D1107. [CrossRef] [PubMed]

43. Kim, S.; Thiessen, P.A.; Bolton, E.E.; Chen, J.; Fu, G.; Gindulyte, A.; Han, L.; He, J.; He, S.; Shoemaker, B.A.; et al. PubChem Substance and Compound databases. *Nucleic Acids Res.* **2016**, *44*, D1202–D1213. [CrossRef] [PubMed]

44. Team, R.S. *RStudio: Integrated Development for R*; RStudio, Inc.: Boston, MA, USA, 2015; Volume 42. Available online: http://www.rstudio.com (accessed on April 2018).

45. Martin, E.J.; Blaney, J.M.; Siani, M.A.; Spellmeyer, D.C.; Wong, A.K.; Moos, W.H. Measuring diversity: Experimental design of combinatorial libraries for drug discovery. *J. Med. Chem.* **1995**, *38*, 1431–1436. [CrossRef] [PubMed]

46. Edgar, R.; Domrachev, M.; Lash, A.E. Gene Expression Omnibus: NCBI gene expression and hybridization array data repository. *Nucleic Acids Res.* **2002**, *30*, 207–210. [CrossRef] [PubMed]

47. Albertsson, P.A.; Basse, P.H.; Hokland, M.; Goldfarb, R.H.; Nagelkerke, J.F.; Nannmark, U.; Kuppen, P.J.K. NK cells and the tumour microenvironment: Implications for NK-cell function and anti-tumour activity. *Trends Immunol.* **2003**, *24*, 603–609. [CrossRef] [PubMed]

48. Vitale, M.; Cantoni, C.; Pietra, G.; Mingari, M.C.; Moretta, L. Effect of tumor cells and tumor microenvironment on NK-cell function. *Eur. J. Immunol.* **2014**, *44*, 1582–1592. [CrossRef] [PubMed]

49. Reeves, E.; James, E. Antigen processing and immune regulation in the response to tumours. *Immunology* **2016**, *150*, 16–24. [CrossRef] [PubMed]

50. Cerezo-Wallis, D.; Soengas, M. Understanding Tumor-Antigen Presentation in the New Era of Cancer Immunotherapy. *Curr. Pharm. Des.* **2016**, *22*, 6234–6250. [CrossRef] [PubMed]

51. Xu, J.; Song, Z.; Guo, Q.; Li, J. Synergistic Effect and Molecular Mechanisms of Traditional Chinese Medicine on Regulating Tumor Microenvironment and Cancer Cells. *BioMed Res. Int.* **2016**, *2016*, 1490738. [CrossRef] [PubMed]

52. Weber, D.A.; Wheat, J.M.; Currie, G.M. Cancer stem cells and the impact of Chinese herbs, isolates and other complementary medical botanicals: A review. *J. Chin. Integr. Med.* **2012**, *10*, 493–503. [CrossRef]

53. Fan, H.; Lin, H. Research Status of Fuzheng Herbs for Tumor Treating. *World Chin. Med.* **2014**, *9*, 825–832.

54. Xiong, L.; Tian, S.X. A concept of regulating tumor microenvironment immune and normalizing angiogenesis by Chinese medicine drug therapy for supporting zheng-qi to prop up root. *Chin. J. Integr. Tradit. West. Med.* **2010**, *30*, 201–204.

55. Qi, Q.; Li, R.; Li, H.; Cao, Y.; Bai, M.; Fan, X.; Wang, S.; Zhang, B.; Li, S. Identification of the anti-tumor activity and mechanisms of nuciferine through a network pharmacology approach. *Acta Pharmacol. Sin.* **2016**, *37*, 963–972. [CrossRef] [PubMed]

56. Wu, G.; Yu, G.; Li, J.; Xiong, F. Short term therapeutic effect on treatment of postoperational large intestine carcinoma by Fupiyiwei decoction combined with chemotherapy and it's effect on immune function. *China J. Chin. Mater. Med.* **2010**, *35*, 782–785.

57. Huang, Y.S.; Shi, Z.M. Intervention effect of Feiji Recipe on immune escape of lung cancer. *Chin. J. Integr. Tradit. West. Med.* **2007**, *27*, 501–504.

58. Madlener, S.; Illmer, C.; Horvath, Z.; Saiko, P.; Losert, A.; Herbacek, I.; Grusch, M.; Elford, H.L.; Krupitza, G.; Bernhaus, A.; et al. Gallic acid inhibits ribonucleotide reductase and cyclooxygenases in human HL-60 promyelocytic leukemia cells. *Cancer Lett.* **2007**, *245*, 156–162. [CrossRef] [PubMed]

59. Xu, H.Y.; Chen, Z.W.; Wu, Y.M. Antitumor activity of total paeony glycoside against human chronic myelocytic leukemia K562 cell lines in vitro and in vivo. *Med. Oncol.* **2012**, *29*, 1137–1147. [CrossRef] [PubMed]

60. Vanneman, M.; Dranoff, G. Combining immunotherapy and targeted therapies in cancer treatment. *Nat. Rev. Cancer* **2012**, *12*, 237. [CrossRef] [PubMed]

61. Gotwals, P.; Cameron, S.; Cipolletta, D.; Cremasco, V.; Crystal, A.; Hewes, B.; Mueller, B.; Quaratino, S.; Sabatos-Peyton, C.; Petruzzelli, L.; et al. Prospects for combining targeted and conventional cancer therapy with immunotherapy. *Nat. Rev. Cancer* **2017**, *17*, 286. [CrossRef] [PubMed]

62. Chen, D.S.; Mellman, I. Elements of cancer immunity and the cancer-immune set point. *Nature* **2017**, *541*, 321–330. [CrossRef] [PubMed]

63. Willett, P.; Winterman, V.; Bawden, D. Implementation of nearest-neighbor searching in an online chemical structure search system. *J. Chem. Inf. Comput. Sci.* **1986**, *26*, 36–41. [CrossRef]

64. Su, S.B.; Jia, W.; Lu, A.; Li, S. Evidence-based ZHENG: A traditional Chinese medicine syndrome. *Evid.-Based Complement. Altern. Med.* **2012**, *2012*, 246538. [CrossRef] [PubMed]

65. Chen, Z.; Chen, L.Y.; Wang, P.; Dai, H.; Gao, S.; Wang, K. Tumor microenvironment varies under different TCMZHENG models correlates with treatment response to herbal medicine. *Evid.-Based Complement. Altern. Med.* **2012**, *2012*. [CrossRef] [PubMed]

66. Shao, W.; Li, S.; Li, L.; Lin, K.; Liu, X.; Wang, H.; Wang, H.; Wang, D. Chemical genomics reveals inhibition of breast cancer lung metastasis by Ponatinib via c-Jun. *Protein Cell.* **2018**, 1–17. [CrossRef] [PubMed]

67. The MathWorks. *MATLAB (2016a)*; The MathWorks Inc.: Natick, MA, USA, 2016.

68. Law, V.; Knox, C.; Djoumbou, Y.; Jewison, T.; Guo, A.C.; Liu, Y.; Maciejewski, A.; Arndt, D.; Wilson, M.; Neveu, V.; et al. DrugBank 40: Shedding new light on drug metabolism. *Nucleic Acids Res.* **2014**, *42*, D1091–D1097. [CrossRef] [PubMed]

69. Smoot, M.E.; Ono, K.; Ruscheinski, J.; Wang, P.; Ideker, T. Cytoscape 28: New features for data integration network visualization. *Bioinformatics* **2010**, *27*, 431–432. [CrossRef] [PubMed]

70. Hamosh, A.; Scott, A.F.; Amberger, J.S.; Bocchini, C.A.; McKusick, V.A. Online Mendelian Inheritance in Man, (OMIM), a knowledgebase of human genes genetic disorders. *Nucleic Acids Res.* **2005**, *33*, D514–D517. [CrossRef] [PubMed]

71. Wu, X.; Jiang, R.; Zhang, M.Q.; Li, S. Network-based global inference of human disease genes. *Mol. Syst. Biol.* **2008**, *4*, 189. [CrossRef] [PubMed]

72. Yao, X.; Hao, H.; Li, Y.; Li, S. Modularity-based credible prediction of disease genes and detection of disease subtypes on the phenotype-gene heterogeneous network. *BMC Syst. Biol.* **2011**, *5*, 79. [CrossRef] [PubMed]

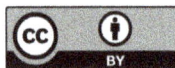

cancers

MDPI

Review

Bioinformatics Analysis for Circulating Cell-Free DNA in Cancer

Chiang-Ching Huang [1],*, Meijun Du [2] and Liang Wang [2],*

[1]   Zilber School of Public Health, University of Wisconsin, Milwaukee, WI 53205, USA
[2]   Department of Pathology and MCW Cancer Center, Medical College of Wisconsin, Milwaukee, WI 53226, USA; mdu@mcw.edu
*   Correspondence: huangcc@uwm.edu (C.-C.H.); liwang@mcw.edu (L.W.);
    Tel.: +1-414-227-5006 (C.-C.H.); +1-414-955-2574 (L.W.)

Received: 22 April 2019; Accepted: 6 June 2019; Published: 11 June 2019

Abstract: Molecular analysis of cell-free DNA (cfDNA) that circulates in plasma and other body fluids represents a "liquid biopsy" approach for non-invasive cancer screening or monitoring. The rapid development of sequencing technologies has made cfDNA a promising source to study cancer development and progression. Specific genetic and epigenetic alterations have been found in plasma, serum, and urine cfDNA and could potentially be used as diagnostic or prognostic biomarkers in various cancer types. In this review, we will discuss the molecular characteristics of cancer cfDNA and major bioinformatics approaches involved in the analysis of cfDNA sequencing data for detecting genetic mutation, copy number alteration, methylation change, and nucleosome positioning variation. We highlight specific challenges in sensitivity to detect genetic aberrations and robustness of statistical analysis. Finally, we provide perspectives regarding the standard and continuing development of bioinformatics analysis to move this promising screening tool into clinical practice.

Keywords: bioinformatics; copy number variation; cell-free DNA; methylation; mutation; next generation sequencing

1. Introduction

To date, tissue biopsy samples are widely used to characterize tumors. Although tissues allow the histological definition of the disease and can reveal details of the genetic profile of the tumor, enabling prediction of disease progression and response to therapies, the applications are limited on tissue availability, sampling frequency, and their genetic heterogeneity [1]. Therefore, attention is turning to liquid biopsies, which enable the analysis of tumor components, including circulating tumor cells (CTC) [2] and circulating tumor nucleic acids from various biological fluids, mostly blood but also other easily accessible fluids such as urine [3]. Compared to conventional tissue biopsy from a single tumor site, the main advantages of liquid biopsies include their non-invasive characteristics, multiple sampling capability, and comprehensive coverage to address issues of tumor heterogeneity [4,5].

Circulating cell-free DNA (cfDNA) is defined as extracellular DNA occurring in blood or other body fluids. It is usually released as small fragments (150–200 bp in length [6]) from normal or tumor cells by apoptosis and necrosis [7], or shed from viable cells [8]. Levels of cfDNA are higher in diseased than healthy individuals [9]. cfDNA can track the evolutionary dynamics and heterogeneity of tumors and detect the early emergence of therapy resistance, residual disease, and recurrence [10–12]. Therefore, analysis of cfDNA has been considered as a potential screening approach for tumor diagnosis and prognosis by detecting tumor-associated aberrations in peripheral blood [13,14].

Next generation sequencing (NGS) has emerged as a powerful tool for cfDNA analysis, which allows the detection of cancer-related genetic and epigenetic alterations such as mutations, copy number variations (CNVs), and DNA methylation changes across wider genomic regions in many cancer types [15,16]. However, detection of cancer with high specificity and sensitivity is still challenging, especially in early-stage cancers, as there exist many barriers to the utilization of cfDNA in clinical applications, including lack of well-accepted sample collection protocol and sensitive detection approaches. Furthermore, analysis of cfDNA sequencing data requires specialized bioinformatics tools to identify robust biomarkers for clinical practice. In this review, we will discuss specific challenges in sensitivity to detect genetic aberrations and provide information on cfDNA bioinformatics approaches. We conclude with a perspective regarding future development in this rapidly evolving area. A simplified workflow of blood-based liquid biopsy is shown in Figure 1.

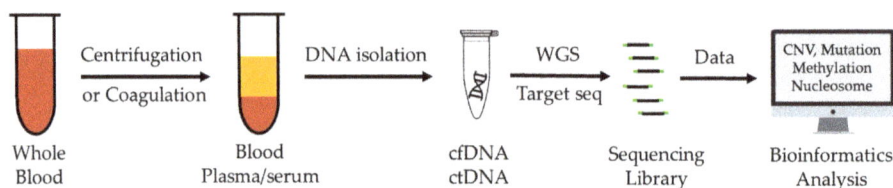

Figure 1. Workflow of blood-based liquid biopsy.

2. Characteristics of Circulating Tumor DNA (ctDNA)

The ctDNA is released from tumor cells only. The ctDNA can be derived from primary or metastatic tumors [17]. Most circulating ctDNA are 160–180 base pair fragments, roughly the size of a mononucleosomal unit [18,19]. However, recent studies have shown that ctDNA tends to be shorter than cfDNA from normal cells [20,21]. Therefore, ctDNA may be enriched by excising smaller DNA fragments from cfDNA on polyacrylamide gels [22]. Currently, cfDNA fragmentation patterns and their applications in liquid biopsy are an emerging research field. Although ctDNA can be used to detect the presence of cancer-related genetic and epigenetic changes, such changes usually vary from case to case, which makes the development of sensitive and generalizable approaches extremely challenging. One major challenge is low ctDNA fraction. In most cases, ctDNA accounts for a small fraction of total cfDNA since most cfDNA is derived from non-cancer cells, especially blood cells. In early-stage cancer patients, ctDNA fraction could be lower than 0.1%. To detect such a rare event with high specificity and sensitivity, a variety of approaches have been developed, which include droplet digital PCR (ddPCR) and molecular index-based next generation sequencing technologies [23,24].

3. Detection and Analysis of Somatic Mutations

Somatic mutations are involved in cancer development and progression. The presence or absence of a single genetic alteration in tumor DNA is currently employed to guide clinical decision making for a number of targeted agents [25–28]. Ever-increasing numbers of genomic alterations are being tested as putative predictive biomarkers in clinical trials of novel anticancer therapies [29]. To detect the cancer-associated alleles in the blood, real-time PCR (RT-PCR) and ddPCR "targeted" methods have been extensively adopted in most clinical trials [30]. Till now, clinical utility has been demonstrated for two FDA-approved cfDNA-based tests: the cobas epidermal growth factor receptor (EGFR) mutation test V2 (Roche Molecular Diagnostics), which detects EGFR mutation in plasma cfDNA from patients with lung cancer [31,32], and Epi proColon (Epigenomics AG), which reports on the methylation status of the Septin 9 promoter in plasma cfDNA from patients undergoing screening for colorectal cancer [33]. ddPCR is particularly useful to sensitively detect well-characterized mutations. The system can partition cfDNA into 20,000 nanoliter-sized droplets, where PCR amplification is carried out simultaneously. It is reported that the sensitivity of ddPCR can reach a limit of detection of 0.0005% BRAF V600E and V600K [34]. Another study reported that ddPCR can reliably detect AR-V7 expression from one spiked cell into 4000 lymphocytes (0.025%) [35]. Compared to the traditional NGS method, ddPCR is easier to use, has lower cost, and provides higher sensitivity and specificity. Although molecular barcoding technology has significantly increased the sensitivity and specificity of NGS, the low cost and easy-to-use features will make ddPCR widely accepted in clinical practice.

Although PCR-based assays can detect known mutations, the assay requires previous knowledge of target genes. In addition, the assay does not cover whole spectrum mutations in specific genes. Restriction of multiplexing capacity limits the simultaneous analysis of a large number of gene targets. Therefore, it may fail to identify less common but clinically relevant mutations. On the other hand, NGS, based on massive parallel sequencing of millions of different DNA molecules, allows the detection of multiple mutations in multiple genes. By using focused gene panels on clinically relevant targets, each nucleotide of interest can be sequenced thousands of times, ensuring a high degree of sensitivity. However, the requirement for such a high degree of sensitivity can easily lead to false positive results due to potential errors of PCR amplification and sequencing. To address this challenge, new data analysis approaches have been developed, among which is a new unique molecular identifier (UMI) strategy [36]. Another challenge related to mutation detection in cfDNA is to differentiate tumor mutations from background somatic mutations. Somatic mutations are common in healthy individuals with a rate between 2–6 mutations per 1 Mb [37]. Given the fact that the majority of cfDNA is from blood cells and ctDNA fraction in cancer patients is generally low, it is likely that most of the mutations identified in cfDNA could be irrelevant to cancer development, thereby impeding their clinical application [38–40]. This challenge points to the need for a large experiment to systematically investigate the mutation spectrum from both cfDNA and white blood cells in healthy and cancer patients.

4. Unique Molecular Identifier (UMI)-Based Target Sequencing

Target enrichment is a critical component of targeted deep sequencing for cost-effective, accurate, and sensitive detection of mutations, CNVs, and methylations in cfDNA. Common bioinformatics workflows allow sensitive and specific variant identification down to 2–5% allele frequency. This provides a sound methodology for identifying somatic mutations from solid tumor biopsies [41]. However, low ctDNA content in the blood and sequencing artifacts currently limit analytical sensitivity. In analyzing cfDNA from healthy controls, background errors are increasingly evident below allele fractions of ~0.2%. It is reported that under an allele fraction of 0.02%, >50% of sequenced genomic positions had artifacts [42]. In addition, common NGS assays involve multiple steps, including end repair, ligation, PCR, and sequencing. These steps often introduce technical biases, limiting accurate quantification and, therefore, hindering the robust and clinically valid detection of biomarkers [43]. Furthermore, PCR-based target enrichment cannot distinguish PCR duplicates from copies of unique fragments generated by a pair of PCR primers.

To overcome these limitations, UMIs (also known as molecular barcodes) have been added into the adaptors to tag individual DNA molecules [44–47]. Such barcodes enable the precise tracking of individual molecules. UMIs can accurately distinguish PCR duplicates from copies of unique fragments generated by PCR amplification [36]. Moreover, UMIs can reduce quantitative bias during experimental processes to detect true ultra-rare variants by distinguishing authentic somatic mutations arising in vivo from artifacts introduced ex vivo. This is largely due to the fact that errors arising from artifacts during library construction and sequencing runs could be eliminated by comparing the sequences of PCR duplicates identified with a UMI sequence [42,48]. Figure 2 illustrates the basic principle of UMI application in the detection of true somatic mutations. Dedicated bioinformatics software packages (Table 1) have been developed for the UMI-tagged targeted resequencing data to improve ultra-rare variant calling by removing errors arising from the first cycle PCR [49,50].

Incorporation of molecular barcoding into a bioinformatics algorithm has significantly increased sensitivity of mutation detection in NGS data. The detection sensitivity can be down to 0.01% [57]. However, recent advances in statistical modeling has also increased sensitivity of variant detection without molecular barcoding. A method ERAS-Seq (Elimination of Recurrent Artifacts and Stochastic Errors) that utilizes technical replicates in conjunction with background error modelling has shown an increased sensitivity of variant detection between 0.05% and 1% allele frequency [58]. By physically extracting and individually amplifying the DNA clones of erroneous reads, another barcoding-free method is reported to distinguish true variants of frequency >0.003% from the systematic NGS error. This method uses 10 times less sequencing reads compared to those from previous studies and achieved a PCR-induced error rate of 2.5×10^{-6} per base per doubling event [59].

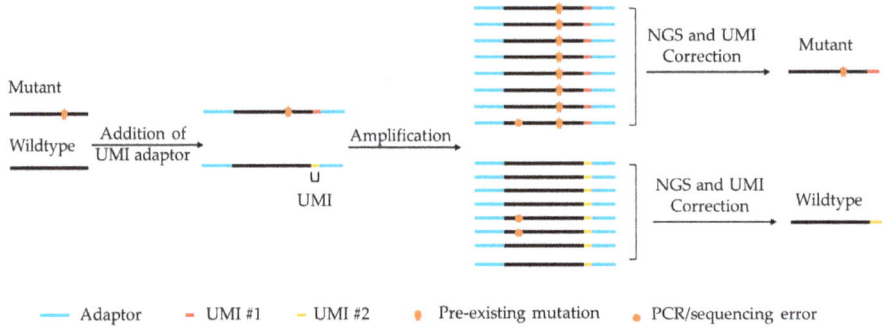

Figure 2. Principle of unique molecular identifiers (UMI) application in the detection of somatic mutations.

Table 1. Bioinformatics programs for detecting genetic and epigenetic changes in cancers.

Program	Website	Key Features	Reference
Mutation			
UMI-tools	https://GitHub.com/CGATOxford/UMI-tools	identifies sequencing errors in the UMI sequence to improve quantification accuracy	[49]
MAGERI	https://github.com/mikessh/mageri	provides an efficient analysis pipeline for UMI-encoded data	[50]
Copy Number			
QDNA-seq	https://github.com/ccagc/QDNAseq	simultaneously corrects for GC and mappability bias	[51]
WisecondorX	https://github.com/CenterForMedicalGeneticsGhent/WisecondorX	optimizes segmentation by reducing noise from problematic bins	[52]
BIC-seq2	http://compbio.med.harvard.edu/BIC-seq/	Avoids high variability of reads in bins	[53]
CNVkit	https://github.com/etal/cnvkit	uses both the targeted reads and the nonspecifically captured off-target reads to infer copy number	[54]
Methylation			
CancerLocator	https://github.com/jasminezhoulab/CancerLocator	simultaneously infers the proportion and tissue of origin of ctDNA	[55]
CancerDetector	https://zhoulab.dgsom.ucla.edu/pages/CancerDetector	Improves ctDNA fraction estimation and identifies outlier markers	[56]

5. Detection of DNA Copy Number Alterations

Currently, most cfDNA applications in cancer screening have focused on somatic point mutations [23,24]. However, methods that interrogate other genomic aberrations should be incorporated to improve detection and characterization of early-stage cancers. One of such genomic abnormalities is CNVs that contribute significantly to genome instability [60,61]. Large-scale cancer genome studies have identified CNVs across various types of cancer and a majority of the CNVs are shared among several cancer types [62,63]. Recently, several lines of investigation have demonstrated the potential of CNVs from cfDNA as sensitive cancer biomarkers [64–66]. Both targeted and whole genome sequencing (WGS) have been employed to identify specific CNVs or genome-wide DNA copy number patterns in cancer patients. Extension of statistical and bioinformatics methods developed from microarray-based comparative genomic hybridization (aCGH) array or NGS are suitable for the detection of CNVs from cfDNA.

For the WGS-based CNV analysis, depth of coverage (DOC) methods (Table 1) are the most used techniques to estimate copy number from the sequence depth in the genome [51–54]. Other methods such as assembly-based, split-read, and read-pair methods [67] can be used to infer copy number changes and chromosomal rearrangement. However, these methods may require high sequence coverage or specific molecular size and thus may not be practical in diagnostic application. The DOC methods can be divided into two major categories depending on whether a reference signal is required. In general, the pseudo-autosomal region on the Y chromosome and genomic regions with low mappability should be removed before the sequencing alignment procedure. This step is especially critical for reference free methods to ensure that the short reads can be mapped to a unique genomic location instead of multiple possible locations. The GEM (GEnome Multitool) mappability algorithm [68] is an efficient program that provides mappability information for multiple genomes. In addition, it is important to filter genomic regions that tend to show artificially high signal (i.e., excessive unstructured anomalous reads mapping). These blacklisted regions in the human genome are often found in highly variable regions (e.g., alternative haplotypes overrepresented on chromosome 19) or at specific types of problematic repeats such as centromeres, telomeres, and satellite repeats. The ENCODE and modENCODE consortia have identified these regions and made them available online [69] at https://sites.google.com/site/anshulkundaje/projects/blacklists. However, empirical data analysis indicates that the ENCODE blacklist may not be sufficient to remove all problematic regions. As such, the QDNAseq algorithm [51] provides a data-driven approach to identify additional regions that should be removed before downstream analysis.

Due to the high cost of WGS assay, current cfDNA-based approaches to CNVs detection normally have low-sequence coverage (e.g., 0.1×~0.5× coverage depth) [64,70,71]. As such, the binning procedure is generally required to aggregate reads mapped to a genomic window. After removing the low mappability reads and blacklisted regions, reads in different genomic windows are counted and normalized by the total number of reads. Depending on the read depth, a fixed bin size is normally chosen such that sufficient detection resolution can be achieved while excessive variation of read counts between adjacent windows can be reduced, thereby enhancing the detection sensitivity for CNVs. Although simple, using a fixed bin size may lead to high variability of read counts among bins with a substantially different number of mappable positions. To overcome this problem, the BIC-seq2 algorithm [53] normalizes read counts at a nucleotide level rather than at the bin level. It calculates the expected number of mapped reads for every position in the mappability map. The ratio of the observed read number and expected number of mappable reads is thus used to infer copy number for a specific genomic region. The normalized read counts can be further subject to GC content correction using smoothing techniques such as LOWESS [72]. The GC-corrected read counts are then normalized to the GC-corrected read counts of cfDNA from a group of reference samples (e.g., healthy controls or patient's own germline DNA) and expressed as $\log_2$ ratio values. For reference-free methods, median normalization can be used to obtain $\log_2$ ratio values.

Segmentation on the $\log_2$ ratio values is generally performed to identify the genomic areas with potential CNVs. The purpose of segmentation is to merge adjacent data points with the same copy number into one segment and divide regions with different copy numbers into different segments. Several statistical techniques and tools have been developed. Two of the most popular methods are circular binary segmentation (CBS) [73,74] and the hidden Markov model (HMM) [75,76]. Thorough review and systematic evaluation of CNV detection methods and software resources have been documented previously [52,77–79]. Researchers may use the information therein to choose appropriate algorithms for their projects. After the segmentation, aberration calling will be made to infer DNA regions with abnormal copy number (e.g., >2 or <2 DNA copies for gain or loss). A commonly used method for determining CNVs from the cfDNA of cancer patients using high throughput sequencing is the Z-score based approach [64,80–82]. These methods identify CNV segments by determining regions in the cfDNA that are significantly different from the reference panel (e.g., Z-score distribution from normal control). Other methods that make formal statistical inference for copy number are available [83,84]. For example, CGHcall [83] uses a two-level hierarchical mixture model to infer for each segment the likelihood of being one of six states of copy number: double deletion, single deletion, normal, gain, double gain, and amplification. This method uses $\log_2$ ratio data to estimate the proportion of different copy number states at the chromosome arm level. Therefore, it may require a large number of samples for robust inference, especially for chromosomes in which abnormal DNA copy numbers are rare. A summary of the bioinformatics procedure for WGS-based CNV analysis in cfDNA is shown in Figure 3.

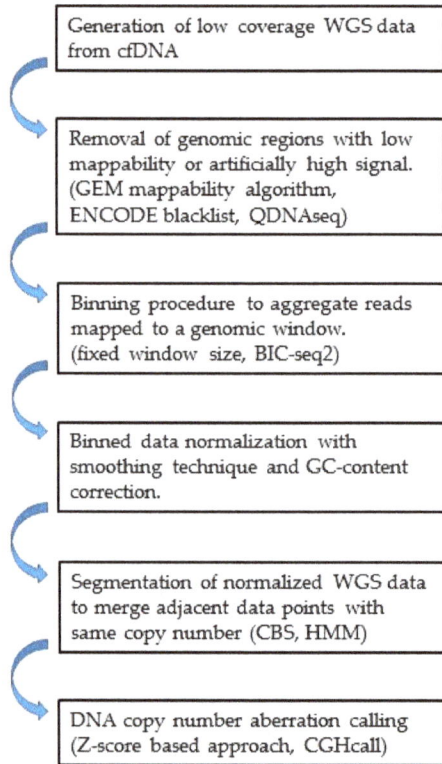

Figure 3. Bioinformatics procedure and techniques/resources used to detect copy number variations (CNVs) from low coverage whole genome sequencing (WGS) data.

One of the challenges to infer CNVs from the cfDNA sequencing data is attributable to the ctDNA content and tumor heterogeneity. In a large portion of cfDNA samples with low ctDNA content (i.e., <2%), especially in the early stages of cancer, sequencing reads are dominated by the DNA from non-cancer cells. Therefore, the signals of CNVs from cancer cells are almost entirely masked, leading to very little statistical power for any segmentation algorithms to detect CNVs, especially for focal amplifications or deletions. In addition, multiple clones of cancer cells could coexist in a cfDNA sample. This will make it even more difficult to detect CNVs due to genetic heterogeneity. To overcome this obstacle, Kirkizar et al. [85] developed a method that employs single-nucleotide polymorphism (SNP)-targeted massively multiplexed PCR (mmPCR) followed by NGS (mmPCR-NGS). Haplotype information is then obtained from the experiment to identify both single nucleotide variants (SNVs) and CNVs with high sensitivity and an average allelic imbalance as low as 0.5%. This method can also detect both clonal and subclonal CNVs in ctDNA.

6. Identification of DNA Methylation Changes from cfDNA

DNA methylation is essential for normal development and plays an important role in epigenetic control of gene activity. Changes in DNA methylation have been recognized as one of the most common molecular alterations in tumorigenesis [86,87]. It is well known that each tissue possesses unique methylation signatures and a genome-wide methylation pattern is distinguished between cancer and normal cells [16,88,89]. Therefore, whole genome methylation profiling from cfDNA could be a potentially powerful tool to detect the presence of specific cancer. Lehmann-Werman et al. [90] first demonstrated the feasibility to identify tissue origin using cfDNA. By leveraging whole genome methylation data sets from The Cancer Genome Atlas (TCGA) and Gene Expression Omnibus (GEO) repositories, they identified individual CpG dinucleotides that were unmethylated in the tissue of interest but methylated in other tissues. By comparing genome-wide methylation data from 35 human tissues generated using the Illumina Infinium HumanMethylation450k BeadChip, tissue-specific DNA methylation markers were selected. Subsequently, Moss et al. [91] generated a reference methylation atlas of 25 human tissues including major organs and cells involved in common diseases. For each tissue or cell type, both uniquely hypermethylated and uniquely hypomethylated CpG sites were identified. Additional CpG sites were further identified to differentiate any two cell types that were found to be most similar in the atlas.

With the data for tissue-specific and cancer methylation signatures, deconvolution algorithms [92], a commonly used algorithm to recover the original signal from a mixture of signal sources, can be used to map tumor tissue of origin from cfDNA. Sun et al. [93] used optimization programming to calculate the methylation densities of 5820 methylation markers in cfDNA from bisulfite sequencing data for 14 human tissues. To improve the selection of informative methylation markers, Guo et al. [94] identified 147,888 blocks of tightly coupled CpG sites, called methylation haplotype blocks, after a comprehensive analysis of a large amount of whole-genome bisulfite sequencing data, reduced-representation bisulfite sequencing data, and methylation array data. The deconvolution algorithm was then applied for tissue-specific methylation analysis at the block level. This method was successfully applied to estimate ctDNA content and differentiate among clinical plasma samples from normal individuals and patients of lung cancer and colorectal cancer.

Recently, probabilistic models have been formulated to identify specific cancer types from cfDNA. Kang et al. developed a method, termed CancerLocator [55], to simultaneously infer the proportion and tissue of origin of ctDNA using whole-genome DNA methylation data. By using TCGA Infinium HumanMethylation450 microarray data from both normal and tumor samples, CancerLocator identified as feature input a large number of CpG clusters that have high inter-individual methylation variation across all normal and cancer types. Since cfDNA from the peripheral blood is a mixture of normal and tumor DNA if a cancer cell is present, the methylation level for each CpG cluster, one for normal and the other one for a cancer type, can be estimated and the ctDNA fraction and the likelihood of the presence of a specific cancer type can be inferred based on the methylation data of informative

CpG clusters. CancerLocator demonstrated a superior prediction performance over popular machine learning algorithms (i.e., random forest and support vector machine) on low-coverage sequencing data, especially for samples with low to moderate ctDNA fraction. However, a challenge facing this method is that the classification accuracy depends substantially on the estimated ctDNA fraction of a specific tumor type.

A variation of CancerLocator was developed later by Li et al. [56]. This method, called CancerDetector, differs slightly from CancerLocator in genomic marker selection and estimation. To identify sensitive genomic markers, CpG clusters were identified such that the level of methylation in a specific cancer tissue differs from matched normal tissue as well as normal plasma samples. This procedure ensures that selected markers are not tissue specific and the methylation signal can be detected in the blood. With selected CpG clusters, a similar probabilistic model to CancerLocator was implemented to predict cancer types and ctDNA fraction. To improve the estimation of ctDNA fraction, an iteration procedure was developed to remove outlier markers whose estimated ctDNA fraction are far from the estimated ctDNA fraction when all markers were used. CancerDetector demonstrated substantial improvement over CancerLocator with high sensitivity and specificity in detecting tumor cfDNAs on real plasma data. Figure 4 illustrates the major principle of the bioinformatics approach for tumor tissue-specific methylation analysis.

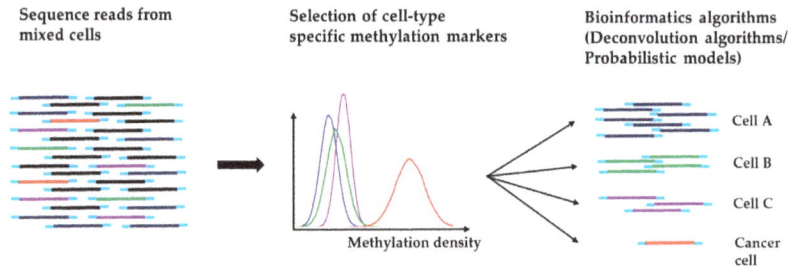

Figure 4. Schematic approach to map cancer tissue of origin from WGS methylation analysis.

7. Association of Nucleosome and Fragmentation Pattern with Tissue of Origin in cfDNA

In addition to DNA methylation, cfDNA fragmentation and/or nucleosome occupancy patterns are another epigenetic feature to trace gene activity and tissue origin [95]. Compaction of nucleosomal structures creates a barrier for DNA-binding transcription factors to access their cognate *cis*-regulatory elements. Usually, active promoters lack nucleosomes, while inactive promoters have densely packed nucleosomes. Nucleosome positioning through genome-wide mapping is shown to be associated with gene activation and expression in a development-dependent and tissue-specific manner [95,96]. Therefore, investigation of nucleosome positioning in a patient's cfDNA may reveal the existence of a specific cancer type.

As cfDNA is preferentially released from apoptotic cells, the size distribution of cfDNA fragments (160–180 bp) can resemble the size of mononucleosome-protected DNA. Specifically, peak sizes correspond to nucleosomes (~147 bp) and chromatosomes (nucleosome + linker histone; ~167 bp), suggesting they could bear the information of the cell type of origin [97]. Based on the expectation that fragment endpoints should cluster next to nucleosome boundaries and should be depleted at sites of nucleosome occupancy, Snyder et al. showed that nucleosome spacing patterns can inform the cell type of origin from cfDNA [98]. The study showed that nucleosome spacing inferred from cfDNA in healthy individuals correlated strongly with epigenetic features of lymphoid and myeloid cells, consistent with hematopoietic cell death as a major source of cfDNA, while the patterns of nucleosome spacing in late-stage cancer patients match the anatomical origin of the patient's cancer. Therefore, different nucleosome footprints between the tumor and the normal source of cfDNA may enable the noninvasive monitoring of a much broader set of clinical conditions than currently possible [98].

8. Conclusions and Future Direction

cfDNA molecules have emerged as promising biomarkers for cancer detection and monitoring due to the easy access to clinical samples from blood or urine. The advent of NGS technology provides an unprecedented opportunity to systematically examine the characteristics of cfDNA for tumor-specific changes. However, the massive amount of sequencing data requires sophisticated bioinformatics analysis to accurately identify genomic abnormalities in cancer. This review discussed major bioinformatics applications of cfDNA in oncological research to identify point mutations, copy number abnormalities, DNA methylation changes, and nucleosome positioning patterns. Using sophisticated bioinformatics analysis, advances have been made to better understand the property of cfDNA through fragmentation and nucleosome spacing patterns. Analysis by leveraging large-scale cancer genomic databases in conjunction with state-of-the-art statistical algorithms demonstrates the great potential of using methylation biomarkers for identification of cancer cell origin. Moreover, patterns of CNV through the WGS analysis can further reveal the extent of tumor heterogeneity. Nevertheless, to move cfDNA into routine clinical practices for better patient management, future studies will need to address several issues. First, studies need to focus more on detection sensitivity in early-stage cancer because there are many barriers to utilizing cfDNA for such applications. For example, most studies that demonstrated the feasibility of cfDNA in cancer detection used samples form late-stage cancer patients. However, the fraction of ctDNA in the plasma from early-stage cancer patients is generally very low. Although a range of NGS-based approaches have been used to characterize tumor genomes in detail and new bioinformatics techniques and analysis tools are rapidly evolving, current technologies and bioinformatics algorithms are not sensitive enough to detect such low level of genetic or epigenetic abnormalities. How to develop advanced technologies to detect mutations, CNVs, and epigenetic changes at the low ctDNA level is likely to be one of the most challenging issues to resolve. Another issue is related to cfDNA contaminations by the lysed blood cells and significant variation into cfDNA due to DNA isolation protocols and choice of instrument. Therefore, a standard protocol for quality control and bioinformatics analysis procedures need to be developed before these technologies can be successfully and reliably used in clinical practice and regulatory decision -making. A joint effort from the scientific community for the MicroArray Quality Control (MAQC) project [99] is an excellent example to follow to attain this goal. Finally, other biomarkers should be further explored for liquid biopsy in addition to genetic and epigenetic markers and nucleosome spacing patterns discussed in this review. For example, recent studies have shown that circulating cell-fee RNA (cfRNA), which encompasses miRNAs, lncRNAs, and mRNAs, could also serve as valuable biomarkers for liquid biopsy [100,101]. Given the finding that transcriptome profiling alone from tissue biopsies can robustly determine cancerous status and tissue origin [102], the multiparameter analyses incorporating the molecular profiles at cfDNA, cfRNA, and protein will result in an improved understanding of molecular aberrations and their functional roles across tumor types, as well as facilitate the identification of novel tumor subtypes [103]. As most of the cfDNA interrogations to date are proof-of-principle studies, large-scale, multi-site cohort studies that systematically investigate all these aspects of molecular profiles are needed to evaluate the complementary nature of their screening power so that liquid biopsy signatures can be refined, validated, and utilized in clinical practice. Eventually, these efforts will lead to the identification of new oncological biomarkers for early detection and outcome prediction, which is a prerequisite for realizing the promise of precision medicine.

Author Contributions: Conceptualization, C.-C.H. and L.W.; Writing—original draft preparation, C.-C.H. and M.D.; Writing—review and editing, L.W. and C.-C.H.; Supervision, L.W.; funding acquisition, C.-C.H. and L.W.

Funding: This research was supported by National Institute of Health (R01CA212097) to L.W. and by National Institutes of Health (NIH) CTSA award (UL1TR001436) to C.-C.H.

Conflicts of Interest: The authors declare no conflict of interest.

References

1. Gerlinger, M.; Rowan, A.J.; Horswell, S.; Math, M.; Larkin, J.; Endesfelder, D.; Gronroos, E.; Martinez, P.; Matthews, N.; Stewart, A.; et al. Intratumor heterogeneity and branched evolution revealed by multiregion sequencing. *N. Engl. J. Med.* **2012**, *366*, 883–892. [CrossRef] [PubMed]
2. Millner, L.M.; Linder, M.W.; Valdes, R., Jr. Circulating tumor cells: A review of present methods and the need to identify heterogeneous phenotypes. *Ann. Clin. Lab. Sci.* **2013**, *43*, 295–304.
3. Xia, Y.; Huang, C.C.; Dittmar, R.; Du, M.; Wang, Y.; Liu, H.; Shenoy, N.; Wang, L.; Kohli, M. Copy number variations in urine cell free DNA as biomarkers in advanced prostate cancer. *Oncotarget* **2016**, *7*, 35818–35831. [CrossRef] [PubMed]
4. Ilie, M.; Hofman, P. Pros: Can tissue biopsy be replaced by liquid biopsy? *Transl. Lung Cancer Res.* **2016**, *5*, 420–423. [CrossRef] [PubMed]
5. Gonzalez-Billalabeitia, E.; Conteduca, V.; Wetterskog, D.; Jayaram, A.; Attard, G. Circulating tumor DNA in advanced prostate cancer: Transitioning from discovery to a clinically implemented test. *Prostate Cancer Prostatic Dis.* **2019**, *22*, 195–205. [CrossRef] [PubMed]
6. Fleischhacker, M.; Schmidt, B. Circulating nucleic acids (CNAs) and cancer—A survey. *Biochim. Biophys. Acta* **2007**, *1775*, 181–232. [CrossRef] [PubMed]
7. Jahr, S.; Hentze, H.; Englisch, S.; Hardt, D.; Fackelmayer, F.O.; Hesch, R.D.; Knippers, R. DNA fragments in the blood plasma of cancer patients: Quantitations and evidence for their origin from apoptotic and necrotic cells. *Cancer Res.* **2001**, *61*, 1659–1665.
8. Alix-Panabieres, C.; Pantel, K. Challenges in circulating tumour cell research. *Nat. Rev. Cancer* **2014**, *14*, 623–631. [CrossRef] [PubMed]
9. Koffler, D.; Agnello, V.; Winchester, R.; Kunkel, H.G. The occurrence of single-stranded DNA in the serum of patients with systemic lupus erythematosus and other diseases. *J. Clin. Investig.* **1973**, *52*, 198–204. [CrossRef]
10. Abbosh, C.; Birkbak, N.J.; Wilson, G.A.; Jamal-Hanjani, M.; Constantin, T.; Salari, R.; Le Quesne, J.; Moore, D.A.; Veeriah, S.; Rosenthal, R.; et al. Phylogenetic ctDNA analysis depicts early-stage lung cancer evolution. *Nature* **2017**, *545*, 446–451. [CrossRef]
11. Qin, Z.; Ljubimov, V.A.; Zhou, C.; Tong, Y.; Liang, J. Cell-free circulating tumor DNA in cancer. *Chin. J. Cancer* **2016**, *35*, 36. [CrossRef] [PubMed]
12. Tie, J.; Wang, Y.; Tomasetti, C.; Li, L.; Springer, S.; Kinde, I.; Silliman, N.; Tacey, M.; Wong, H.L.; Christie, M.; et al. Circulating tumor DNA analysis detects minimal residual disease and predicts recurrence in patients with stage II colon cancer. *Sci. Transl. Med.* **2016**, *8*, 346ra92. [CrossRef] [PubMed]
13. Crowley, E.; Di Nicolantonio, F.; Loupakis, F.; Bardelli, A. Liquid biopsy: Monitoring cancer-genetics in the blood. *Nat. Rev. Clin. Oncol.* **2013**, *10*, 472–484. [CrossRef] [PubMed]
14. Diaz, L.A., Jr.; Bardelli, A. Liquid biopsies: Genotyping circulating tumor DNA. *J. Clin. Oncol.* **2014**, *32*, 579–586. [CrossRef] [PubMed]
15. Zehir, A.; Benayed, R.; Shah, R.H.; Syed, A.; Middha, S.; Kim, H.R.; Srinivasan, P.; Gao, J.; Chakravarty, D.; Devlin, S.M.; et al. Mutational landscape of metastatic cancer revealed from prospective clinical sequencing of 10,000 patients. *Nat. Med.* **2017**, *23*, 703–713. [CrossRef] [PubMed]
16. Saghafinia, S.; Mina, M.; Riggi, N.; Hanahan, D.; Ciriello, G. Pan-Cancer Landscape of Aberrant DNA Methylation across Human Tumors. *Cell Rep.* **2018**, *25*, 1066–1080. [CrossRef] [PubMed]
17. Heitzer, E.; Auer, M.; Hoffmann, E.M.; Pichler, M.; Gasch, C.; Ulz, P.; Lax, S.; Waldispuehl-Geigl, J.; Mauermann, O.; Mohan, S.; et al. Establishment of tumor-specific copy number alterations from plasma DNA of patients with cancer. *Int. J. Cancer* **2013**, *133*, 346–356. [CrossRef] [PubMed]
18. Jung, K.; Fleischhacker, M.; Rabien, A. Cell-free DNA in the blood as a solid tumor biomarker—A critical appraisal of the literature. *Clin. Chim. Acta* **2010**, *411*, 1611–1624. [CrossRef] [PubMed]
19. Jiang, P.; Chan, C.W.; Chan, K.C.; Cheng, S.H.; Wong, J.; Wong, V.W.; Wong, G.L.; Chan, S.L.; Mok, T.S.; Chan, H.L.; et al. Lengthening and shortening of plasma DNA in hepatocellular carcinoma patients. *Proc. Natl. Acad. Sci. USA* **2015**, *112*, E1317–E1325. [CrossRef]
20. Jiang, P.; Lo, Y.M.D. The Long and Short of Circulating Cell-Free DNA and the Ins and Outs of Molecular Diagnostics. *Trends Genet.* **2016**, *32*, 360–371. [CrossRef]

21. Lo, Y.M.; Chan, K.C.; Sun, H.; Chen, E.Z.; Jiang, P.; Lun, F.M.; Zheng, Y.W.; Leung, T.Y.; Lau, T.K.; Cantor, C.R.; et al. Maternal plasma DNA sequencing reveals the genome-wide genetic and mutational profile of the fetus. *Sci. Transl. Med.* **2010**, *2*, 61ra91. [CrossRef] [PubMed]

22. Underhill, H.R.; Kitzman, J.O.; Hellwig, S.; Welker, N.C.; Daza, R.; Baker, D.N.; Gligorich, K.M.; Rostomily, R.C.; Bronner, M.P.; Shendure, J. Fragment Length of Circulating Tumor DNA. *PLoS Genet.* **2016**, *12*, e1006162. [CrossRef] [PubMed]

23. Volik, S.; Alcaide, M.; Morin, R.D.; Collins, C. Cell-free DNA (cfDNA): Clinical Significance and Utility in Cancer Shaped by Emerging Technologies. *Mol. Cancer Res.* **2016**, *14*, 898–908. [CrossRef] [PubMed]

24. Wood-Bouwens, C.; Lau, B.T.; Handy, C.M.; Lee, H.; Ji, H.P. Single-Color Digital PCR Provides High-Performance Detection of Cancer Mutations from Circulating DNA. *J. Mol. Diagn.* **2017**, *19*, 697–710. [CrossRef] [PubMed]

25. Allegra, C.J.; Jessup, J.M.; Somerfield, M.R.; Hamilton, S.R.; Hammond, E.H.; Hayes, D.F.; McAllister, P.K.; Morton, R.F.; Schilsky, R.L. American Society of Clinical Oncology provisional clinical opinion: Testing for KRAS gene mutations in patients with metastatic colorectal carcinoma to predict response to anti-epidermal growth factor receptor monoclonal antibody therapy. *J. Clin. Oncol.* **2009**, *27*, 2091–2096. [CrossRef]

26. Shaw, A.T.; Engelman, J.A. ALK in lung cancer: Past, present, and future. *J. Clin. Oncol.* **2013**, *31*, 1105–1111. [CrossRef] [PubMed]

27. Gonzalez, D.; Fearfield, L.; Nathan, P.; Taniere, P.; Wallace, A.; Brown, E.; Harwood, C.; Marsden, J.; Whittaker, S. BRAF mutation testing algorithm for vemurafenib treatment in melanoma: Recommendations from an expert panel. *Br. J. Derm.* **2013**, *168*, 700–707. [CrossRef]

28. Marchetti, A.; Palma, J.F.; Felicioni, L.; De Pas, T.M.; Chiari, R.; Del Grammastro, M.; Filice, G.; Ludovini, V.; Brandes, A.A.; Chella, A.; et al. Early Prediction of Response to Tyrosine Kinase Inhibitors by Quantification of EGFR Mutations in Plasma of NSCLC Patients. *J. Thorac. Oncol.* **2015**, *10*, 1437–1443. [CrossRef] [PubMed]

29. Simon, R.; Roychowdhury, S. Implementing personalized cancer genomics in clinical trials. *Nat. Rev. Drug Discov.* **2013**, *12*, 358–369. [CrossRef]

30. Gevensleben, H.; Garcia-Murillas, I.; Graeser, M.K.; Schiavon, G.; Osin, P.; Parton, M.; Smith, I.E.; Ashworth, A.; Turner, N.C. Noninvasive detection of HER2 amplification with plasma DNA digital PCR. *Clin. Cancer Res.* **2013**, *19*, 3276–3284. [CrossRef]

31. Sacher, A.G.; Paweletz, C.; Dahlberg, S.E.; Alden, R.S.; O'Connell, A.; Feeney, N.; Mach, S.L.; Janne, P.A.; Oxnard, G.R. Prospective Validation of Rapid Plasma Genotyping for the Detection of EGFR and KRAS Mutations in Advanced Lung Cancer. *JAMA Oncol.* **2016**, *2*, 1014–1022. [CrossRef]

32. Leighl, N.B.; Rekhtman, N.; Biermann, W.A.; Huang, J.; Mino-Kenudson, M.; Ramalingam, S.S.; West, H.; Whitlock, S.; Somerfield, M.R. Molecular testing for selection of patients with lung cancer for epidermal growth factor receptor and anaplastic lymphoma kinase tyrosine kinase inhibitors: American Society of Clinical Oncology endorsement of the College of American Pathologists/International Association for the study of lung cancer/association for molecular pathology guideline. *J. Clin. Oncol.* **2014**, *32*, 3673–3679. [PubMed]

33. Warren, J.D.; Xiong, W.; Bunker, A.M.; Vaughn, C.P.; Furtado, L.V.; Roberts, W.L.; Fang, J.C.; Samowitz, W.S.; Heichman, K.A. Septin 9 methylated DNA is a sensitive and specific blood test for colorectal cancer. *BMC Med.* **2011**, *9*, 133. [CrossRef] [PubMed]

34. Reid, A.L.; Freeman, J.B.; Millward, M.; Ziman, M.; Gray, E.S. Detection of BRAF-V600E and V600K in melanoma circulating tumour cells by droplet digital PCR. *Clin. Biochem.* **2015**, *48*, 999–1002. [CrossRef] [PubMed]

35. Ma, Y.; Luk, A.; Young, F.P.; Lynch, D.; Chua, W.; Balakrishnar, B.; de Souza, P.; Becker, T.M. Droplet Digital PCR Based Androgen Receptor Variant 7 (AR-V7) Detection from Prostate Cancer Patient Blood Biopsies. *Int. J. Mol. Sci.* **2016**, *17*, 1264. [CrossRef] [PubMed]

36. Kivioja, T.; Vaharautio, A.; Karlsson, K.; Bonke, M.; Enge, M.; Linnarsson, S.; Taipale, J. Counting absolute numbers of molecules using unique molecular identifiers. *Nat. Methods* **2011**, *9*, 72–74. [CrossRef] [PubMed]

37. Martincorena, I.; Roshan, A.; Gerstung, M.; Ellis, P.; Van Loo, P.; McLaren, S.; Wedge, D.C.; Fullam, A.; Alexandrov, L.B.; Tubio, J.M.; et al. Tumor evolution. High burden and pervasive positive selection of somatic mutations in normal human skin. *Science* **2015**, *348*, 880–886. [CrossRef] [PubMed]

38. Liu, J.; Chen, X.; Wang, J.; Zhou, S.; Wang, C.L.; Ye, M.Z.; Wang, X.Y.; Song, Y.; Wang, Y.Q.; Zhang, L.T.; et al. Biological background of the genomic variations of cf-DNA in healthy individuals. *Ann. Oncol.* **2019**, *30*, 464–470. [CrossRef] [PubMed]

39. Bauml, J.; Levy, B. Clonal Hematopoiesis: A New Layer in the Liquid Biopsy Story in Lung Cancer. *Clin. Cancer Res.* **2018**, *24*, 4352–4354. [CrossRef] [PubMed]

40. Chin, R.I.; Chen, K.; Usmani, A.; Chua, C.; Harris, P.K.; Binkley, M.S.; Azad, T.D.; Dudley, J.C.; Chaudhuri, A.A. Detection of Solid Tumor Molecular Residual Disease (MRD) Using Circulating Tumor DNA (ctDNA). *Mol. Diagn. Ther.* **2019**, *23*, 311–331. [CrossRef] [PubMed]

41. Frampton, G.M.; Fichtenholtz, A.; Otto, G.A.; Wang, K.; Downing, S.R.; He, J.; Schnall-Levin, M.; White, J.; Sanford, E.M.; An, P.; et al. Development and validation of a clinical cancer genomic profiling test based on massively parallel DNA sequencing. *Nat. Biotechnol.* **2013**, *31*, 1023–1031. [CrossRef] [PubMed]

42. Newman, A.M.; Lovejoy, A.F.; Klass, D.M.; Kurtz, D.M.; Chabon, J.J.; Scherer, F.; Stehr, H.; Liu, C.L.; Bratman, S.V.; Say, C.; et al. Integrated digital error suppression for improved detection of circulating tumor DNA. *Nat. Biotechnol.* **2016**, *34*, 547–555. [CrossRef] [PubMed]

43. Wan, J.C.M.; Massie, C.; Garcia-Corbacho, J.; Mouliere, F.; Brenton, J.D.; Caldas, C.; Pacey, S.; Baird, R.; Rosenfeld, N. Liquid biopsies come of age: Towards implementation of circulating tumour DNA. *Nat. Rev. Cancer* **2017**, *17*, 223–238. [CrossRef] [PubMed]

44. Kennedy, S.R.; Schmitt, M.W.; Fox, E.J.; Kohrn, B.F.; Salk, J.J.; Ahn, E.H.; Prindle, M.J.; Kuong, K.J.; Shen, J.C.; Risques, R.A.; et al. Detecting ultralow-frequency mutations by Duplex Sequencing. *Nat. Protoc.* **2014**, *9*, 2586–2606. [CrossRef] [PubMed]

45. Schmitt, M.W.; Fox, E.J.; Prindle, M.J.; Reid-Bayliss, K.S.; True, L.D.; Radich, J.P.; Loeb, L.A. Sequencing small genomic targets with high efficiency and extreme accuracy. *Nat. Methods* **2015**, *12*, 423–425. [CrossRef] [PubMed]

46. Chung, J.; Lee, K.W.; Lee, C.; Shin, S.H.; Kyung, S.; Jeon, H.J.; Kim, S.Y.; Cho, E.; Yoo, C.E.; Son, D.S.; et al. Performance evaluation of commercial library construction kits for PCR-based targeted sequencing using a unique molecular identifier. *BMC Genom.* **2019**, *20*, 216. [CrossRef] [PubMed]

47. Teder, H.; Koel, M.; Paluoja, P.; Jatsenko, T.; Rekker, K.; Laisk-Podar, T.; Kukuskina, V.; Velthut-Meikas, A.; Fjodorova, O.; Peters, M.; et al. TAC-seq: Targeted DNA and RNA sequencing for precise biomarker molecule counting. *NPJ Genom. Med.* **2018**, *3*, 34. [CrossRef]

48. Phallen, J.; Sausen, M.; Adleff, V.; Leal, A.; Hruban, C.; White, J.; Anagnostou, V.; Fiksel, J.; Cristiano, S.; Papp, E.; et al. Direct detection of early-stage cancers using circulating tumor DNA. *Sci. Transl. Med.* **2017**, *9*, eaan2415. [CrossRef]

49. Smith, T.; Heger, A.; Sudbery, I. UMI-tools: Modeling sequencing errors in Unique Molecular Identifiers to improve quantification accuracy. *Genome Res.* **2017**, *27*, 491–499. [CrossRef]

50. Shugay, M.; Zaretsky, A.R.; Shagin, D.A.; Shagina, I.A.; Volchenkov, I.A.; Shelenkov, A.A.; Lebedin, M.Y.; Bagaev, D.V.; Lukyanov, S.; Chudakov, D.M. MAGERI: Computational pipeline for molecular-barcoded targeted resequencing. *PLoS Comput. Biol.* **2017**, *13*, e1005480. [CrossRef]

51. Scheinin, I.; Sie, D.; Bengtsson, H.; van de Wiel, M.A.; Olshen, A.B.; van Thuijl, H.F.; van Essen, H.F.; Eijk, P.P.; Rustenburg, F.; Meijer, G.A.; et al. DNA copy number analysis of fresh and formalin-fixed specimens by shallow whole-genome sequencing with identification and exclusion of problematic regions in the genome assembly. *Genome Res.* **2014**, *24*, 2022–2032. [CrossRef] [PubMed]

52. Raman, L.; Dheedene, A.; De Smet, M.; Van Dorpe, J.; Menten, B. WisecondorX: Improved copy number detection for routine shallow whole-genome sequencing. *Nucleic Acids Res.* **2019**, *47*, 1605–1614. [CrossRef] [PubMed]

53. Xi, R.; Lee, S.; Xia, Y.; Kim, T.M.; Park, P.J. Copy number analysis of whole-genome data using BIC-seq2 and its application to detection of cancer susceptibility variants. *Nucleic Acids Res.* **2016**, *44*, 6274–6286. [CrossRef] [PubMed]

54. Talevich, E.; Shain, A.H.; Botton, T.; Bastian, B.C. CNVkit: Genome-Wide Copy Number Detection and Visualization from Targeted DNA Sequencing. *PLoS Comput. Biol.* **2016**, *12*, e1004873. [CrossRef] [PubMed]

55. Kang, S.; Li, Q.; Chen, Q.; Zhou, Y.; Park, S.; Lee, G.; Grimes, B.; Krysan, K.; Yu, M.; Wang, W.; et al. CancerLocator: Non-invasive cancer diagnosis and tissue-of-origin prediction using methylation profiles of cell-free DNA. *Genome Biol.* **2017**, *18*, 53. [CrossRef]

56. Li, W.; Li, Q.; Kang, S.; Same, M.; Zhou, Y.; Sun, C.; Liu, C.C.; Matsuoka, L.; Sher, L.; Wong, W.H.; et al. CancerDetector: Ultrasensitive and non-invasive cancer detection at the resolution of individual reads using cell-free DNA methylation sequencing data. *Nucleic Acids Res.* **2018**, *46*, e89. [CrossRef] [PubMed]

57. Schmitt, M.W.; Kennedy, S.R.; Salk, J.J.; Fox, E.J.; Hiatt, J.B.; Loeb, L.A. Detection of ultra-rare mutations by next-generation sequencing. *Proc. Natl. Acad. Sci. USA* **2012**, *109*, 14508–14513. [CrossRef]

58. Kamps-Hughes, N.; McUsic, A.; Kurihara, L.; Harkins, T.T.; Pal, P.; Ray, C.; Ionescu-Zanetti, C. ERASE-Seq: Leveraging replicate measurements to enhance ultralow frequency variant detection in NGS data. *PLoS ONE* **2018**, *13*, e0195272. [CrossRef]

59. Yeom, H.; Lee, Y.; Ryu, T.; Noh, J.; Lee, A.C.; Lee, H.B.; Kang, E.; Song, S.W.; Kwon, S. Barcode-free next-generation sequencing error validation for ultra-rare variant detection. *Nat. Commun.* **2019**, *10*, 977. [CrossRef]

60. Andor, N.; Maley, C.C.; Ji, H.P. Genomic Instability in Cancer: Teetering on the Limit of Tolerance. *Cancer Res.* **2017**, *77*, 2179–2185. [CrossRef]

61. Hanahan, D.; Weinberg, R.A. Hallmarks of cancer: The next generation. *Cell* **2011**, *144*, 646–674. [CrossRef]

62. Beroukhim, R.; Mermel, C.H.; Porter, D.; Wei, G.; Raychaudhuri, S.; Donovan, J.; Barretina, J.; Boehm, J.S.; Dobson, J.; Urashima, M.; et al. The landscape of somatic copy-number alteration across human cancers. *Nature* **2010**, *463*, 899–905. [CrossRef] [PubMed]

63. Zack, T.I.; Schumacher, S.E.; Carter, S.L.; Cherniack, A.D.; Saksena, G.; Tabak, B.; Lawrence, M.S.; Zhsng, C.Z.; Wala, J.; Mermel, C.H.; et al. Pan-cancer patterns of somatic copy number alteration. *Nat. Genet.* **2013**, *45*, 1134–1140. [CrossRef] [PubMed]

64. Heitzer, E.; Ulz, P.; Belic, J.; Gutschi, S.; Quehenberger, F.; Fischereder, K.; Benezeder, T.; Auer, M.; Pischler, C.; Mannweiler, S.; et al. Tumor-associated copy number changes in the circulation of patients with prostate cancer identified through whole-genome sequencing. *Genome Med.* **2013**, *5*, 30. [CrossRef]

65. Dawson, S.J.; Tsui, D.W.; Murtaza, M.; Biggs, H.; Rueda, O.M.; Chin, S.F.; Dunning, M.J.; Gale, D.; Forshew, T.; Mahler-Araujo, B.; et al. Analysis of circulating tumor DNA to monitor metastatic breast cancer. *N. Engl. J. Med.* **2013**, *368*, 1199–1209. [CrossRef] [PubMed]

66. Leary, R.J.; Sausen, M.; Kinde, I.; Papadopoulos, N.; Carpten, J.D.; Craig, D.; O'Shaughnessy, J.; Kinzler, K.W.; Parmigiani, G.; Vogelstein, B.; et al. Detection of chromosomal alterations in the circulation of cancer patients with whole-genome sequencing. *Sci. Transl. Med.* **2012**, *4*, 162ra154. [CrossRef]

67. Pirooznia, M.; Goes, F.S.; Zandi, P.P. Whole-genome CNV analysis: Advances in computational approaches. *Front. Genet.* **2015**, *6*, 138. [CrossRef]

68. Derrien, T.; Estelle, J.; Marco Sola, S.; Knowles, D.G.; Raineri, E.; Guigo, R.; Ribeca, P. Fast computation and applications of genome mappability. *PLoS ONE* **2012**, *7*, e30377. [CrossRef] [PubMed]

69. Kundaje, A. A Comprehensive Collection of Signal Artifact Blacklist Regions in the Human Genome. Available online: https://personal.broadinstitute.org/anshul/projects/encode/rawdata/blacklists/hg19-blacklist-README.pdf (accessed on 3 June 2019).

70. Xia, S.; Huang, C.C.; Le, M.; Dittmar, R.; Du, M.; Yuan, T.; Guo, Y.; Wang, Y.; Wang, X.; Tsai, S.; et al. Genomic variations in plasma cell free DNA differentiate early stage lung cancers from normal controls. *Lung Cancer* **2015**, *90*, 78–84. [CrossRef]

71. Hovelson, D.H.; Liu, C.J.; Wang, Y.; Kang, Q.; Henderson, J.; Gursky, A.; Brockman, S.; Ramnath, N.; Krauss, J.C.; Talpaz, M.; et al. Rapid, ultra low coverage copy number profiling of cell-free DNA as a precision oncology screening strategy. *Oncotarget* **2017**, *8*, 89848–89866. [CrossRef]

72. Benjamini, Y.; Speed, T.P. Summarizing and correcting the GC content bias in high-throughput sequencing. *Nucleic Acids Res.* **2012**, *40*, e72. [CrossRef] [PubMed]

73. Olshen, A.B.; Venkatraman, E.S.; Lucito, R.; Wigler, M. Circular binary segmentation for the analysis of array-based DNA copy number data. *Biostatistics* **2004**, *5*, 557–572. [CrossRef] [PubMed]

74. Venkatraman, E.S.; Olshen, A.B. A faster circular binary segmentation algorithm for the analysis of array CGH data. *Bioinformatics* **2007**, *23*, 657–663. [CrossRef] [PubMed]

75. Shah, S.P.; Xuan, X.; DeLeeuw, R.J.; Khojasteh, M.; Lam, W.L.; Ng, R.; Murphy, K.P. Integrating copy number polymorphisms into array CGH analysis using a robust HMM. *Bioinformatics* **2006**, *22*, e431–e439. [CrossRef] [PubMed]

76. Lai, D.; Ha, G.; Shah, S. HMMcopy: Copy number prediction with correction for GC and mappability bias for HTS data. R Package Version 1.26.0. 2019. Available online: http://bioconductor.org/packages/release/bioc/html/HMMcopy.html (accessed on 3 June 2019).

77. Liu, B.; Morrison, C.D.; Johnson, C.S.; Trump, D.L.; Qin, M.; Conroy, J.C.; Wang, J.; Liu, S. Computational methods for detecting copy number variations in cancer genome using next generation sequencing: Principles and challenges. *Oncotarget* **2013**, *4*, 1868–1881. [CrossRef] [PubMed]

78. Eckel-Passow, J.E.; Atkinson, E.J.; Maharjan, S.; Kardia, S.L.; de Andrade, M. Software comparison for evaluating genomic copy number variation for Affymetrix 6.0 SNP array platform. *BMC Bioinform.* **2011**, *12*, 220. [CrossRef] [PubMed]

79. Zhang, X.; Du, R.; Li, S.; Zhang, F.; Jin, L.; Wang, H. Evaluation of copy number variation detection for a SNP array platform. *BMC Bioinform.* **2014**, *15*, 50. [CrossRef] [PubMed]

80. Mohan, S.; Heitzer, E.; Ulz, P.; Lafer, I.; Lax, S.; Auer, M.; Pichler, M.; Gerger, A.; Eisner, F.; Hoefler, G.; et al. Changes in colorectal carcinoma genomes under anti-EGFR therapy identified by whole-genome plasma DNA sequencing. *PLoS Genet.* **2014**, *10*, e1004271. [CrossRef]

81. Xu, H.; Zhu, X.; Xu, Z.; Hu, Y.; Bo, S.; Xing, T.; Zhu, K. Non-invasive Analysis of Genomic Copy Number Variation in Patients with Hepatocellular Carcinoma by Next Generation DNA Sequencing. *J. Cancer* **2015**, *6*, 247–253. [CrossRef] [PubMed]

82. Ulz, P.; Belic, J.; Graf, R.; Auer, M.; Lafer, I.; Fischereder, K.; Webersinke, G.; Pummer, K.; Augustin, H.; Pichler, M.; et al. Whole-genome plasma sequencing reveals focal amplifications as a driving force in metastatic prostate cancer. *Nat. Commun.* **2016**, *7*, 12008. [CrossRef]

83. Van de Wiel, M.A.; Kim, K.I.; Vosse, S.J.; van Wieringen, W.N.; Wilting, S.M.; Ylstra, B. CGHcall: Calling aberrations for array CGH tumor profiles. *Bioinformatics* **2007**, *23*, 892–894. [CrossRef] [PubMed]

84. Engler, D.A.; Mohapatra, G.; Louis, D.N.; Betensky, R.A. A pseudolikelihood approach for simultaneous analysis of array comparative genomic hybridizations. *Biostatistics* **2006**, *7*, 399–421. [CrossRef] [PubMed]

85. Kirkizlar, E.; Zimmermann, B.; Constantin, T.; Swenerton, R.; Hoang, B.; Wayham, N.; Babiarz, J.E.; Demko, Z.; Pelham, R.J.; Kareht, S.; et al. Detection of Clonal and Subclonal Copy-Number Variants in Cell-Free DNA from Patients with Breast Cancer Using a Massively Multiplexed PCR Methodology. *Transl. Oncol.* **2015**, *8*, 407–416. [CrossRef] [PubMed]

86. Baylin, S.B.; Herman, J.G. DNA hypermethylation in tumorigenesis: Epigenetics joins genetics. *Trends Genet.* **2000**, *16*, 168–174. [CrossRef]

87. Jones, P.A.; Laird, P.W. Cancer epigenetics comes of age. *Nat. Genet.* **1999**, *21*, 163–167. [CrossRef] [PubMed]

88. Chen, Y.; Breeze, C.E.; Zhen, S.; Beck, S.; Teschendorff, A.E. Tissue-independent and tissue-specific patterns of DNA methylation alteration in cancer. *Epigenet. Chromatin* **2016**, *9*, 10. [CrossRef] [PubMed]

89. Zhang, B.; Zhou, Y.; Lin, N.; Lowdon, R.F.; Hong, C.; Nagarajan, R.P.; Cheng, J.B.; Li, D.; Stevens, M.; Lee, H.J.; et al. Functional DNA methylation differences between tissues, cell types, and across individuals discovered using the M&M algorithm. *Genome Res.* **2013**, *23*, 1522–1540. [PubMed]

90. Lehmann-Werman, R.; Neiman, D.; Zemmour, H.; Moss, J.; Magenheim, J.; Vaknin-Dembinsky, A.; Rubertsson, S.; Nellgard, B.; Blennow, K.; Zetterberg, H.; et al. Identification of tissue-specific cell death using methylation patterns of circulating DNA. *Proc. Natl. Acad. Sci. USA* **2016**, *113*, E1826–E1834. [CrossRef]

91. Moss, J.; Magenheim, J.; Neiman, D.; Zemmour, H.; Loyfer, N.; Korach, A.; Samet, Y.; Maoz, M.; Druid, H.; Arner, P.; et al. Comprehensive human cell-type methylation atlas reveals origins of circulating cell-free DNA in health and disease. *Nat. Commun.* **2018**, *9*, 5068. [CrossRef] [PubMed]

92. Teschendorff, A.E.; Breeze, C.E.; Zheng, S.C.; Beck, S. A comparison of reference-based algorithms for correcting cell-type heterogeneity in Epigenome-Wide Association Studies. *BMC Bioinform.* **2017**, *18*, 105. [CrossRef]

93. Sun, K.; Jiang, P.; Chan, K.C.; Wong, J.; Cheng, Y.K.; Liang, R.H.; Chan, W.K.; Ma, E.S.; Chan, S.L.; Cheng, S.H.; et al. Plasma DNA tissue mapping by genome-wide methylation sequencing for noninvasive prenatal, cancer, and transplantation assessments. *Proc. Natl. Acad. Sci. USA* **2015**, *112*, E5503–E5512. [CrossRef] [PubMed]

94. Guo, S.; Diep, D.; Plongthongkum, N.; Fung, H.L.; Zhang, K.; Zhang, K. Identification of methylation haplotype blocks aids in deconvolution of heterogeneous tissue samples and tumor tissue-of-origin mapping from plasma DNA. *Nat. Genet.* **2017**, *49*, 635–642. [CrossRef] [PubMed]

95. Kelly, T.K.; Liu, Y.; Lay, F.D.; Liang, G.; Berman, B.P.; Jones, P.A. Genome-wide mapping of nucleosome positioning and DNA methylation within individual DNA molecules. *Genome Res.* **2012**, *22*, 2497–2506. [CrossRef] [PubMed]

96. Ye, Z.; Chen, Z.; Sunkel, B.; Frietze, S.; Huang, T.H.; Wang, Q.; Jin, V.X. Genome-wide analysis reveals positional-nucleosome-oriented binding pattern of pioneer factor FOXA1. *Nucleic Acids Res.* **2016**, *44*, 7540–7554. [CrossRef] [PubMed]

97. Fan, H.C.; Blumenfeld, Y.J.; Chitkara, U.; Hudgins, L.; Quake, S.R. Noninvasive diagnosis of fetal aneuploidy by shotgun sequencing DNA from maternal blood. *Proc. Natl. Acad. Sci. USA* **2008**, *105*, 16266–16271. [CrossRef] [PubMed]

98. Snyder, M.W.; Kircher, M.; Hill, A.J.; Daza, R.M.; Shendure, J. Cell-free DNA Comprises an In Vivo Nucleosome Footprint that Informs Its Tissues-Of-Origin. *Cell* **2016**, *164*, 57–68. [CrossRef] [PubMed]

99. Consortium, M.; Shi, L.; Reid, L.H.; Jones, W.D.; Shippy, R.; Warrington, J.A.; Baker, S.C.; Collins, P.J.; de Longueville, F.; Kawasaki, E.S.; et al. The MicroArray Quality Control (MAQC) project shows inter- and intraplatform reproducibility of gene expression measurements. *Nat. Biotechnol.* **2006**, *24*, 1151–1161. [CrossRef] [PubMed]

100. Heitzer, E.; Perakis, S.; Geigl, J.B.; Speicher, M.R. The potential of liquid biopsies for the early detection of cancer. *NPJ Precis. Oncol.* **2017**, *1*, 36. [CrossRef]

101. Koh, W.; Pan, W.; Gawad, C.; Fan, H.C.; Kerchner, G.A.; Wyss-Coray, T.; Blumenfeld, Y.J.; El-Sayed, Y.Y.; Quake, S.R. Noninvasive in vivo monitoring of tissue-specific global gene expression in humans. *Proc. Natl. Acad. Sci. USA* **2014**, *111*, 7361–7366. [CrossRef] [PubMed]

102. Sun, K.; Wang, J.; Wang, H.; Sun, H. GeneCT: A generalizable cancerous status and tissue origin classifier for pan-cancer biopsies. *Bioinformatics* **2018**, *34*, 4129–4130. [CrossRef] [PubMed]

103. Hodara, E.; Morrison, G.; Cunha, A.; Zainfeld, D.; Xu, T.; Xu, Y.; Dempsey, P.W.; Pagano, P.C.; Bischoff, F.; Khurana, A.; et al. Multiparametric liquid biopsy analysis in metastatic prostate cancer. *JCI Insight* **2019**, *4*. [CrossRef] [PubMed]

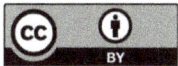

cancers

MDPI

Review

Insights into Telomerase/hTERT Alternative Splicing Regulation Using Bioinformatics and Network Analysis in Cancer

Andrew T. Ludlow *, Aaron L. Slusher and Mohammed E. Sayed

School of Kinesiology, University of Michigan, Ann Arbor, MI 48109, USA; alslush@umich.edu (A.L.S.);
mosayed@umich.edu (M.E.S.)
* Correspondence: atludlow@umich.edu

Received: 27 April 2019; Accepted: 13 May 2019; Published: 14 May 2019

Abstract: The reactivation of telomerase in cancer cells remains incompletely understood. The catalytic component of telomerase, *hTERT*, is thought to be the limiting component in cancer cells for the formation of active enzymes. *hTERT* gene expression is regulated at several levels including chromatin, DNA methylation, transcription factors, and RNA processing events. Of these regulatory events, RNA processing has received little attention until recently. RNA processing and alternative splicing regulation have been explored to understand how *hTERT* is regulated in cancer cells. The *cis-* and *trans*-acting factors that regulate the alternative splicing choice of *hTERT* in the reverse transcriptase domain have been investigated. Further, it was discovered that the splicing factors that promote the production of full-length *hTERT* were also involved in cancer cell growth and survival. The goals are to review telomerase regulation via alternative splicing and the function of *hTERT* splicing variants and to point out how bioinformatics approaches are leading the way in elucidating the networks that regulate *hTERT* splicing choice and ultimately cancer growth.

Keywords: *hTERT*; telomerase; telomeres; alternative splicing; network analysis; hierarchical clustering analysis; differential gene expression analysis

1. Introduction

Telomeres are specialized DNA and protein structures found at the ends of linear chromosomes made up of the hexameric repeat DNA 5′-TTAGGG$_n$ [1]. The main function of telomeres is to protect the ends of linear chromosomes from inappropriate recognition as broken DNA by cellular DNA damage response proteins [2]. Telomeres prevent the recognition of chromosome ends by DNA damage response proteins by being bound by a six-protein complex called shelterin. Thus, telomeres and the shelterin complex overcome the "end protection problem". Telomeres are also involved in determining the maximal number of times a cell can divide. Due to the inability of DNA polymerase to completely replicate the lagging strand of telomere DNA, a small (30–150 nucleotides) piece of DNA is lost with each round of replication (Figure 1). This phenomenon, known as the "end replication problem", results in telomere shortening overtime. Upon reaching a critically shortened length, telomere uncapping and DNA damage sensing of telomeres by p53 results in growth arrest [1–3]. Growth arrest is triggered when one or a few telomeres become short enough to be sensed as damaged DNA, resulting in replicative senescence [4]. The limited proliferative capacity, also known as the "Hayflick limit", of cells can act as a 'cellular aging/timing' mechanism in humans and other large long-lived organisms. By having a counting mechanism, cells can prevent unlimited cell growth (i.e., telomeres are short and thus sensed as DNA damage). Without such a mechanism, cells could accumulate mutations associated with cancer development. Thus, telomere shortening and replicative senescence is thought to act as a potent inhibitor of progression to malignancy [1,5].

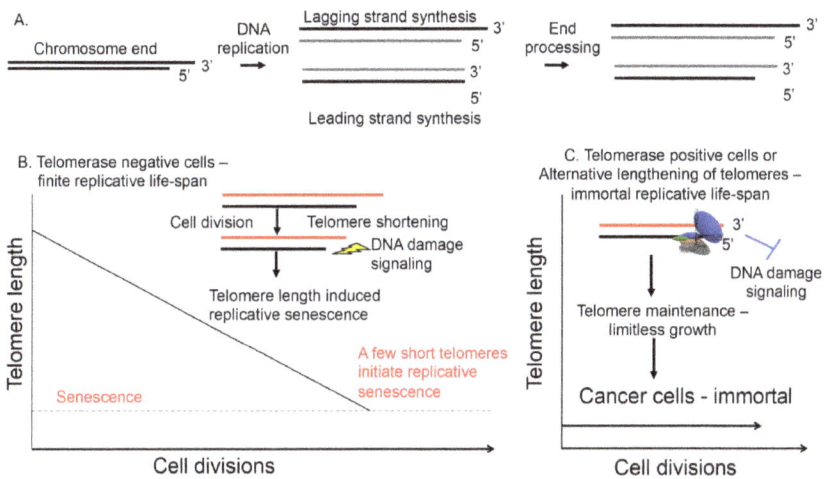

Figure 1. Telomere biology. (**A**) Telomeres are replicated during cell division (mitosis). A set of enzymes process the end of replicated chromosomes so that a 3′ G-rich overhang is produced. The single stranded 3′ end displaces the double-stranded structure to form a three-stranded structure (D-loop). Shelterin binds to both the single- and double-stranded portion of the telomere, protecting it from being recognized by the DNA damage machinery, solving the "end-protection" problem. (**B**) Telomerase negative cells or cells without a telomere maintenance mechanism. Due to the "end-replication" problem, a small piece of DNA at the lagging strand end of DNA is not replicated and is lost from the chromosome that is passed on to the daughter cells. Over time, this slow erosion results in the loss of telomere length. When a few telomeres have DNA damage at chromosome ends, deprotection occurs and cellular senescence is initiated. This removes cells with critically short telomeres from the replicating population of cells and acts as a potent block to tumor progression. (**C**) Cells become replicatively immortal by adopting a telomere maintenance mechanism. Telomeres are maintained by two mechanisms, telomerase RNP or a homology-directed mechanism called alternative lengthening of telomeres. Telomerase is the mechanism that approximately 90% of human cancer cells use to maintain telomeres and immortality. In male germline cells, telomeres are also maintained or elongated by the ribonucleoprotein telomerase.

In order to achieve immortality, cancer cells need a telomere length maintenance mechanism [6]. Nearly all cancer cells up-regulate telomerase to re-elongate or maintain telomeres by de novo synthesis of telomere repeats on to chromosome ends [1,7,8]. Although most cancer cells have detectable telomerase activity, enzyme levels vary considerably between tumors and individual cells within tumors [9]. Telomere length is also heterogenous between tumor types and within tumors [10]. Telomerase is a ribonucleoprotein (RNP) with reverse transcriptase activity that consists of two main components and several accessory proteins. The core RNP is composed of the catalytic protein subunit telomerase reverse transcriptase (hTERT) and an RNA template component (human telomerase RNA component; *hTERC, hTR*) that when assembled and recruited can elongate or maintain telomeres [7,11]. Telomerase is active during embryonic development but is rapidly repressed in most somatic tissues [12]. Only specialized subpopulations of transit amplifying stem/ progenitor cells are capable of transient telomerase expression post-development [1,13].

Telomerase is subject to a myriad of gene expression regulatory mechanisms. Little consensus exists in the field about chromatin environment, DNA methylation, DNA looping, promoter mutations, and transcription factor binding [14,15]. Despite the vast amount of research that has focused on transcriptional and epigenetic regulation of *hTERT*, little research has focused on the regulation of the resultant RNA molecules and co/post-transcriptional gene expression regulation [16,17]. hTERT mRNA levels are highest in embryonic stem cells, induced pluripotent stem cells and transit-amplifying adult progenitors, and lower in normal cells. Contrary to the dogma in the field, recent evidence indicates that there may or may not be a slight increase in *hTERT* mRNA abundance in cancer cells [18–20]. Full-length (FL) *hTERT* mRNA is the limiting factor for the formation of telomerase activity. Despite the presence of active telomerase enzymes in cancer cells and stem cells, the mRNA copy number or mRNA abundance is very low compared to other genes [21–23]. For instance, quantification of telomerase components has shown 5000–10,000 molecules of *hTR* in cells, while *hTERT* mRNA is expressed between 1–40 molecules per cell [21–23]. Although the general paradigm is that the *hTERT* is limiting for active telomerase, either component can be limiting in the formation of active telomerase [23,24]. In most normal cells, *hTR* is present in excess and thus *hTERT* is limiting. Evidence for this is the observation that *hTERT* expression is sufficient for immortalization (but not transformation) of fibroblast cells [25]. Recent evidence has demonstrated that there is a subpopulation of *hTERT* protein that is not assembled into the telomerase complexes that could be capable of maintaining telomeres. Estimates indicate that there are anywhere from 100–700 hTERT protein molecules that can interact with *hTR* in a telomerase active cell at any given time [26,27]. In order to develop better telomerase inhibitors, a more thorough understanding of hTERT gene expression regulation and function is necessary to gain insights into possible therapeutic avenues.

Due to the lack of telomerase activity in most normal cells, besides transit-amplifying stem cells and germ line cells, and the fact that the majority (~90%) of cancer cells have telomerase activity, telomerase has been a highly sought-after cancer therapeutic target. While both public and private efforts have attempted to develop inhibitors of this enzyme, the most clinically progressed drug is an anti-sense RNA (Imeltelstat, GRN163L) of the template RNA, *hTR* [10,28–30]. Other small molecule drugs and vaccine-like approaches to target telomerase positive cancer cells have been attempted but have failed due to dose-limiting toxicities and other off target effects on normal cells [30–33]. Further, clinical trials of Imetlestat are still underway and this drug may be best for cancers with already very short telomeres [10]. Thus, the potential therapeutic benefits of targeting telomerase have not been realized with current strategies. The major issue with direct inhibition of telomerase activity is the long lag period that it takes to treat cells with inhibitors before telomeres are critically shortened and cancer cells begin to die [1]. Recent advances in the field, however, have led to a resurgence in interest towards finding a therapeutic window and means to inhibit telomerase/target telomere biology as a cancer therapy. For instance, the observations that certain cancer cells/tumors appear to be addicted to hTERT/telomerase as indicated by rapid telomere length-independent apoptosis, suggests that there may be other strategies to target cancer cells [34]. *hTERT* promoter somatic mutations in cancer cells also provide a new approach to targeting hTERT/telomerase positive cancer cells with minimal off target effects. Additionally, a new class of drugs called telomere uncapping drugs are showing significant benefits in pre-clinical studies. Leading the way in this class is a nucleotide analogue, 6-thio-deoxyguanosine (6-thio-dG) [35]. This nucleotide is preferentially incorporated by telomerase into telomeres, which is hypothesized to generate a mutant telomere sequence. Shelterin components cannot bind to mutant (6-thio-dG containing) telomeres which contributes to rapid telomere uncapping, DNA damage signaling at the telomeres, and cell death in telomerase-expressing cancer cells [35]. Thus, a more thorough biochemical analysis of the *hTERT* regulatory mechanisms is being sought to find new and more potent telomerase/TERT/telomere biology drugs.

One area of gene expression regulation that has mostly been ignored is alternative RNA splicing of *hTERT*. Alternative RNA splicing has recently been observed to impact at least 95% of human multi-exon genes and serves as a mechanism to control gene expression in several evolutionary conserved ways [36]. For example, alternative splicing generates proteome diversity by making several proteins from the same transcriptional unit/gene, allowing ~20,000 genes to code for more than 100,000 proteins [37]. While gene number does not scale with organism complexity, intron number and thus splicing, does scale with organism complexity [38]. Alternative splicing of a gene can lead to proteins with similar function or even opposing functions (dominant-negative isoforms). Alternative splicing can also regulate the abundance of functional gene products by splicing to isoforms that have premature stop codons (degraded by non-sense mediated mRNA decay [39]). Ultimately, alternative splicing offers a biological mechanism utilized by cells to regulate the functional outcomes of each gene. hTERT/telomerase offers a good model gene that utilizes alternative splicing as part of its regulatory repertoire, which is of particular importance in cancer biology and stem cells.

2. Alternative Splicing is Dysregulated in Cancer Leading to the Re-Emergence of Splice Variants Normally Found in Development but Silenced in Normal Cells

Alternative splicing is dysregulated in cancers [40]. Alternative splicing is regulated by the combination of cellular context, *cis*-elements, and *trans*-factor/RNA binding proteins [41]. Alternative splicing is also co-transcriptionally regulated according to the kinetic coupling model [42]. As RNA polymerase II transcribes a new pre-mRNA molecule, the spliceosome is recruited to the pre-mRNA, even docking on the C-terminal domain of RNA polymerase II and dictating the inclusion and exclusion of exons [43]. Further, the rate of RNA polymerase across a gene body, along with the chromatin environment, DNA methylation patterns, and other unknown factors, can significantly impact the alternative splicing pattern of a gene [44]. The spliceosome is a megadalton molecular machine that is composed of five small nuclear ribonucleic particle (snRNP) core components (U1, U2, U4, U5 and U6) and an additional ~700 proteins [45]. The spliceosome components are recruited with RNA polymerase II to the growing pre-mRNA and assembled in a step-wise manner at the 5′ and 3′ splice sites, branch point, and polypyrimidine tract in order to complete intron lariat formation and removal, and joining of exons in the processed transcript [45] (Figure 2). Exon joining may be constitutive, meaning the exons are always included in the mRNA of a gene or alternative (only included sometimes in the mRNA of a gene), giving rise to alternative splice variants (ASVs; [45]). Other types of splicing events can occur such as intron retention, alternative 5′ or 3′ splicing sites, alternative promoters/first exons, and alternative polyadenylation/3′ exon (Figure 2). Splice site selection is a complex process but generally the proximity of local sequence elements (*cis*) such as exonic splicing enhancers/silencers (ESE/ESI) and intronic splicing enhancers/silencers (ISE/ISI) and the RNA binding proteins in the cell at any given time dictate splicing choice (Figure 2; [46]). There are at least 700 known splicing factors/RNA binding proteins that can participate in alternative splicing [47]. We are only at the beginning of understanding the roles and regulation of splicing in normal cells and the many ways cancer cells utilize dysregulated splicing to promote growth and survival. Nearly all of the hallmarks of cancer cells have dysregulated splicing products that have been identified, including hTERT and cellular immortality [48]. These mechanistic insights may pave the way for new therapeutic avenues into treating cancer, or specific aspects of cancer cells.

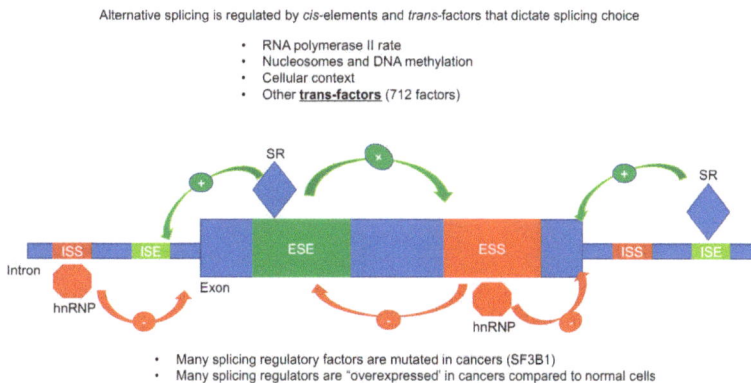

Alternative splicing is regulated by *cis*-elements and *trans*-factors that dictate splicing choice

- RNA polymerase II rate
- Nucleosomes and DNA methylation
- Cellular context
- Other **trans-factors** (712 factors)

- Many splicing regulatory factors are mutated in cancers (SF3B1)
- Many splicing regulators are "overexpressed" in cancers compared to normal cells

Figure 2. Alternative splicing regulation. A cartoon image of important sequence (*cis*) and protein (*trans*) regulatory features that result in exon inclusion or exclusion. The majority of the splicing information is contained in intronic and exonic sequences that are called intronic splicing silencers/enhancers (ISS/ISE) and exonic splicing silencers/enhancers (ESS/ESE). Specialized RNA binding proteins bind to these sequence elements and recruit in the megadalton spliceosome. Serine/Arginine-Rich (SR) proteins are typically splicing enhancers (enhanced exon inclusion) while hnRNP proteins are typically splicing silencers (repress exon inclusion, promote exon skipping/alternative RNA splicing). There are at least 700 RNA binding proteins in the human genome that can act as splicing *trans* factors, thus the repertoire of splicing regulatory features is vast.

3. Alternative Splicing of hTERT

The reverse transcriptase component of telomerase, hTERT, is subjected to regulation by alternative splicing. It is important to note that the murine TERT (mTERT) gene is not alternatively spliced in the same fashion as human TERT (hTERT) [20]. Thus, we will focus solely on the splicing of human TERT in this review. There are 22 known splice isoforms of hTERT that have been detected in a variety of cell types [49]. hTERT is a 16 exon (15 intron) gene (Figure 3 and Table 1). hTERT consists of four major protein domains (TEN domain, RNA binding domain, reverse transcriptase domain, and C-terminal domain; Figure 3). Only the full-length 16 exon isoform of TERT that codes for a protein that can be assembled into telomerase ribonucleoproteins is capable of maintaining or elongating telomeres (Table 1; [17]). hTERT is spliced into active and inactive forms simultaneously in telomerase positive cells (i.e., cancer cells, embryonic stem cells, iPS cells, male germ line precursor cells, transit-amplifying adult stem cells, and activated immune T cells). The full-length protein coding hTERT mRNA is expressed in the range of 1–90% of the steady state transcripts depending on cell line/tissue studied [19,21,22].

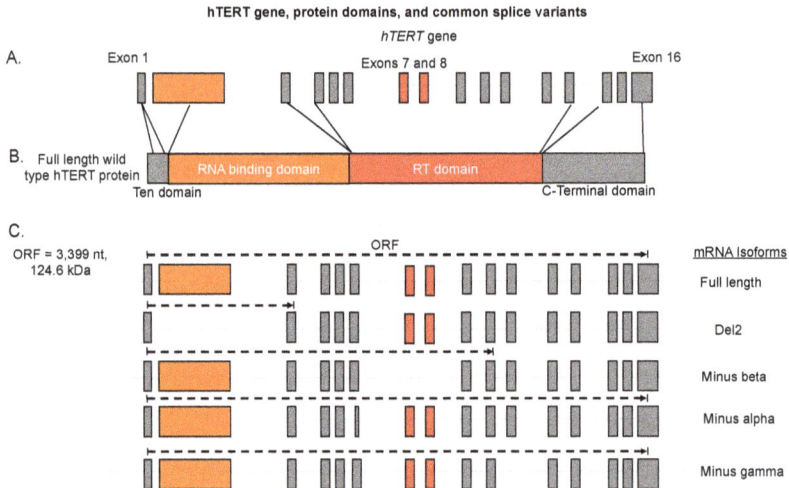

Figure 3. hTERT gene, protein domains and commonly studied splice variants. (**A**) Cartoon image of hTERT exons and introns. hTERT is a 16 exon/15 intron gene that generates the reverse transcriptase component of the telomerase enzyme. Exon 2 is highlighted in orange as it is the major contributor to the telomerase RNA binding domain (TRBD). Exons 7 and 8 are highlighted in red as these two exons represent one of the most commonly studied splicing events in the hTERT gene and they encode for critical residues in the reverse transcriptase domain (RT). (**B**) Protein domains of hTERT. Lines linking exons to the domains they encode are shown. Critical domains are the TEN (exon 1), RNA binding (exons 2 and 3), RT (exons 4–13), and c-terminal (exons 14–16). All four of these domains are essential for telomerase activity, processivity, recruitment, and function. (**C**) Open reading frames of abundant hTERT alternative RNA splicing isoforms.

Table 1. Description of major *hTERT* splice isoforms.

Isoform	Exon Structure	Intron Retention?	Biochemical Function
Full-length	1–16. Original ORF.	No	Functional hTERT protein, maintains telomeres when in active telomerase holoenzyme (RNP)
Minus beta	1–6, 9, and 10; PTC in 10. Skipping of exons 7 and 8.	No	Mostly degraded by non-sense mediated decay, some translated into protein and may play a role in DNA damage repair/ protection from apoptosis, may bind *hTERC (hTR)*
Minus alpha	1–16, alternative 3′ splice acceptor site in exon 6 generates in frame shift of 36 nucleotides. Original ORF.	No	Dominant-negative, binds *hTERC (hTR)*
INS3	1–16 plus, PTC in intron 14.	Retention of intron 14 nucleotide 623 to end of intron 14.	Dominant-negative, binds *hTERC (hTR)*
INS4	1–14, and alternative exon 16 3′ splice site NT492, PTC in exon 14.	Retention of intron 14 nucleotides 1–600.	Dominant-negative, binds *hTERC (hTR)*
DEL2	1,3–16, PTC in exon 3.	No	Proposed mitochondrial *hTERT* variant, retains *hTERT* MLS in exon 1.
Delta4–13	1–3, 14–16, original ORF.	No	Proposed to stimulate proliferation. Interacts with WNT/Beta catenin.
Minus Gamma	Skipping of exon 11. Original ORF.	No	Tissue specific and may inhibit telomerase action at the telomeres.

PTC—premature termination codon. RNP—ribonucleoprotein. NT—nucleotide.

The alternative RNA splicing isoforms that are expressed in each cell type are not well described but are likely to be tissue- and cell line-specific. The most commonly studied isoforms of hTERT result from alternative splicing in the reverse transcriptase domain (RT) between exons 5 and 9 [19,50]. Alternative splicing in the RT domain consists of splicing in regions called the alpha and beta regions (Table 1; Figure 3). The hTERT alpha region is a cryptic splice site within exon 6 that results in deletion of the 5′ 36 nucleotides resulting in the minus alpha variant [51]. This alternative variant is in the canonical hTERT reading frame and codes for a dominant-negative protein that can interact with hTR, and when overexpressed, results in telomere shortening in telomerase positive cells [51]. However, this variant is not very abundant, accounting for less than 5% of the steady state transcripts in cancer cells [22]. The beta region consists of exons 7 and 8 of hTERT and these exons are skipped in the minus beta variant of hTERT. The skipping of exons 7 and 8 of hTERT puts a premature stop codon in exon 10 in frame and thus results in the majority of the steady state mRNA of this transcript being targeted for non-sense-mediated decay [22,51]. However, recent evidence in certain cancer cells indicates that not all of this transcript is degraded and some may interact with polyribosomes and be translated into truncated hTERT proteins [50]. The suspected function of minus beta truncated hTERT proteins is similar to that of minus alpha in that it would contain exon 2 and the RNA binding domain, and thus could interact with hTR and compete with full-length telomerase for telomere binding [26]. Other evidence indicates that minus beta may be interacting with DNA damage and repair complexes and be protecting cells that express this variant from certain types of genotoxic stressors [50,52]. However, these results are controversial since an antibody to minus beta hTERT does not exist. The abundance of minus beta varies from cell type to cell type but can be anywhere from 10% to 90% of the steady state transcript levels [19,50]. The combination of minus alpha and minus beta splicing also occurs in some cell types. The abundance of minus alpha minus beta can range from 1% to 15% depending on cell type [22]. The function of this variant is assumed to be null as it should be degraded by non-sense-mediated decay pathways.

Several other variants outside of these have been described in the literature such as the minus gamma variant, Del2, INS3, INS4, and delta4–13 (Table 1) [49,53]. The gamma deletion variant results from skipping of exon 11 and is in the original reading frame of hTERT [16]. This splicing event impacts the RT domain, is highly tissue-specific, and may act as a dominant-negative protein if it is expressed at sufficient levels in cells. Recently, the Del2 (deletion of exon 2) alternative splicing variant (ASV) of TERT was quantified in several cancer cell lines [21]. Exon 2 codes for part of the RNA binding domain of hTERT. ASVs lacking this exon would be unable to interact with hTR and thus would not have canonical telomerase activity. This variant was estimated at 40 copies per cell in certain cell lines investigated but was absent in other lines, thus its expression is tissue- and cell line-specific [44]. The authors also went on to show that this ASV could indeed code for a protein of 12 kDa; however, no function or physiological studies were performed so the function of this protein is unknown [36]. Several intron retention variants exist in hTERT as well. Many of these variants contain premature stop codons, but two variants, INS3 and INS4, have been defined to function as dominant-negative inhibitors of telomerase activity [53]. INS3 contains a 159 bp insertion of intron 14 (622–781 nucleotides) at the end of exon 14, encoding for 44 amino acids, followed by a stop codon [52]. INS4 contains a 600 bp insertion of the entire intron 14, encoding for 17 amino acids, followed by a stop codon [12]. The expression of INS3 and INS4 is tissue-specific and when expressed may account for 1–15% of the total steady state levels of hTERT mRNAs. Another recent study exploring the identity of hTERT ASVs in a variety of human cell lines discovered several new variants including delta4–13 [49]. The authors demonstrated that hTERT was transcribed in all lines investigated, even telomerase negative lines, but that the transcript in the negative lines was alternatively spliced to the delta4–13 ASV which lacks the RT domain and thus cannot produce active telomerase. The delta4–13 ASV codes for a truncated hTERT protein that seemingly interacts with WNT/beta-catenin pathway and stimulates the proliferation of cells in culture. While hTERT alternative splicing variants have been documented in various tissues and cell lines to date, technological and methodological limitations make some of the above conflicting findings difficult to interpret. Moving forward and as described below, RNA sequencing technologies and new informatic techniques will pave the way for a more thorough understanding of hTERT ASVs.

3.1. hTERT Alternative Splicing during Human Embryogenesis and Development Indicates that Telomerase Activity is Regulated by Alternative Splicing

hTERT is regulated by alternative splicing during human embryonic development. During tissue development and the first phases of differentiation, hTERT is transcribed and spliced to multiple forms [54,55]. The most commonly studied isoforms arising from exons 5–9 have been documented. For example, full-length (FL) hTERT and minus beta hTERT are present along with telomerase activity during kidney development. At about week 17 of development, there is a massive shift in hTERT splicing where the full-length (exon 7/8 containing) transcript is eliminated and only minus beta remains. This shift in splicing coincides with a complete loss of telomerase activity [54]. These observations can be interpreted to indicate that alternative splicing regulates telomerase activity. However, the splicing factors that regulate the turning off of telomerase activity during tissue differentiation and specification are completely unknown. Further, the expression and splicing of other hTERT ASVs is not well studied during the differentiation and development of human tissues. This area deserves further investigation as telomerase halopinsufficiency leads to stem cell diseases and risk of early cancers in patients. Thus, further characterization of hTERT regulation in stem cells may lead to early interventions and cancer prevention.

3.2. A Paradigm Shift: hTERT Is Regulated by Alternative Splicing in Cancers

A long-held paradigm in the telomere/telomerase field was and still is that hTERT and telomerase is regulated by transcription. It appeared that hTERT was transcriptionally silenced following fetal development and this was the mechanism that prevented hTERT expression and thus telomerase activity, and allowed for progressive telomere shortening that is observed in the soma [16,17]. However, recent evidence from several groups indicates that this may have been a mis-interpretation of the assays used to measure hTERT steady state transcripts. The most common assays to measure hTERT transcripts are designed to detect exons 5–9 in the RT domain, however, we now know that those exons are spliced out of most transcripts of hTERT [20,49]. Thus, previous research using primers in exons 5–9 led to missing transcripts that contained other regions of hTERT mRNA and the interpretation that hTERT is transcriptionally silenced in normal somatic cells. We and others have reported that hTERT is indeed transcribed in all cells but it is spliced to forms that do not encode for reverse transcriptase activity [18,49]. Further, exon 1 of hTERT is extremely G/C rich making it difficult to detect without using PCR additives and modified polymerases at higher than normal annealing temperatures. We have quantitated that normal cells and tissues express between 50–90% of the abundance of hTERT transcripts as cancer cells and that ultimately an upregulation of transcription of hTERT in cancer cells is minimal in terms of overall transcripts [18]. The major regulatory mechanism that leads to active telomerase and full-length hTERT production is a shift in splicing. Thus, the new working model going forward should be to understand how hTERT alternative splicing is regulated in normal cells and becomes dysregulated during the progression to malignancy, leading to tumor cell immortality.

3.3. RNA Sequencing and Other Technologies to Detect hTERT Splice Variants in Cancer

The abundance and splicing of hTERT makes it difficult to detect using standard techniques. Using short read sequencing and RT-PCR to quantify and identify splicing variants leads to bias and the potential for mis-interpretations of the data [56]. The coverage and sequencing depth of short read RNA sequencing experiments can significantly mislead research concerning hTERT splicing and must be interpreted and validated carefully. New and emerging sequencing technologies and informatics tools have significantly advanced the detection and quantification of full-length cDNAs [57]. For instance, Sayed et al. 2018 demonstrated using third generation single molecule sequencing of hTERT-specific cDNA libraries that HeLa cells splice hTERT into several variants [20]. This sequencing technology was combined with informatics analysis that allowed the authors to define the identity of full-length transcripts in cells [20]. The most common variants in the libraries were identified as a very short transcript-containing exons 1, 15 and 16, a transcript splicing from exon 4 to exon 16. Other variants where detected using this method such as full-length being the second most abundant transcript identified. Interestingly, minus beta as well as Del2 were detected but these variants in their full-length context were not as abundant as previously estimated by other techniques. These newer sequencing technologies and informatics have their own sets of caveats. Improvements in reagent chemistry, library generation techniques, and analysis software that allows mapping and quantification of detected transcripts of third generation sequencing will prove advantageous over other methods for splice isoform measures.

3.4. Regulation of hTERT Alternative Splicing by cis-Elements and trans-Factors

The general rules of splicing regulation or the splicing code are still being elucidated; several recent efforts to understand the role of *cis*-and-*trans* elements of hTERT alternative splicing regulation have been published. Two seminal studies investigated the reverse transcriptase domain alternative splicing of hTERT [17,50]. Both groups generated minigene constructs including exons 5–9 to determine what sequence elements and *trans*-factors were responsible for the formation of full-length (containing all five exons) versus the minus beta splice variants containing only exons 5, 6, and 9. In breast cancer cells, Listerman et al. focused on the formation of minus beta. Using their minigene construct they observed that the majority of the product when in the context of breast cancer cells was the full-length variant (90%) with about 10% of the observed transcripts being minus beta [50]. Next, they undertook a small-scale cDNA screen of common splicing enhancers (Serine/Arginine-rich (SR) proteins) and splicing repressors (hnRNP proteins; Figure 4). They observed that SRSF11 promoted the alternative splicing (repressed full-length splicing; Figure 4) and formation of minus beta in their minigene. They also observed that hnRNPH2 and hnRNPL promoted full-length splicing of their hTERT minigene [29].

This study also observed that not all of the minus beta transcript was degraded by non-sense mediated decay and may make a dominant-negative protein of telomerase. Further the authors demonstrated that minus beta may protect breast cancer cells from chemotherapeutic insults [29]. Thus, future research is needed to more carefully explore the role of minus beta in cancer cells.

In a study by Wong et al., an hTERT minigene was generated and an interesting observation was made that the initial construct only formed full-length hTERT transcripts containing exons 5–9 when placed in the context of HeLa cells [58]. To determine what sequence elements may be missing in the minigene construct, the authors performed a self-blast of hTERT exons 5–10 and observed highly repetitive sequences in these exons and introns of hTERT. To determine if these repeat regions might be important in regulation, they looked at the conservation of these repeats in species that regulate TERT similar to humans (i.e., old world primates) compared to species that regulate TERT differently (i.e., rodents). The authors found several conserved repeat regions shared between old world primates and human TERT gene loci, but these elements were lacking/missing in rodents and other shorter-lived primates. Utilizing this information, the authors inserted three of the conserved elements into the hTERT minigene and observed the expected ratio of full-length to minus beta steady state expression (i.e., recapitulating the endogenous hTERT isoform expression ratio). These *cis*-elements were termed block 6 repeats (a variable number tandem repeat in intron 6), direct repeat 6 (DR6), and direct repeat 8. The direct repeats are 256 nucleotides within intron 6 and 285 nucleotides within intron 8 respectively, and consist of 85% homologous sequences [58]. Through deletion analysis, the authors determined the impact of each element on steady state hTERT isoform expression. It was observed that the 1.1 kb VNTR (38 nucleotide repeat) termed block 6 repeats was essential for exclusion/skipping of exons 7 and 8 and production of the minus beta deletion containing transcripts. Further, DR8 was important for the formation of exon 7- and 8-containing transcripts, or potential full-length transcripts. To follow up these observations, the authors went on to show that a minimal number of VNTR block 6 repeats were needed to promote minus beta splicing (skipping of exons 7 and 8) and that blocking DR8 with an anti-sense oligonucleotide could promote skipping of exons 7 and 8, indicating that DR8 is likely a docking site for *trans*-factors [58]. In a second study, Wong et al. utilized RNA secondary structure modeling to predict how the pre-mRNA could be folding following transcription [59]. They then utilized a modified mutation complementation assay to demonstrate that the VNTR block 6 repeats could potentially form RNA:RNA pairing, making the splicing of the exon 6 5′ splice site be in closer proximity to the exon 9 3′ splice site [59]. Combined, these foundational data indicate that alternative splicing of hTERT, which is a very low abundant transcript, does not follow the typical splicing rules of more abundant transcripts. These studies determined a few *trans*-factors and the pivotal sequence elements in determination of the splicing choice of exons 7 and 8 of hTERT.

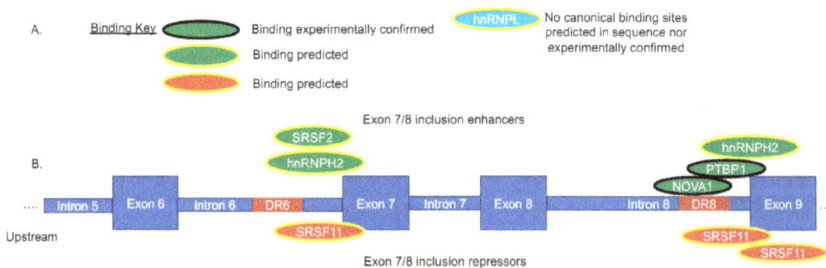

Figure 4. Reverse transcriptase alternative splicing regulation of hTERT. (**A**) Key of RNA binding proteins associated with hTERT. Enhancers are depicted in green. Repressors in red. Blue indicates a likely indirect impact on TERT splicing caused by the manipulation of a splicing factor. (**B**) Cartoon image of introns 5 through exon 9 of hTERT in the reverse transcriptase domain (RT). On top of the cartoon image are the hTERT exon 7/8 enhancers. On the bottom are the proteins that repress the inclusion of exons 7/8.

To begin to elucidate additional *trans*-factors, Ludlow et al. used a dual-reporter minigene loss of the function screen focused on 516 splicing factors [19]. The list of RNA binding proteins was derived based on both empirically determined RNA binding proteins via literature searches and searching protein data bases (Genecards, etc.) that resulted in the curation of a list of 516 putative RNA binding proteins. Following the screen, there were 110 individual genes that resulted in a two-fold change in reporter activity. Since the goal of this initial study was to understand splicing factors/RNA binding proteins involved in the promotion of full-length TERT and telomerase activity, they focused on 93 genes that resulted in a two-fold change in minus beta to full length splicing. A systematic approach utilizing bioinformatics techniques and network analysis was then utilized to focus the analysis and narrow down the list of candidate genes (detailed below in Section 4).

4. Using Bioinformatics to Discover hTERT Alternative Splicing Regulation in Cancers

Following high throughput screening, target identification is an important yet difficult process. Several approaches can be taken to narrow down candidates. To begin to narrow down our list of candidate genes, we utilized a panel of well characterized lung cancer cells and developed highly quantitative droplet digital PCR measures of hTERT exon inclusion/exclusion events [19]. From these measures, we were able to segregate cell lines into high hTERT full length (FL) lines and low hTERT FL lines. Using publicly available gene expression data from the same lung cancer cell lines, we used hierarchical clustering analysis based on the expression level of the 516 splicing factors. We then compared and overlapped the minigene hits to the differential expression analysis. This analysis narrowed down the list from 93 potential candidate genes to 12 genes that were differentially expressed between high and low TERT FL lines. This led us to identify one gene, NOVA1, that was related to hTERT FL splicing in non-small cell lung cancer cells that express NOVA1. We then hypothesized that NOVA1, hTERT FL, telomerase activity, and telomere length interacted to define subsets of lung cancer cells that may be more or less similar in terms of splicing factor expression. Again, we utilized hierarchical clustering analysis based on the expression of NOVA1, hTERT FL, telomerase activity, and telomere length, and clustered lung cancer cell lines into categories expressing high and low levels of these variables. We then used differential expression analysis focusing on the expression of the 516 splicing factors and found a set of splicing genes that were differentially expressed between these high and low cell lines [19]. This analysis identified a network of genes that are related to the alternative splicing of hTERT and may lead to the identification of potential lead candidate genes for targeted therapies given hTERT/telomerase specificity to cancer. These analyses were done with a combination of in-laboratory measures and publicly available data. Other studies have done similar analyses to try to understand hTERT alternative splicing in cancer.

Investigating the genetic landscape at the hTERT locus, a group utilized largescale analysis and fine mapping to elucidate the relationships between single nucleotide polymorphisms (SNPs) and telomere length, hTERT expression, and alternative splicing [60]. The authors combined cohorts to generate a large study population that had data on 110 SNPs in hTERT and correlated these SNPs to telomere length, hTERT expression and splicing from available RNA sequencing data. Further, the SNPs were also correlated (step-wise regression analysis) to cancer risk for specific cancers. Interestingly, an SNP in intron 4 was found to impact the alternative splicing of hTERT. The minor allele of this SNP was found to impact the splicing choice of hTERT by introducing the use of a novel alternative splice donor. In a follow up study, it was observed that this SNP generated a new splice variant termed INS1B which is a variant of a known hTERT ASV called INS1 [61]. The expression of INS1B reduced telomerase activity when the authors used oligonucleotides to switch the splicing to favor INS1B. The authors concluded that this SNP results in subtle inadequacies in telomerase activity in normal cells, which over time results in an increased risk for genome instability and cancer [61].

Other research has used The Cancer Genome Atlas or Pan Cancer Atlas to study telomere and telomerase biology including hTERT alternative splicing. Barthel et al. utilized these public resources to analyze a variety of regulatory features that lead to the expression of hTERT in cancer cells [62].

Concerning the alternative splicing of hTERT, the authors reported that the full length transcript was the most abundant in the samples with detectable levels of hTERT. This is in contrast to the common thought paradigm that the minus beta transcript is most abundant in cancer cells. However, more recent data and improved reagents and techniques are providing more evidence that FL may indeed be more abundant compared to commonly measured alternatively spliced transcripts. Several technical limitations should be mentioned briefly. hTERT is an extremely low abundant transcript making it difficult to detect and quantify accurately. RNA sequencing technologies are limited in the sensitivity for low abundance targets and thus caution must be taken when interpreting hTERT expression estimates from large consortia RNA sequencing data. Furthermore, predicting the functional outcome of full-length hTERT must also be interpreted cautiously. hTERT protein can be assembled into active telomerase molecules but it also has telomere-independent roles in cells [26,63]. That being said, this group attempted to derive a gene expression signature to predict telomerase activity levels [62]. This expression signature generated a telomerase activity score and was correlated to expression levels of hTERT and hTERC (telomerase RNA component) in the Pan-cancer analysis [62]. Overall, this paper utilized a wide variety of bioinformatic tools and public data to make inferences about the activation of telomerase in cancer and how hTERT and hTERT splicing may be related to cellular immortality of tumors. Very recently, a group published an additional *trans*-factor that may bind hTERT pre-mRNA to regulate the splicing choice of exons 7/8 of hTERT. Wang et al. reported that an antisense oligonucleotide aimed at the intronic cluster of SRSF2 binding sites in intron 6 of hTERT results in reduced FL hTERT splicing and increased alternative splicing [64]. These data combined indicate that alternative splicing is an emerging important regulatory paradigm for hTERT and telomerase and that it may indeed be targetable for cancer therapeutics.

5. Utilizing Predictive Models of RNA Folding and RNA *trans*-Factor Binding

Alternative splicing is regulated by the combination of *cis*- and *trans*-acting factors along with the combination and competition of *trans*-RNA binding proteins available in a given cell or tissue at a given time (i.e., context). Many computational biology groups have attempted to model and predict both RNA folding in vivo and RNA *trans*-factor binding (recently reviewed in References [65,66]). There are many programs that have resulted from such efforts. Groups have utilized these programs to predict the hTERT RNA secondary structure to help explain alternative RNA splicing. Wong et al. in 2013 and 2014 utilized RNAfold to predict the potential structure of hTERT exons and introns 5–9 [59]. They observed the potential for RNA:RNA pairing within intron 6 and between introns 6 and 8. They inferred that this model could explain why cancer cells tend to skip exons 7 and 8 and allow for the joining of exons 6 and 9. Many tools have since evolved from these initial predictive models, and as machine learning capabilities improve, better and more accurate secondary structure prediction tools will become available.

Another important consideration in the regulation of alternative splicing is the contribution of RNA *trans*-acting factors or RNA binding proteins' involvement in site choice. Given its importance in gene expression regulation, many tools have been developed to predict RNA–protein interactions [66]. We used a series of freely available webtools to predict where NOVA1 may be interacting with hTERT. NOVA1 is an RNA binding protein involved in neuronal development [67–69]. It was initially described in small cell lung cancer patients with neurological complications [67]. NOVA1 was later associated with breast and lung cancers in general. The binding motif of NOVA1 is YCAY (where Y is a C or a U in RNA) and NOVA1 has been extensively characterized in neurons [70]. We experimentally determined that NOVA1 in fact interacts with hTERT pre-mRNAs at DR8 [19]. Experimental confirmation of RNA binding–protein interaction predictions is critical as RNA:protein interactions are not completely understood and are difficult to predict. Since a number of prediction models exist, utilizing several predictive models could provide a higher level of confidence of interaction when experimental techniques are not available. Overall, the RNA biologist tool kit continues to grow and many of these tools are freely available and can be found at Galaxy, RNA Galaxy workbench 2.0.

6. Conclusions

Telomerase regulation in cancer cell progression is incompletely understood. The emergence of hTERT full length mRNA and telomerase activity is a multi-step process that leads to telomere length maintenance and survival of cancer cells. The role of alternative RNA splicing in the production of full-length hTERT mRNA is not completely defined. Understanding how cells choose to splice hTERT pre-mRNAs to either functional telomerase-generating mRNAs or to alternatively spliced products will inform tumor progression models of cancer. Further, hTERT is a low abundant gene with several regulatory features that make it an interesting model gene for understanding non-canonical splicing processes. Elucidating the role of alternative RNA splicing in telomerase biology will take a combination of molecular and cellular studies coupled with bioinformatics, network analysis, the generation of new tools potentially involving machine learning, and access to large cohorts of patient samples. Overall, the knowledge gained by studying the role of hTERT alternative RNA splicing in cancer cells and during cancer progression may lead to new therapeutic targets of telomere biology and could lead to novel paradigms of gene expression regulation of low abundance genes.

Author Contributions: Conceptualization, A.T.L.; writing—original draft preparation, A.T.L.; writing—review and editing, M.E.S., A.L.S.

Funding: This review was funded by National Institutes of Health/National Cancer Institute, grant number: 5R00CA197672-04.

Conflicts of Interest: The authors declare no conflict of interest.

References

1. Shay, J.W.; Wright, W.E. Telomeres and telomerase: Three decades of progress. *Nat. Rev. Genet.* **2019**, *20*, 299–309. [CrossRef]
2. De Lange, T. How shelterin solves the telomere end-protection problem. *Cold Spring Harb. Symp. Quant. Biol.* **2010**, *75*, 167–177. [CrossRef]
3. Blackburn, E.H.; Epel, E.S.; Lin, J. Human telomere biology: A contributory and interactive factor in aging, disease risks, and protection. *Science* **2015**, *350*, 1193–1198. [CrossRef] [PubMed]
4. Zou, Y.; Sfeir, A.; Gryaznov, S.M.; Shay, J.W.; Wright, W.E. Does a sentinel or a subset of short telomeres determine replicative senescence? *Mol. Biol. Cell* **2004**, *15*, 3709–3718. [CrossRef]
5. Wright, W.E.; Shay, J.W. The two-stage mechanism controlling cellular senescence and immortalization. *Exp. Gerontol.* **1992**, *27*, 383–389. [CrossRef]
6. Hanahan, D.; Weinberg, R.A. Hallmarks of cancer: The next generation. *Cell* **2011**, *144*, 646–674. [CrossRef]
7. Greider, C.W.; Blackburn, E.H. Identification of a specific telomere terminal transferase activity in Tetrahymena extracts. *Cell* **1985**, *43*, 405–413. [CrossRef]
8. Kim, N.W.; Piatyszek, M.A.; Prowse, K.R.; Harley, C.B.; West, M.D.; Ho, P.L.; Coviello, G.M.; Wright, W.E.; Weinrich, S.L.; Shay, J.W. Specific association of human telomerase activity with immortal cells and cancer. *Science* **1994**, *266*, 2011–2015. [CrossRef] [PubMed]
9. Ludlow, A.T.; Robin, J.D.; Sayed, M.; Litterst, C.M.; Shelton, D.N.; Shay, J.W.; Wright, W.E. Quantitative telomerase enzyme activity determination using droplet digital PCR with single cell resolution. *Nucleic Acids Res.* **2014**, *42*, e104. [CrossRef]
10. Frink, R.E.; Peyton, M.; Schiller, J.H.; Gazdar, A.F.; Shay, J.W.; Minna, J.D. Telomerase inhibitor imetelstat has preclinical activity across the spectrum of non-small cell lung cancer oncogenotypes in a telomere length dependent manner. *Oncotarget* **2016**, *7*, 31639–31651. [CrossRef]
11. Greider, C.W.; Blackburn, E.H. The telomere terminal transferase of Tetrahymena is a ribonucleoprotein enzyme with two kinds of primer specificity. *Cell* **1987**, *51*, 887–898. [CrossRef]
12. Wright, W.E.; Piatyszek, M.A.; Rainey, W.E.; Byrd, W.; Shay, J.W. Telomerase activity in human germline and embryonic tissues and cells. *Dev. Genet.* **1996**, *18*, 173–179. [CrossRef]
13. Hiyama, K.; Hirai, Y.; Kyoizumi, S.; Akiyama, M.; Hiyama, E.; Piatyszek, M.A.; Shay, J.W.; Ishioka, S.; Yamakido, M. Activation of telomerase in human lymphocytes and hematopoietic progenitor cells. *J. Immunol.* **1995**, *155*, 3711–3715. [PubMed]

14. Avin, B.A.; Umbricht, C.B.; Zeiger, M.A. Human telomerase reverse transcriptase regulation by DNA methylation, transcription factor binding and alternative splicing (Review). *Int. J. Oncol.* **2016**, *49*, 2199–2205. [CrossRef] [PubMed]

15. Leao, R.; Apolonio, J.D.; Lee, D.; Figueiredo, A.; Tabori, U.; Castelo-Branco, P. Mechanisms of human telomerase reverse transcriptase (hTERT) regulation: Clinical impacts in cancer. *J. Biomed. Sci.* **2018**, *25*, 22. [CrossRef] [PubMed]

16. Liu, X.; Wang, Y.; Chang, G.; Wang, F.; Wang, F.; Geng, X. Alternative Splicing of hTERT Pre-mRNA: A Potential Strategy for the Regulation of Telomerase Activity. *Int. J. Mol. Sci.* **2017**, *18*. [CrossRef] [PubMed]

17. Wong, M.S.; Wright, W.E.; Shay, J.W. Alternative splicing regulation of telomerase: A new paradigm? *Trends Genet.* **2014**, *30*, 430–438. [CrossRef]

18. Kim, W.; Ludlow, A.T.; Min, J.; Robin, J.D.; Stadler, G.; Mender, I.; Lai, T.P.; Zhang, N.; Wright, W.E.; Shay, J.W. Regulation of the Human Telomerase Gene TERT by Telomere Position Effect-Over Long Distances (TPE-OLD): Implications for Aging and Cancer. *PLoS Biol.* **2016**, *14*, e2000016. [CrossRef] [PubMed]

19. Ludlow, A.T.; Wong, M.S.; Robin, J.D.; Batten, K.; Yuan, L.; Lai, T.-P.; Dahlson, N.; Zhang, L.; Mender, I.; Tedone, E.; et al. NOVA1 regulates hTERT splicing and cell growth in non-small cell lung cancer. *Nat. Commun.* **2018**, *9*, 3112. [CrossRef]

20. Sayed, M.E.; Yuan, L.; Robin, J.D.; Tedone, E.; Batten, K.; Dahlson, N.; Wright, W.E.; Shay, J.W.; Ludlow, A.T. NOVA1 directs PTBP1 to hTERT pre-mRNA and promotes telomerase activity in cancer cells. *Oncogene* **2019**, *38*, 2937–2952. [CrossRef]

21. Withers, J.B.; Ashvetiya, T.; Beemon, K.L. Exclusion of exon 2 is a common mRNA splice variant of primate telomerase reverse transcriptases. *PLoS ONE* **2012**, *7*, e48016. [CrossRef]

22. Yi, X.; Shay, J.W.; Wright, W.E. Quantitation of telomerase components and hTERT mRNA splicing patterns in immortal human cells. *Nucleic Acids Res.* **2001**, *29*, 4818–4825. [CrossRef] [PubMed]

23. Yi, X.; Tesmer, V.M.; Savre-Train, I.; Shay, J.W.; Wright, W.E. Both transcriptional and posttranscriptional mechanisms regulate human telomerase template RNA levels. *Mol. Cell. Biol.* **1999**, *19*, 3989–3997. [CrossRef] [PubMed]

24. Greider, C.W. Telomerase RNA levels limit the telomere length equilibrium. *Cold Spring Harb. Symp. Quant. Biol.* **2006**, *71*, 225–229. [CrossRef]

25. Bodnar, A.G.; Ouellette, M.; Frolkis, M.; Holt, S.E.; Chiu, C.P.; Morin, G.B.; Harley, C.B.; Shay, J.W.; Lichtsteiner, S.; Wright, W.E. Extension of life-span by introduction of telomerase into normal human cells. *Science* **1998**, *279*, 349–352. [CrossRef]

26. Akincilar, S.C.; Low, K.C.; Liu, C.Y.; Yan, T.D.; Oji, A.; Ikawa, M.; Li, S.; Tergaonkar, V. Quantitative assessment of telomerase components in cancer cell lines. *FEBS Lett.* **2015**, *589*, 974–984. [CrossRef] [PubMed]

27. Xi, L.; Cech, T.R. Inventory of telomerase components in human cells reveals multiple subpopulations of hTR and hTERT. *Nucleic Acids Res.* **2014**, *42*, 8565–8577. [CrossRef] [PubMed]

28. Burchett, K.M.; Yan, Y.; Ouellette, M.M. Telomerase inhibitor Imetelstat (GRN163L) limits the lifespan of human pancreatic cancer cells. *PLoS ONE* **2014**, *9*, e85155. [CrossRef] [PubMed]

29. Chiappori, A.A.; Kolevska, T.; Spigel, D.R.; Hager, S.; Rarick, M.; Gadgeel, S.; Blais, N.; Von Pawel, J.; Hart, L.; Reck, M.; et al. A randomized phase II study of the telomerase inhibitor imetelstat as maintenance therapy for advanced non-small-cell lung cancer. *Ann. Oncol.* **2015**, *26*, 354–362. [CrossRef]

30. Marian, C.O.; Cho, S.K.; McEllin, B.M.; Maher, E.A.; Hatanpaa, K.J.; Madden, C.J.; Mickey, B.E.; Wright, W.E.; Shay, J.W.; Bachoo, R.M. The telomerase antagonist, imetelstat, efficiently targets glioblastoma tumor-initiating cells leading to decreased proliferation and tumor growth. *Clin. Cancer Res.* **2010**, *16*, 154–163. [CrossRef]

31. Jafri, M.A.; Ansari, S.A.; Alqahtani, M.H.; Shay, J.W. Roles of telomeres and telomerase in cancer, and advances in telomerase-targeted therapies. *Genome Med.* **2016**, *8*, 69. [CrossRef]

32. Holohan, B.; Hagiopian, M.M.; Lai, T.P.; Huang, E.; Friedman, D.R.; Wright, W.E.; Shay, J.W. Perifosine as a potential novel anti-telomerase therapy. *Oncotarget* **2015**, *6*, 21816–21826. [CrossRef]

33. Buseman, C.M.; Wright, W.E.; Shay, J.W. Is telomerase a viable target in cancer? *Mutat. Res.* **2012**, *730*, 90–97. [CrossRef]

34. Reyes-Uribe, P.; Adrianzen-Ruesta, M.P.; Deng, Z.; Echevarria-Vargas, I.; Mender, I.; Saheb, S.; Liu, Q.; Altieri, D.C.; Murphy, M.E.; Shay, J.W.; et al. Exploiting TERT dependency as a therapeutic strategy for NRAS-mutant melanoma. *Oncogene* **2018**, *37*, 4058–4072. [CrossRef] [PubMed]

35. Mender, I.; Gryaznov, S.; Dikmen, Z.G.; Wright, W.E.; Shay, J.W. Induction of telomere dysfunction mediated by the telomerase substrate precursor 6-thio-2′-deoxyguanosine. *Cancer Discov.* **2015**, *5*, 82–95. [CrossRef]

36. Wang, E.T.; Sandberg, R.; Luo, S.; Khrebtukova, I.; Zhang, L.; Mayr, C.; Kingsmore, S.F.; Schroth, G.P.; Burge, C.B. Alternative isoform regulation in human tissue transcriptomes. *Nature* **2008**, *456*, 470–476. [CrossRef] [PubMed]

37. Black, D.L. Protein diversity from alternative splicing: A challenge for bioinformatics and post-genome biology. *Cell* **2000**, *103*, 367–370. [CrossRef]

38. Taft, R.J.; Pheasant, M.; Mattick, J.S. The relationship between non-protein-coding DNA and eukaryotic complexity. *Bioessays* **2007**, *29*, 288–299. [CrossRef] [PubMed]

39. Hillman, R.T.; Green, R.E.; Brenner, S.E. An unappreciated role for RNA surveillance. *Genome Biol.* **2004**, *5*, R8. [CrossRef]

40. Oltean, S.; Bates, D.O. Hallmarks of alternative splicing in cancer. *Oncogene* **2014**, *33*, 5311–5318. [CrossRef]

41. Fu, X.D.; Ares, M., Jr. Context-dependent control of alternative splicing by RNA-binding proteins. *Nat. Rev. Genet.* **2014**, *15*, 689–701. [CrossRef] [PubMed]

42. Schor, I.E.; Gomez Acuna, L.I.; Kornblihtt, A.R. Coupling between transcription and alternative splicing. *Cancer Treat. Res.* **2013**, *158*, 1–24. [CrossRef] [PubMed]

43. Nojima, T.; Rebelo, K.; Gomes, T.; Grosso, A.R.; Proudfoot, N.J.; Carmo-Fonseca, M. RNA Polymerase II Phosphorylated on CTD Serine 5 Interacts with the Spliceosome during Co-transcriptional Splicing. *Mol. Cell* **2018**, *72*, 369–379. [CrossRef] [PubMed]

44. Robert, C.; Watson, M. The incredible complexity of RNA splicing. *Genome Biol.* **2016**, *17*, 265. [CrossRef] [PubMed]

45. Shi, Y. Mechanistic insights into precursor messenger RNA splicing by the spliceosome. *Nat. Rev. Mol. Cell Biol.* **2017**, *18*, 655–670. [CrossRef] [PubMed]

46. Wang, Z.; Burge, C.B. Splicing regulation: From a parts list of regulatory elements to an integrated splicing code. *RNA* **2008**, *14*, 802–813. [CrossRef] [PubMed]

47. Dominguez, D.; Freese, P.; Alexis, M.S.; Su, A.; Hochman, M.; Palden, T.; Bazile, C.; Lambert, N.J.; Van Nostrand, E.L.; Pratt, G.A.; et al. Sequence, Structure, and Context Preferences of Human RNA Binding Proteins. *Mol. Cell* **2018**, *70*, 854–867. [CrossRef]

48. El Marabti, E.; Younis, I. The Cancer Spliceome: Reprograming of Alternative Splicing in Cancer. *Front. Mol. Biosci.* **2018**, *5*, 80. [CrossRef]

49. Hrdlickova, R.; Nehyba, J.; Bose, H.R., Jr. Alternatively spliced telomerase reverse transcriptase variants lacking telomerase activity stimulate cell proliferation. *Mol. Cell. Biol.* **2012**, *32*, 4283–4296. [CrossRef]

50. Listerman, I.; Sun, J.; Gazzaniga, F.S.; Lukas, J.L.; Blackburn, E.H. The major reverse transcriptase-incompetent splice variant of the human telomerase protein inhibits telomerase activity but protects from apoptosis. *Cancer Res.* **2013**, *73*, 2817–2828. [CrossRef]

51. Yi, X.; White, D.M.; Aisner, D.L.; Baur, J.A.; Wright, W.E.; Shay, J.W. An alternate splicing variant of the human telomerase catalytic subunit inhibits telomerase activity. *Neoplasia* **2000**, *2*, 433–440. [CrossRef]

52. Fleisig, H.B.; Hukezalie, K.R.; Thompson, C.A.; Au-Yeung, T.T.; Ludlow, A.T.; Zhao, C.R.; Wong, J.M. Telomerase reverse transcriptase expression protects transformed human cells against DNA-damaging agents, and increases tolerance to chromosomal instability. *Oncogene* **2016**, *35*, 218–227. [CrossRef]

53. Zhu, S.; Rousseau, P.; Lauzon, C.; Gandin, V.; Topisirovic, I.; Autexier, C. Inactive C-terminal telomerase reverse transcriptase insertion splicing variants are dominant-negative inhibitors of telomerase. *Biochimie* **2014**, *101*, 93–103. [CrossRef]

54. Ulaner, G.A.; Hu, J.F.; Vu, T.H.; Giudice, L.C.; Hoffman, A.R. Telomerase activity in human development is regulated by human telomerase reverse transcriptase (hTERT) transcription and by alternate splicing of hTERT transcripts. *Cancer Res.* **1998**, *58*, 4168–4172.

55. Teichroeb, J.H.; Kim, J.; Betts, D.H. The role of telomeres and telomerase reverse transcriptase isoforms in pluripotency induction and maintenance. *RNA Biol.* **2016**, *13*, 707–719. [CrossRef]

56. Hansen, K.D.; Brenner, S.E.; Dudoit, S. Biases in Illumina transcriptome sequencing caused by random hexamer priming. *Nucleic Acids Res.* **2010**, *38*, e131. [CrossRef]

57. Bayega, A.; Wang, Y.C.; Oikonomopoulos, S.; Djambazian, H.; Fahiminiya, S.; Ragoussis, J. Transcript Profiling Using Long-Read Sequencing Technologies. *Methods Mol. Biol.* **2018**, *1783*, 121–147. [CrossRef]

58. Wong, M.S.; Chen, L.; Foster, C.; Kainthla, R.; Shay, J.W.; Wright, W.E. Regulation of telomerase alternative splicing: A target for chemotherapy. *Cell Rep.* **2013**, *3*, 1028–1035. [CrossRef]

59. Wong, M.S.; Shay, J.W.; Wright, W.E. Regulation of human telomerase splicing by RNA:RNA pairing. *Nat. Commun.* **2014**, *5*, 3306. [CrossRef]

60. Bojesen, S.E.; Pooley, K.A.; Johnatty, S.E.; Beesley, J.; Michailidou, K.; Tyrer, J.P.; Edwards, S.L.; Pickett, H.A.; Shen, H.C.; Smart, C.E.; et al. Multiple independent variants at the TERT locus are associated with telomere length and risks of breast and ovarian cancer. *Nat. Genet.* **2013**, *45*, 371–384. [CrossRef]

61. Killedar, A.; Stutz, M.D.; Sobinoff, A.P.; Tomlinson, C.G.; Bryan, T.M.; Beesley, J.; Chenevix-Trench, G.; Reddel, R.R.; Pickett, H.A. A Common Cancer Risk-Associated Allele in the hTERT Locus Encodes a Dominant Negative Inhibitor of Telomerase. *PLoS Genet.* **2015**, *11*, e1005286. [CrossRef]

62. Barthel, F.P.; Wei, W.; Tang, M.; Martinez-Ledesma, E.; Hu, X.; Amin, S.B.; Akdemir, K.C.; Seth, S.; Song, X.; Wang, Q.; et al. Systematic analysis of telomere length and somatic alterations in 31 cancer types. *Nat. Genet.* **2017**, *49*, 349–357. [CrossRef] [PubMed]

63. Khattar, E.; Kumar, P.; Liu, C.Y.; Akincilar, S.C.; Raju, A.; Lakshmanan, M.; Maury, J.J.; Qiang, Y.; Li, S.; Tan, E.Y.; et al. Telomerase reverse transcriptase promotes cancer cell proliferation by augmenting tRNA expression. *J. Clin. Invest.* **2016**, *126*, 4045–4060. [CrossRef] [PubMed]

64. Wang, F.; Cheng, Y.; Zhang, C.; Chang, G.; Geng, X. A novel antisense oligonucleotide anchored on the intronic splicing enhancer of hTERT pre-mRNA inhibits telomerase activity and induces apoptosis in glioma cells. *J. Neurooncol.* **2019**, *143*, 57–68. [CrossRef] [PubMed]

65. Fallmann, J.; Will, S.; Engelhardt, J.; Gruning, B.; Backofen, R.; Stadler, P.F. Recent advances in RNA folding. *J. Biotechnol.* **2017**, *261*, 97–104. [CrossRef] [PubMed]

66. Si, J.; Cui, J.; Cheng, J.; Wu, R. Computational Prediction of RNA-Binding Proteins and Binding Sites. *Int. J. Mol. Sci.* **2015**, *16*, 26303–26317. [CrossRef]

67. Buckanovich, R.J.; Posner, J.B.; Darnell, R.B. Nova, the paraneoplastic Ri antigen, is homologous to an RNA-binding protein and is specifically expressed in the developing motor system. *Neuron* **1993**, *11*, 657–672. [CrossRef]

68. Jensen, K.B.; Dredge, B.K.; Stefani, G.; Zhong, R.; Buckanovich, R.J.; Okano, H.J.; Yang, Y.Y.; Darnell, R.B. Nova-1 regulates neuron-specific alternative splicing and is essential for neuronal viability. *Neuron* **2000**, *25*, 359–371. [CrossRef]

69. Saito, Y.; Miranda-Rottmann, S.; Ruggiu, M.; Park, C.Y.; Fak, J.J.; Zhong, R.; Duncan, J.S.; Fabella, B.A.; Junge, H.J.; Chen, Z.; et al. NOVA2-mediated RNA regulation is required for axonal pathfinding during development. *eLife* **2016**, *5*. [CrossRef]

70. Dredge, B.K.; Stefani, G.; Engelhard, C.C.; Darnell, R.B. Nova autoregulation reveals dual functions in neuronal splicing. *EMBO J.* **2005**, *24*, 1608–1620. [CrossRef]

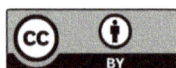

cancers

MDPI

Review

A Review on a Deep Learning Perspective in Brain Cancer Classification

Gopal S. Tandel [1], Mainak Biswas [2,3], Omprakash G. Kakde [4], Ashish Tiwari [1], Harman S. Suri [5], Monica Turk [6], John R. Laird [7], Christopher K. Asare [8], Annabel A. Ankrah [9], N. N. Khanna [10], B. K. Madhusudhan [11], Luca Saba [12] and Jasjit S. Suri [13,*]

1   Department of Computer Science and Engineering, Visvesvaraya National Institute of Technology, Nagpur 440012, India; gtandel@gmail.com (G.S.T.); atiwari.rcs@gmail.com (A.T.)
2   Department of Computer Science and Engineering, Marathwada Institute of Technology, Aurangabad 431010, India; mainakmani@gmail.com
3   Global Biomedical Technologies Inc., Roseville, CA 95661, USA
4   Indian Institute of Information Technology, Nagpur 440012, India; ogkakde25@gmail.com
5   Brown University, Providence, RI 02912, USA; harman_suri@brown.edu
6   Department of Neurology, University Medical Centre Maribor, 2000Maribor, Slovenia; monika.turk84@gmail.com
7   Department of Cardiology, St. Helena Hospital, St. Helena, CA 94574, USA; lairdjr@ah.org
8   Department of Neurosurgery, Greater Accra Regional Hospital, Ridge, Accra233, Ghana; drchristopher.asare@yahoo.com
9   Department of Radiology, Greater Accra Regional Hospital, Ridge, Accra233, Ghana; aaankrah@yahoo.com
10 Department of Cardiology, Apollo Hospitals, New Delhi 110076, India; drnnkhanna@gmail.com
11 Neuro and Epileptology, BGS Global Hospitals, Bangaluru 560060, India; drmadhubk@gmail.com
12 Department of Radiology, A.O.U., Cagliari 09128, Italy; lucasaba@tiscali.it
13 Stoke Monitoring and Diagnostic Division, AtheroPoint™, Roseville, CA 95661, USA
*   Correspondence: Jasjit.Suri@AtheroPoint.com

Received: 29 November 2018; Accepted: 10 January 2019; Published: 18 January 2019

Abstract: A World Health Organization (WHO) Feb 2018 report has recently shown that mortality rate due to brain or central nervous system (CNS) cancer is the highest in the Asian continent. It is of critical importance that cancer be detected earlier so that many of these lives can be saved. Cancer grading is an important aspect for targeted therapy. As cancer diagnosis is highly invasive, time consuming and expensive, there is an immediate requirement to develop a non-invasive, cost-effective and efficient tools for brain cancer characterization and grade estimation. Brain scans using magnetic resonance imaging (MRI), computed tomography (CT), as well as other imaging modalities, are fast and safer methods for tumor detection. In this paper, we tried to summarize the pathophysiology of brain cancer, imaging modalities of brain cancer and automatic computer assisted methods for brain cancer characterization in a machine and deep learning paradigm. Another objective of this paper is to find the current issues in existing engineering methods and also project a future paradigm. Further, we have highlighted the relationship between brain cancer and other brain disorders like stroke, Alzheimer's, Parkinson's, and Wilson's disease, leukoriaosis, and other neurological disorders in the context of machine learning and the deep learning paradigm.

Keywords: cancer; brain; pathophysiology; imaging; machine learning; extreme learning; deep learning; neurological disorders

1. Introduction

The fatality rate due to brain cancer is the highest in Asia [1]. Brain cancer develops in the brain or spinal cord [2]. The various symptoms of brain cancer include coordination issues, frequent headaches, mood swings, changes in speech, difficulty in concentration, seizures and memory loss. Brain cancer is a form of tumor which stays in the brain or central nervous system [2]. Brain tumors are categorized into various types based on their nature, origin, rate of growth and progression stage [3,4]. Brain tumors can be either benign or malignant. Benign brain tumor cells rarely invade neighboring healthy cells, have distinct borders and a slow progression rate (e.g., meningiomas, pituitary tumors and astrocytomas (WHO Grade-I)). Malignant brain tumor cells (e.g., oligodendrogliomas, high-grade astrocytomas, etc) readily attack neighboring cells in the brain or spinal cord, have fuzzy borders and rapid progression rates. Brain tumors can be further classified into two types based on their origin: primary brain tumors and secondary brain tumors. A primary tumor originates directly in the brain. If the tumor emerges in the brain due to cancer existing in some other body organ such as lungs, stomach etc., then it is known as a secondary brain tumor or metastasis. Further, grading of brain tumors is done as per the rate of growth of cancerous cells, i.e., from low to high grade. WHO categorizes brain tumors into four grades (I, II, III and IV) as per the rate of growth [2,5–9] (discussed later). Brain tumors are also characterized by their progression stages (Stage-0, 1, 2, 3 and 4). Stage-0 refers to cancerous tumor cells which are abnormal, but do not spread to nearby cells. Stages-1, 2 and 3 denote cells which are cancerous and spreading rapidly. Finally in Stage-4 the cancer spreads throughout the body. It is for sure that many lives could be saved if cancer were detected at an early stage through fast and cost-effective diagnosis techniques. However, it is very difficult to treat cancer at higher stages where survival rates are low.

Brain cancer diagnosis can be either invasive or non-invasive. Biopsy is the invasive approach where an incision is done to collect a tumor sample for examination. It is considered the gold standard for cancer diagnosis where the pathologists observe various features of cells of the tumor sample under a microscope to confirm malignancy. The physical examination of the body and brain scanning using imaging modalities constitute non-invasive approaches. The various imaging modalities such as computed tomography (CT), or magnetic resonance imaging (MRI) of brain are faster and safer techniques than biopsy. These imaging modalities help radiologists locate brain disorders, observe disease progression and in surgical planning [10]. Brain scans or brain image reading to rectify disorders is however subject to inter-reader variability and accuracy which depends on the proficiency of the medical practitioner [11].

The advent of powerful computing machines and decreased hardware costs has led to the development of many computer-assisted tools (CAT) for cancer diagnosis by the research community. It is projected that CAT may help radiologists in improving the precision and consistency of the diagnostic results. In this study, various CAT-based intelligent learning methods i.e., machine learning (ML) and deep learning (DL) for automatic tissue characterization and tumor segmentation has been discussed. The basic objective of this paper is to highlight state-of-the-art of brain tumor classification methods, current achievements, challenges, and find the future scope.

The paper is organized as follows: Section 2 provides an overview of the pathophysiology of brain cancer. Sections 3–6 discuss various imaging modalities, the WHO guidelines on brain cancer grading, brain cancer tests and characterization methodologies, respectively. Section 7 briefly introduces different brain diseases and finally, Section 8 provides an overall discussion.

2. Pathophysiology of Brain Cancer

The pathophysiology of brain cancer is discussed here. The reasons of occurrence of brain cancer are given from the perspective of cellular architecture and its functioning within the human body.

2.1. Cellular Level Architecture

The cell is the basic building block of the human body. It also defines the function of each organ within the body such as oxygen flow, blood flow and waste materials management. Each cell has a central control system known as the nucleus which contains 23 pairs of chromosomes consisting of millions of genes. The instructions for these genes are contained within deoxyribonucleic acid (DNA) [12], which is like a blueprint for genes and defines their behavior. The protein of the gene is like a messenger that communicates between the cells or between the genes themselves. The message conveyed is defined by its 3D structure [13]. Genes control the continuous process of the death of unhealthy or unwanted cells besides reproduction of healthy cells. The main cause of a cancer is uncontrolled growth of cells. A mutation alters this DNA sequence, which is the root cause of malfunctioning of the genes. There are many factors involved in DNA mutations such as environmental, lifestyle, and eating habits.

The genes responsible for cancer are divided into three categories. We introduce and define each category in detail:

(i)   The first category is known as tumor suppressors that controls the cell death cycle (apoptosis) [14]. This process has two signaling pathways. In the first pathway, the signal is generated by a cell to kill itself while in the second, the cell receives the death signal from nearby cells. This process of cell death is slowed down by a mutation in one of the pathways. It stops completely if this mutation happens in both pathways, leading to unstoppable cell growth [14,15]. Some examples of cell suppressor genes are RB1, PTEN, which are responsible for cell death [16].

(ii) The second category of genes is responsible for the repair of the DNA. Example of DNA repair genes are MGMT and p53 protein. Any malfunctioning in them may trigger cancer.

(iii) The third group known as proto-oncogenes, are in opposition to the function of the tumor suppressor genes and are responsible for the production of the protein fostering the division process and inhibiting the normal cell death [17,18]. In healthy cells, the cell division cycle is controlled by proto-oncogenes via protein signals which are generated by the cell itself or the connected cells. Once the signal is generated, it goes through a series of different steps, which is called signal transduction cascade or pathway as shown in Figure 1. This signal may be generated by the cell itself or from the nearby cells that are directly connected to it. In this pathway, many proteins are involved to carry the signal from the cell membrane to nucleus through the cytoplasm. In this process the cell membrane receptor accepts the signal and carries the message to nucleolus through various intermediate factors. Once, the signal reaches to the nucleus, the responsible genes for transcription is activated and performs the cell division task. One of the known proto-oncogenes responsible for the transcription is RAS which acts as a switch to turn 'on' or 'off' the cell division process [19]. Mutation alters its functionality which leads to transform this gene into an oncogene. In this situation the gene is unable to switch off the cell division signal and unstoppable growth of the cells may begin.

If cancer starts in the body due to any of the above-mentioned reasons, it is known as a primary tumor which invades other organs directly. If the cancer starts through blood vessels then it known as secondary tumor or metastasis [20]. Even though the secondary tumor is formed, it needs oxygen, nutrients and a blood supply to survive. Many genes exist in the body to detect these needs and start establishing a vascular network for them to satisfy their needs. This process is known as angiogenesis and is another cause of cancer explosion [21]. The genes discussed above as well as their expended form has given in Table 1.

About 15 percent of cancers worldwide are caused by viruses [22]. The viruses infect cells by altering DNA in the chromosomes which are responsible for converting proto-oncogenes into oncogenes. Only a few cancer causing viruses have been identified i.e., DNA virus and retroviruses or oncorna viruses (an RNA virus). The four basic DNA viruses responsible for human cancers are human papillomavirus, Epstein-Barr, Hepatitis B and human herpes virus. The RNA viruses which cause cancer are Human T lymphotropic type1 and hepatitis C. Several environmental factors also affect the cells. X-rays, UV light, viruses, tobacco products, pollution and many other daily use chemicals carry carcinogenic agents. Sunlight may also alter tumor suppressor genes in skin cells leading to skin cancer. Further, the carcinogenic compounds in smoke alters the lung cells causing lung cancer [23].

Many studies have shown that tumor cells have unique molecular signatures and characteristics [24]. Hyperplasia, metaplasia, anaplasia, dysplasia, and neoplasia are the various stages of the cells that define the cellular abnormality during microscopic analysis. Hyperplasia is the stage, where abnormal growth of the cell starts but the cell continues to appear normal. The cell first begins to appear abnormal in metaplasia. In the anaplasia state, cells lose their morphological features and are difficult to discriminate. The cell appears to be abnormal and little aggressive in dysplasia. Anaplasia is the most aggressive stage of this abnormal cell growth, where they seem quite abnormal and invade the surrounding tissues or start flowing through the bloodstream, which is one of the leading causes of metastasis [25]. The physical changes in cells due to cancer can be captured using high resolution imaging such as MRI or CT imaging, which are the focus of the next section.

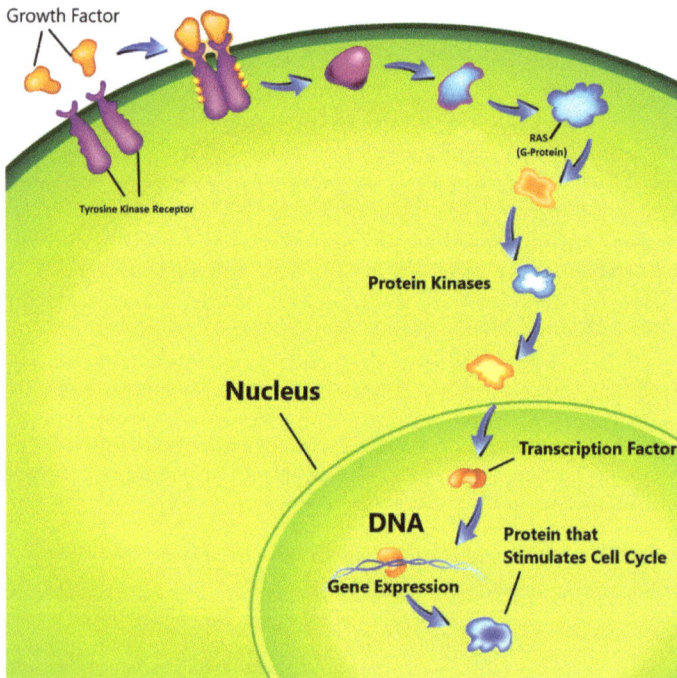

Figure 1. Cell cycle proliferation. (image courtesy: AtheroPoint^{TM}, Roseville, CA, USA).

Table 1. Genomics relevance with Brain Tumor, RKT: Receptor Tyrosine Kinase, TP53 (p53): Tumor Protein53, RB1: Retino Blastoma1, EGFR: Epidermal Growth Factor Receptor, PTEN: Phosphatase and Tensin Homolog, IDH1/DH2: Isocitrate Dehydrogenase 1/2, 1p and 19 co-deletion, MGMT: O6-methylguanine DNA methyltransferase, BRAF: B-Raf proto-oncogene, ATRX: The α-thalassemia-mental retardation syndrome X-linked, HGG: High-Grade Gliomas, GBM: Glioblastoma.

Gene Type	Function	Mutation Effect	Relevancy Between Brain Tumor and Genes [Degree of Mutation]
TP53(p53) [26]	DNA repair Initiating Apoptosis	• Genetic Instability • Reduced Apoptosis • Angiogenesis	• More relevant to HGG • Brain Tumor (80%)

Table 1. *Cont.*

Gene Type	Function	Mutation Effect	Relevancy Between Brain Tumor and Genes [Degree of Mutation]
RB1 [26]	Tumor Suppressor	• Blocks cell cycle progression • Unchecked cell cycle progression	• More relevant to GBM • Brain Tumor (75%)
EGFR [27]	Trans-Membrane Receptor In (RTK)	• Increased Proliferation • Increased Tumor Cell Survival	• Primary GBM (Approx. 40%)
PTEN [27]	Tumor Suppressor	• Increased Cell Proliferation • Reduced Cell Death	• Primary GBM (15–40%) • GBM (up to 80%)
IDH1 and DH2 [28]	Control citric acid cycle	• Inhibits the function of enzymes	IDH1 • Primary GBM (5%) • GBM Grade II-III (70–80%) • IDH1 longer survival. IDH2 • Relevant to oligodendroglial tumors
1p and 19q [29]	Prognosis of the disease or treatment assessment	• Poor prognosis	• Oligodendrogliomas (80%) • Anaplastic Oligodendrogliomas (60%) • Oligoastrocytomas (30–50%) • Anaplastic Oligoastrocytomas (20–30%)
MGMT [30]	DNA repair predict patient survival	• Cell proliferation	• GBM (35–75%)
BRAF [26]	Proto-oncogene	• Cell Proliferation • Apoptosis	• Pilocyticastrocytomas (65–80%) • Pleomorphic Xanthoastrocytomas and Gangliogliomas (25%)
ATRX [26]	Deposition of Genomic Repeats.	• Genital Anomalies, • Hypotonia, • Intellectual Disability • Mild-To-Moderate Anemia • Secondary To α-Thalassemi	• Relevent to oligodendroglial

2.2. Relevancy between Brain Tumor and Genes

As discussed in the last section, mutations in certain types of genes define the cancer. In various studies, some connection is found between degree of mutation in genes and type of brain tumor, which we have summarized in Table 1. Tumor protein-53 (TP53) is involved in DNA repair and initiating apoptosis. Tp53 level is found to be quite abnormal in high-grade gliomas and mutations have been found in more than 80% of tumors [26]. The retinoblastoma (RB1) gene is a tumor suppression gene. RB1 mutation is found in approximately 75% of brain tumors and it is more relevant to glioblastoma [26]. EGFR is a trans-membrane receptor in the receptor tyrosine kinase (RTK) family. Mutation in EGFR will lead to increased cell cycle proliferation and increased tumor cell survival. It is generally associated with primary glioblastomas and approximately 40% of the mutations that caused them are found within it [27]. PTEN is a tumor suppressor gene and are responsible for about 15–40% of mutations found in primary glioblastomas. The degree of mutation may be up to 80%, indifferent glioblastoma [27]. IDH1 and IDH2 are enzymes that control the citric acid cycle. Mutations in them inhibit enzyme activity. Generally, IDH1 mutation is found less in primary glioblastoma patients (5%), but more in high grade glioblastomas (70–80%). IDH2 mutations are generally seen in oligodendroglial tumors [28]. Co-deletion of chromosomes 1p and 19q is indicative of oligodendroglial lineage and mainly seen in anaplastic oligoastrocytomas (20–30%), oligoastrocytomas (30–50%), anaplastic oligodendrogliomas (60%) and oligodendrogliomas (80%). 1p/19q helps in prognosis and treatment assessment [29]. MGMT protein is another DNA repair gene, for which 35–75% abnormality is found in glioblastomas [30]. BRAF is a proto-oncogene encoded as BRAF protein, which is involved in the cell proliferation cycle, apoptosis process and treatment assessment. BRAF mutations are generally found in pilocyticastrocytomas (65–80%), pleomorphic xanthoastrocytomas (about 80%) and gangliogliomas (25%) [26]. A-Thalassemia-mental retardation syndrome X-linked (ATRX) is a gene that encodes a protein and is associated with TP53 and IDH1 mutations. It is use as a prognostic indicator when tumors have anIDH1 mutation and it distinguishes between the tumors of oligodendroglial origin [26].

3. Imaging Modality

Medical imaging techniques help doctors, medical practitioners and researchers view inside the human body and analyze internal activities without incisions. Cancer diagnosis, grade estimation, treatment response assessment, patient prognosis and surgery planning are the main steps and challenges in cancer treatment. There are a number of medical imaging techniques used by hospitals across the world for different treatments. The brain imaging techniques can be categorized into two types: *i.e.*, structural and functional imaging [31,32]. Structural imaging consists of different measures related to brain structure, tumor location, injuries and other brain disorders. The functional imaging techniques detect metabolic changes, lesions on a finer scale and visualize brain activities. This activity visualization is possible due to metabolic changes in a certain part of the brain which are reflected in the scans. CT and MRI are used for brain tumor analysis and are able to capture different cross-sections of the body without surgery [33,34].

3.1. Computed Tomography Imaging

In a CT scan, an X-ray beam circulates around specific part of the body and a series of images captured from various angles. The computer uses this information to create a series of two-dimensional (2D) cross-sectional image of the organ and combines them to make a three-dimensional (3D) image, which provides a better view of the organs. Positron emission tomography (PET) is a variant of CT where a contrast agents is injected into the body in order to highlight abnormal regions. CT scans are recommended by doctors in many conditions such as hemorrhages, blood clots or cancer. However, CT scans use X-rays which emit ionizing radiation and have the potential to affect living tissues, thereby increasing the risk of cancer. In one study, it is shown that the risk of radiation in CT is 100 times higher than in a normal X-ray diagnosis [35].

3.2. Magnetic Resonance Imaging

MRI is a radiation free and therefore a safer imaging technique than CT and provides finer details of the brain, spinal cord and vascular anatomy due to its good contrast. Axial, sagittal, and coronal are the basic planes of MRI to visualize the brain's anatomy as shown in Figure 2. The most commonly used MRI sequences for brain analysis are Tl-weighted, T2-weighted, and FLAIR [36]. Tl-weighted scan provides gray and white matter contrast. T2-weighted is sensitive to water content and therefore well suited to diseases where the water accumulates inside brain tissues. T1- and T2-weighted images are also used to differentiate cerebrospinal fluid (CSF). The CSF is colorless and found in the brain and spinal cord. It looks dark in T1-weighted imaging and bright on T2-weighted imaging. The third sequence is fluid attenuated inversion recovery (FLAIR) which is similar to T2-weighted image except for its acquisition protocol. FLAIR is used in pathology to distinguish between CSF and brain abnormalities. FLAIR can locate an edema region from CSF by suppressing free water signals, and hence periventricular hyperintense lesions are clearly visible in the images.

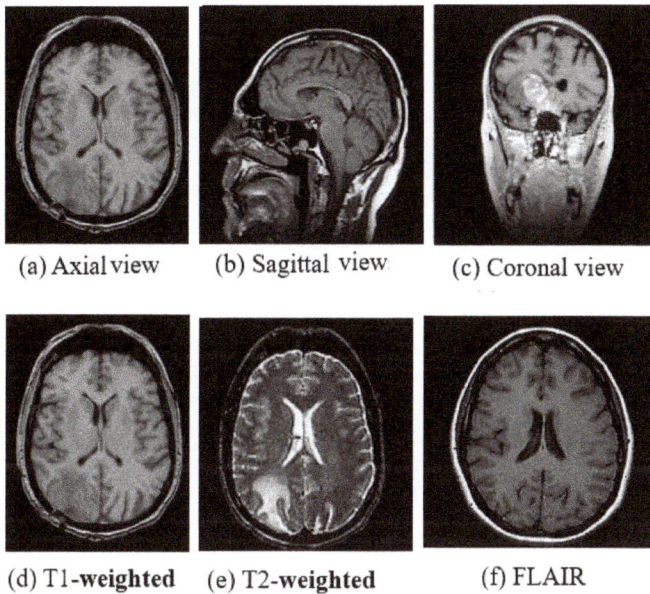

Figure 2. (**a**) Axial view, (**b**) Sagittal view, (**c**) Coronal view and (**d**) T1-weighted, (**e**) T2-weighted and (**f**) FLAIR Images of MRI. (image courtesy: AtheroPoint^TM).

The comparison between the above three sequences is shown in Figure 2. Diffusion-weighted imaging (DWI) [37] is another MRI sequence that helps to detect the random movements of water particles inside the brain. As the water movement becomes restricted, an extremely bright signal on the DWI is reflected, thus the DWI technique is mostly used for acute stroke detection. Perfusion-weighted MRI (PWI) highlights the specific part of the brain where the blood flow has been altered. Diffusion-tensor MRI (DTMRI) detects water motion in tissues through a microscopic image which helps during surgical removal of the brain tumor. Functional magnetic resonance imaging (fMRI) [38] is another variant of MRI that is used for measuring the changes in blood oxygenation in order to interpret the neural activity. When a certain part of the brain is more active, it starts consuming more oxygen and blood. Consequently, an fMRI maps the ongoing activity of the brain by correlating the mental process and location. Although MRI is very useful for brain image analysis, it has some limitations compared to CT. The motion artifact effect is inferior in MRI which helps in acute hemorrhage and brain injury detection, but also causes it to require a greater acquisition time than many other imaging techniques.

3.3. Biopsy

Biopsies are the gold standard for all cancer diagnosis and grade estimation. In a biopsy, the color, shape, and size of the cell nuclei of tumor sample are observed. This brings complexity in manual microscopic biopsy image analysis. The accuracy depends on the experience and expertise of the pathologist and therefore, computer assisted tools can help pathologist in Digital Pathological Image (DPI) analysis and may provide better results than manual approach [39]. Hematoxylin & Eosin (H&E) staining is the most commonly used method for a biopsy sample analysis. Cytopathology is used to know the cell structure, function and their chemistry. Tissue proteins are assessed by using immuno-fluorescence imaging.

3.4. Hyperstereoscopy Imaging

High-grade tumors invade the surrounding normal tissues, which makes them extremely difficult to differentiate from each other through the naked eyes of surgeon (especially glioma). Incorrect resection leads to reduced survival rate of the brain cancer patients [40,41]. In this case, hyperspectral imaging (HSI) can be used. HSI is a minimally invasive, non-ionizing sensing technique. HSI uses a wider range of the electromagnetic spectrum compared to normal three channel Red, Green and Blue (RGB) image type [41], which provides detailed information about tissues in the captured scene [42].

Recently, scientists have proposed a novel visualization system based on HSI, which can assist surgeons to detect the brain tumor boundaries during neurosurgical procedures [40]. This model uses both supervised (SVM and KNN) and unsupervised (K-Means) machine learning techniques to differentiate cell classes such as normal, cancerous, blood vessels/hyper-vascularized tissue and background in the spectral image. The brain cancer detection algorithm is divided into off-line (training process) and in situ (online) process. In the off-line process, the samples are labeled by experts and in the in situ process, the HSI are directly acquired from the patient for real-time image analysis in the operation theater. SVM is adapted for classification during the in situ process to get a supervised classification map, while the kNN algorithm is used to find the spatial-spectral classification map. To get the final definitive classification map, image fusion is performed between spatial-spectral classification map (derived from KNN-supervised) and hierarchical K-means map (unsupervised strategy). Finally, a majority voting (MV) method is used to fuse both images for superior results. For dimensionality reduction, a principal component analysis (PCA) algorithm is adapted in the above settings.

Another study utilizing the hyperspectral paradigm is [43], where, head and neck cancer classification was done using a deep learning (DL) technique. In this study, the authors demonstrated that DL techniques have the potential to be used as a real-time tissue classifier (tissue labeling process) using HS images to identify boundaries of the cancerous and non-cancerous tissues during surgery. A CNN network was proposed consisting of six convolution layers and three fully connected layers to classify three types of classes such as head and neck tissue, squamous-cell carcinoma and thyroid cancer. The database consisted of 50 subjects. The network was trained for 25,000 iterations using a batch size of 250. Performance was evaluated using leave-one-out cross-validation protocol while computing the performance parameters giving the accuracy, sensitivity, specificity as 80%, 81% and 78%, respectively. The CNN strategy was benchmarked against conventional ML methods such as SVM, kNN, logistic regression (LR), decision tree (DT), linear discriminant analysis (LDA) demonstrating its superiority.

3.5. MR Spectroscopy

MRI is able to visualize the anatomical structure of the brain, whereas, Magnetic Resonance spectroscopy (MRS) is able to detect small biochemical changes in the brain. This property is useful for the brain tissue classification in brain tumor, stroke and epilepsy. Here, several metabolites and their products such as amino acids, lactate, lipids, alanine, etc., where, the frequency can be measured in parts per million (ppm). There are unique metabolic signatures associated with each tumor type and their grades [44], therefore, the neurologist measures the changes between normal and cancerous tissues by the frequency map of ppm of each metabolite. In [45], the authors had proposed a deep learning-based model for brain tumor diagnosis using MRS imaging techniques. The authors proposed three deep models for brain tumor classification into healthy, low or high grade tissue types. In another study [46], the authors proposed a brain tumor grading method using MR spectroscopy. The proposed method showed that metabolite values/ratios could provide better classification/grading of brain tumors using, short and long echo times (TEs). A machine learning method was proposed by authors in [47] for glioma classification into benign and malignant types. Features were extracted from MR spectroscopy and then classified using popular ML methods such as SVM, random forest, multilayer perceptron, and locally weighted learning (LWL). The best performance was achieved by random forest, giving an AUC of 0.91, while a sensitivity of 86.1% was achieved using the LWL-based method.

Each imaging modality has its own merits and demerits. Occasionally we need to combine the merits of more than one imaging modality for accurate diagnosis and assessment of various severe diseases. Combining multiple image modalities is called image fusion which helps in better diagnosis than when using a single imaging technique. Image fusion improves the image quality and may reduce randomness and redundancy of the medical images. Some of the popular methods of image fusions are [48] based on morphology, knowledge, wavelets and fuzzy logic methods.

4. World Health Organization Guidelines for Tumor Grading

Cancer identification and correct grade estimation are crucial part of the diagnosis process. It helps doctors decide on a personalized treatment plan which may increase the survival expectancy of the patients. Medical practitioners or histopathologists use WHO guidelines for brain tumor grading. The WHO proposed five amendments or editions since 1979 for tumor classification, presented in Table 2. In 1979, the WHO first proposed miotic activity, necrosis and infiltration for the tumor classification. In 1993, the WHO came up with another amendment, where immune histochemistry was considered for tumor assessment. After that, a genetic profile was included in the year of 2000. In the 4th amendment, a genetic profile and histological variation were combined for the tumor analysis in the year of 2007.Recently, on May 9, 2016 the WHO published an official fifth amendment to the central nervous system (CNS) tumor classification, which may precisely define the tumor cells and helps in better tumor classification [49]. All the studies have shown that tumor cells have unique molecular signatures and characteristics which define their grade and group [50]. The WHO classifies brain tumors using four basic features such as mitoses, necrosis, nuclear atypia, and microvascular proliferation [51]. The assigned grades from the least aggressive to the most aggressive (malignant) tumors are in the range of I to IV [49–52]. Grade-I cells look nearly normal and spread slowly. Grade-II cells look slightly abnormal and grow slowly and may invade nearby tissues. These are more life-threatening than Grade-I but can be cured by a suitable treatment. In Grade-III, tumor cells seem abnormal and invade the nearby healthy brain tissues. These tumors may be treated. Grade-IV cells look completely abnormal and grow and very rapidly. Eventually, it is very difficult to sub-grade tumor due to the fuzzy difference in cell structure microscopically. Therefore, grade estimation of tumor is challenging for a pathologist.

Table 2. WHO recommendations for tumor assessment in different editions.

Edition	Year	Recommended Parameters for Tumor Assessment
I	1979	Miotic Activity, Necrosis and Infiltration
II	1993	Immunohistochemistry (IHC)
III	2000	Genetic Profile
IV	2007	Genetic Profile and Histological Variation
V	2016	Molecular Features and Histology

5. Brain Tumor Tests

In neurological examination, the doctor asks about the patient's health and checks vision, hearing, alertness, muscle strength and reflexes. The doctor may also examine the eyes of a patient to see any swelling. Brain scans, tumor biopsy and biomarkers are major tests to confirm cancer and its grade. If the doctor finds any symptoms of brain cancer then they may suggest any one of them depending on the patient condition to confirm the malignancy of the brain tumor. Some of the tests are given in the following subsections.

5.1. Biomarker Test

Mutation in the genes is the root cause of cancer and the degree of this mutation in specific genes can be measured through biomarker tests. Some of the genes responsible for specific brain cancers are given in Table 1. This test diagnoses tumors, helps to find its type and may help in tumor growth measurement, treatment response and personalized treatment therapy [53].

5.2. Biopsy

Biopsy is the primary test for diagnosis and stage conformation [54] for all types of cancer. This is an invasive cancer diagnosis approach. In this test, a sample of the brain tumor is taken out through surgery and the procedure may take several hours. The collected biopsy samples go through a laboratory test where the histopathologists look for the cellular patterns and characteristics to estimate the grade of the brain tumor. The low and high-grades of tumor are difficult to differentiate as their cellular structures are similar. Accurate diagnosis is an important step to analyze the behavior of the tumor and make the correct treatment plan. The estimation of the grade of the tumor is subject to inter-reader variability and correct analysis of the DPI depends on the training and experience of the histopathologists [55]. Image features that grade tumors are not always clear or difficult to determine by different observers. The computerized image analysis can partially overcome these shortcomings [56]. Complexity in clinical features representation, large size single histopathology image and insufficient images for training are the major barriers in the automatics classification techniques development [56]. Computerized image analysis include image registration, preprocessing, feature selection, the region of interest (ROI) identification, segmentation and image classification which are discussed later.

For many years, The Medical Image Computing and Computer Assisted Intervention (MICCAI) Society has been organizing many conferences and open challenges that foster to develop computer assisted tools or medical inventions in medical image analysis. Recently, many digital histopathology image analysis challenges were organized worldwide to boost the tumor histopathology among researchers community. We have summarized some of the MICCA challenges in Table 3.

Table 3. Overview of some open challenges in digital pathology images analysis worldwide.

Year	Challenges	Reference
2012	ICPR Mitosis Detection Competition	[57]
2012	EM segmentation challenge 2012 2D segmentation of neuronal processes	[58]
2013	MICCAI Grand Challenge on Mitosis Detection	
2014	MICCAI Brain Tumor Digital Pathology Challenge	[59]
2014	MICCAI Brain Tumor Digital Pathology Challenge	
2015	MICCAI Gland Segmentation Challenge Contest	
2016	Tumor Proliferation Assessment Challenge 2016	[60]
2017	CAMELYON17 challenge	[61]
2018	Medical Imaging with Deep Learning (MIDL-2018)	[62]

5.3. Imaging Test

Imaging modalities such as CT, MRI, PET, and SPECT are popular brain imaging techniques to confirm the presence of tumors without using surgery. Amongst them, MRI is the most popular diagnostic imaging modality. MRI is mainly used for neural disorder or abnormality detection because of its good contrast resolution for different tissues and lack of radiation. Automatic brain tumor detection and classification is a challenging task due to overlapping intensities, anatomical inconsistency in shape, size and orientation, noise perturbations and low contrast of images [63]. Some of the open challenges proposed worldwide for brain image analysis have been summarized in Table 4. Our main focus of this review is to highlight the challenges involved and find the future scope in a non-invasive procedure of brain tumor detection and classification using the ML and DL approaches. In the next section, we have discussed various ML and DL methods for the brain image segmentation, tumor detection, and classification and point out limitations and future scope for the enhancements.

Table 4. Overview open challenges of brain image analysis worldwide.

Challenge	Objective	Modality	Reference
BraTS 2012	Brain Tumor Segmentation	MRI	[64]
BraTS 2013	Brain Tumor Segmentation	MRI	[65]
BraTS 2014	Brain Tumor Segmentation	MRI	[66]
BraTS 2015	Brain Tumor Segmentation	MRI	[67]
BraTS 2016	Quantifying longitudinal changes: evaluate the accuracies of the volumetric changes between any two time points.	MRI	[68]
BraTS 2017	Segmentation of gliomas in pre-operative scans. Prediction of patient overall survival (OS) from pre-operative scans.	MRI	[69]
BraTS 2018	Segmentation of gliomas in pre-operative MRI scans. Prediction of patient overall survival (OS) from pre-operative scans.	MRI	[70]
MICCAI 2018	The segmentation ofgray matter, white matter, cerebrospinal fluid, andother structureson multi-sequence brain MR images with and without (large) pathologies. (large) pathologies on segmentation and volumetry.	MRI	[71]
HC-18	To design an algorithm that can automatically measure the fetal head circumference given a 2D ultrasound image.	Ultrasound Image	[72]

6. Classification Methods

Machine learning can be defined as a situation where a machine is given a task in which the machine performance improves with experience [73]. ML algorithms are divided into two types: supervised learning and unsupervised learning [74,75]. In supervised learning, ML algorithms learn from already labeled data. In unsupervised learning, the ML algorithms try to understand the inter-data relationship from unlabeled data. In the case of brain image analysis, ML has been used in characterizing brain tumors [75,76]. The inner workings of ML algorithms consist of two stages: feature extraction and application of ML algorithm for characterization. The process model is shown in Figure 3.

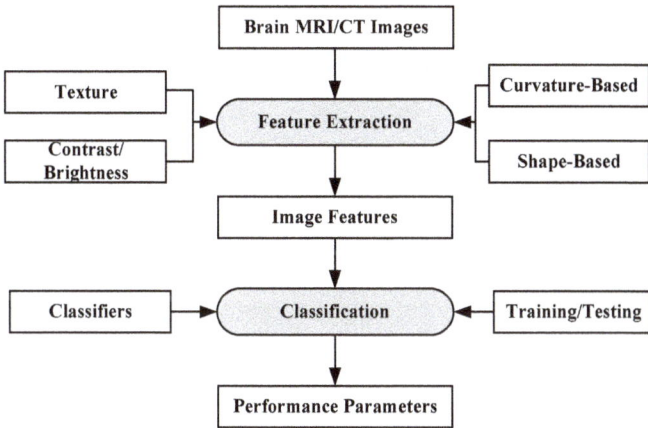

Figure 3. Working of ML-based algorithms.

The feature extraction algorithms are generally mathematical models based on various image properties such as texture, brightness, contrast. Sometimes, several features from different extraction models are fused together to increase the discrimination power of ML algorithms [77]. Some of the most common algorithms for classification and segmentation of brain images are: K-Nearest Neighbors (KNN) [78], Support Vector Machines (SVM) [79], Artificial Neural Networks (ANN) [80] etc. The KNN classification is based on the premise that features of the same class cluster together. The KNN assigns an unknown instance the most common label amongst its K nearest neighbors. The SVM applies two approaches for characterization: at first it tries to find the largest separating hyper-plane between two classes. In the second approach, if the features are not separable in one dimension, they are mapped to higher dimension where they are linearly separable, by using the kernel approach. ANN forms hierarchical network of computing nodes capable of learning from features. ANNs are classified into many types depending on their architecture, number of hidden layers, connection weight updating algorithms, etc. The most common ANN models are extreme learning machines (ELMs) [81], recurrent neural networks (RNN) [82], restricted Boltzmann machine (RBN) [83] etc. ELM is single-layer feed-forward neural network (SLFFNN), RNNs apply feedback mechanism in the network connections and RBN is a stochastic neural network.

The advent of high performance computers, as well as lower hardware costs have led to the emergence of models with multiple layers of abstraction and millions of computing nodes which has enabled characterization/segmentation with a high degree of accuracy. These models are collectively called DL methodologies [84]. The most common DL models for brain image characterization are convolution neural networks (CNN) [85], auto encoders [86] and deep belief networks (DBNs) [87]. DL-based tools for brain images are rapidly finding interest amongst the research community.

6.1. Machine Learning

KNN, SVM, DT, the naive Bayes (NB) classifier, expectation maximization (EM), random forest (RF) etc. are the most popular ML techniques for medical image analysis. Many of them were used alone or in combination by various researchers for brain image analysis. Some of them are discussed in Table 4. We provide different brain cancer classification techniques using ML in the following subsections.

6.1.1. ANN-Based MRI Brain Tumor Classification Using Genetic Features

The artificial neural network (ANN)-based approach for brain tumor classification using MRI was proposed in [63]. The method is able to characterize normal (N), benign (B) and malignant (M) tumor. The N, B and image example is shown in Figure 4.

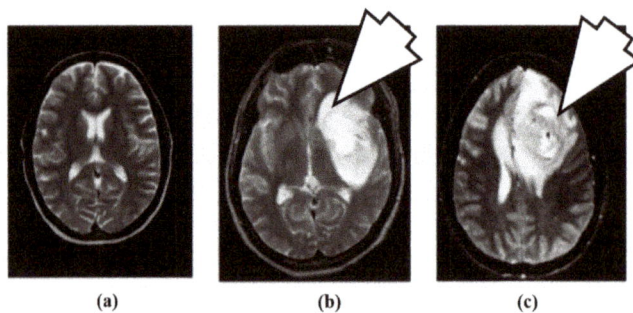

(a)   (b)   (c)

Figure 4. Brain MR images: (**a**) normal brain, (**b**) benign tumor (7 O' clock arrow) and (**c**) malignant tumor (7 O' clock arrow) (reproduced from [63] with permission).

For the purpose of characterization, 100 brain MR images ($N = 35$, $B = 35$, $M = 30$) were collected. A semi-automatic method was applied to extract the region-of-interest (ROI). A wavelet-based feature selection was performed to extract the features. A genetic-based feature selection algorithm along with principal component analysis (PCA) and classical sequential algorithm was applied for feature selection. Finally, all the features are input into the ANN. The ANN classifier is a three-layer feed forward neural network with a single hidden layer. The process model of the approach is shown in Figure 5. It's found that the genetic approach using only four of the available 29 features attained a classification accuracy of 98%. Similar approaches such as PCA and other classical algorithms required a large feature set to achieve a similar accuracy level.

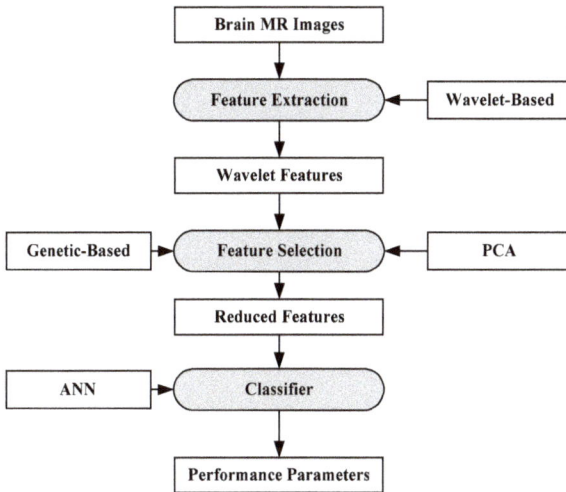

Figure 5. Process model of ANN-based classification model [63].

6.1.2. A Hybrid Characterization System for Brain Cancer Tumors

In [88], a hybrid system consisting of two ML algorithms has been proposed for brain cancer tumor characterization. A total of 70 brain MRI images (abnormal: 60, normal: 10) were considered for this purpose. The features were extracted from the images using DWT [89]. The total numbers of features were reduced using PCA [90]. After feature extraction, two classifiers were used separately on the reduced features (i.e., feed forward back propagation based artificial neural network (FP-ANN) and KNN). FP-ANN applies to the back-propagation learning algorithm for weight updating [91]. KNN is discussed earlier. This method achieves 97% and 98% accuracy using FP-ANN and KNN, respectively. The process model of the proposed method is shown in Figure 6.

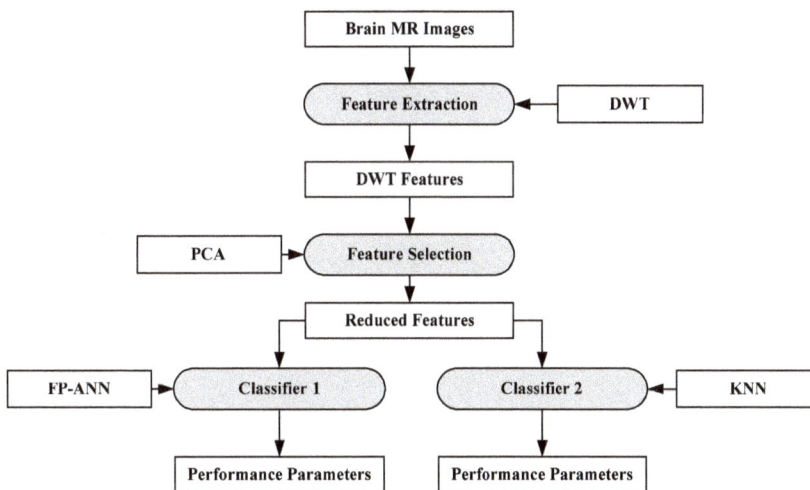

Figure 6. Hybrid characterization system for brain cancer characterization [88].

6.1.3. A Characterization System for Grading Brain Cancer Tumors

A fully automated brain tumor classification scheme using conventional MRI and rCBV maps calculated from perfusion MRI was proposed in [92]. The method classifies meningioma, glioma grades (II, III, IV), and metastasis brain images as shown in Figure 7. Earlier, researchers used linear discriminant analysis (LDA) as a model based on principle component regression (PCR) [93]. In this method, a linear SVM model is used for characterization. A total of 102 MRI brain scans were used for the purpose of characterization. The images were pre-processed and ROIs were extracted. Several features were extracted such as tumor shape characteristics, image intensity characteristics and Gabor features. In order to reduce the features, selection algorithms were applied (i.e., Ranking-based and SVM-recursive feature elimination (SVM-RFE)). Finally, SVM is applied. A process model of the methodology is shown in Figure 8. The highest classification accuracy obtained for metastasis was 91.7%, while for low-grade gliomas it was 90.9%. The highest accuracy of 97.8% was achieved when distinguishing grade II gliomas from metastasis. The lowest accuracy of 75% is obtained when distinguishing grade II from grade III gliomas. This showed that grade II and III gliomas are difficult to distinguish.

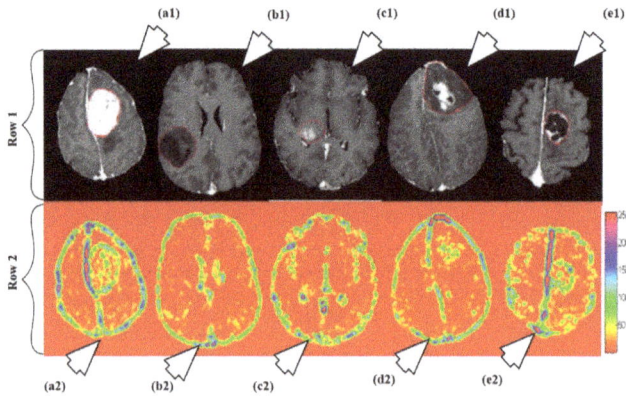

Figure 7. Illustration of different types as per their grades: row 1 and row 2 consists of T1ce brain images and its corresponding texture images, respectively. The images are pointed to by arrow are as follows: a1 (T1ce) and a2 (Texture): meningioma; b1 (T1ce) and b2 (Texture): Grade-II; c1 (T1ce), c2 (Texture): Grade-III; d1 (T1ce) and d2 (Texture): Grade-IV; e1 (T1ce) and e2 (Texture): metastasis (reproduced from [92] with permission).

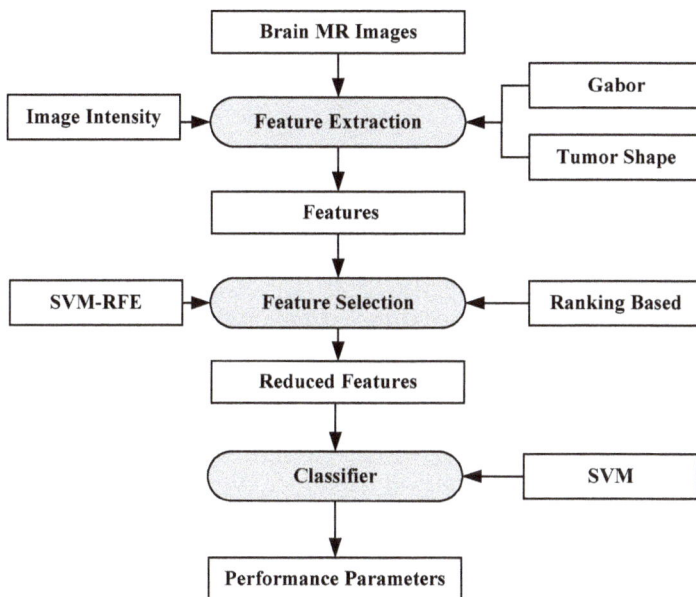

Figure 8. Process model using SVM-based grade estimation method [92].

6.1.4. A Multi-Parametric Tissue Characterization System for Brain Neoplasm

A characterization system was developed for identifying neoplastic tissue from healthy tissue, as well as the classification of different tumor components and edema-like areas [94]. Data was collected from 14 patients recently diagnosed with brain cancer. The images were pre-processed and voxel-wise intensity feature vectors were collected. Bayesian [95–97] and SVM were used to distinguish neoplastic tissue from healthy tissue, as well as the classification of different tumor components and edema-like areas. The results show that the Bayesian classifier obtains higher accuracy for classifying edema, enhancing neoplasm and non-enhancing neoplasm at 97.03%, 96.39% and 93.05%, respectively. SVM obtained highest accuracy for cerebrospinal fluid at 91.34%. The process model is shown in Figure 9.

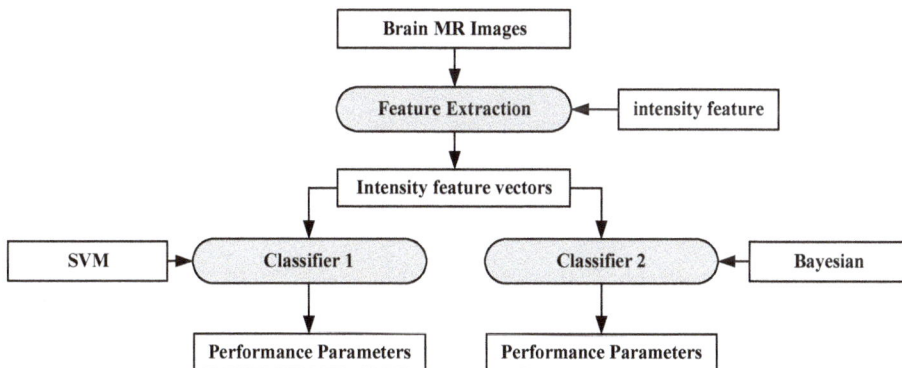

Figure 9. Process model of SVM-based grade estimation method [92].

6.1.5. Extreme Learning Machine

Extreme learning machine (ELM) is another emerging area which is less computationally expensive compared to neural networks. It is based on the single-layer feed-forward neural network (SLFFNN) which is used for real-time classification or regression. ELM chooses randomly initialized weights in the input-to-hidden layer, whereas, hidden-to-output layer weights are trained using Moore-Penrose inverse form [97] to generate least square solution. This feature minimizes network complexity, training time, learning speed, and improves classification accuracy. Moreover, the weights in the hidden layer give a multi-tasking capability to the network as in other ML methods like SVM, KNN and Bayesian network. The ELM network consists of three layers as shown in Figure 10 and all the layers are fully connected. The weight between input and hidden layer are fixed at random initially and unchanged throughout the training process and weights between hidden and output are only allowed to change. Therefore it learns the weights in a single pass and reaches a global optimum [98]. There is a claim of researchers [98,99] that due to its simpler architecture and one shot training makes this network better and faster as compared to SVM.

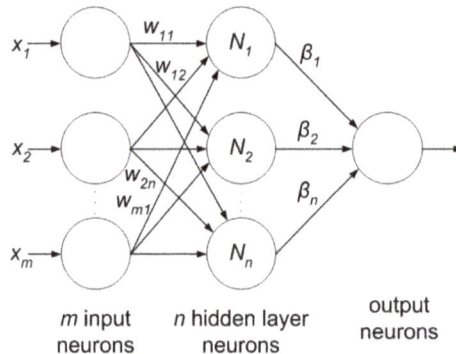

Figure 10. Extreme learning machine.

6.2. Deep Learning

DL is most extensively used for the brain image analysis in several applications such as normal or abnormal brain tumor classification, segmentation (edema, enhancing and non-enhancing tumor region), stroke lesion segmentation, Alzheimer diagnosis, etc. A convolution neural network (CNN) is the most popular DL model used widely for classification and segmentation of medical images. The CNN learns the spatial relationship between pixels in a hierarchical manner. This is done by using convolving the images using learned filters to build a hierarchy of feature maps. This convolution function is done in several layers such that the features obtained are translation and distortion invariant resulting in high degree of accuracy. The basic layers of CNN network are described below.

6.2.1. Input Image Format

The input image is considered as an array of pixel values which depends on the resolution and size of the image. For example, a sample colored input image is represented by a $3 \times m \times n$ array of numbers (the 3refers to red, green and blue color values in case of color image with the pixel value for each color ranging from 0–255; m and n are the dimensions of the image). In the case of a grayscale image, the image size is defined by 2D array (m × n), where the intensity of the pixels also ranges from 0–255.

6.2.2. Convolution Layer

The first layer of CNN architecture is the convolution layer, which extracts features from the given input image using the convolution filters. The filter is a square array of numbers which are weights or parameters. These filters can loosely be thought of as the neurons of an ANN or the kernel. The first position of the filter corresponds to the top left corner of the image in the convolution operation. This operation is described in Equation (1), which shows an example of an image (R) being convolved with the kernel (S), where $\otimes$ denotes the convolution operation. Essentially operation can be thought of as a series of multiplications of the image pixel matrix and the filter matrix and then a summing of these multiplications. Important to note in Equation (1) is that the kernel is size of m $\times$ m and the operation is performed at the center pixel (x, y), and nearby, where the p and q are the dummy variables. This process repeated by sliding filter to the right. The number of cell shifts to the right in each step defines the stride (number of cells sliding right in each step). The CNN architecture is shown in Figure 11. CNN learns and updates filters or kernel values during the training.

$$f(x,y) = R(x,y) \otimes S(p,q) = \sum_{p=-m/2}^{m/2} \sum_{q=-m/2}^{m/2} R(x+p, y+q) \times S(p,q) \tag{1}$$

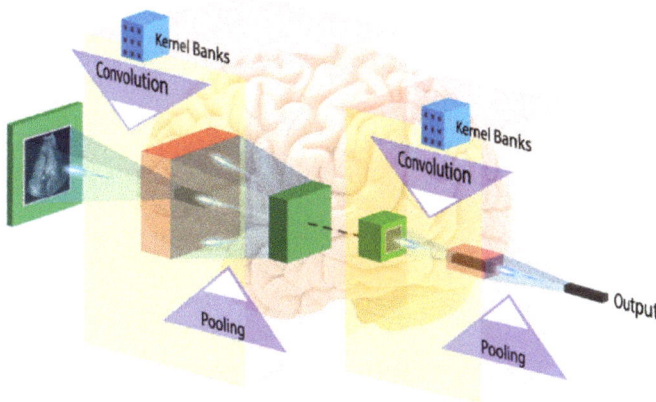

Figure 11. CNN architecture (image courtesy: AtheroPoint^{TM}).

6.2.3. Activation Function

In ANNs, the training progress is measured by gradient-based methods where the gradient is considered as a learning parameter, which reflects the changes in the training process. Since the changes in gradient are very small during training then learning is not effective and this phenomenon is known as vanishing gradient problem. This problem is more severe in DL because of large number of layers. It can be avoided by using suitable activation function which, don't have this property of suppressing the input space into a small region. ReLu is very simple and computationally inexpensive activation function which performs the non-linear operation and replaces all negative values in the feature map by zero using a simple formula [max (0, x)], whereas, x is an input parameter [100].

6.2.4. Pooling Layer

To make the method computational inexpensive, a pooling layer is introduced between convolution layers to reduce the dimensionality of each feature maps but retain the most important feature information. Average pooling and max-pooling are the two popular pooling operations.

In average pooling; selected patch features are replaced by the single average value of patch in next layer, whereas, for max pooling only maximum value of patch features move further.

6.2.5. Fully Connected Layer

The first three operations i.e., convolution, ReLu, and pooling are used for extracting high-level image features. For features classification, a fully connected network appended at the end of the CNN, which convert last 2D layers into a one-dimensional feature vector. The output of the FC layer defines by N-dimensional vector which refers to the number of output classes. Only one of the output class chosen from the vector by using probabilistic methods such as softmax.

6.3. Brain Image Analysis Using Deep Learning

As discussed earlier, DL algorithms are used in brain image analysis in different application domains like Alzheimer's disease identification, segmentation of lesion (e.g., tumors, white matter lesions, lacunes, micro-bleeds) and brain tissue classification [101]. Much of the ongoing research is limited to brain segmentation and only little work has been done for the tumor grading. Hence, there are a lot of potentials to explore the grade estimation for brain tumor using ML and DL approaches. In this section, we have discussed some recently existing DL based brain image segmentation methods.

6.3.1. DL-Based Inter-Institutional Brain Tumor Segmentation

A CNN-based brain tumor segmentation method was proposed in [102]. In the experiment, three CNNs were used for training on multi-institutional data. Each CNN consisted of four convolution layers followed by two fully connected layers. Data of 68 patients were collected from two institutes. Patching-based segmentation was used. The equal sized patches extracted from images were annotated into three classes: tumor patches, healthy patches surrounding the tumor and other healthy patches. The tumor images were further divided into five classes based on patient data i.e, class-0: normal, class-2: enhancing region, class-3: necrotic region, class-4: T1-abnormality, class-5: FLAIR abnormality, class-1: ground truth region based on combination of classes 2–5. The various classes of tumor are shown in Figure 12.

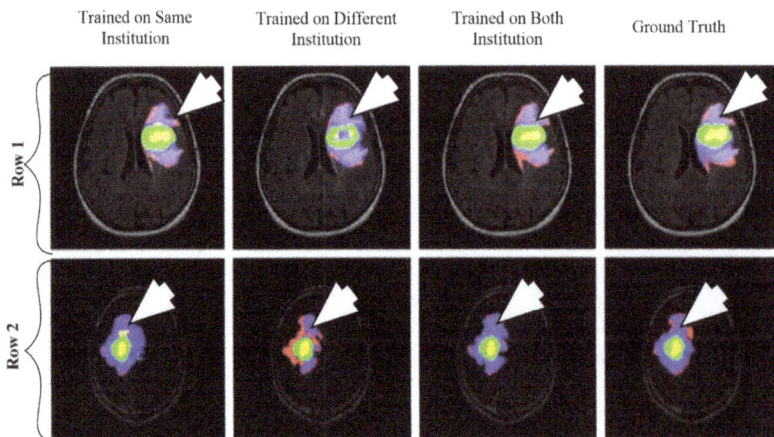

Figure 12. Segmentation results from two different patients. Class1: ground truth; Class 2 (enhancing region): green; Class 3 (necrotic region): yellow, Class 4 (T1abnormality-hypointensity region on T1, excluding enhancing and necrotic regions): red, and Class 5 (FLAIR abnormality excluding classes 2-4): blue (reproduced from [102] with permission).

The first CNN was trained for the institution-1 data set, second for the institute-2 dataset and third CNN was trained for patients from both institutions. Dice similarity coefficients and Hausdorff distance were used for the assessment between the ground truth and automatic segmentation. Ten-fold cross-validation scheme was applied to compare the performance between different approaches. They observed that performance of the model decreased when network is trained and tested on different institutional data (dice coefficients: 0.68 ± 0.19 and 0.59 ± 0.19) in comparison with same institutional data (dice coefficients: 0.72 ± 0.17 and 0.76 ± 0.12) and concluded that the reasons behind this effect require extra comprehensive investigation. The process model is shown in Figure 13.

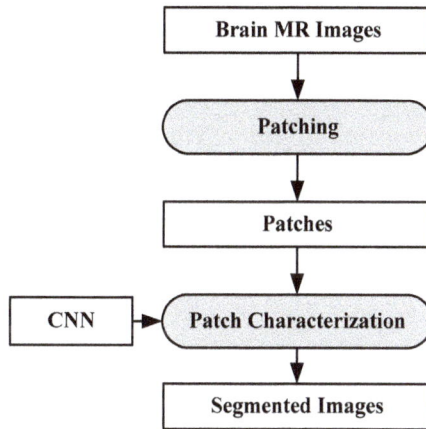

Figure 13. Process model for segmentation [102].

6.3.2. Brain Tumor Segmentation Using Two-Pathway CNN

Two-pathway based fully automated segmentation method was proposed for brain tumors [103]. The method segments glioblastomas (low grade glioma/LGG and high grade glioma/HGG) from MR images. The two pathways are executed using a small convolution filter for local segmentation and large filter for global segmentation. At last the feature maps from both pathways are concatenated to give us the segmented image. Based on this approach three cascaded networks were developed: Input Cascade CNN, MF Cascade CNN and Local Cascade CNN. The Input Cascade CNN obtained the highest Dice similarity of 0.89. The segmented results are shown in Figure 14. The architecture of the model is shown in Figure 15.

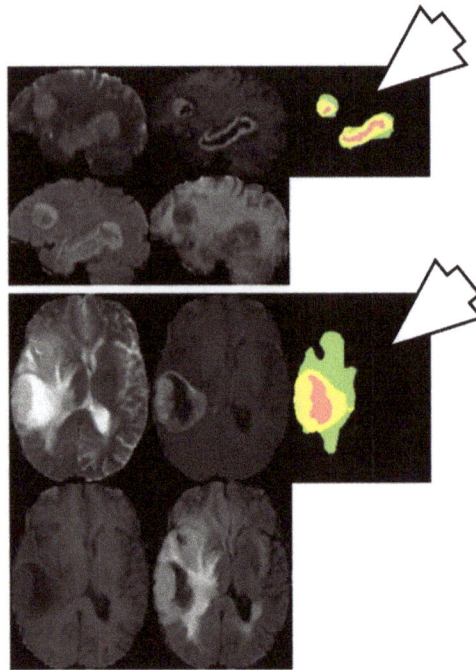

Figure 14. Segmentation results from two different patients. Green: edema, yellow: enhanced tumor, pink: necrosis, blue: non-enhanced tumor (reproduced from [103] with permission).

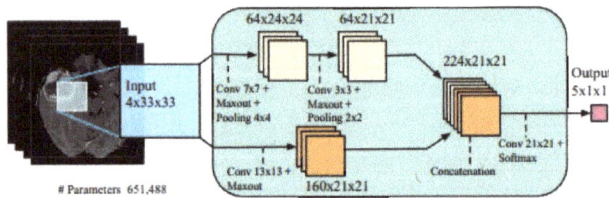

Figure 15. Model Architecture (reproduced from [103] with permission).

6.4. Plausible Solution for Brain Cancer Classification

Gliomas are the most common brain tumor in adults, and are generally divided into two categories: HGG and LGG. The WHO further divides LGG into I-II grade tumors and HGG into III-IV grade. Features such as shape and size of cell and its nuclei and cellular distribution are used to measure the degree of malignancy of the tumor microscopically. Differentiating HGG and LGG is somewhat easier than further sub-classification between LGG grade-I and II or HGG grade-III and IV, due to their uneven structure of the cell in this state. Grade estimation of the cancer is a very important parameter to decide targeted therapy and assessment of prognosis. Although biopsy is the gold standard, it is inherently invasive, along with its sampling errors and variability in interpretation, therefore, most doctors prefer MRI (T1, T2, and FLAIR) test in case surgical resection is difficult due to the location of tumor or patient condition, because of its good contrast and radiation-free nature from brain scans (MRI, CT, etc.). Most of the medical practitioners manually measure the degree of aggressiveness (grade) of the tumor. The accuracy of grade estimation depends on the proficiency of the practitioners and subjected to inter-reader variability studies. In this case, computer-assisted tools may help for better accuracy.

There are some automatic brain tumor grading methods which were proposed by researchers based on texture analysis using ML techniques [92,104,105]. Most of them use MRI (T1, T2, FLAIR, etc.). Recently many DL architectures (especially CNN) have shown remarkable performance in medical image analysis such as brain tumor segmentation and tissue classification on brain MRI. However, tumor grading utilizing DL methods is unexplored so far and there is a lot of research scope to explore further. We have provided a plausible solution for the tumor grading as shown in Figure 16. The model is described vividly in the discussion section.

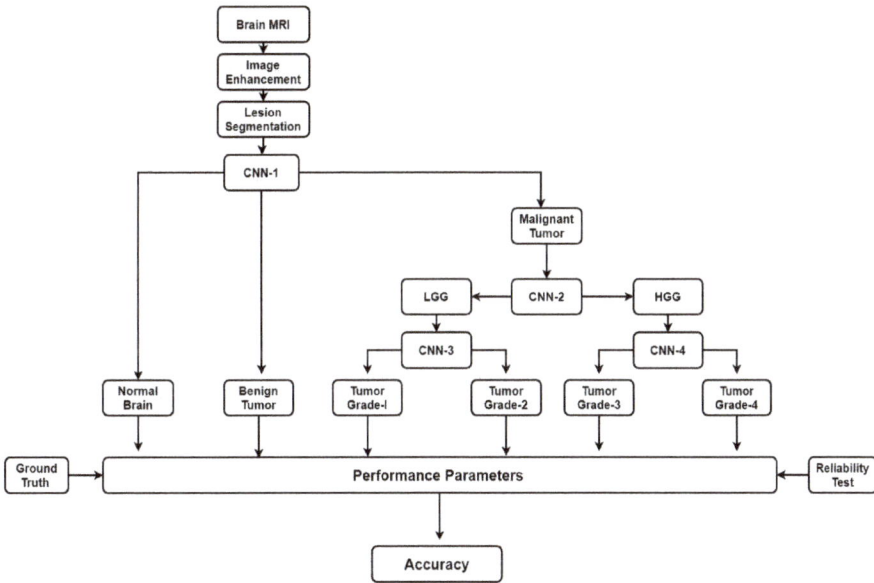

Figure 16. Plausible solution for brain tumor grading.

7. Brain Cancer and Other Brain Disorders

7.1. Stroke

There are two major classes of stroke: ischemic and hemorrhagic stroke [106]. Ischemic strokes happen when blood supply is interrupted in the brain, while hemorrhagic strokes results from blood vessel damage or abnormal vascular structure. Although stroke and brain cancer are two different diseases, the relationships between them have been examined by some researchers. A study was done on longitudinal risk of developing brain cancer in stroke patients [107]. For this study, they have selected 35 cases of malignant gliomas with or without stroke cases using brain MRI. They observed that the stroke patients have a higher risk of developing brain cancer than other forms of cancers with a hazard ratio of 3.09 (95% Confidence Interval (CI): 1.80–5.30). Another interesting finding of the study is that the old stroke patients and females between 40–60 age groups have more risk of developing brain cancer.

7.2. Alzheimer's Disease

Alzheimer's disease (AD) is a chronic neurodegenerative disease, where the short term memory loss is an initial symptom which may become worse over the time as disease advances i.e., language problem, behavioral issues, and the inability of self-care, etc [107]. Although, AD and cancer are two different diseases there is relationship between them in some studies. It is found that there is an inverse relationship between cancer and Alzheimer's disease in their study. Over a mean follow-up of 10 years of patients, they found that the cancer survivors have a 33% decreased risk of Alzheimer's disease as compared to the people without cancer. Another interesting outcome came out of the study is that the patients who have AD had risk of cancer decreased by 61%.

7.3. Parkinson's Disease

Parkinson's disease (PD) mainly affects the motor system of the brain resulting in tremors, rigidity, and slowness in movement and difficulty in walking. Sometimes thought process and behavioral changes are also observed [108]. A meta-analysis for demonstrating the relationship between PD and brain found a positive connection between them. Eight groups were involved in the study where 329,276 patients had participated. The study revealed that occurrence of brain tumor was relatively higher after the diagnosis of PD (odds ratio 1.55, 95% CI 1.18 ± 2.05), but not statistically significant before PD diagnosis (odds ratio 1.21, 95% CI 0.93 ± 1.58).

7.4. Leukoaraiosis

Leukoaraiosis is an abnormal change in the appearance of white matter near the lateral ventricles. It is often seen in old age, but sometimes also found in young adults. Leukoaraiosis may be the initial stage of Binswanger's disease but this may not always happen [109]. We cannot find any direct relation between brain cancer and Leukoaraiosis.

7.5. Multiple Sclerosis

Multiple sclerosis (MS) is a brain and spinal cord disease. In this disease, the immune system attacks the protective sheath (myelin) that covers nerve fibers which hampers communication system from the brain to rest of the body. The severity of the disease is measured by the quantity of nerve damage. Signs and symptoms of the disease may differ person to person. The symptoms are partial or complete loss of vision, double vision, speech slur, tingling in different parts of the body and losing walking ability at a higher stage. There is no permanent cure available for MS. In a recent study, it was shown that the MS patients have an increased risk of brain cancer [110,111].

7.6. Wilson's Disease

Wilson's Disease (WD) is caused by genetic disorder which is inherited from the parents. In this disease, copper builds up in the body and generally affects the brain and liver. Vomiting, weakness, fluid buildup in the abdomen, swelling of the legs, yellowish skin, and itchiness are some common liver related symptoms. Brain-related symptoms are tremors, muscle stiffness, trouble in speaking, personality changes, anxiety and seeing or hearing things [112]. A comparison of the differences in brain diseases is shown in Figure 17.

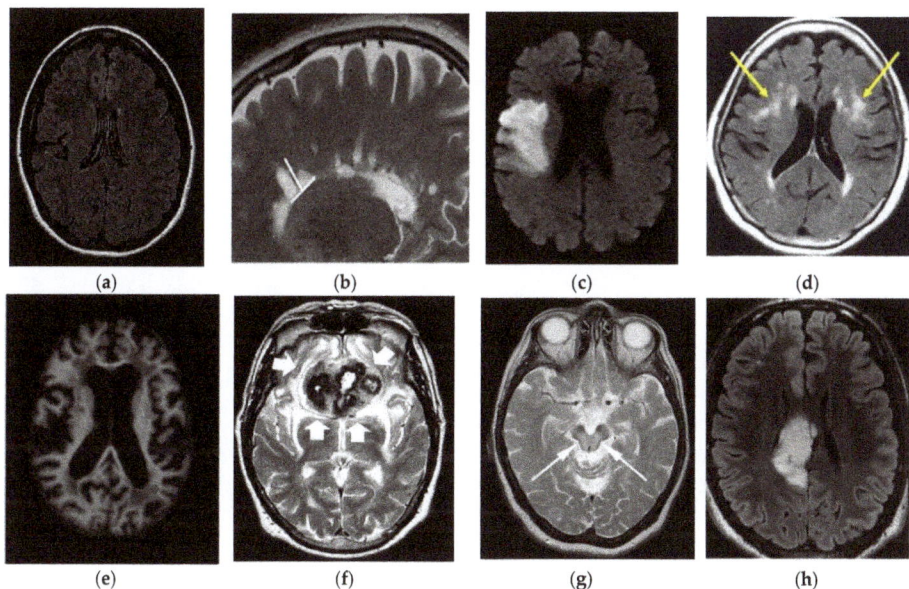

Figure 17. Comparison of brain tumor with other brain disorders (image permission requested from sources). (**a**) Normal Brain [AtheroPoint^{TM}]; (**b**) Multiple Sclerosis [113]; (**c**) Stroke [114]; (**d**) Leukoaraiosis [115]; (**e**) Alzheimer's Disease [116]; (**f**) Parkinson's Disease [117]; (**g**) Wilson'sDisease [118]; (**h**) Brain Tumor [119].

8. Discussion

Brain tumor analysis using medical imaging is a complicated and challenging task, which can be broadly categorized into pre-processing, classification and post-processing steps. There are many challenges associated with the aforementioned steps, which make this task complicated. No ideal computer assisted tools available so far to conform, tumor malignancy and its degree of aggressiveness. Thus doctors rely on the biopsy test [54,55] only for all types of cancer. The manual microscopic biopsy image analysis is done by pathologists and medical practitioners by observing cell or tissue structure under the microscope. The analysis is a challenging issue for them and subject to inter-reader variability tests. Therefore, DPI analysis is a growing area of research. In DPI, some common features include the shape and size of cells, shape and size of cell nuclei and distribution of the cells which are used to measure the degree of malignancy of the tumor. Characterizing benign and malignant cells is easier than sub-classifying malignant tumor due to uneven structure of the cell in this state. Staining variations, usage of different scanners and colors variations of the tissues may appear in DPI which may lead to wrong interpretation. Another challenge with DPI is that most of the whole slide image (WSI) scanner generates only 2D image, whereas the depth information is unavailable in 2D image, which is an important parameter for pathologists to confirm certain tissue class. It is anticipated that the design of 3D WSI scanners may be available soon [120]. Since biopsies are time-consuming and more risk-prone in the case of the brain tumor, therefore, various brain scans such as CT, MRI, etc. are used to confirm tumors and the degree of malignancy. Again, this analysis depends on the proficiency of the medical practitioners and is subject to inter-reader variability.

As discussed above, many automatic brain image analysis methods were proposed by various researchers for brain segmentation and tissue classification. Most of them use MRI (T1, T2, and FLAIR), due to its good contrast and radiation-free nature. As discussed earlier, brain image analysis consists of image registration, image enhancement, features reduction, feature extraction and classification. The image registration is the first and most important step in medical imaging. Image acquisition is not always consistent because of the effects of noise and blurring due to organ movements. The performance of the medical image analysis highly depends on several parameters such as modality, similarity measures, transformation, image contents, optimization of algorithm and implementation mechanism. Generally medical images suffer from low contrast which leads to deterioration of image quality. Gaussian (high-pass, low-pass) filter, histogram equalization, contrast starching are most commonly used image enhancement techniques for medical images. Large numbers of features are computationally expensive and make classification complex. Therefore, principal component analysis (PCA), linear discriminant analysis (LDA), and genetic algorithm (GA) are the most popular methods for feature reduction. SVM, DT, naive Bayes classifier, Bayesian classifier, KNN, ANNs etc. are the most commonly used ML methods for brain image classification and have achieved high-level accuracy in classification. In ML, features are first extracted by using hand-made techniques and then input to the ML-based characterization system. The difficulty of image classification using ML-based algorithms is that there lies continuous variability within image classes. Further, the contemporary distance measures used by feature extraction methods are unable to compute similarity between images. Nowadays, DL methods (CNN's, ResNets) are gaining more popularity than ML techniques for the brain image classification. In DL, the images are directly input to the system. DL models such as CNN produce features from images which are translation invariant and stable to deformations leading to more accurate characterization/segmentation. In addition to characterization/segmentation of brain, it is suggested to utilize DL models for grading of brain tumor. A proposed DL-based model is already shown in Figure 16. There are four CNNs (CNN-1, 2, 3 and 4) employed for brain cancer characterization and grading. Brain MR Images are first pre-processed and tumor part is segregated. The tumor part is characterized as normal, benign or malignant. If the tumor is malignant CNN2 is employed to characterize it as LGG or HGG. LGG is further characterized as tumor grade-I or grade-II using CNN3. Similarly, HGG is classified as tumor grade-III and grade-IV by CNN4. This model can effectively diagnose brain cancer and do its grading.

Although DL methods are widely popular among the research community, there are many challenges involved with DL architectures. DL models are quite computationally expensive because of additional hardware (GPUs) requirements to run the models. The memory and processing requirement of DL models are huge. It is also not necessary that increasing the number of layers in DL architecture will improve the performance of the architecture.

8.1. A Note on Biomarkers for Cancer Detection

Various tests have been suggested for diagnosing brain cancer: (a) including the one stated earlier in the section of imaging modalities, such as MRI, MRS, CT, etc., and (b) laboratory sampling of brain tumor i.e., biopsy. The inclusion of intelligence-based techniques such as ML or DL for imaging modalities are very likely to increase the effectiveness of the diagnosis and enhance the radiologists' capability towards accurate diagnosis for brain cancer in a timely manner. In addition to the computer-aided diagnosis using imaging modalities and biopsy methodologies, spread of cancer in the nervous system can be detected using a sample of cerebrospinal fluid from the spinal cord. This technique is called lumbar puncture or spinal tap [121]. In this methodology, several biomarkers related to brain tumor were detected [122]. In addition, molecular tests on brain tumor sample can be carried out to identify specific genes, proteins, and cells related to the particular tumor. Doctors can look into these biomarkers to assess the grade, type of tumor and decide treatment options. Further, examining these biomarkers can help in early treatment before the symptoms begin. Inclusion of ML and DL techniques in assessing these biomarkers can lead to accurate diagnosis that can save both time and cost, proving to be more economical.

8.2. Benchmarking

The benchmarking of several ML-based brain cancer classification system has been provided in Table 5. Sasikal et al. (Row #1) applied ANN-based classifier on featured extracted using DWT from

100 T2W MRI images. The accuracy obtained is 98%. In 2008, Verma et al. (Row #2) applied Bayesian and SVM on 14 DWI, B), FLAIR, T1 and GAD images and achieved sensitivity of 91.84% and specificity of 99.57% for SVM. Zacharaki et al. achieved 97.8% accuracy using NL-SVM on SVM-RFE features from 102 T1,2 FLAIR, rCBV images (Row #3). EL Dahashanet al. (Row #4) in 2009, applied FP-ANN and KNN on features extracted using DWT from 70 MR images and obtained highest accuracy of 98.0%. Similarly, Ryu et al. (Row #5) applied entropy histogram techniques on GLCM features extracted from 42 DWI, ADC images and achieved accuracy of 84.4%. Further, Skogen et al. (Row #6) applied standard deviation on 95 patients from 95 T1W, T2 and FLAIR images and also achieved an accuracy of 84.4%.

Table 5. Overview of Brain Tumor Classification Methods.

Sno	Reference	Tissue Classes	MRI Subtype	Data Size	Feature Processing	Feature Reduction	Architecture for Classification	Highest Performance
1	Sasikala et al. 2008 [63]	N, ABN, B, M	T2W	100, (N = 35, B = 35, M = 30)	DWT	GA	ANN	ACC = 98%; SEN = NA; SPC = NA; AUC = NA
2	Verma et al. 2008 [94]	Neoplasms, edema, and healthy tissue	DWI, B0, FLAIR, T1, and GAD	14 (G-3 = 8, G-4 = 7)			Bayesian, and SVM	ACC = NA; SEN = 91.84; SPC = 99.57; AUC = NA
3	Zacharaki et al. 2009 [92]	Metastasis, meningiomas gliomas (G-2,3) GBM	T1W, T2W, FLAIR, rCBV	102 (Metastasis (24), meningiomas (4), gliomas (G-2) (22), gliomas (G-3) (18), GBM (34))	SVM, RFE	Feature Ranking	LDA, KNN, NL-SVM	ACC = 97.8%; SEN = 100%; SPC = 95%; AUC = 98.6%
4	El-Dahshan et al. 2010 [88]	N, ABN	T2W	60, (N = 60, ABN = 10)	DWT	PCA	FP-ANN, KNN	ACC = 98.6%; SEN = 100; SPC = 90; AUC = NA
5	Ryu et al. 2014 [123]	Glioma (G-2,3,4)	DWI, ADC	42 Glioma (G2(N = 8)), G-3 (N = 10) and G-4 (N = 22))	GLCM		Entropy, Histogram	ACC = 84.4%; SEN = 81.8%; SPC = 90%; AUC = 94.1%
6	Skogenet al. 2016 [105]	LGG (G-2), HGG (G-3-4)	T1W, T2W, FLAIR	95 (LGG = 27 (G-2I) HGG = 68 (G-3 = 34 and G-4 = 34)	Statistical Analysis		Standard Deviation	ACC = 84.4%; SEN = 93%; SPC = 81%; AUC = 91%

GLCM: Gray Level Co-Occurrence Matrix, NL-SVM: Nonlinear SVM, MDF: Most Discriminent Factor, LDA: Linear Discriminant Analysis, ADC: Apparent Diffusion Coefficient, GLCM: Gray Level Co Occurrence Matrix, GA: Genetic Algorithm, DWT: Discrete Wavelet Transform, SVM: Support Vector Machines, RFE: Recursive Feature Elimination, N: Normal, ABN: Abnormal, GBM: Glioblastomas, HGG: High Grade Glioma, B: Benign, M: Malignant, T1W: T1-Weighted, T2W: T2 Weighted, FLAIR: Fluid-attenuated inversion recovery, rCBV: Relative cerebral blood volume, G: Grade, ANN: Artificial Neural Network, DWT: Discrete Wavelet Transform, FP-ANN: Feedforward, Back Propagation-ANN, ACC: Accuracy, SEN: Sensitivity, SPC: Specificity, AUC: Area Under Curve, ROC: Receiver Operating Characteristic.

9. Conclusions

Our main focus of the review is to provide state of art in brain cancer area that includes pathophysiology of cancer, imaging modality, WHO guidelines for tumor classification, primary diagnosis methods, and existing computer-assisted algorithms for brain cancer classifications using the machine and deep learning techniques. Finally, we have compared brain tumor with other brain disorders. We have concluded that due to automatic feature extraction capability of DL based methods, recently it is getting more attention and accuracy compared to conventional classification techniques for medical imaging. It is for sure that many lives can be saved if cancer detected and suitable grade estimated through fast and cost-effective diagnosis techniques. Therefore, there is dare need to develop fast, non-invasive and cost effective diagnosis techniques. Here, DL methods can play a major role for the same. In best of our knowledge, very less work has done for the automatic tumor grading using DL techniques and their full potential, yet to be explored.

Funding: This research received no external funding.

Conflicts of Interest: The authors declare no conflict of interest.

References

1. International Agency for Research on Cancer. Available online: https://gco.iarc.fr/ (accessed on 1 November 2018).
2. Brain Tumor Basics. Available online: https://www.thebraintumourcharity.org/ (accessed on 1 November 2018).
3. American Cancer Society website. Available online: www.cancer.org/cancer.html (accessed on 1 November 2018).
4. Brain Tumor Diagnosis. Available online: https://www.cancer.net/cancer-types/brain-tumor/diagnosis (accessed on 1 November 2018).
5. WHO Statistics on Brain Cancer. Available online: http://www.who.int/cancer/en/ (accessed on 1 November 2018).
6. Shah, V.; Kochar, P. Brain Cancer: Implication to Disease, Therapeutic Strategies and Tumor Targeted Drug Delivery Approaches. *Recent Pat. Anti-Cancer Drug Discov.* **2018**, *13*, 70–85. [CrossRef] [PubMed]
7. Ahmed, S.; Iftekharuddin, K.M.; ArastooVossoug. Efficacy of texture, shape, and intensity feature fusion for posterior-fossa tumor segmentation in MRI. *IEEE Trans. Inf. Technol. Biomed.* **2011**, *15*, 206–213. [CrossRef] [PubMed]
8. Behin, A.; Hoang-Xuan, K.; Carpentier, A.F.; Delattre, J. Primary brain tumoursinadults. *Lancet* **2003**, *361*, 323–331. [CrossRef]
9. Deorah, S.; Lynch, C.F.; Sibenaller, Z.A.; Ryken, T.C. Trends in brain cancer incidence and survival in the United States: Surveillance, Epidemiology, and End Results Program, 1973 to 2001. *Neurosurg. Focus* **2006**, *20*, E1. [CrossRef] [PubMed]
10. Mahaley, M.S., Jr.; Mettlin, C.; Natarajan, N.; Laws, E.R., Jr.; Peace, B.B. National survey of patterns of care for brain-tumor patients. *J. Neurosurg.* **1989**, *71*, 826–836. [CrossRef]
11. Hayward, R.M.; Patronas, N.; Baker, E.H.; Vézina, G.; Albert, P.S.; Warren, K.E. Inter-observer variability in the measurement of diffuse intrinsic pontine gliomas. *J. Neuro-Oncol.* **2008**, *90*, 57–61. [CrossRef]
12. Griffiths, A.J.F.; Wessler, S.R.; Lewontin, R.C.; Gelbart, W.M.; Suzuki, D.T.; Miller, J.H. *An Introduction to Genetic Analysis*; Macmillan: New York, NY, USA, 2005.
13. Shinoura, N.; Chen, L.; Wani, M.A.; Kim, Y.G.; Larson, J.J.; Warnick, R.E.; Simon, M.; Menon, A.G.; Bi, W.L.; Stambrook, P.J. Protein and messenger RNA expression of connexin43 in astrocytomas: Implications in brain tumor gene therapy. *J. Neurosurg.* **1996**, *84*, 839–845. [CrossRef] [PubMed]
14. Evan, G.I.; Vousden, K.H. Proliferation, cell cycle and apoptosis in cancer. *Nature* **2001**, *411*, 342. [CrossRef]
15. Burch, P.R. *The Biology of Cancer: A New Approach*; Springer Science & Business Media: New York, NY, USA, 2012.
16. Song, M.S.; Salmena, L.; Pandolfi, P.P. The functions and regulation of the PTEN tumoursuppressor. *Nat. Rev. Mol. CellBiol.* **2012**, *13*, 283. [CrossRef]
17. Rak, J.; Filmus, J.; Finkenzeller, G.; Grugel, S.; Marme, D.; Kerbel, R.S. Oncogenes as inducers of tumor angiogenesis. *Cancer Metastasis Rev.* **1995**, *14*, 263–277. [CrossRef]

18. Yarden, Y.; Kuang, W.-J.; Yang-Feng, T.; Coussens, L.; Munemitsu, S.; Dull, T.J.; Chen, E.; Schlessinger, J.; Francke, U.; Ullrich, A. Human proto-oncogene c-kit: A new cell surface receptor tyrosine kinase for an unidentified ligand. *EMBO J.* **1987**, *6*, 3341–3351. [CrossRef]

19. Greenberg, M.E.; Greene, L.A.; Ziff, E.B. Nerve growth factor and epidermal growth factor induce rapid transient changes in proto-oncogene transcription in PC12 cells. *J. Biol. Chem.* **1985**, *260*, 14101–14110. [PubMed]

20. Sneed, P.K.; Suh, J.H.; Goetsch, S.J.; Sanghavi, S.N.; Chappell, R.; Buatti, J.M.; Regine, W.F.; Weltman, E.; King, V.J.; Breneman, J.C.; et al. A multi-institutional review of radiosurgery alone vs. radiosurgery with whole brain radiotherapy as the initial management of brain metastases. *Int. J. Radiat. Oncol. Biol. Phys.* **2002**, *53*, 519–526. [CrossRef]

21. Bertram, J.S. The molecular biology of cancer. *Mol. Asp. Med.* **2000**, *21*, 167–223. [CrossRef]

22. Liao, J.B. Cancer issue: Viruses and human cancer. *Yale J. Biol. Med.* **2006**, *79*, 115–122.

23. Golemis, E.A.; Scheet, P.; Beck, T.N.; Scolnick, E.M.; Hunter, D.J.; Hawk, E.; Hopkins, N. Molecular mechanisms of the preventable causes of cancer in the United States. *Genes Dev.* **2018**, *32*, 868–902. [CrossRef] [PubMed]

24. Swartling, F.J.; Čančer, M.; Frantz, A.; Weishaupt, H.; Persson, A.I. Deregulated proliferation and differentiation in brain tumors. *Cell Tissue Res.* **2015**, *359*, 225–254. [CrossRef]

25. Montes-Mojarro, I.; Steinhilber, J.; Bonzheim, I.; Quintanilla-Martinez, L.; Fend, F. The Pathological Spectrum of Systemic Anaplastic Large Cell Lymphoma (ALCL). *Cancers* **2018**, *10*, 107. [CrossRef]

26. Mabray, M.C.; Barajas, R.F.; Cha, S. Modern brain tumor imaging. *Brain tumor research and treatment* **2015**, *3*, 8–23. [CrossRef]

27. Hegi, M.E.; Murat, A.; Lambiv, W.L.; Stupp, R. Brain tumors: Molecular biology and targeted therapies. *Ann. Oncol.* **2006**, *17*, x191–x197. [CrossRef]

28. Yan, H.; Parsons, D.W.; Jin, G.; McLendon, R.; Rasheed, B.A.; Yuan, W.; Kos, I.; Batinic-Haberle, I.; Jones, S.; Riggins, G.J.; et al. IDH1 and IDH2 mutations in gliomas. *N. Engl. J. Med.* **2009**, *360*, 765–773. [CrossRef] [PubMed]

29. Hu, N.; Richards, R.; Jensen, R. Role of chromosomal 1p/19q co-deletion on the prognosis of oligodendrogliomas: A systematic review and meta-analysis. *Interdiscip. Neurosurg.* **2016**, *5*, 58–63. [CrossRef]

30. Lee, E.; Yong, R.L.; Paddison, P.; Zhu, J. Comparison of glioblastoma (GBM) molecular classification methods. In *Seminars in Cancer Biology*; Academic Press: New York, NY, USA, 2018. [CrossRef]

31. Amyot, F.; Arciniegas, D.B.; Brazaitis, M.P.; Curley, K.C.; Diaz-Arrastia, R.; Gandjbakhche, A.; Herscovitch, P.; Hindsll, S.R.; Manley, G.T.; Pacifico, A.; et al. A review of the effectiveness of neuroimaging modalities for the detection of traumatic brain injury. *J. Neurotrauma* **2015**, *32*, 1693–1721. [CrossRef] [PubMed]

32. Pope, W.B. Brain metastases: Neuroimaging. *Handb. Clin. Neurol.* **2018**, *149*, 89–112. [CrossRef] [PubMed]

33. Morris, Z.; Whiteley, W.N.; Longstreth, W.T.; Weber, F.; Lee, Y.; Tsushima, Y.; Alphs, H.; Ladd, S.C.; Warlow, C.; Wardlaw, J.M.; et al. Incidental findings on brain magnetic resonance imaging: Systematic review and meta-analysis. *BMJ* **2009**, *339*, b3016. [CrossRef] [PubMed]

34. Lagerwaard, F.; Levendag, P.C.; Nowak, P.J.C.M.; Eijkenboom, W.M.H.; Hanssens, P.E.J.; Schmitz, P.M. Identification of prognostic factors in patients with brain metastases: A review of 1292 patients. *Int. J. Radiat. Oncol. Biol. Phys.* **1999**, *43*, 795–803. [CrossRef]

35. Smith-Bindman, R.; Lipson, J.; Marcus, R.; Kim, K.P.; Mahesh, M.; Gould, R.; de González, A.B.; Miglioretti, D.L. Radiation dose associated with common computed tomography examinations and the associated lifetime attributable risk of cancer. *Arch. Intern. Med.* **2009**, *169*, 2078–2086. [CrossRef] [PubMed]

36. Dong, Q.; Welsh, R.C.; Chenevert, T.L.; Carlos, R.C.; Maly-Sundgren, P.; Gomez-Hassan, D.M.; Mukherji, S.K. Clinical applications of diffusion tensor imaging. *J. Magn. Reson. Imaging* **2004**, *19*, 6–18. [CrossRef]

37. Khoo, M.M.Y.; Tyler, P.A.; Saifuddin, A.; Padhani, A.R. Diffusion-weighted imaging (DWI) in musculoskeletal MRI: A critical review. *Skelet. Radiol.* **2011**, *40*, 665–681. [CrossRef]

38. Savoy, R.L. Functional magnetic resonance imaging (fMRI). In *Encyclopedia of Neuroscience*; Elsevier: Charlestown, MA, USA, 1999.

39. Gurcan, M.N.; Boucheron, L.; Can, A.; Madabhushi, A.; Rajpoot, N.; Yener, B. Histopathological image analysis: A review. *IEEE Rev. Biomed. Eng.* **2009**, *2*, 147. [CrossRef]

40. Fabelo, H.; Ortega, S.; Lazcano, R.; Madroñal, D.; M Callicó, G.; Juárez, E.; Salvador, R.; Bulters, D.; Bulstrode, H.; Szolna, A.; et al. An intraoperative visualization system using hyperspectral imaging to aid in brain tumor delineation. *Sensors* **2018**, *18*, 430. [CrossRef] [PubMed]

41. Petersson, H.; Gustafsson, D.; Bergstrom, D. Hyperspectral image analysis using deep learning—A review. In Proceedings of the IEEE 2016 6th International Conference on Image Processing Theory Tools and Applications (IPTA), Oulu, Finland, 12–15 December 2016; pp. 1–6. [CrossRef]

42. Lu, G.; Fei, B. Medical hyperspectral imaging: A review. *J. Biomed. Opt.* **2014**, *19*, 010901. [CrossRef] [PubMed]

43. Halicek, M.; Lu, G.; Little, J.V.; Wang, X.; Patel, M.; Griffith, C.C.; El-Deiry, M.W.; Chen, A.Y.; Fei, B. Deep convolutional neural networks for classifying head and neck cancer using hyperspectral imaging. *J. Biomed. Opt.* **2017**, *22*, 060503. [CrossRef] [PubMed]

44. Nelson, S.J. Multivoxel magnetic resonance spectroscopy of brain Tumors1. *Mol. Cancer Ther.* **2003**, *2*, 497–507. [PubMed]

45. Olliverre, N.; Yang, G.; Slabaugh, G.; Reyes-Aldasoro, C.C.; Alonso, E. Generating Magnetic Resonance Spectroscopy Imaging Data of Brain Tumours from Linear, Non-linear and Deep Learning Models. In *International Workshop on Simulation and Synthesis in Medical Imaging*; Springer: Cham, Switzerland, 2018; pp. 130–138.

46. Hamed, S.A.I.; Ayad, C.E. Grading of Brain Tumors Using MR Spectroscopy: Diagnostic value at Short and Long. *IOSR J. Dent. Med. Sci.* **2017**, *16*, 87–93. [CrossRef]

47. Ranjith, G.; Parvathy, R.; Vikas, V.; Chandrasekharan, K.; Nair, S. Machine learning methods for the classification of gliomas: Initial results using features extracted from MR spectroscopy. *Neuroradiol. J.* **2015**, *28*, 106–111. [CrossRef]

48. James, A.P.; Dasarathy, B.V. Medical image fusion: A survey of the state of the art. *Inf. Fusion* **2014**, *19*, 4–19. [CrossRef]

49. Louis, D.N.; Perry, A.; Reifenberger, G.; Von Deimling, A.; Figarella-Branger, D.; Cavenee, W.K.; Ellison, D.W. The 2016 World Health Organization classification of tumors of the central nervous system: A summary. *Acta Neuropathol.* **2016**, *131*, 803–820. [CrossRef]

50. DeAngelis, L.M. Brain tumors. *N. Engl. J. Med.* **2001**, *344*, 114–123. [CrossRef]

51. Louis, D.N.; Ohgaki, H.; Wiestler, O.D.; Cavenee, W.K.; Burger, P.C.; Jouvet, A.; Scheithauer, B.W.; Kleihues, P. The 2007 WHO classification of tumours of the central nervous system. *Acta neuropathol.* **2007**, *114*, 97–109. [CrossRef]

52. Collins, V.P. Brain tumours: Classification and genes. *J. Neurol. Neurosurg. Psychiatry* **2004**, *75*, ii2–ii11. [CrossRef] [PubMed]

53. Ludwig, J.A.; Weinstein, J.N. Biomarkers in cancer staging, prognosis and treatment selection. *Nat. Rev. Cancer* **2005**, *5*, 845–856. [CrossRef]

54. Sharma, H.; Alekseychuk, A.; Leskovsky, P.; Hellwich, O.; Anand, R.S.; Zerbe, N.; Hufnagl, P. Determining similarity in histological images using graph-theoretic description and matching methods for content-based image retrieval in medical diagnostics. *Diagn. Pathol.* **2012**, *7*, 134. [CrossRef] [PubMed]

55. Bardou, D.; Zhang, K.; Ahmad, S.M. Classification of Breast Cancer Based on Histology Images Using Convolutional Neural Networks. *IEEE Access* **2018**, *6*, 24680–24693. [CrossRef]

56. Xu, Y.; Jia, Z.; Wang, L.B.; Ai, Y.; Zhang, F.; Lai, M.; Chang, C. Large scale tissue histopathology image classification, segmentation, and visualization via deep convolutional activation features. *BMC Bioinform.* **2017**, *18*, 281. [CrossRef] [PubMed]

57. ICPR 2012 - Mitosis Detection Contest. Available online: http://www.ipal.cnrs.fr/event/icpr-2012 (accessed on 1 November 2018).

58. Segmentation of neuronal structures in EM stacks challenge-ISBI 2012. Available online: https://imagej.net/Segmentation_of_neuronal_structures_in_EM_stacks_challenge_-_ISBI_2012 (accessed on 1 November 2018).

59. GlaS@MICCAI'2015: Gland Segmentation Challenge Contest. Available online: https://warwick.ac.uk/fac/sci/dcs/research/tia/glascontest/ (accessed on 1 November 2018).

60. Tumor Proliferation Assessment Challenge 2016. Available online: http://tupac.tue-image.nl/ (accessed on 1 November 2018).

61. CAMELYON17. Available online: https://camelyon17.grand-challenge.org/ (accessed on 1 November 2018).

62. Medical Imaging with Deep Learning. Available online: https://midl.amsterdam/ (accessed on 1 November 2018).

63. Sasikala, M.; Kumaravel, N. A wavelet-based optimal texture feature set for classification of brain tumours. *J. Med. Eng. Technol.* **2008**, *32*, 198–205. [CrossRef] [PubMed]

64. Multimodal Brain Tumor Segmentation. Available online: http://www2.imm.dtu.dk/projects/BRATS2012/index.html (accessed on 1 November 2018).

65. The Quantitative Translational Imaging in Medicine Lab at the Martinos Center. Available online: https://qtim-lab.github.io/ (accessed on 1 November 2018).

66. MICCAI-BRATS 2014. Available online: https://sites.google.com/site/miccaibrats2014/ (accessed on 1 November 2018).

67. BraTS 2015. Available online: https://sites.google.com/site/braintumorsegmentation/home/brats2015 (accessed on 1 November 2018).

68. BraTS 2016. Available online: https://sites.google.com/site/braintumorsegmentation/home/brats_2016 (accessed on 1 November 2018).

69. 20th International Conference on Medical Image Computing and Computer Assisted Intervention 2017. Available online: http://www.miccai2017.org/ (accessed on 1 November 2018).

70. Multimodal Brain Tumor Segmentation Challenge 2018. Available online: https://www.med.upenn.edu/sbia/brats2018.html (accessed on 1 November 2018).

71. MRBrainS18. Available online: http://mrbrains18.isi.uu.nl/ (accessed on 1 November 2018).

72. Automated Measurement of Fetal Head Circumference. Available online: https://hc18.grand-challenge.org/ (accessed on 1 November 2018).

73. Haykin, S.S. *Neural Networks and Learning Machines*; Pearson: Upper Saddle River, NJ, USA, 2009; Volume 3.

74. Nasrabadi, N.M. Pattern recognition and machine learning. *J. Electron. Imaging* **2007**, *16*, 049901. [CrossRef]

75. Wernick, M.N.; Yang, Y.; Brankov, J.G.; Yourganov, G.; Strother, S.C. Machine learning in medical imaging. *IEEE Signal Process. Mag.* **2010**, *27*, 25–38. [CrossRef] [PubMed]

76. Erickson, B.J.; Korfiatis, P.; Akkus, Z.; Kline, T.L. Machine learning for medical imaging. *Radiographics* **2017**, *37*, 505–515. [CrossRef]

77. Vasantha, M.; SubbiahBharathi, V.; Dhamodharan, R. Medical image feature, extraction, selection and classification. *Int. J. Eng. Sci. Technol.* **2010**, *2*, 2071–2076.

78. Altman, N.S. An introduction to kernel and nearest-neighbor nonparametric regression. *Am. Stat.* **1992**, *46*, 175–185. [CrossRef]

79. Cortes, C.; Vapnik, V. Support vector machine. *Mach. Learn.* **1995**, *20*, 273–297. [CrossRef]

80. Yegnanarayana, B. *Artificial Neural Networks*; PHI Learning Pvt. Ltd.: Delhi, India, 2009.

81. Huang, G.-B.; Zhu, Q.-Y.; Siew, C.-K. Extreme learning machine: Theory and applications. *Neurocomputing* **2006**, *70*, 489–501. [CrossRef]

82. Grossberg, S. Recurrent neural networks. *Scholarpedia* **2013**, *8*, 1888. [CrossRef]

83. Hinton, G.E. A practical guide to training restricted Boltzmann machines. In *Neural Networks: Tricks of the Trade*; Springer: Berlin/Heidelberg, Germany, 2012; pp. 599–619.

84. LeCun, Y.; Bengio, Y.; Hinton, G. Deep learning. *Nature* **2015**, *521*, 436. [CrossRef] [PubMed]

85. Krizhevsky, A.; Sutskever, I.; Hinton, G.E. Imagenet classification with deep convolutional neural networks. In *Advances in Neural Information Processing Systems*; NIPS: Nevada, USA, 2012; pp. 1097–1105.

86. Hinton, G.E.; Salakhutdinov, R.R. Reducing the dimensionality of data with neural networks. *Science* **2006**, *313*, 504–507. [CrossRef] [PubMed]

87. Hinton, G.E. Deep belief networks. *Scholarpedia* **2009**, *4*, 5947. [CrossRef]

88. El-Dahshan, E.S.A.; Hosny, T.; Salem, A.B.M. Hybrid intelligent techniques for MRI brain images classification. *Dig. Signal Process* **2010**, *20*, 433–441. [CrossRef]

89. Yang, G.; Nawaz, T.; Barrick, T.R.; Howe, F.A.; Slabaugh, G. Discrete wavelet transform-based whole-spectral and subspectral analysis for improved brain tumor clustering using single voxel MR spectroscopy. *IEEE Trans. Biomed. Eng.* **2015**, *62*, 2860–2866. [CrossRef]

90. Jolliffe, I. Principal component analysis. In *International Encyclopedia of Statistical Science*; Springer: Berlin/Heidelberg, Germany, 2011; pp. 1094–1096.

91. Rumelhart, D.E.; Hinton, G.E.; Williams, R.J. *Learning Internal Representations by Error Propagation. No. ICS-8506. California Univ. San Diego La Jolla Inst for Cognitive Science*; OCLC Number: 20472667; Defense Technical Information Center: Fort Belvo, VA, USA, 1985.

92. Zacharaki, E.I.; Wang, S.; Chawla, S.; Yoo, D.S.; Wolf, R.; Melhem, E.R.; Davatzikos, C. MRI-based classification of brain tumor type and grade using SVM-RFE. *IEEE Int. Symp. Biomed. Imaging Nano Macro* **2009**, 1035–1038. [CrossRef]

93. Barker, M.; Rayens, W. Partial least squares for discrimination. *J. Chemometr.* **2003**, *17*, 166–173. [CrossRef]

94. Verma, R.; Zacharaki, E.I.; Ou, Y.; Cai, H.; Chawla, S.; Lee, S.; Melhem, E.R.; Wolf, R.; Davatzikos, C. Multiparametric tissue characterization of brain neoplasms and their recurrence using pattern classification of MR images. *Acad. Radiol.* **2008**, *15*, 966–977. [CrossRef] [PubMed]

95. Murphy, K.P. *Naïve Bayes Classifiers*; University of British Columbia: Vancouver, BC, Canada, 2006; Volume 18.

96. Leung, K.M. *Naïve Bayesian Classifier*; Polytechnic University Department of Computer Science/Finance and Risk Engineering: New York, NY, USA, 2007.

97. John, G.H.; Langley, P. Estimating continuous distributions in Bayesian classifiers. In Proceedings of the Eleventh Conference on Uncertainty in Artificial Intelligence, Montreal, QC, Canada, 18–20 August 1995; Morgan Kaufmann Publishers Inc.: San Francisco, CA, USA, 1995; pp. 338–345.

98. Huang, G.B.; Zhu, Q.Y.; Siew, C.K. Extreme learning machine: Theory and applications. *Neurocomputing* **2006**, *70*, 489–501. [CrossRef]

99. Kuppili, V.; Biswas, M.; Sreekumar, A.; Suri, H.S.; Saba, L.; Edla, D.R.; Marinhoe, R.T.; Sanches, J.M.; Suri, J.S. Extreme learning machine framework for risk stratification of fatty liver disease using ultrasound tissue characterization. *J. Med. Syst.* **2017**, *41*, 152. [CrossRef] [PubMed]

100. Biswas, M.; Kuppili, V.; Edla, D.R.; Suri, H.S.; Saba, L.; Marinho, R.T.; Sanches, J.M.; Suri, J.S. Symtosis: A liver ultrasound tissue characterization and risk stratification in optimized deep learning paradigm. *Comput. Methods Programs Biomed.* **2018**, *155*, 165–177. [CrossRef] [PubMed]

101. Litjens, G.; Kooi, T.; Bejnordi, B.E.; Setio, A.A.A.; Ciompi, F.; Ghafoorian, M.; van der Laak, J.A.W.M.; Ginneken, B.; Sánchez, C.I. A survey on deep learning in medical image analysis. *Med. Image Anal.* **2017**, *42*, 60–88. [CrossRef]

102. AlBadawy, E.A.; Saha, A.; Mazurowski, M.A. Deep learning for segmentation of brain tumors: Impact of cross-institutional training and testing. *Med. Phys.* **2018**, *45*, 1150–1158. [CrossRef]

103. Havaei, M.; Davy, A.; Warde-Farley, D.; Biard, A.; Courville, A.; Bengio, Y.; Larochelle, H. Brain tumor segmentation with deep neural networks. *Med. Image Anal.* **2017**, *35*, 18–31. [CrossRef] [PubMed]

104. Erickson, B.J.; Korfiatis, P.; Akkus, Z.; Kline, T.; Philbrick, K. Toolkits and libraries for deep learning. *J. Dig. Imaging* **2017**, *30*, 400–405. [CrossRef] [PubMed]

105. Skogen, K.; Schulz, A.; Dormagen, J.B.; Ganeshan, B.; Helseth, E.; Server, A. Diagnostic performance of texture analysis on MRI in grading cerebral gliomas. *Eur. J. Radiol.* **2016**, *85*, 824–829. [CrossRef]

106. Kreisl, T.N.; Toothaker, T.; Karimi, S.; DeAngelis, L.M. Ischemic stroke in patients with primary brain tumors. *Neurology* **2008**, *70*, 2314–2320. [CrossRef] [PubMed]

107. Burns, A.; Iliffe, S. Alzheimer's disease. *BMJ* **2009**, *338*, b158. [CrossRef] [PubMed]

108. Ye, R.; Shen, T.; Jiang, Y.; Xu, L.; Si, X.; Zhang, B. The relationship between parkinson disease and brain tumor: A meta-analysis. *PLoS ONE* **2016**, *11*, e0164388. [CrossRef] [PubMed]

109. Wardlaw, J.M.; Sandercock, P.A.G.; Dennis, M.S.; Starr, J. Is breakdown of the blood brain barrier responsible for lacunar stroke, leukoaraiosis, and dementia. *Stroke* **2003**, *34*, 806–812. [CrossRef] [PubMed]

110. Plantone, D.; Renna, R.; Sbardella, E.; Koudriavtseva, T. Concurrence of multiple sclerosis and brain tumors. *Front. Neurol.* **2015**, *6*, 40. [CrossRef] [PubMed]

111. Bahmanyar, S.; Montgomery, S.M.; Hillert, J.; Ekbom, A.; Olsson, T. Cancer risk among patients with multiple sclerosis and their parents. *Neurology* **2009**, *72*, 1170–1177. [CrossRef] [PubMed]

112. Reitan, R.M.; Wolfson, D. *The Halstead-Reitan Neuropsychological Test Battery: Theory and Clinical Interpretation*; Reitan Neuropsychology: Tucson, AZ, USA, 1985; Volume 4.

113. Cahalane, A.M.; Kearney, H.; Purcell, Y.M.; McGuigan, C.; Killeen, R.P. MRI and multiple sclerosis—the evolving role of MRI in the diagnosis and management of MS: The radiologist's perspective. *Ir. J. Med. Sci.* **2018**, *187*, 781–787. [CrossRef] [PubMed]

114. Wikipedia. Available online: https://www.wikipedia.org/ (accessed on 23 December 2018).

115. Nakano, K.; Park, K.; Zheng, R.; Fang, F.; Ohori, M.; Nakamura, H.; Irimajiri, A. Leukoaraiosissignificantly worsens driving performance of ordinary older drivers. *PLoS ONE.* **2014**, *9*, e108333. [CrossRef]

116. Islam, J.; Zhang, Y. Brain MRI analysis for Alzheimer's disease diagnosis using an ensemble system of deep convolutional neural networks. *Brain informatics* **2018**, *5*, 2. [CrossRef]

117. Heim, B.; Krismer, F.; De Marzi, R.; Seppi, K. Magnetic resonance imaging for the diagnosis of Parkinson's disease. *J. Neural. Transm.* **2017**, *124*, 915–964. [CrossRef]

118. Bandmann, O.; Weiss, K.H.; Kaler, S.G. Wilson's disease and other neurological copper disorders. *Lancet Neurol.* **2015**, *14*, 103–113. [CrossRef]

119. Villanueva-Meyer, J.E.; Mabray, M.C.; Cha, S. Current Clinical Brain Tumor Imaging. *Neurosurgery* **2017**, *81*, 397–415. [CrossRef] [PubMed]

120. Madabhushi, A.; Lee, G. Image analysis and machine learning in digital pathology: Challenges and opportunities. *Med. Image Anal.* **2016**, *33*, 170–175. [CrossRef] [PubMed]

121. Quincke, H.I. *Lumbar Puncture. Diseases of the Nervous System*; Church, A., Ed.; Appleton: New York, NY, USA, 1909; p. 223.

122. Lynch, H.T.; Lynch, J.F.; Shaw, T.G.; Lubiński, J. HNPCC (Lynch Syndrome): Differential Diagnosis, Molecular Genetics and Management—A Review. *Hereditary Cancer Clin. Pract.* **2003**, *1*, 7. [CrossRef]

123. Ryu, Y.J.; Choi, S.H.; Park, S.J.; Yun, T.J.; Kim, J.H.; Sohn, C.H. Glioma: Application of whole-tumor texture analysis of diffusion-weighted imaging for the evaluation of tumor heterogeneity. *PLoS ONE* **2014**, *9*, e108335. [CrossRef] [PubMed]

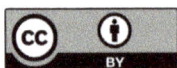

MDPI

St. Alban-Anlage 66

4052 Basel

Switzerland

Tel. +41 61 683 77 34

Fax +41 61 302 89 18

www.mdpi.com

Cancers Editorial Office

E-mail: cancers@mdpi.com

www.mdpi.com/journal/cancers

www.ingramcontent.com/pod-product-compliance
Lightning Source LLC
Chambersburg PA
CBHW051706210326
41597CB00032B/5386